Palpation Techniques

Surface Anatomy for Physical Therapists

Third Edition

Bernhard Reichert, MScPT, MT
Practicing Massage Therapist, Physical Therapist, and Manual Therapist
Fellbach, Germany

With the collaboration of
Wolfgang Stelzenmüller and Omer Matthijs

877 illustrations

Thieme
Stuttgart • New York • Delhi • Rio de Janeiro

Library of Congress Cataloging-in-Publication Data
is available from the publisher.

This book is a new updated edition based on the authorized translation of both volumes of the German editions of 'Anatomie in vivo', published and copyrighted 2012 and 2007 by Georg Thieme Verlag, Stuttgart, Germany, and merged with the authorized translation of parts from the German edition of 'Palpations-Techniken', published and copyrighted 2018 by Georg Thieme Verlag, Stuttgart, Germany.

Original translation by: Gertrud G. Champe, Surry, Maine, USA; Michelle Hertrich, Nettetal, Germany
New parts translated by: Karen Leube, PhD
Leube Translation and Language Services
Aachen, Germany

Photos: Oskar Vogl, Affalterbach, Germany; Benjamin Stollenberg, Ludwigsburg, Germany; Kirsten Oborny, Thieme Group

Illustrations: Martin Hoffmann, Neu-Ulm, Germany; Markus Voll, München, Germany

© 2021. Thieme. All rights reserved.

Georg Thieme Verlag KG
Rüdigerstraße 14, 70469 Stuttgart, Germany
www.thieme.de
+49 [0]711 8931 421, customerservice@thieme.de

Cover design: Thieme Publishing Group
Typesetting by DiTech, India

Printed in Germany by Beltz Grafische Betriebe

ISBN 978-3-13-242987-1

Also available as e-book:
eISBN 978-3-13-242988-8

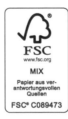

FSC
www.fsc.org
MIX
Papier aus ver-
antwortungsvollen
Quellen
FSC® C089473

Contents

Foreword to the First English Edition

The clinical practice community has been left wanting for a textbook dedicated to the precise execution of in-vivo anatomical examination, and this excellent text emerges in a timely fashion. Healthcare professionals have witnessed an escalation in the need for relevant clinical examinations and the use of manual therapeutic interventions, both of which rely on a thorough understanding and execution of precise in-vivo surface anatomy skills. Because surgical exposure may not be readily available, the clinician must rely on nonsurgical measures for identifying relevant anatomical structures. Thus, surface anatomy skillsets become indispensable for localizing structures and landmarks. This text can serve as a roadmap for locating relevant structures with exactitude. The clear means with which this text instructs the clinician in tactile localization will complement essential knowledge in structural and functional anatomy.

The authors have organized the approach to identifying structures by both layer and region. This process of organization can guide the clinician to visualizing a particular structure's relative depth and relationship to surrounding structures. Moreover, the text is complete, offering a thorough and methodical approach to all major musculoskeletal areas of the human body. This will assist the clinician in developing a musculoskeletal surface anatomy approach to the entire human body, allowing for the identification of patterns, similarities, and differences between structures in the different regions. Finally, the clinician is cued on how the information can be directly applied to clinical examination, which bridges the gap between knowledge and implementation. When used in accompaniment to a thorough, systematic clinical examination, precise structural localization can help to confirm a suspicion of that structure's involvement in the patient's condition.

Surface anatomy is essentially manual in nature. Thus, this text can serve as a segue for accurate localization of structures involved in manual therapeutic intervention. Moreover, because a patient's response to manual therapeutic interventions could be influenced by a clinician's confidence in technique execution, the clinician's thorough knowledge of structural architecture that is accompanied by accurate tactile localization could serve to enhance the patient's response to treatment.

The knowledge and skills gained from this text can provide a foundation for increased clinical confidence, as it can reduce the clinician's guesswork when navigating to a particular structure. The authors offer practical guidance for enhancing the clinician's success with an in-vivo surface anatomy experience. So not only are clinicians instructed on what skills to utilize, they are additionally guided on how to best implement them. This text can join the top ranks of a clinician's library and serve as a bridge between foundational science, clinical knowledge, and practical skills. With these features in mind, the text can support an individual's development and progress as a master manual clinician.

Phillip S. Sizer Jr., PT, PhD, OCS, FAAOMPT
Professor and Program Director
ScD Program in Physical Therapy;
Director, Clinical Musculoskeletal Research Laboratory
Center for Rehabilitation Research
School of Allied Health Sciences, Texas Tech University
Health Sciences Center
Lubbock, Texas, USA

Preface

This book is the result of years of teaching anatomy and practical experience with diagnostics and therapy. Proficiency in targeted palpation is the key to a number of local applications, ranging from physical therapy to local injection.

My realization that practitioners do not really learn anatomy until they have translated theoretical knowledge into tactile familiarity led me to reassess the importance of surface anatomy.

I also realized that experienced therapists and even physicians themselves may still find it challenging to locate certain anatomical structures, even after years of working in the medical profession. My work in training future medical and health professionals has shown me that they must have orientation toward local anatomy to gain the confidence required to apply specific manual techniques.

In this vein, teaching surface anatomy is very satisfying. Identifying the structures being sought, feeling the different types of tissue resistance, and recognizing details is genuinely exciting for students and course participants. Suddenly, the anatomical interconnections become clear, and the learner starts viewing the musculoskeletal system three-dimensionally.

What's New?

Some of the tests and approaches based on palpation have been substituted with those based on scientific evaluation and practical relevance. For learners to be able to rely on palpation results, emphasis on both reliability and validity is indispensable. Keeping in view the trend for a stronger focus on scientific publications, this edition features a separate list of references for each chapter.

One may think that when it comes to topographic and morphological anatomy, there is nothing new to learn. Nothing is further from the truth. New, high-quality anatomical studies are helping us in locating clinically relevant structures more efficiently. One example of this is the discussion about the origin and course of the medial collateral ligament of the knee joint in the revised chapter "Knee Joint." Findings from studies conducted at the Institute of Anatomical Sciences, Texas Tech University Health Sciences Center, Texas, USA, are presented in various chapters of this book.

A new chapter "Abdominal Region" focuses on palpation of the abdomen and groin. This anatomical region is less familiar to therapists and is thus characterized by a high degree of uncertainty. This chapter offers simple and practical access to this region.

In addition to the content changes and updates, the book design has been refreshed, which enhances its look and feel and makes it easier to understand.

What Has Remained the Same?

This book targets individuals working towards the diagnosis and treatment of musculoskeletal disorders and diseases.

It intends to enable experienced students in training for careers in physical therapy. Participants in various continuing professional education courses, medical students and physicians, as well as experienced therapists can orient themselves with the musculoskeletal system using this book.

The only way to learn palpation is through practice. This book encourages its readers to simulate the palpation activities presented.

The book aims to present instructions for beginners presented in clear, easy-to-understand language. Research findings and anatomical studies help therapists and instructors become more secure in dealing with the results of specific palpation.

Choice of Structures

Surface anatomy discussed in this book focuses on the key parts of the musculoskeletal system that lead to complaints in the extremities, in many cases, irritated joints and tendons, and their insertions and tendon sheaths. Muscle bellies, bursae, and ligaments are also the target of specific palpations.

The structures selected for this book are the most important sites on which examination and treatment techniques are applied in daily practice.

The instructions are oriented toward "normal" structures of the musculoskeletal system or, in other words, those that are not pathologically altered. To be able to identify pathological changes, the examiner must be well versed in the palpation of normal structures.

Applicability of Surface Anatomy

Surface anatomy is undeniably important for diagnosis and treatment. Several examples illustrate its significance:
• During the examination, the practitioner attempts to precisely locate a diseased structure or perform pain testing by applying pressure or transverse friction (provocative palpation).

- In most cases, the joint space is the crucial factor. Thus, in many cases, local identification of certain bony points and palpation of the course of the joint space is dependent on correct execution of tests and treatment techniques as part of manual therapy.
- The palpation of peripheral nerves is also a key element of surface anatomy. However, only a few examiners are familiar with them in terms of palpation, despite the fact that several peripheral nerves of the arm and leg are quite thick structures and are very easy to find in some places.
- Deep frictions of soft tissue structures constitute another mode of therapy; they are primarily used for pain relief.

Bernhard Reichert, MScPT, MT

Acknowledgments

Revising, refining, and compiling existing material requires the same care and prudence as writing a new text and only works in a team. I am very grateful to Angelika-Marie Findgott, who has proven to be a highly experienced, competent, and composed project manager in the publishing house. She guided the team through this project in a finely coordinated and reliable manner. She and Deborah Cecere executed the editorial fine-tuning of the new and revised text with utmost precision and style. Dr. Karen Leube also deserves thanks for translating the new parts of the text and integrating them into the existing second edition with a great deal of finesse. My gratitude goes to illustrator Markus Voll for his outstanding work with adapting and recreating various graphics. Dennis Wagner, the model for my massage therapy book, also kindly posed for some new photographs that were expertly photographed by Kirsten Oborny.

Dr. Brigitte Klett, a general practitioner specializing in internal and psychosomatic medicine and an expert in Traditional Chinese Medicine (ida-therapiezentrum.de), advised me on developing the chapter on palpation of the abdomen and groin.

I would especially like to thank Dr. Omer Matthijs, ScD PT, for his collaboration on the subject matter of the book. As a research director at the International Academy of Orthopedic Medicine (IAOM.eu), collaborator in research projects at Texas Tech University, Lubbock, Texas, USA, and through his work as a practitioner of physical therapy, he promotes the continuity of the development of specialized practical knowledge, which greatly benefits therapists in practice. Dr. Matthijs contributed to this project by sharing specialized skills and knowledge he developed and gathered and has been a true asset for assuring the high quality of the book's content.

Bernhard Reichert, MScPT, MT

Chapter 1

Basic Principles

1

1 Basic Principles

"You must be relaxed to have a good tactile sense"
(A. Vleeming, Berlin, 2003)

1.1 Why Do Clinicians Need Surface Anatomy?

The need to locate anatomical features on living subjects for the purpose of assessment and treatment has existed since the beginning of professional training for massage therapists, physical therapists, and physicians.

In medical and health care training programs, information on the position, appearance, and function of musculoskeletal structures is mostly communicated verbally, with the support of two-dimensional illustrations.

Due to the enormous flood of information, students of anatomy quickly find study material dry and abstract. Didactic-style training programs demonstrate the functional importance of a specific structure within a kinematic complex or a complicated motion sequence. Using a large number of illustrations, they also convey only an *approximate* three-dimensional idea of that structure, which quickly exhausts the amount of time and materials available to students.

In addition, students are often unable to recognize anatomical features on specimens, for example, when they visit a pathological institute during basic professional training or continuing education courses. It is likewise rare that theoretical knowledge is successfully transferred onto living bodies. Surface anatomy (anatomy on living subjects) becomes a part of professional training that is mentioned in passing; a coincidence during the assessment and treatment of patients; the object of troublesome self-learning; and the content of expensive continuing education courses.

The anatomical images used for training and further education are often drawings demonstrating an idealistic norm. These drawings breach a basic principle of anatomy: variation (Aland and Kippers, 2005). The concept of the anatomical norm cannot be standardized. Rather, it has to include inter-individual (between two people) and intra-individual (left-right) variations in position and shape. Old anatomy books teach us about possible variations in certain topographical and morphological properties, something that modern anatomy books often lack. For example, the classic anatomy book by von Lanz and Wachsmuth *Praktische Anatomie* (2004a), describes the percentage of the population who have differently shaped or nonexistent structures; for example in 5 to 20% of the population the lumbar spine does not possess a fifth lumbar vertebra (depending on which anatomical study is cited). Töndury (1968, in von Lanz and Wachsmuth 2004a) wrote about the abundance of variation in all spinal section boundaries: "Only approximately 40% of all people have their boundaries [of the sections of the spine] in the normal location."

What should we do when we lose our confidence in topographic orientation—the knowledge gained from our training—when coming across a variation? First of all, it is important to keep an open mind and be prepared to accept anatomical anomalies when palpating. Experience in palpating and faith in anatomical facts found in every individual take on an even greater significance. Certain structures remain constant in position and shape and can be identified without a large degree of variation; for example, the iliac crests, the scapula, the sternum, and the 1st to 10th ribs. Recognizing variants takes experience.

The palpation procedure starts with the therapist assuming the topographic standard and transferring this knowledge to the situation in the living body. The first step involves therapists attempting to locate a certain structure. They then imagine the structure's approximate position and shape and start palpating with these details in mind. With the right technique and proper expectation of what you should feel, along with sufficient experience, you will soon become successful.

Memorize

The less confident you are using concrete structural details for orientation, the more helpful technical tricks, guiding structures, or drawings become in confirming that the correct structure has been palpated.

It is highly likely, therefore, that in the treatment setting, important anatomical features cannot be located, and the error rate in local treatment becomes inevitably high. This is something that neither physicians nor therapists can really afford.

1.2 What Is Understood by Surface Anatomy in this Book?

This book deals with both clinically relevant structures in the musculoskeletal system and accessible conductive pathways (blood vessels and peripheral nerves). It uses precise palpation to systematically transfer topographical anatomical knowledge onto living bodies. Therapists should be provided with a logical system to locate relevant structures quickly and reliably. This toolbox of techniques not only includes the actual palpation, it also gives therapists indications of what to expect when searching for a structure and the difficulties they may encounter.

This book is not about reinventing palpatory techniques, but about the clarification of procedures and the detailed documentation of techniques in words and pictures. The substantial number of illustrations allows therapists to monitor their execution of the techniques. The descriptions allow even visually impaired clinicians to reliably locate each structure after hearing the text.

Some authors who have also dealt with surface anatomy (e.g., Winkel, 2004) incorporate the following in their books:
- Surface topography (dividing the body into different regions).
- Anthropometric methods (e.g., measurements of length and circumference).
- General and local observation of regions of the body.

These aspects have been deliberately left out of this book, and readers should understand the term "surface anatomy" as a system used for palpation only.

1.3 When Can Surface Anatomy Be Used?

The precise palpation of structures is used in physical therapy assessment and treatment.

1.3.1 Physical Therapy Assessment

A physical therapy assessment comprises the following:
- Defining the areas to be treated.
- Confirming the presumed location.
- Examining the consistency of skin and muscles.
- Extremities: The provocation of ligaments, tendons, insertions, joint capsules, etc.
- Spinal column: The provocation of local segmental parts and assessment of segmental mobility.
- Examining the craniomandibular joint.

One of the aims of assessment is to identify the affected structure by applying a specific test to provoke the patient's current symptoms. The accuracy of tests and the interpretation of their findings are quite refined nowadays; nevertheless, it is not always possible to differentiate a painful tendon from a group of synergistic muscles, for example.

Often, the possible causes of pain in a structure are spread over only a few centimeters. For example, in one muscle the cause could be located at the site of insertion, the tendon, or the junction between the muscle and the tendon. Only provocative precise palpation is of help in these instances.

1.3.2 Basic Principles of Regional or Local Treatment

Treatment is based on the following methods:
- *Regional treatment:* Swedish massage, functional massage, connective tissue massage, electrotherapy, hydrotherapy, heat therapy, balneotherapy, and manual therapy techniques.
- *Local treatment:* segmental oscillations for pain relief, local segmental manual therapeutic mobilization techniques to maintain or improve mobility, cross-frictions according to Cyriax, and colon massage.

Disorders of the musculoskeletal soft tissue usually appear in very localized areas. Only large traumas or inflammation spread over larger areas. Physical therapy interventions for the treatment of soft-tissue conditions also include local, thermic, electrotherapeutic, and mechanical interventions. Local application of these treatments can only be effective if applied precisely to the affected structure.

Accurate location of an affected site is ensured only through the experienced and reliable use of palpatory techniques.

1.4 Workflow for Palpation

"You cannot feel what you do not know."

This simple phrase illustrates the necessity of a solid background in topographical and morphological anatomy for local palpation. It does not make sense to look for a specific transverse process if you are unable to visualize its shape, position, and spatial relationship to its surroundings.

It is always a difficult task to recall the exact anatomy of a clinically relevant structure. A lot of time and motivation are needed to deal with this considerable amount of information. For this reason, two short theoretical sections can be found at the start of each topic:
- The significance and functional importance of each region and its individual parts. This acts as an introduction to the topic and refers to current knowledge about the fascinating interplay between individual parts.
- Required basic anatomical and biomechanical knowledge. It is extremely useful to recall topographical relationships again before searching for specific structures. Important anatomical details required for palpation are therefore mentioned in the text and highlighted in the figures.

▶ Fig. 1.1 shows the procedure to be used for palpation.

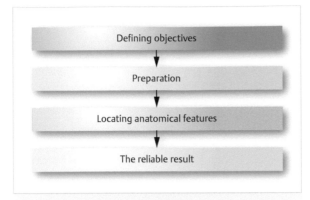

Fig. 1.1 General workflow in palpation.

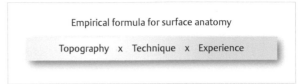

Fig. 1.2 The formula for successful palpation.

1.4.1 Objective and Location

The objective of precise palpation of detailed structures is to obtain local orientation for assessment and treatment based on the reasons described above.

The therapist should start with the areas that they know best. The description of the palpatory process generally starts with the palpation of known and easy-to-reach bony structures (e.g., sacrum, occiput) and muscles (erector spinae, semispinalis).

Memorize

Precise palpation always requires the appropriate technique. There is a specific technique especially suited to each structure.

1.4.2 The Reliable Result

Certain measures (tensing specific muscles, passive vertebral movement, etc.) can be applied to test whether the structure in question has actually been found. It is also helpful to draw the structure or its borders on the skin. This obliges the therapist to determine and then document that the structure is actually located where indicated by palpation and drawing. This is even more interesting when students are palpating in a small study group and comparing their results.

In his courses, Vleeming (personal communication), the founder of the Rotterdam Spine and Joint Centre and pioneer of targeted palpation, recommends drawing the palpated structure for each palpation session, including palpation carried out on patients.

Every author on precise palpation writes about the importance of practical experience. The author of this textbook believes that each structure should be deliberately and correctly palpated at least 10 times to achieve

an approximate idea of the technique to be applied and the location and shape of the structure.

▶ Fig. 1.2 summarizes the prerequisites for surface anatomy in an empirical formula.

Memorize

Experience is ultimately the deciding factor in obtaining the necessary confidence.

1.4.3 Central Aspects of the Procedure

Three essential features characterize the palpatory process:
- The application of the appropriate palpatory technique.
- The expected consistency of tissue.
- Differentiating the resistance felt in palpated structures.

As explained above, topographical and morphological knowledge and experience in precise palpation are crucial. Each structure requires a certain palpatory technique, and it is necessary to have an idea about what the structure should feel like. Before palpating, it is also important to know exactly what type of resistance the palpating finger will encounter when it exerts pressure or slides over the structure being sought.

For example, the exact location of a bony edge is found by palpating at a right angle to the edge being sought. The structure is expected to have a hard consistency. The position and shape of a structure can be correctly found among the surrounding tissue when the therapist is able to differentiate between the different types of consistencies found in the different tissues.

Memorize

Soft, elastic tissue is examined slowly to perceive the elasticity.
Hard tissue is examined with a quick movement to feel the hardness.

These principles are also recommended when assessing the end-feel using angular tests (passive functional tests) and translation tests (joint play tests).

1.4.4 Pressure Applied during Palpation

The palpation pressure is usually selected by applying a given technique in a downward direction.

It is definitely incorrect to insist that palpation is always conducted with minimal pressure. The amount of pressure applied depends on the following:

- The expected **consistency of the targeted structure.** For example, if you are searching for a bony edge or prominence, it is correct to assume that it will feel hard when direct pressure is applied to it. In this case, the palpation tends to be performed with more intensity so that the hard tissue response can be felt. Soft tissue is detected using less pressure. It is impossible to perceive its resilience if too much pressure is applied.
- The **firmness and thickness of the more superficial tissue.** Deeply located bony landmarks covered by a strong muscular layer or a layer of fat cannot be reached by palpating lightly.

A dexterous therapist can easily locate the structure sought and the expected consistency by using the appropriate technique and the suitable palpation pressure.

1.5 Palpatory Techniques

1.5.1 Palpating the Skin

▶ **Example.** Posterior trunk.

▶ **Technique**
- Skin quality: the palm of the hand strokes the skin.
- Skin temperature: the back of the hand strokes the skin.
- Skin consistency: displacement test, skin lifting test, skin rolling.

▶ **Expectations**
- Skin quality: smooth, pliable skin. Light hair growth is sometimes present.
- Skin temperature: uniform body temperature.
- Skin consistency: soft and very elastic. The skin becomes firmer when more tension is placed on it.

▶ **Commentary.** The skin qualities described above represent the ideal situation for young patients. Needless to say, age-related changes to the skin should not be immediately classified as pathological.

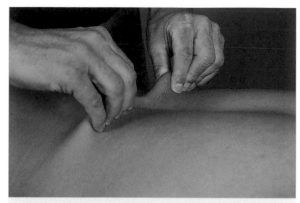

Fig. 1.3 Using the lifting test to check skin consistency.

The skin's consistency is determined by the balance of fluid in the skin. Elasticity tests are used to assess the consistency of skin and include the displacement test, lifting test (▶ Fig. 1.3), and skin rolling. All three tests should provide identical results. The same amount of elasticity, sensitivity, and changes in these parameters should be found. If this is not the case, techniques should be reassessed or patients questioned again. These tests place different tensile stresses on the skin. The displacement test can be used to find a sensitive or significantly inflamed region; small changes in consistency can be detected especially well using skin rolling with a large amount of stretch.

1.5.2 Palpating Bony Edges

▶ **Examples.** Spine of the scapula (▶ Fig. 1.4), edge of the acromion, joint line of the wrist, a variety of joint spaces, iliac crest, rib shaft, spinous process, mastoid process, mandibular arch.

▶ **Technique.** The fingertip palpates perpendicular to the edge of the bone.

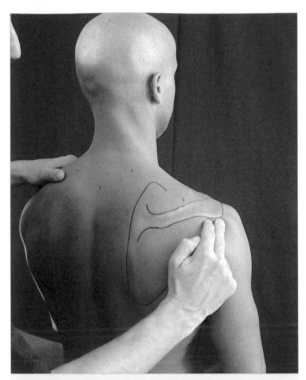

Fig. 1.4 Palpating the edge of bone, demonstrated here on the scapular spine.

▶ **Expectations.** Hard consistency and a clearly defined border.

▶ **Commentary.** This technique enables the therapist to accurately locate the outer boundaries of a bone. The palpating finger must always be positioned perpendicular to the edge of the structure. All other techniques are less reliable. This is particularly important when looking for the component bones of small joints and for delineation of the intra-articular space.

> **Tip**
>
> To feel the hard consistency and palpate the bony edge distinctly, the therapist should palpate the soft tissue first and then gradually move toward the presumed location of the bony edge.

It becomes increasingly difficult to locate bony contours when superficial tissue is tense. Muscles tense up when patients are seated in an unsupported position. Tension increases in all soft tissue when the SP alters the normal curvature of the spine, and tissue is stretched, for example, when padding is placed under the abdomen in the prone position or when sitting patients place their arms in front of them on a treatment table.

Arthritic swelling and bone deformations change the expected consistency and contour of the target structure at the affected joint.

1.5.3 Palpating Bony Prominences

▶ **Examples.** Medial epicondyle of the femur, Lister tubercle, anterior superior iliac spine, tibial tuberosity, Gerdy tubercle.

▶ **Technique.** Circular palpation using the finger pads and a minimal amount of pressure.

▶ **Expectations.** The bony prominence protrudes from the surrounding bone. The structure itself feels hard when direct pressure is applied to it.

▶ **Commentary.** The iliac spines are usually distinctly elevated from the surrounding structures and can be clearly discerned (▶ Fig. 1.5). The borders are not always so easy to detect as in ▶ Fig. 1.5. This technique can also be used to palpate smaller elevations in the extremities referred to as tubercles or tuberosities. Moving the palpating finger over the area makes it possible to discern the shape, but too much pressure makes palpation difficult because the differences in the shape and position can no longer be clearly felt. Direct pressure on the structure is used only to confirm that the structure is a bone.

> **Tip**
>
> Therapists can gain an idea about the shape of the raised bony structure from their knowledge of morphological anatomy. However, variations are common; see, for example, the external occipital protuberance, which may be distinctly elevated or very flat.

1.5.4 Palpating Muscle Bellies

▶ **Examples.** Infraspinatus, deltoid, and gluteal muscles (▶ Fig. 1.6).

▶ **Technique.** Slow palpation over the area with the finger pads positioned perpendicular to the muscle fibers little pressure.

▶ **Expectations.** Soft consistency. Tissue yields slightly to pressure. Deeper structures can frequently be palpated.

▶ **Commentary.** The muscles are palpated using one or several finger pads. Pressure should target the muscle directly. The tissue's soft, elastic consistency can only be felt by proceeding slowly.

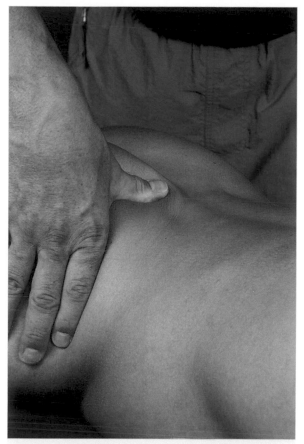

Fig. 1.5 Locating the superior posterior iliac spine.

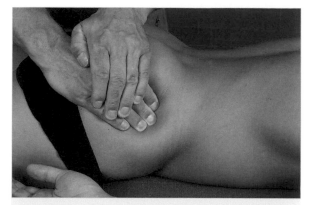

Fig. 1.6 Palpating muscle bellies, demonstrated here on the small gluteal muscles.

Tension in the Fasciae

Thickness of the Fasciae

Fasciae can be very soft on the anterior and lateral sides of the trunk, in the neck, along the throat, in the medial forearm, the calf, or the medial aspect of the thigh, for example. Muscles yield easily to the pressure of precise palpation here and have an especially soft, elastic consistency. In contrast, extremely hard fasciae feel significantly firmer during palpation, even when the active muscle tension is normal. Typical examples of this are the thoracolumbar fascia superficial to the lumbar erector spinae and the rectus sheath. Therapists may easily conclude that muscles are tense when increased resistance is felt in the tissues. Once they are aware of the qualities fasciae possess, however, they will have correct expectations regarding the consistency of muscle tissue.

Approximation or lengthening occurs *in the limbs* due to the angular position of joints. It is very difficult to palpate local quadriceps induration when the knee is bent at 90°.

Positioning can influence muscle length *in the trunk* considerably. The changes to palpation become obvious when the lumbar and thoracic trunk extensors in the sitting SP are palpated and this is compared with palpation in the prone position. Even when resting the upper body on a treatment table and other supportive surfaces, muscles are stretched by the flexion/kyphosis of the lumbar spine in a sitting position and by the forward bend of the body. Tissue feels significantly firmer when pressure is applied. Therapists may interpret this as a pathological increase in muscle tension. The amount of tension in the back muscles is also altered when the therapist places padding underneath the abdomen in the prone position, lowers the head end of the treatment table, and elevates the arms. It is not always possible to avoid approximating or stretching muscles during the positioning or skillful examination of patients while keeping symptoms to a minimum. It is important that the therapist takes this into account when looking at the expected consistency of the muscles to be palpated and does not reach the wrong conclusion when interpreting results.

The following exercises should clarify how differences in fascial tension can affect the interpretation of palpatory results on the posterior aspect of the body:

- **Exercise 1:** The gluteal region is palpated, starting at the sacrum and moving systematically in a lateral direction. A hardened area is frequently palpated between the greater trochanter and the iliac crests. The iliotibial tract is located here (thickening of the fascia in the buttocks and the thigh), running from the iliac crest toward the greater trochanter and the lateral thigh. The therapist changes the hip joint's SP by moving it into more abduction or adduction and attempts to feel how the tract changes under direct palpation (different consistencies due to the muscle being stretched or approximated).
- **Exercise 2:** Firm fascia already restricts direct pressure from being applied to the lumbar trunk extensors. The patient's pelvis is moved toward or away from the therapist. This causes lumbar lateral flexion. The therapist palpates the trunk extensors and attempts to find out how their consistency changes (→ different consistencies due to the muscle being stretched or approximated). Lumbar tension is also increased when patients raise their arms over their heads.

1.5.5 Palpating the Edge of Muscles

▶ **Examples.** Sartorius, adductor longus (▶ Fig. 1.7), hand extensors, semispinalis capitis, erector spinae, sternocleidomastoid.

▶ **Technique.** A muscle edge is usually palpated with the muscle slightly tensed. The palpating fingers can be positioned using all possible variations (fingertips, finger pads, sides of the fingers) and should be placed against the edge of the muscle as best as possible. Once the edge of the muscle has been located, it is steadily followed so that the course and the length of the muscle can be perceived.

▶ **Expectations.** When tensed, the edge of the muscle has a firm consistency and a uniform, smooth contour. Large and small gaps differentiate the edges of the muscle from neighboring muscles.

▶ **Commentary.** Many neighboring muscles and borders cannot be differentiated from one another or identified without selective activation of the muscle. Well-trained muscles with low fat content as well as muscles with pathologically increased tension are exceptions and project themselves from their surroundings.

> **Tip**
>
> A muscle and its edges can be quickly identified in difficult situations by alternating muscular tension. The patient is instructed how to quickly alternate between tensing and relaxing the muscle. Reciprocal inhibition is sometimes an option to help switch off neighboring muscles. Often the muscle edges can be followed along their further course, as tendons, as far as their insertion onto a bone.

1.5.6 Palpating Tendons

▶ **Examples.** Tendons in the extensor compartments of the wrist, flexors of the wrist and fingers (▶ Fig. 1.8), biceps brachii tendon, ankle plantar flexors and toe flexors, and hamstring tendons. The trunk muscles rarely attach onto the bone via a tendon. A fleshy insertion is more common. Limb muscles near the trunk are more likely to have insertions that feel like tendons when palpated, for example, the common head of the hamstrings.

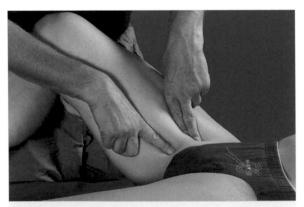

Fig. 1.7 Palpating the edges of muscles, demonstrated here on the adductor longus muscle.

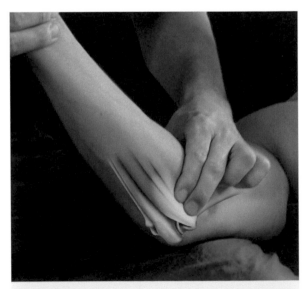

Fig. 1.8 Palpating tendons, demonstrated here on the wrist and finger flexors.

▶ **Technique.** The choice of technique depends on how difficult it is to find the target tissue and the aim of palpation:
- Tendon that is difficult to locate: place the finger pads flatly and directly onto the point where you suspect the tendon to be, then alternately tense and relax the muscle.
- Tendon that is easy to locate: place the tip of the finger alongside the edge of the tendon. Tense the muscle when necessary.
- For pain provocation: administer transverse friction massage using the finger pads, applying firm pressure on the presumably affected site.

▶ **Expectations.** Firm consistency and, when the muscle is tensed, very firm consistency. A tendon remains somewhat elastic when direct pressure is applied to it, even when under a large amount of tension. In most cases, the tendon is a rounded structure with a clearly defined contour.

▶ **Commentary.** Tendons and their insertions belong to the soft-tissue structures in the musculoskeletal system that most frequently present with local lesions. It is therefore imperative to familiarize oneself with the different techniques used for this taut connective tissue.

Tip

The treating finger should not slip off the tendon while Cyriax transverse friction is being applied to the tendon for treatment or pain provocation. The tendon is kept stable by positioning the muscle in a stretched position, thus placing the tendon under tension.

1.5.7 Palpating Ligaments

▶ **Examples.** Medial collateral ligament or the patellar ligament at the knee joint (▶ Fig. 1.9), talofibular ligament at the ankle. With very few exceptions the precise palpation of spinal ligaments is rarely possible. The pelvic ligamental structures, e.g., the sacrotuberous ligament (▶ Fig. 1.9, as

Excursus: Using Friction to Treat Tendinopathy
The techniques of transverse friction of soft tissue structures developed by James Cyriax can also be used as provocative palpation in settings other than examinations. They can also be used to treat inflammation in the junctions between muscles and tendons, tendons, insertions, tendon sheaths, and joint capsules, as well as for painful degenerative tendinopathy. This excursus will present methods for implementing the techniques to be used for the examples discussed in subsequent chapters. For more detailed information, see Reichert (2015).

Transverse/Longitudinal Friction in Tendons with Inflammation
Pain relief from the treatment can be expected in a matter of minutes. Once this has set in, the intensity can either be applied again, at a higher level, or an adjacent—now more painful—area may be sought. Since the assessment of the pain-relieving effect is dependent on what the patient reports, at the outset of treatment the patient should deliberately register the intensity with which the transverse frictions are executed.
- Direction: Transverse or longitudinal to the course of the fibers of the affected structure.
- Submaximal intensity: Transverse frictions may be distinctly perceived by the patient, but should not be excessively painful. The patient should not perceive pain higher than level 2 to 3 out of 10 on the visual analog scale (VAS) for pain.
- Pressure emphasis is in only one direction.
- Duration is around 5 to 10 minutes.
- Additional treatment methods: Ointment dressings with anti-inflammatory agents, relaxation of the affected muscle bellies, functional tape dressings, and thermal and electrotherapeutic physiotherapy methods.

Transverse Friction for Treating Chronic Painful Tendinopathy
For strenuous eccentric exercise, an established method for treating tendonitis, it takes several weeks for pain relief to set in. Before the model for influencing neovascularization of tendinosis through the successful application of transverse frictions, many therapists followed the notion of Prentice (1994) that the effect was a result from conversion of a chronic inflammation to an acute inflammation which would then heal. The latter model to explain tendonitis is now obsolete, since during the healing of tendonitis no signs of inflammation are observed (Alfredson and Lorentzon, 2002).
- Direction: Transverse or longitudinal to the course of the fibers of the affected structure.
- High intensity: For this method to be indicated, the patient must report pain of at least 5 out of 10 on the VAS in order to influence neovascularization.
- Pressure emphasis is in both directions.
- Duration is around 10 to 20 minutes.
- Pain relief during treatment cannot be expected.
- Additional training methods: Eccentric exercise and night splints.

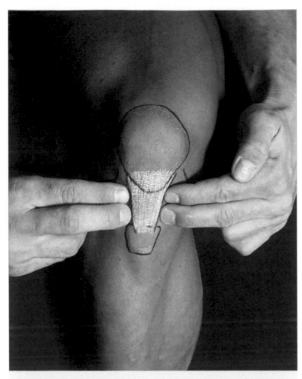

Fig. 1.9 Palpating ligaments, demonstrated here on the patellar ligament.

well as the supraspinosus and the nuchal ligaments, are the only ligaments on the trunk that can be palpated well.

▶ **Technique**
- Ligament that is easy to locate: The tip of the finger is positioned on the edge of the ligament, for example, sacrotuberous ligament.
- Ligament that is difficult to locate: Initially place the ligament under tension and use direct pressure to palpate the firm, elastic consistency, for example, nuchal ligament.
- For pain provocation: Administer transverse friction using the finger pads, applying firm, direct pressure onto the ligament, for example, supraspinous ligament.

▶ **Expectations.** Firm consistency. Very firm consistency when stretched. A ligament remains somewhat elastic, even when placed under a large amount of tension. Clearly defined contours are seldom found for the rest of the capsule.

▶ **Commentary.** Capsular ligaments consisting of dense connective tissue act as mechanical reinforcements. In contrast to tendons, most ligaments are not easily distinguishable from the unreinforced capsule or other tissues. As components of the fibrous membrane of the articular capsule, they very rarely exhibit distinct edges. Two exceptions are the patellar ligament and the medial

collateral ligament of the knee joint. For other ligaments, one must know the characteristic course and the associated bony landmarks in order to visualize their location.

1.5.8 Palpating Capsules

▶ **Examples**
- Test for large effusions in the knee joint, effusions at the elbow joint.
- Pain provocation: Cervical facet joints (▶ Fig. 1.10).

▶ **Technique**
- The palpation is performed at a slow pace with the entire surface of the finger pads palpating directly over the capsule. The finger pads move repeatedly over the capsule, applying minimal pressure.
- Pain provocation: The palpation is performed at a slow pace with the entire surface of the finger pads palpating directly over the capsule. The finger pads move repeatedly over the capsule, applying minimal pressure.

▶ **Expectations**
- Test for swelling: A very soft consistency and fluctuation of synovial fluid inside the swollen capsule is to be expected.
- Pain provocation: During the objective of pain provocation in arthritis, the consistency of the capsule may feel softer than an unaffected capsule.

▶ **Commentary.** The palpatory findings, that is, the identification of swelling, must match the results of observation at a local level. Palpation for an increase in temperature is also usually positive.

The sacroiliac joints, the lumbar and thoracic facet joints, and the atlanto-occipital joints cannot be directly reached using palpation. It is not customary to palpate for warmth or swelling as there is too much soft tissue overlying these joints. The focus is the provocation of pain using palpation to locate the level of the cervical facet

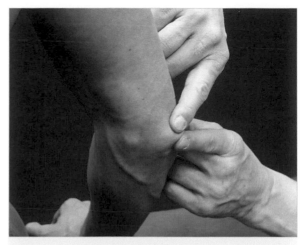

Fig. 1.11 Palpating bursae, demonstrated here with the olecranon bursa.

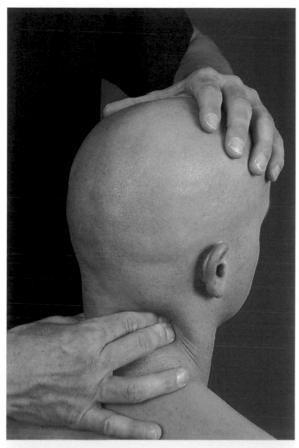

Fig. 1.10 Palpating the capsules of the cervical facet joints.

joints. The result of this palpation, that is, the discovery of sensitivity to pressure and possible associated swelling, must be accompanied by a functional assessment (end-of-range combined movement).

Tip

In addition to searching for lesions on an injured capsule-reinforcing ligament of the joint of an extremity, confirming capsular swelling constitutes another important reason for palpating the joint capsule when arthritis is expected.

1.5.9 Palpating Bursae

▶ **Examples.** Olecranon bursa (▶ Fig. 1.11), trochanteric bursa.

▶ **Technique.** The palpation is performed at a slow pace with the entire surface of the finger pads palpating directly over the bursa. The palpatory movements are repeated several times, applying minimal pressure.

▶ **Expectations.** The normal expectation: no exceptional palpation result. When a bursitis is present, it is expected that the bursa will have a soft consistency and that the fluid in the inflamed bursa will fluctuate with repeated palpation.

▶ **Commentary.** One reason for wanting to feel the fluctuation in a bursa is local pain. This pain arises in tests of the basic joint examination, which cause compression of the bursa. Another reason is the presence of clearly visible local swelling. With bursitis of the trochanter, activity against resistance in the direction of abduction and passive adduction of the hip joint is painful.

Tip

Local swelling can be clearly seen in a superficially located bursa. The fluctuation of fluid can be felt well when two finger pads are used for the palpation and pressure is alternately applied using one finger and then the other. Muscular or tendinous structures located superficial to the affected bursa (iliotibial tract over the trochanteric bursa) should not be tensed or stretched during the palpation. The consistency naturally changes when palpating through these tissues. They may lose the softness, and fluctuations can no longer be palpated. In this case, the technique serves only to provoke pain in cases of suspected bursitis.

1.5.10 Palpating Peripheral Nerves

▶ **Examples.** Median nerve, ulnar nerve, tibial nerve, common peroneal nerve, and superficial peroneal nerve (▶ Fig. 1.12).

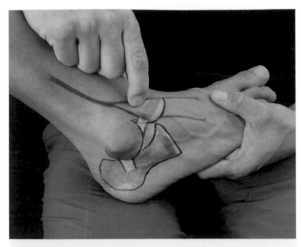

Fig. 1.12 Palpating peripheral nerves, demonstrated here on the superficial peroneal nerve.

- In most cases, it is not possible to palpate and locate neural structures without initially placing the neural structures under tension.
- The important peripheral nerves for the upper and lower limbs are especially thick near the trunk.
- Nerves can tolerate direct pressure and short-term adjustments in their pathway quite well. Extreme caution is not necessary. The nerves have to be stretched past their physiological boundaries, undergo repeated frictioning, or experience long-lasting pressure before they show signs of intolerance. Sensitive people report a "pins and needles" sensation when the preliminary tension on a nerve is uncomfortable.
- Accessory lines often help make the position of a neural structure more distinct (e.g., sciatic nerve at the pelvis).

▶ **Technique.** The fingertips palpate at a right angle to the path of the neural structure sought. It is possible to slide over the nerve if the nerve is placed under tension beforehand. This is similar to plucking a tightened guitar string. Do not use too little pressure and do not proceed too slowly.

▶ **Expectations.** The nerve feels very firm and has an elastic consistency when it has been placed under tension beforehand and direct pressure is applied to it.

▶ **Commentary.** The number of peripheral nerve compressions identified during patient assessment is increasing. These conditions sometimes give the impression that a lesion is present in a muscle or tendon. For example, irritation of the ulnar nerve at the medial epicondyle of the humerus in the elbow joint imitates a "golfer's elbow," while irritation of the radial nerve appears to be an inflammation of the synovial sheath in the first extensor tendon compartment. In addition to further indications, good palpatory differentiation is very useful.

Compressions and stretching of neural structures play a major role when examining patients with spinal complaints. Sometimes, local irritations suggest the appearance of a lesion of a muscle or tendon.

For example, an irritation of the sciatic nerve on the sciatic tubercle causes hamstring syndrome, such as bursitis, or the ischiocrural muscles may be affected.

However, it is possible to discern neural structures well only by palpating at the transition between the trunk and the extremities and in the further course of the extremities.

1.5.11 Palpating Blood Vessels (Arteries)

▶ **Examples.** Brachial artery, femoral artery, anterior tibial artery, occipital artery (▶ Fig. 1.13).

▶ **Technique.** A finger pad is placed flat and with very little pressure over the presumed position of the artery.

▶ **Expectations.** Location of contours or different consistencies is not being addressed here and pain is not being provoked as a test. Instead, the palpation of arteries involves detection of a pulse, how the artery knocks on the finger pad. This can only be achieved when the applied pressure is minimal. The finger pad receptors are unable to discriminate between the pulsation and the consistency of the surrounding tissues when too much pressure is applied. Excessive pressure can also compress small arteries, making it more difficult to feel the pulse.

▶ **Commentary.** Knowledge of position and course of the vessels in the examination of internal medicine patients are helpful in the palpatory evaluation of peripheral arterial circulation in arms and legs.

Furthermore, in performing manual techniques, compression of neural structures and vessels should be avoided if possible. However, it is still important to be familiar with the vessels that can be palpated and their location. Arteries on the thoracic wall can rarely be palpated. They can only be distinctly palpated on the back of the head, the throat, and the face.

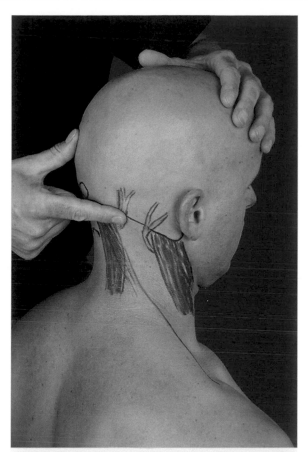

Fig. 1.13 Palpating arteries, demonstrated here on the occipital artery.

1.6 Palpation Aids

It is sometimes necessary to enlist the help of guiding structures and spatial relationships to locate the structure in question.

1.6.1 Guiding Structures

It is sometimes extremely difficult or even impossible to find the exact location of an anatomical structure using direct palpation. In these cases, other anatomical structures are used that guide the palpating finger to the point being sought. Guiding structures can be tendons that make the position of a structure clearer. The edge of muscles or certain bony points (reference points or landmarks) can also be used for orientation.

▶ **Examples**
- The tendon of the sternocleidomastoid guides the palpating finger to the sternoclavicular (SC) joint space (see ▶ Fig. 2.40).
- The tendon of the palmaris longus reveals the position of the median nerve in the forearm (see ▶ Fig. 4.82).
- The scaphoid can be found in the anatomical snuffbox. The snuffbox is formed by two tendons (see ▶ Fig. 4.42).
- The distal radioulnar joint space lies immediately beneath the tendon of the extensor digiti minimi (see ▶ Fig. 4.34).
- The tip of the patella is always found at the same level as the joint space of the knee (see ▶ Fig. 6.16).
- The common peroneal nerve is found in the popliteal fossa, running parallel to the biceps femoris, approximately 1 cm away from it (see ▶ Fig. 6.69).
- The 12th rib and the transverse process of T12 are at the level of the spinous process of T11 (see ▶ Fig. 1.14).

1.6.2 Connecting Lines

It is also possible to use a line connecting two bony landmarks for safe orientation without having to palpate directly. This aid is used in particular when the anatomical structures from which the connecting lines start do not vary widely.

▶ **Examples**
- The palpatory differentiation of individual carpal bones using direct palpation is difficult or, in some cases, even impossible. Connecting lines are of great assistance (see ▶ Fig. 4.53). For example, the therapist can assume that the joint space between the scaphoid and lunate is halfway along the line connecting the head of the ulna and the Lister tubercle on the posterior aspect. Initially, this still appears to be quite complicated. However, if the therapist is able to accurately find these bony landmarks, it is easy to use the connective line.

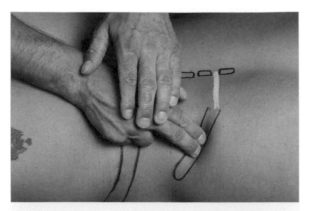

Fig. 1.14 Guiding structures. The 12th rib leads to the T11 spinal process.

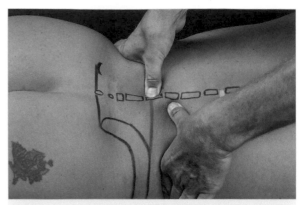

Fig. 1.15 Connecting lines at the pelvis and lumbar spine.

The sciatic nerve is located at the halfway point of the line connecting the tip of the sciatic tubercle and the tip of the greater trochanter (see ▶ Fig. 5.10).
- The line connecting the two posterior superior iliac spines is found at the same level as the S2 spinous process (see ▶ Fig. 1.15).
- The sciatic nerve is located at the halfway point of the line connecting the tip of the sciatic tubercle and the tip of the greater trochanter.

1.6.3 Supporting Measures for Confirming a Palpation

Several measures can be used to confirm the location of a structure when the clinician is not sure what structure is being palpated:
- The successful palpation of a cervical facet joint gap is best confirmed by passively moving one side of the joint.
- The successful palpation of an intervertebral space is best confirmed by passively moving one of the vertebrae involved (see ▶ Fig. 1.16).
- The insertions of a muscle belly into a bone or the edge of a muscle can be palpated by tensing the muscle in several short repetitions.
- If a therapist feels they are palpating a peripheral nerve, they can position the joints differently in order to place the nerve under tension or to relax it.
- Palpable ligaments (e.g., medial collateral ligament at the knee joint) can be tightened using a wide-range movement to allow the change in consistency to be felt.

If therapists think they have palpated a peripheral nerve, they can use different joint positions to tense or relax the nerve.

These measures thus cause a change in the resistance felt, indicating exactly where the structure is to be found. It is, however, the aim of routine palpation to find structures without these aids. Some measures cannot be used

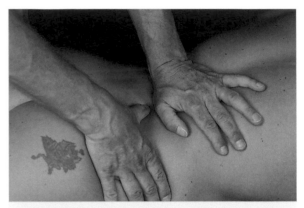

Fig. 1.16 Movement of the superior vertebra to confirm the location of an interspinous space.

on the patient. For instance, with a painfully swollen joint, it may happen that a movement to confirm the intra-articular space being sought cannot be used without causing even more difficulties for the patient.

1.6.4 Marking Structures

Marking anatomical structures is not imperative and therefore tends to be rarely done on patients. However, marking the position or course of a structure when practicing can be very helpful. Drawing clarifies the location of different anatomical shapes and develops spatial orientation abilities.

A drawing can also ensure that a third person can examine the findings and check whether they are correct. Drawing a structure is a moment of truth.

In this book, the structures found during palpation are marked on the skin. Bony borders, edges of muscles and tendons, etc. are illustrated exactly where they have been felt. This helps to visualize where the specific structure can be found.

Marking an anatomical structure on the skin means tracing a palpated three-dimensional structure onto an almost two-dimensional surface. Hence a drawing always appears more extensive and wider than the palpated structure actually is. A drawing is more reliable in demonstrating the actual size of a structure when the structure is more superficial.

1.6.5 Starting Positions for Practice (Practice SPs)

Generally it is necessary to practice palpatory techniques on a study partner in appropriate SPs. It is permissible to use SPs that do not always correspond to the clinical situation when practicing.

Once the techniques can be confidently performed in the practice SPs, the study partner should be placed in more difficult positions that mirror clinical practice and an attempt made to locate the structure again.

Bibliography

Aland RC, Kippers V. Addressing Interindividual Variation within a Science Dissection based Anatomy Course. In: Abstracts of the ANZACA 2005: 2nd Annual Conference of the Australian and New Zealand Association of Clinical Anatomists. Dunedin, Otago, N.Z. (Abstract No. 1). 2–3 September 2005

Alfredson H, Lorentzon R. Chronic tendon pain: no signs of chemical inflammation but high concentrations of the neurotransmitter glutamate. Implications for treatment? Curr Drug Targets. 2002; 3(1):43–54

Lanz T von, Wachsmuth W. Praktische Anatomie, Rücken. Berlin: Springer; 2004

Prentice W. Therapeutic Modalities in Sports Medicine. 3. Aufl. St. Louis: Mosby; 1994: 336–349

Reichert B. Massage-Therapie. Stuttgart: Thieme; 2015

Winkel D. Nichtoperative Orthopädie und Manualtherapie. Anatomie in vivo. 3. Aufl. München: Urban & Fischer bei Elsevier; 2004

Chapter 2

Shoulder Complex

2

2 Shoulder Complex

2.1 Introduction

2.1.1 Significance and Function of the Shoulder Region

This chapter will consider the function and pathology of the shoulder region, or shoulder complex.

The shoulder complex is one of the largest movement complexes in the musculoskeletal system. It includes the following:

- The glenohumeral or GH joint.
- The bony parts and joints in the shoulder girdle (acromioclavicular and sternoclavicular joints).
- The sliding scapulothoracic articulation.
- The cervicothoracic transition to the cranial rib joints.
- Costal joints 1 to 6.

The **most important principle of function** of the shoulder complex is the optimization of arm movements with the greatest radius possible and to provide a mobile and stable base for the arm movements. End-range arm elevation is one of the most complex movements of our body.

The intricate interplay between the individual components of the shoulder complex can lead to a variety of dysfunctions. A cause of restricted shoulder elevation, for example, can be found in every single mobile articulation in the cervicobrachial region.

There are a comparatively large **number of causes** for shoulder/arm pain. Pain may be referred or projected from the cervical spine and the thoracic outlet, or may be due to several other possible causes ranging from arthritis, ligamentous laxity and instability to soft-tissue lesions such as internal or external impingement or labral lesions and ruptures of the rotator cuff muscles.

When presented with a "shoulder patient," the therapist is often compelled to thoroughly assess all components of the shoulder complex and frequently finds it quite difficult to interpret results.

2.1.2 Common Applications for Treatment in this Region

Techniques used in this region that require knowledge of palpation include the following:

- Joint play tests and manual therapy techniques (e.g., glenohumeral, acromioclavicular, and sternoclavicular).
- Laxity and instability tests of shoulder joints.
- Local cross-frictions according to Cyriax, for example, on tendons and at insertion sites of the rotator cuff muscles.
- Local application of electrotherapy and thermotherapy on the muscles and articular structures.

2.1.3 Required Basic Anatomical and Biomechanical Knowledge

Therapists should be familiar with the location and form of the articular structures in all shoulder joints, as well as the location, course, and attachments of clinically important muscles, for example, the subscapularis. A good spatial sense is of advantage as the clinically important structures are found close to each other, especially in the GH joint. Knowledge of the shape of the spine of the scapula and the acromion, of the proximal humerus, the dimensions of the clavicle, and the position of the joint spaces is especially important (▶ Fig. 2.1, ▶ Fig. 2.2, ▶ Fig. 2.3).

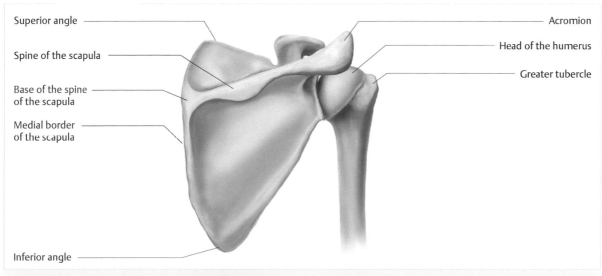

Fig. 2.1 Overview of the topography on the posterior aspect.

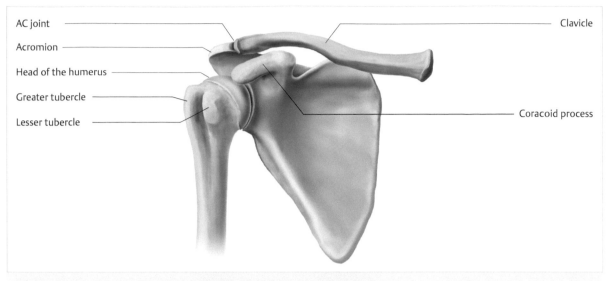

AC joint

Acromion

Head of the humerus

Greater tubercle

Lesser tubercle

Clavicle

Coracoid process

Fig. 2.2 Overview of the topography on the anterior aspect.

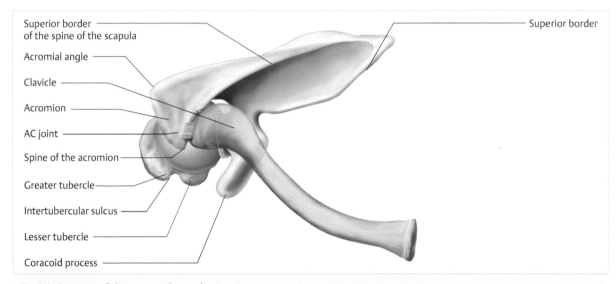

Superior border
of the spine of the scapula

Acromial angle

Clavicle

Acromion

AC joint

Spine of the acromion

Greater tubercle

Intertubercular sulcus

Lesser tubercle

Coracoid process

Superior border

Fig. 2.3 Overview of the topography on the superior aspect.

Glenohumeral Joint

The glenoid cavity or glenoid fossa is the socket of the humeral head. Its concavity is directed laterally, forward, and somewhat upward as an extension of the scapular spine. Since the scapula adapts itself to the shape of the thorax as a relatively flat bone, the socket tips in an anterior direction in the sagittal plane so that the anteroposterior surface of the cavity is not transverse. The head of the humerus is almost spherical; in the transverse plane it exhibits a retrotorsion of approximately 30° to the line connecting the epicondyles of the humerus. This retrotorsion determines the range of motion in outward and inward rotation. A slight retrotorsion leads to a smaller outward rotation. In the frontal plane, the humeral head is angled at 45° to the shaft of the humerus. Since the insertion of the capsule lies at the anatomical neck, directly adjacent to the head of the humerus, the superior portions of the capsule are stretched when the arm is allowed to hang. For equal tension on the superior and inferior portions of the capsule, the arm must be abducted by about 45°. This is the resting position.

On the basis of the anatomy seen in radiographs, it was claimed that the shoulder joint was incongruent and that the radii of curvature of the two members of the joint provided a poor fit. According to this finding, the socket would hardly be able to contribute to the stability of the shoulder joint. However, studies of anatomical preparations and modern imaging techniques (CT and MRI) show a high degree of congruence between head and socket.

The decisive factor is the shape of the cartilaginous lining of the socket and the glenoid labrum. The drawing in ▶ Fig. 2.4 summarizes what is known today about the interrelations of shapes in the glenohumeral joint. The cartilage is thicker at the edges than in the center of the socket. The depth of the socket and the resulting congruence play a decisive role in the stability of the glenohumeral joint. The glenoid labrum is a fibrocartilaginous structure that increases the contact surface and

functions like a suction cup. Furthermore, it is the origin of the long biceps tendon and the capsule of the labrum.

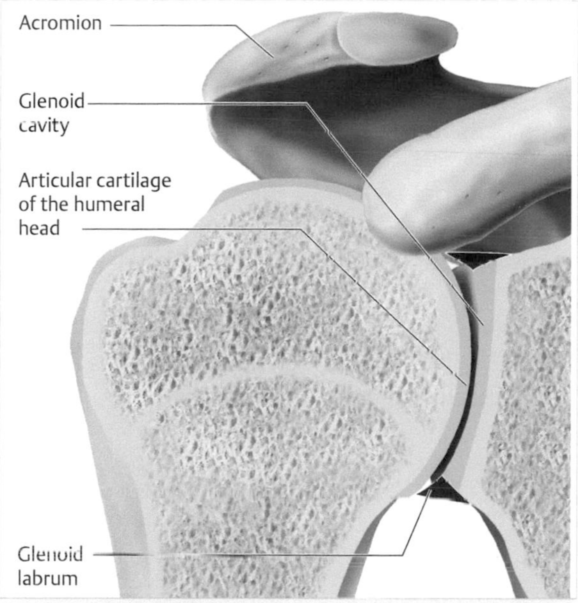

Overall, the high degree of congruence creates such a strong adhesion between the joint surfaces that it is hardly possible to separate the head from the socket in the direction of traction. In 2003, Gokeler et al. were able to demonstrate in a study that it is not possible to separate head and socket with 14 kg of tractive force.

▶ Fig. 2.5 shows a view of the glenoid cavity with the fibrocartilaginous ring (glenoid labrum) and the interior of the capsule with the reinforcing structures as well as the position of the rotator cuff tendons. The capsular fibers are somewhat twisted in their arrangement, in a clockwise direction in the right shoulder, so that the capsule tenses more rapidly in extension than in flexion. Approximately half of the capsular surface is the area of insertion for the rotator cuff muscles, which greatly strengthens the capsule. The subscapularis (SSC) has the broadest tendon; this muscle supports the capsule anteriorly. In the superior part of the capsule there is a gap in the muscle insertion. At this point, the long head of the biceps brachii leaves the capsule and continues in the intertubercular sulcus. The so-called rotator interval is reinforced and overlapped by two bands of the coracohumeral ligament (Werner et al., 2000).

The three glenohumeral ligaments, the superior, middle, and inferior glenohumeral ligaments, arise at the edge of the labrum. They reinforce the anterior inferior capsule and limit certain movements of the humerus by increasing tension. The effect of this increasing tension is to center the head in the socket with increasing extent of motion. The axillary recess runs between the two portions of the inferior ligament. The most important centering function is performed by the anterior portion of the inferior glenohumeral ligament. With increasing abduction and outward

Fig. 2.4 Congruence of the glenohumeral articular surfaces (after Omer Matthijs).

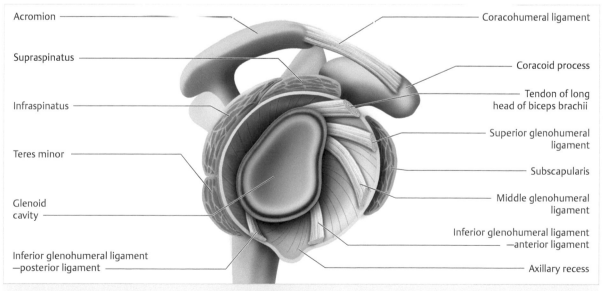

Fig. 2.5 Structure of the glenohumeral capsule (after Omer Matthijs).

rotation (the back-swing phase of the throwing motion) it wraps around the head of the humerus and thus prevents abnormal forward displacement (subluxation) of the head. The subscapular muscle plays a decisive reinforcing role here.

The acromion, the coracoacromial ligament, and the coracoid process form the summit of the shoulder, the fornix humeri. The tendons of the rotator cuff and the subacromial bursa (not illustrated) lie in the subacromial space. In inflammatory processes, the tendons and the bursa can become impinged (clamped) between the tubercula and the fornix humeri. The tendons of the supraspinatus (SSP) and the infraspinatus (ISP) overlap. Only the teres minor (TM) cannot be clamped in this external impingement.

Acromioclavicular Joint

The acromioclavicular (AC) joint has all the characteristics typical of a classical amphiarthrosis:
- It is part of the shoulder girdle motor complex.
- Because it does not have its own muscles it moves only together with the neighboring joints.
- Because of its rather flat joint surface and very tight ligaments it is not very mobile.

However, the joint is very small, with an intra-articular space of only about 1 cm long (▶ Fig. 2.6). Many people have an intra-articular disk. There are numerous variations in the shape of the acromial end of the clavicle in the frontal and transverse planes (De Palma, 1963; Moseley, 1968) and the clavicle is not always convex. Colegate-Stone et al. (2010) describe an even distribution of vertical, oblique, and curved (convex clavicle) shapes in the acromioclavicular joints of the specimens they studied.

One particular shape variation, with sides raised, looks like a volcano and makes precise location of the intra-articular space much harder.

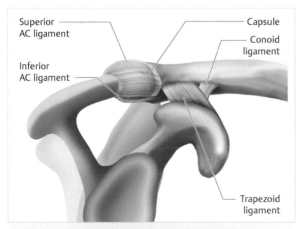

Superior AC ligament
Capsule
Conoid ligament
Inferior AC ligament
Trapezoid ligament

Fig. 2.6 Structure of the AC joint (after Omer Matthijs).

The reinforcing ligaments of the AC joint (Saccomanno et al., 2014) are divided into the following:
- *Intrinsic ligaments:* Superior and inferior acromioclavicular ligaments. The superior ligament is very strong and primarily limits all transverse movements, for instance the translatory tests of manual therapy (see ▶ Fig. 2.36).
- *Extrinsic ligaments:* The coracoclavicular ligaments (conoid and trapezoid ligaments). Except in passive elevation of the shoulder, they are never completely relaxed. They guarantee stability in the face of large, transverse forces (e.g., when the intrinsic ligaments are torn) and limit vertical movements between acromion and clavicle.

Since the AC joint is an amphiarthrosis, it has no motor muscle supply of its own. Nevertheless, fibers in the descending portion of the trapezius muscle and the clavicular portion of the deltoid muscle can extend across the intraarticular space and, at a deep level, make contact with the capsule. For this reason, both muscles are suitable for active stabilization of the joint.

Sternoclavicular Joint

In the sternoclavicular (SC) joint, the movements of the shoulder girdle are facilitated while the forces for the shoulder girdle movements are exerted more on the scapula (▶ Fig. 2.7). During support of the arm and hand, it transfers compression forces on the thorax. Likewise, end-range arm elevations are transmitted via the first rib to the cervicothoracic transition.

It is anatomically classified as a sellar joint. However, the rotation of the clavicle during arm elevation means that it functions as a ball-and-socket joint. The narrow sternal end of the clavicle articulates with the joint surface of the sternal manubrium by means of a disk that subdivides each joint into two compartments. The joint space tilts in the frontal plane by approximately 45° from superomedial to inferolateral.

The joint, which is rather unstable in terms of its bony structure, derives its stability from intrinsic (directly capsule-reinforcing) and extrinsic ligaments (Sewell et al., 2013):
- *Intrinsic ligaments:* Anterior and posterior sternoclavicular ligaments, and interclavicular ligament.
- *Extrinsic ligament:* Costoclavicular ligament.

The costoclavicular ligament is particularly interesting in terms of biomechanics. It is 3 to 10 mm long and is fused directly to the lateral edge of the sternoclavicular (SC) joint (Tubbs et al., 2009). End-range arm elevations are transferred to the first rib via tension of the costoclavicular ligament and further to the cervicothoracic transition. During protraction and retraction, this ligament tenses up and thus becomes a rotational axis. The clavicle therefore behaves consistently with the convex rule during

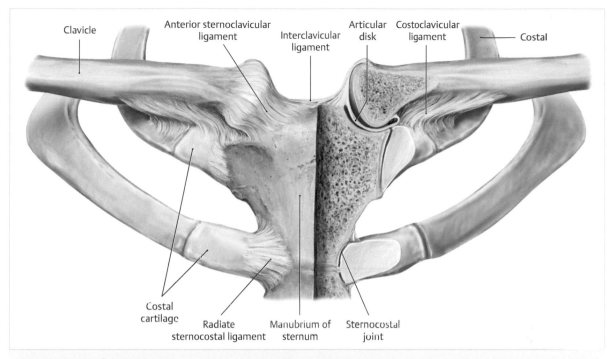

Fig. 2.7 Structure of the SC joint.

movements in both planes. When a patient falls on an arm with a shoulder in protraction, in the worst case the clavicle can become dislocated in a posterior direction.

2.2 General Orientation—Posterior

2.2.1 Summary of the Palpatory Process

Palpation begins dorsally at the scapula, moves toward the acromioclavicular joint and then toward the SC joint, finishing with the anterolateral aspect.

This order has developed from experiences in continuing education courses and is a purely didactic suggestion. Of course, the therapist can begin the palpation at any point.

Starting Position

When the important structures in the shoulder girdle are being located in detail, a practice starting position (SP) is taken: upright-sitting on a stool or a treatment table with the arms hanging loosely by the sides. In this SP, all components of the shoulder complex are usually found in a neutral position and all structures can be reached with ease. Dorsal orientation in this region begins by observing the topographical location of the scapula in relation to the spinal column and the thorax. The position of the most familiar bony landmarks (inferior angle and

acromion) is also checked. To do this, the therapist stands behind the patient.

2.2.2 Topographical Position of the Scapula

According to Winkel (2004), Kapandji (2006), and Williams (2009), the superior angle of the scapula is found at the level of the T1 spinous process and the second rib. The inferior angle of the scapula can be clearly palpated and is found at the same level as the T7 spinous process and the seventh rib. The triangular origin of the spine of the scapula can be located at the level of the T3 spinous process (▶ Fig. 2.8).

> **Tip**
>
> The correlations described above are very constant, but only apply when the shoulder is relaxed and a sitting or upright SP is used. They are no longer reliable, however, if the patient changes position, for example, into side-lying, as the position of the scapula has changed (e.g., there is more elevation or abduction).

Medial Border of the Scapula

When the shoulder joint rotates medially, the scapula follows and the medial border of the scapula moves away

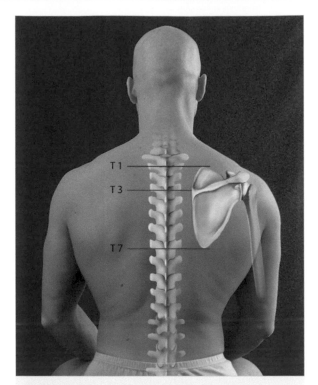

Fig. 2.8 Position of the scapula in relation to the spine.

T 1
T 3
T 7

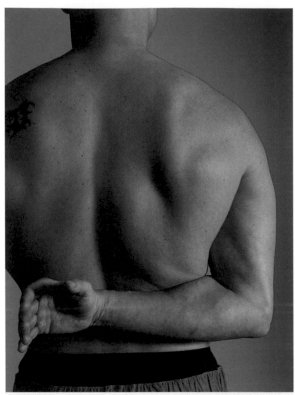

Fig. 2.9 Movement of the scapula with medial rotation of the arm.

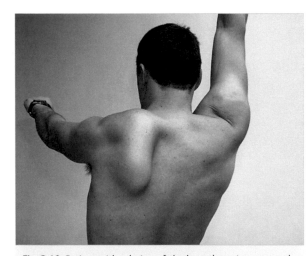

Fig. 2.10 Patient with a lesion of the long thoracic nerve and paresis of the left serratus anterior.

from the thoracic wall (▶ Fig. 2.9). This assists movement of the arm and is normal. It should not be considered pathological. Only the timing and the range of motion allow the therapist to draw conclusions about the ability of the shoulder joint to rotate medially. Extensive outward movement of the scapula indicates a decreased ability of the glenohumeral joint to rotate inward.

The medial border of the scapula is usually only visible when weakness in the rhomboids and serratus anterior results in insufficient thoracic stabilization of the scapula.

Considerable weakness or paralysis in these muscles causes winging of the scapula especially when the arm is raised and is also known as scapula alata (▶ Fig. 2.10).

2.3 Local Palpation—Posterior

2.3.1 Overview of the Structures to be Palpated

- Inferior angle of the scapula.
- Medial border of the scapula.
- Superior angle of the scapula.
- Spine of the scapula—inferior edge.
- Acromial angle.
- Acromion.
- Spine of the scapula—superior edge.
- Supraspinatus—muscle belly.
- Infraspinatus—tendon and insertion.

2.3.2 Summary of the Palpatory Process

Following completion of the introductory orientation on the posterior aspect of the shoulder, first several important bony structures will be located. The palpation starts medially, over the spine of the scapula toward the lateral region of the shoulder. The different sections of the acromion are of special interest here and guide the therapist to two structures of great clinical importance: the supraspinatus and infraspinatus.

Starting Position

The patient's SP is identical to that used in the previous section.

2.3.3 Palpation of Individual Structures

Inferior Angle of the Scapula

The inferior angle of the scapula is an important reference point when assessing movement of the scapula. Therapists use this structure for orientation when they are assessing the range of scapular motion during abduction and inward and outward rotation in relation to the spinal column.

Technique

To assess rotation of the scapula, the therapist first palpates the inferior angle of the scapula in its resting position. The patient is then instructed to raise the arm. With regard to scapular movement, it is of no significance whether this is done through flexion or abduction. Once the arm has been raised as far as possible, the therapist palpates the position of the angle again and assesses the range of motion (▶ Fig. 2.11). This is also compared with the other side. It is more difficult to locate the inferior angle when the latissimus dorsi is well developed.

Range of motion is not the only aspect of interest when analyzing movement of the scapula. Asymmetrical or even jerky movements of the inferior angle as it moves to assist elevation of the arm indicate poor coordination and a possible weakness of the serratus anterior. Two types of movement can be distinguished, particularly at the start and the end of arm elevation—scapular winging and scapular tipping. Scapular winging describes the brief swinging outward of the medial border of the scapula in the transverse plane. Scapular tipping describes the brief lifting of the inferior angle in the sagittal plane. A lack of support by the scapula for arm elevation not only limits the overall movement but can also be the cause of various forms of external or internal impingement of the shoulder joint.

Medial Border of the Scapula

The medial border of the scapula is located using a perpendicular technique and palpating from inferior to superior. This is the first opportunity for students to consciously use this technique and to differentiate between the soft and elastic consistency of the muscles and the hard resistance of the edge of bone.

Technique

The palpating fingertips come from a medial position and push against the border (▶ Fig. 2.12). It is easy to locate the inferior part of the border as relatively few muscles are found here that impede access. If the border is followed in a cranial direction, precise palpation becomes difficult.

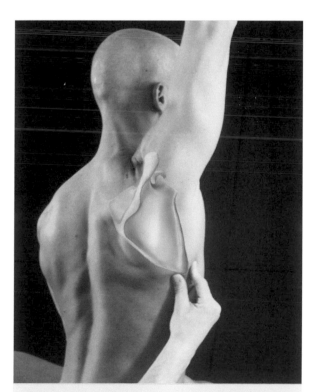

Fig. 2.11 Position of the inferior angle of the scapula in maximal arm elevation.

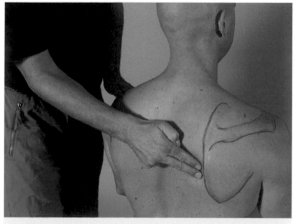

Fig. 2.12 Palpation of the medial border of the scapula.

If circumstances make it difficult to locate the border, it can help to ease the shoulder into medial rotation so that the medial border of the scapula wings out (see also ▶ Fig. 2.9). However, the aim of this palpatory exercise is to be able to find the edge of bone in any shoulder and with different tissue conditions.

Superior Angle of the Scapula

The superior angle lies at the cranial end of the medial border and approximately at the level of the second rib, thus usually lying higher in a cranial direction than expected.

Technique

The finger is placed as an extension of the medial border at the posterior edge of the descending trapezius muscle belly and palpates from cranial toward the angle.

It is very difficult to palpate the superior angle of the scapula. The trapezius that runs past it and the inserting levator scapulae are often very tense, making it difficult for the therapist to differentiate between the elevated muscle tension and the superior angle. Moreover, the first costotransverse joint, which is often sensitive, lies directly cranial. The therapist can avoid this problem by passively elevating the shoulder girdle. This can be done in any SP. The therapist elevates the shoulder girdle by pushing along the axis of the hanging arm. The superior angle is then recognized by its pressure from caudal against the palpating finger (▶ Fig. 2.13).

Spine of the Scapula—Inferior Edge

The spine of the scapula is another important bony reference point when palpating the posterior aspect. From this point, the therapist has reliable access to the acromion to the side and to the bellies of clinically prominent muscles (supraspinatus and infraspinatus). The spine of the scapula points toward the opening of the socket of the shoulder joint (glenoid cavity) and is the direction for manual therapeutic traction at the GH joint. For this reason, before applying traction to the joint, the manual therapist should determine the direction by palpating the spine of the scapula.

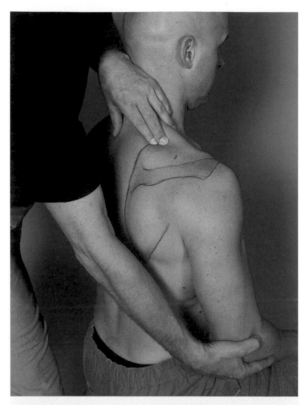

Fig. 2.13 Palpation of the superior angle of the scapula.

Technique

The inferior and superior edges of the spine of the scapula are palpated using the perpendicular technique we are already familiar with. The supraspinatus and infraspinatus are often quite tense, which makes locating the spine of the scapula more difficult than on the medial border of the scapula.

The inferior edge is palpated from medial to lateral. The spine of the scapula has a rolling, undulating shape that has developed as a result of the pull of muscular attachments, for example, the ascending part of the trapezius.

To locate the inferior edge exactly, the therapist uses the finger pads to push against the elastic resistance of the skin and muscles on the posterior side of the scapula and moves the palpating fingers in a superior direction until the finger pads encounter hard resistance (▶ Fig. 2.14).

The muscle belly of the infraspinatus lies in the space between the lower edge of the spine, the inferior angle, and the lateral border of the scapula.

Acromial Angle

Technique

At the lateral end of the inferior edge there is an angle that is distinctly prominent when the arm is hanging down—the acromial angle (▶ Fig. 2.15). At this point, the inferior edge of the spine describes an almost right-angle bend and runs anteromedial as the edge of the acromion.

Acromion

The acromion is also an important reference point. The height of the acromion in the resting position can indicate the presence of an elevated shoulder. During arm elevation, the acromion is also used for orientation to assess the range and speed of shoulder girdle elevation and, when observed from the side, retraction.

Tip

The lateral edge of the acromion is generally aligned anteriorly, medially, and slightly superiorly. The shape and dimensions of the acromion vary greatly among individuals and must be palpated precisely. This will be described later in the text.

Spine of the Scapula—Superior Edge

In the next stage of the palpation, the superior edge of the spine of the scapula is followed from medial to lateral until it meets up with the posterior edge of the clavicle. The therapist will discover that the spine of the scapula is significantly thicker than imagined. When the superior and inferior edges are projected and drawn onto the skin, they are almost parallel to each other, appear very broad, and are approximately 2 cm apart.

Technique

Palpation uses the same technique of perpendicular palpation, this time with the pad of the finger pushing against the edge from cranial and following the edge from the medial origin of the spine in a lateral direction (▸ Fig. 2.16).

The spine of the scapula can be followed from its base to the acromion. The palpation finishes laterally when the fingertips encounter another hard structure. This is the posterior edge of the clavicle. Both of these bony edges (superior edge of the spine of the scapula and the posterior border of the clavicle) taper in toward each other and connect, forming a posterior V (see ▸ Fig. 2.27).

Supraspinatus—Muscle Belly

The muscle belly of the supraspinatus is found in its bony depression between the superior edge of the spine of the scapula and the descending part of the trapezius. Its muscle belly, and further lateral, the muscle-tendon transition, are palpable between the superior angle and the posterior V.

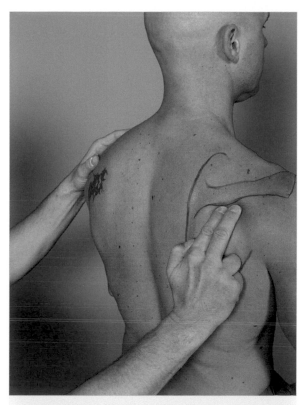

Fig. 2.14 Palpation of the inferior edge of the spine of the scapula.

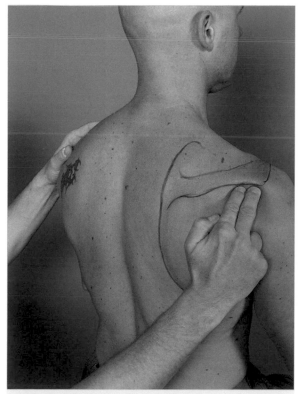

Fig. 2.15 Palpation of the acromial angle.

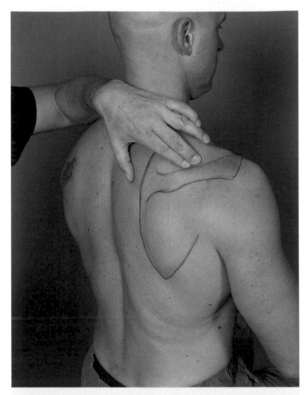

Fig. 2.16 Palpation of the superior edge of the spine of the scapula.

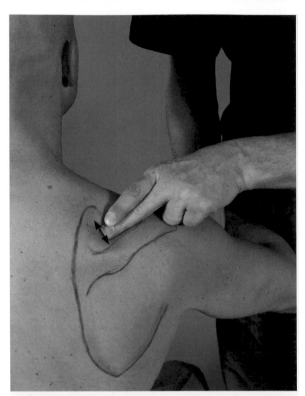

Fig. 2.17 Transverse friction at the muscle belly of the supraspinatus, starting position.

The muscle occasionally causes difficulties in its muscle belly or its insertion at the greater tubercle (external impingement or tendinosis).

Starting Position

To locate the muscle belly, the patient does not have to adopt a certain position and may remain sitting upright. The shoulder should be easily accessible from the side. For better access to the muscle-tendon transition, the muscle can be brought closer to the level of the scapula by passive abduction (scaption) (▶ Fig. 2.17). In this way, the position of the muscle-tendon transition is shifted and becomes more accessible to palpation.

Technique

The muscle belly of the supraspinatus is found deep in the supraspinous fossa and only the slender superficial section of the muscle can be reached directly. The therapist must therefore use a technique that can be applied to tight spaces but is nevertheless intense enough to reach the affected area.

Transverse friction is used for palpation. This technique is used during the assessment to confirm that this structure is symptomatic. It is also used with other techniques to treat tendinitis or tendinosis at the muscle-tendon junction or in injuries to the muscle belly.

The suitable technique here is to come from the side, positioning the middle finger parallel to the muscle fibers and applying pressure. The index finger is placed over the middle finger as support (▶ Fig. 2.17). Transverse friction is performed with deep pressure, moving from posterior to anterior by supination of the underarm. This technique can be used over the entire length of the muscle between the superior angle of the scapula and the posterior V.

The muscle becomes tendinous laterally. Its insertion into the greater tubercle is of clinical interest but is not accessible when the arm is positioned in neutral, as it is then found underneath the acromion. Location of this tendon is discussed in the section "Local Palpation—Anterolateral" below (Chapter 2.7).

Infraspinatus—Tendon and Insertion

Starting Position

The patient must assume a difficult position in order to make the clinically relevant parts of the infraspinatus accessible (muscle-tendon transition, tendon and its insertion). The patient is prone, very close to the edge of the treatment table on the side to be palpated.

The patient supports themselves on the forearms and a cushion is placed under the abdomen to prevent an uncomfortable hyperlordosis. This position produces a 70° flexion in the shoulder joint. In addition, the joint is slightly adducted (approx. 10°, elbows approximately 1 hand width from the edge of the treatment table) with approximately 20° external rotation (the hand has a firm grip on the edge of the treatment table) (▸ Fig. 2.18). Through the flexion the insertion at the greater tubercle, which is otherwise difficult to access under the acromion, is rotated outward and dorsally (▸ Fig. 2.19).

This position was described by Cyriax in 1984 and confirmed by studies of Mattingly and Mackarey in 1996. The tendon of the infraspinatus is tensed by the adduction and the support on the elbows, with a cranial push to the humerus, and acquires a firmer consistency. This makes it easier to define the boundary between the muscle-tendon transition and surrounding structures. During application of this technique as therapeutic transverse friction, the muscle-tendon transition and the tendon remain stable under the treating finger and do not slide away.

Alternative Starting Positions

The usual SP can cause discomfort in the cervical and lumbar spines despite padding in the abdominal area. Many massage therapists and physical therapists use other positions to avoid this problem:

- The patient lies flat on the stomach (not supporting themselves on the forearms). The affected arm hangs down over the side of the treatment table and the forearm rests on a stool. The therapist then attempts to place the GH joint in slight adduction and lateral rotation again (▸ Fig. 2.20).
- The patient sits on a stool at the head-end of the table. The head-end of the treatment table is lowered and the arm is placed in the position described above, resting on the head-end of the table (not illustrated). Mattingly and Mackarey were able to confirm in 1996 that the insertion is accessible in the same way.

> **Tip**
>
> All alternative starting positions are more comfortable for patients but are not particularly conducive to finding the tendon and the insertion site. They have the drawback that insufficient axial pressure is applied to the humerus to tighten up the tendon. The tendon feels less firm underneath the palpating finger and it is more difficult to differentiate it from the surrounding tissue and its insertion into the bone. The tendon gives way under the pressure applied during transverse friction.

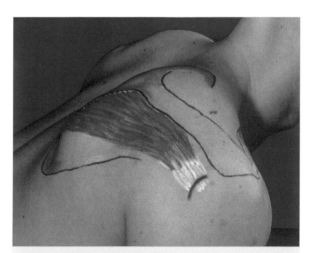

Fig. 2.18 SP—palpation of the infraspinatus.

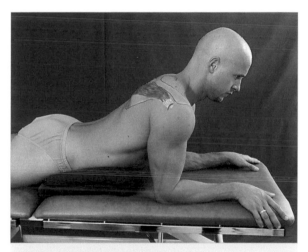

Fig. 2.19 Position of the infraspinatus.

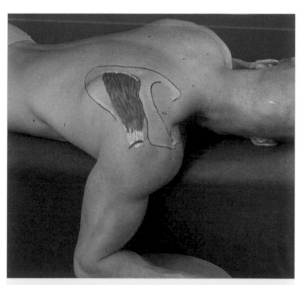

Fig. 2.20 Alternative SP.

Technique

The palpation starts at the already familiar posterior angle of the acromion (acromial angle, see ▶ Fig. 2.15). The location of the broad muscle-tendon transition of the infraspinatus can be found approximately 2 cm from the acromial angle toward the axilla (▶ Fig. 2.21). The palpating finger feels the muscle-tendon transition as a flat, tense structure that offers a firm, but still elastic resistance to transverse palpation. In order to find the tendon, palpation continues along the structure with transverse friction movements approximately 2 cm laterally, parallel to the scapular spine. The resistance felt by the finger is distinctly firmer. To find the insertion at the middle facet of the greater tubercle (see ▶ Fig. 2.60), palpation continues along the tendon, which becomes progressively flatter, further in a lateral direction until a hard resistance is felt. This is the tenoosseous junction, the infraspinatus insertion. This line of palpation can be repeatedly disturbed by coarse fiber bundles of the deltoid muscle. Their course is typically oblique, rising to the superomedial.

The extent of the facet can be precisely determined. If the palpating finger is moved further in a lateral direction, it slips over the edge of the facet onto the humerus. If the finger is moved toward the acromion, it slips approximately 45° anteriorly and arrives at the facet of the supraspinatus (see ▶ Fig. 2.59). If the finger slips to the inferior, it again tips by 45°, onto the facet of the teres minor (see ▶ Fig. 2.61). To treat the more superficial portions of the insertion that can cause difficulties in cases of tendinitis or tendinosis, treatment should be focused on the lateral aspect of the facet.

Comment on the treatment of tendinosis: transverse friction is applied with significant intensity, maintaining pressure in both directions. When treating the deep portions of the tendon at the humerus that can be irritated in the case of an internal impingement, friction should be applied on the medial portion of the facet. Palpation or transverse friction treatment can be performed with two different methods, which will be described below:

Method 1

Two different methods of transverse friction exist that can generally be applied to provoke pain or to treat. In the first method, the therapist stands on the side to be treated. The thumbs are positioned on top of each other and on the muscle-tendon transition (▶ Fig. 2.22). The fingers hold onto the coracoid process anteriorly. The thumbs maintain skin contact, apply almost no pressure, and move in a caudal and somewhat lateral direction. The pressure is increased as the thumbs press deeper. They move in a cranial and somewhat medial direction with this pressure. Both forearms supinate slightly during this movement.

If the insertion is to be treated, the thumb applying the friction should not only push deep into the tissue, it also has to apply pressure laterally against the middle facet of the greater tubercle.

Method 2

As an alternative, the therapist may stand in front of the patient and somewhat toward the contralateral side. The thumbs are now used to stabilize the hands and rest on the coracoid process.

The work is done by the index fingers, placed one over the other (▶ Fig. 2.23). Once again, no pressure is applied when moving down the above-described line. The palpatory or therapeutically effective part of the technique is

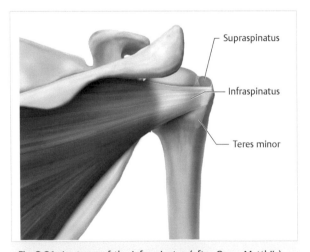

Fig. 2.21 Anatomy of the infraspinatus (after Omer Matthijs).

Supraspinatus

Infraspinatus

Teres minor

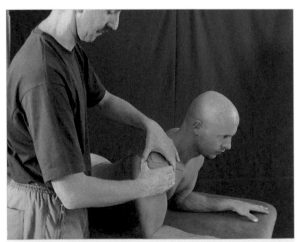

Fig. 2.22 Palpation of the infraspinatus, first method.

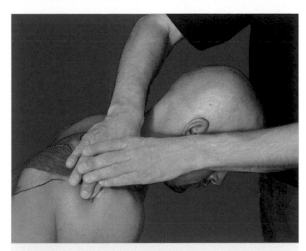

Fig. 2.23 Second method—detailed view.

conducted when pressure is applied during the upward movement.

The main movement here is extension of the wrist. This method is less strenuous and is preferable to techniques that involve finger flexion.

2.4 Local Palpation—Lateral

2.4.1 Overview of the Structures to be Palpated

• Lateral edge of the acromion.
• Acromial spine.
• AC joint—anterior approach.
• AC joint—posterior approach.
• Acromioclavicular joint (AC joint).

2.4.2 Summary of the Palpatory Process

This region also contains important bony reference points that guide the therapist to a variety of clinically pathological structures. The AC joint is the focus of palpation and the anterior and posterior access to this structure will be clarified. The exact position of the AC joint is ascertained by palpating the capsule and depicting the joint's position. This in turn increases confidence in locating the AC joint, as well as the diagnosis and treatment of problems in this region.

Starting Position

The patient sits on a chair or a treatment table with the shoulder girdle relaxed. The lateral region of the shoulder should be easily accessible. This SP is initially used when practicing palpation. Several assessment and treatment techniques require patients to be positioned in supine,

side-lying, or prone position. Later, the therapist should therefore be able to correctly locate important structures in these SPs as well.

Alternative Starting Positions

The patient is not always in a sitting position when the source of shoulder girdle pain is being identified or when the AC joint is being treated. Therefore, it is recommended that the palpation be repeated in other SPs. This knowledge is advantageous when applying manual therapy treatment techniques that require therapists to locate the small joint space in unusual SPs and sometimes even without visual control.

With a little practice, it is not difficult to locate the AC joint space in the sitting position described above. Once the therapist feels confident using this technique, other SPs can be chosen and the palpation repeated:

• Palpation of the AC joint in side-lying position.
• Palpation of the AC joint in supine position.
• In each position with both resting shoulder and complete elevation of the arm.

Arm elevation dramatically changes the joint space alignment. While the joint space has a posterior-anterior alignment when the shoulder is relaxed, concomitant rotation of the scapula during arm elevation changes its alignment so that it points more toward the tip of the chin.

The lateral palpation is continued when the therapist is familiar with the general and special orientation of anterior structures (see ▶ Fig. 2.58).

2.4.3 Palpation of Individual Structures

Lateral Edge of the Acromion

Starting at the angle of the acromion, the therapist attempts to follow the edge of the acromion anteriorly. It is not easy to palpate this edge exactly as it is undulated and jagged and its alignment changes a lot.

Technique

A perpendicular palpation technique is used here. Either the fingertip or the entire length of the finger is placed on the edge of the acromion (▶ Fig. 2.24).

Acromial Spine

The therapist can only follow the edge of the acromion to its anterior border, the acromial spine. This small rounded tip is an important reference point for orientation on the anterolateral aspect of the shoulder.

The therapist uses this point to gain access to the AC joint from anterior and to reliably access the site of

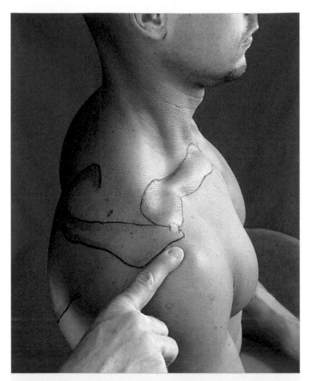

Fig. 2.24 Palpation of the edge of the acromion.

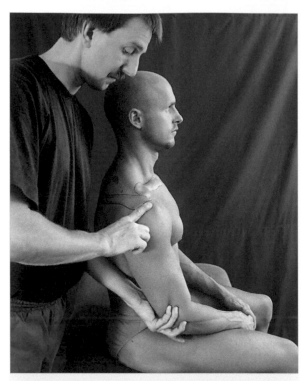

Fig. 2.25 Palpation of the edge of the acromion—with inferior traction of the humerus.

insertion for the supraspinatus when the arm is preposi-tioned in end-range internal rotation (see ▶ Fig. 2.62).

Tip

It is easier to palpate the edge of the acromion and its anterior tip when the therapist pulls inferiorly on the upper arm so that the head of the humerus is distracted from the edge or spine of the acromion (▶ Fig. 2.25). This improves reliability when palpating these structures and differentiating them from the head of the humerus. Manual therapists use the edge of the acromion for orientation when monitoring inferior glide of the humeral head.

AC Joint—Anterior Approach

The palpation continues medially along the acromial spine. A small indentation is felt first, followed by bone. The fingertips encounter the clavicle at this point; the fin-ger pads are resting in the "anterior V." The tip of this V-shaped indentation usually points directly posterior. The anterior section of the AC joint capsule ends here.

Tip

The difficulty of finding the structures lies in being able to feel the acromial spine precisely and follow the contour consistently in a medial direction. The most common mistake—the anterior V is presumed to be too far medially. The palpatory technique that has proven successful involves placing the medial side of the index finger downward on the patient so that the finger pad palpates the tip of the acromial spine and the fingertip the indentation marking the anterior V.

AC Joint—Posterior Approach

The anterior point of access to the AC joint has already been pinpointed. The so-called "posterior V" is needed to mark the further course of the AC joint. The laterally directed pal-pation along the superior border of the spine of the scapula and the posterior edge of the clavicle has already been described. The therapist will notice that the lateral end of the clavicle is significantly larger than generally expected based on the knowledge of topographical anatomy. In addi-tion, the descending part of the trapezius is often quite tense and hinders access to the posterior border.

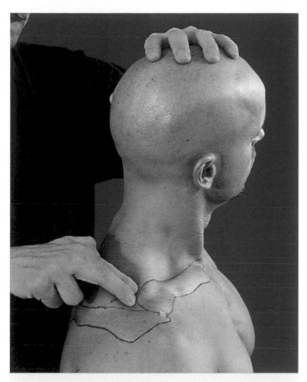

Fig. 2.26 Palpation of the posterior border of the clavicle.

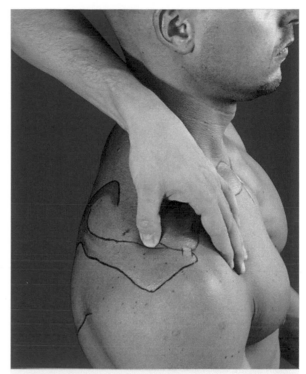

Fig. 2.27 Palpation of the posterior V.

Technique

Step 1: Posterior Border of the Clavicle

The palpation is begun further medial, at the middle of the clavicle. The posterior edge can be felt here; it can be systematically directed laterally with a transverse palpation technique. In this process, palpation is severely hindered by the insertion of the descending trapezius muscle. To decrease the tension of the trapezius muscle and increase the ease of palpation, the patient's head is tipped to the same side and rotated to the opposite side, which brings the muscle closer (▶ Fig. 2.26).

Tip

Another reliable method to locate the posterior border is to palpate in an anterior direction from the superior border of the spine of the scapula. The clavicle must be the next bony structure that offers firm resistance.

Step 2: Posterior V

The posterior V is defined as the point where both palpable edges (superior border of the spine of the scapula and the posterior border of the clavicle) meet. The tip of this V points anterolaterally.

The therapist changes the technique by placing one finger vertically between the border of the spine of the scapula and the border of the clavicle when locating this point exactly (▶ Fig. 2.27).

The posterior V is found exactly at the point where both of these borders prevent the finger from pushing deep into firm-elastic tissue.

The entire dimensions of the lateral clavicle can be determined by following the anterior border of the clavicle from medial to lateral until the anterior V is reached.

Its length is often underestimated. It should be noted that the width of the clavicular borders depicted here results from the two-dimensional representation of the palpated three-dimensional structure (▶ Fig. 2.28).

Acromioclavicular Joint (AC Joint)

The line connecting the tips of the two Vs corresponds to the general alignment of the AC joint space. Only the anterior section of this line (approx. 0.5–1 cm from the anterior V in a posterior direction) is used for orientation when locating the joint. Based on this information, the AC joint space is generally aligned anteriorly and often a little laterally (▶ Fig. 2.29).

The therapist should also keep in mind that intra- and interindividual variations in the alignment of this joint space are highly probable. The degree of variation in alignment depends strongly on posture, the form of the thorax, and the corresponding position of the shoulder girdle. If the vertebral column is hyperkyphotic, the

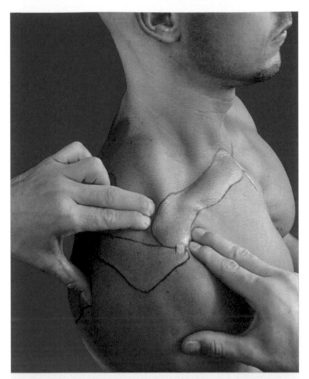

Fig. 2.28 Anterior and posterior borders of the clavicle.

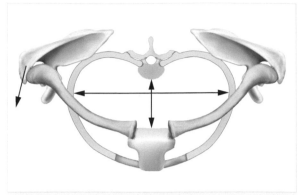

Fig. 2.29 Alignment of the AC joint space when the thorax form is normal.

shoulder girdle hangs down more in protraction and the AC joint is clearly tilted, pointing in a more anteromedial direction.

In a straight thoracic spine (flat back type), the scapulae are often located in a more medial position, toward the spine. The shoulder girdle position also deviates from the norm in these cases. The shoulder girdle seems to be adducted and the AC joint space is positioned more in the sagittal plane.

Technique

Acromioclavicular Joint Capsule

The previously described procedure for finding the AC joint space can be used for rapid orientation and can be performed with even more precise palpation. The therapist starts by palpating the posterior border of the clavicle and following the convex lateral end of the clavicle as it curves anteriorly (▶ Fig. 2.30).

By palpating with the fingertip perpendicular to the border of the clavicle, the therapist will next feel a distinct step. The pad of the finger lies flat on the acromion and the fingertip encounters the clavicle (▶ Fig. 2.31 and ▶ Fig. 2.32).

The palpating finger is located directly over the AC joint space when the edge feels flattened and at a tilt and no longer like a step. This tilted "ramp" is formed by the capsule and its reinforcements filling up the ligamentary step (▶ Fig. 2.33 and ▶ Fig. 2.34).

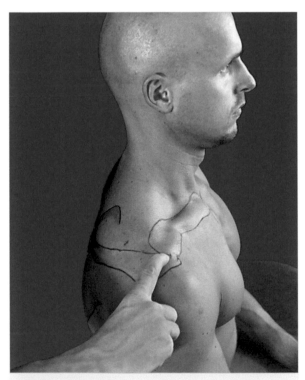

Fig. 2.30 Palpation of the lateral clavicle, near-cranial view.

> ### Tip
>
> This palpatory identification of the AC joint capsule that differentiates between step and ramp is based on the assumption that the superior side of the acromion runs flat in a medial direction toward the clavicle, but this is not always the case.

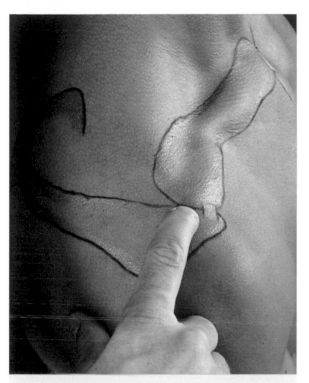

Fig. 2.31 Palpation of the lateral clavicle, detailed view.

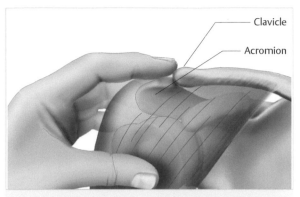

Fig. 2.32 Palpation of the lateral clavicle, anterior view.

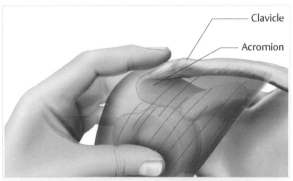

Fig. 2.34 Palpation of the AC joint capsule, anterior view.

Tip

A frequent variant is where the superior surface of the acromion is wavy as it extends toward the clavicle, so that both bones of the AC joint extend toward each other like the tapered sides of a volcano and the articular space looks like the funnel-shaped mouth of the volcano (Da Palma 1963) (see ▶ Fig. 2.35).This variant can also make it more difficult to find the posterior "V" as a location aid for the AC joint space (see technique Spine of the Scapula—Superior Edge and posterior "V"). If the cranial aspect of the scapular spine is followed, the posterior "V" can be erroneously identified where the posterior aspect of the volcano rises up in a cranial direction away from the acromion.

If the ramp model were the only method for confirmation of the AC joint capsule, the AC joint would be assumed to be much too far medial. Therefore, for reliable identification, it is always advisable to select a technique that confirms the position of the joint through movement (▶ Fig. 2.36 and ▶ Fig. 2.37).

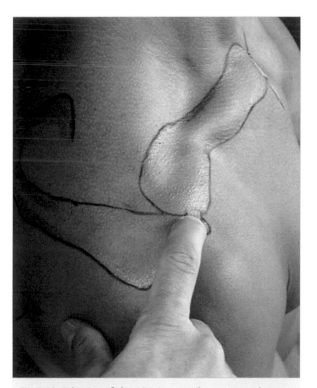

Fig. 2.33 Palpation of the AC joint capsule, near-cranial view.

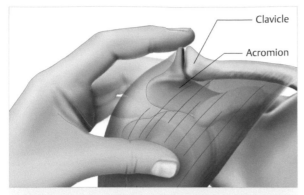

Fig. 2.35 Common variant of the shape of the AC joint space in the frontal plane (after Omer Matthijs).

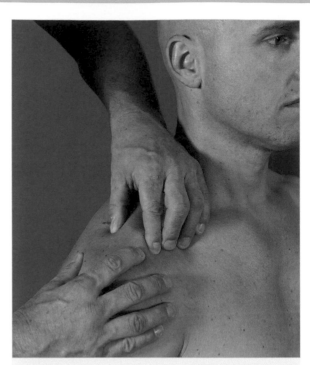

Fig. 2.36 Anterior-posterior clavicular translation.

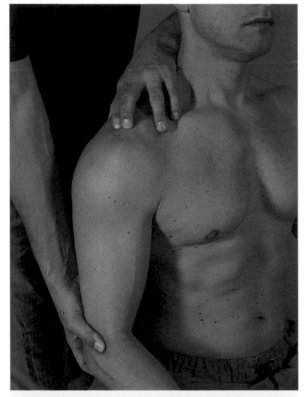

Fig. 2.37 Superior-inferior translation of the acromion.

Tips for Assessment and Treatment

The therapist uses important bony reference points in this region to gain access to a variety of clinically pathological structures:

- The **acromial angle** is another point to start from when determining the dimensions and position of the acromion and is a reliable point to access anterolateral structures of the greater tuberculum. (► Fig. 2.59)
- The **lateral edge of the acromion** is used to differentiate the scapula from the head of the humerus (important for manual therapy techniques).

- Beginning at the **acromial spine,** the point of greatest clinical interest, the insertion of the supraspinatus with prepositioning of the arm (► Fig. 2.63) as well as the anterior access to the AC joint are located.
- The general alignment and exact position of the **AC joint** have to be determined to successfully apply manual therapeutic techniques targeting the joint and Cyriax cross-frictions on the joint capsule. A knowledge of its orientation ensures diagnostically conclusive tests and gentle mobilization.

Joint-specific techniques yield information about the mobility of the AC joint. Transverse translation tests capsular elasticity where there is a question of hypomobility and it tests the stability of the capsule-reinforcing ligaments (see ► Fig. 2.36). To perform this test, the thumb and index finger of the lateral hand grasp and immobilize the acromion at the angle and acromial spine. The thumb and fingertips of the medial hand surround the lateral end of the clavicle and push it in an anterior/posterior direction. With a few trials of different directions, the push that produces the greatest play in the joint is found. This is quite variable, both between individuals and in a given individual. The index finger of the lateral hand, placed on the probable location of the articular space, can feel the movement of the clavicle against the acromion.

Pushing and pulling the hanging upper arm exerts vertical stress on the AC joint (see ► Fig. 2.37). This is first and foremost a test of the integrity of the coracoclavicular ligaments. A positive test result is laxity due to excessive

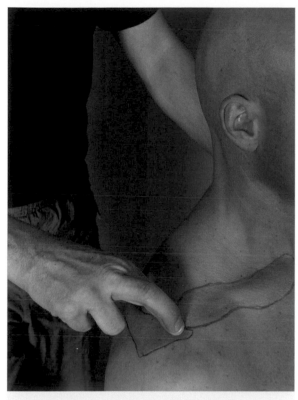

Fig. 2.38 Transverse friction of the AC joint capsule.

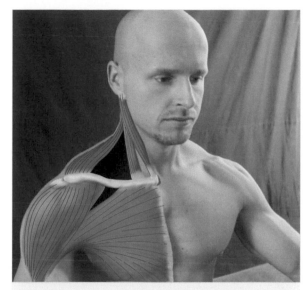

Fig. 2.39 Supraclavicular and infraclavicular fossae.

vertical mobility of the acromion with respect to the stabilized clavicle. Palpating fingers on the probable articular space can ensure the correct location of the AC joint and determine by touch the degree of vertical movement.

Cyriax transverse friction for pain relief has proven effective not only on irritated tendons, insertions, and tendon sheaths but also on various forms of arthritis. In mild forms of arthritis, particularly traumatic arthritis of the AC capsule, transverse friction is helpful. After reliable location of the capsule, the pad of the index finger, under pressure, is placed on the capsule directly from cranial (▶ Fig. 2.38). For stability, the thumb is pressed against the scapular spine from dorsal. The index finger is drawn from anterior to posterior, with and without pressure, with pressure on the capsule, and avoiding friction on the skin.

2.5 General Orientation—Anterior

2.5.1 Starting Position

The patient sits upright with the shoulder girdle relaxed. The therapist initially stands in front of the patient. For optimal orientation before continuing with additional special palpation of specific structures, the therapist should first make a rough division of the anterior shoulder region.

2.5.2 Supraclavicular and Infraclavicular Fossae

The curved length of the clavicle divides this region into depressions on the surface above and below the clavicle (supraclavicular and infraclavicular fossae). The anteriorly curving, convex section of the clavicle forms the inferior boundary of the supraclavicular fossa while its posteriorly curving section forms the superior boundary of the infraclavicular depression (▶ Fig. 2.39).

The following structures form the boundaries for the **supraclavicular fossa:**
- Inferior boundary = posterior border of the clavicle.
- Medial boundary = clavicular head of the sternocleidomastoid and scalene muscles.
- Posterior boundary = descending part of the trapezius.

The following structures are found in the floor of the supraclavicular fossa: the first rib, the subclavian vein and artery as they pass through the anterior scalene gap, the brachial plexus as it passes through the posterior scalene gap, as well as the further course of these vessels and nerves up to the point where they travel beneath the clavicle.

The following structures form the boundaries for the **infraclavicular fossa:**
- Superior boundary = inferior border of the clavicle.
- Medial boundary = lateral edge of the clavicular head of the pectoralis major.
- Lateral boundary = medial edge of the clavicular part of the deltoid muscle.

The boundaries of the supra- and infraclavicular fossae can be well visualized with muscle activity. To visualize the infraclavicular fossa, the patient raises the arm slightly from the null position by means of flexion. This activates the deltoid muscle in particular. From this position, the patient performs horizontal adduction against a slight resistance. In addition, the pectoralis major is activated. Both muscular boundaries of the infraclavicular fossa become distinctly visible. This depression is also called the deltopectoral groove or the clavipectoral triangle. Blood vessels are found in the floor of this fossa medial to the anterior fibers of the deltoid muscle before they travel to the upper arm: the subclavian artery and vein, also named the thoracoacromial artery and vein (Thiel, 2006).

2.6 Local Palpation—Anteromedial

2.6.1 Overview of the Structures to be Palpated

- Sternocleidomastoid.
- Medial end of the clavicle.
- Sternoclavicular joint space.

2.6.2 Summary of the Palpatory Process

Certain structures on the anterior shoulder girdle are located quite medially and are used in particular to correctly locate the SC joint. The therapist then gains access to the anterolateral region where it is important that the infraclavicular fossa and coracoid process are precisely located.

Starting Position

The patient sits with relaxed shoulder girdle on a stool or a treatment table. The therapist stands behind the patient.

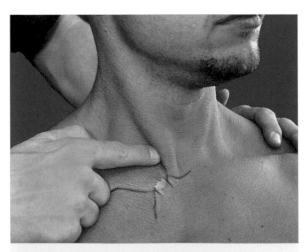

Fig. 2.40 Palpation of the sternal sternocleidomastoid.

2.6.3 Palpation of Individual Structures

Sternocleidomastoid

The therapist first makes the sternal head of the sternocleidomastoid more distinct by having the patient actively rotate the head to the opposite side

If in addition the patient is asked to tip the head to the ipsilateral side against a slight resistance, the clavicular portion of the muscle stands out. This muscle head can be followed until it inserts into the medial third of the clavicle.

As a reminder: this muscle forms the medial boundary of the supraclavicular fossa and the anterior boundary of the anterior scalene gap.

Medial End of the Clavicle

The lateral aspect of the muscular cord and tendon of the sternal head of the sternocleidomastoid is palpated and continually followed until its insertion onto the manubrium (▶ Fig. 2.40).

It inserts directly medial into the SC joint space. A bony structure can be clearly felt lateral to the tendon, just before it inserts onto the manubrium: this is the superior section of the medial end of the clavicle.

Approximately half of the increasingly wider end of the clavicle is found superior to the SC joint space when the shoulder girdle is positioned at rest (with the shoulder hanging down normally, ▶ Fig. 2.41).

These parts of the articular surface first come into contact with the sternal articular surface when the arm is raised. This is due to the inferior gliding of the clavicle when the arm is raised as a result of the applicable arthrokinematic convex rule.

Sternoclavicular Joint Space

Based on this information, it can be seen that the actual SC joint space is found further inferiorly. Its alignment can be described as superomedial to inferolateral.

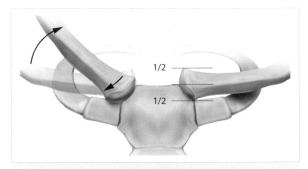

Fig. 2.41 Dimensions of the medial end of the clavicle.

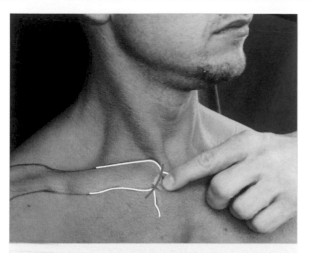

Fig. 2.42 Palpation of the SC joint space.

Technique

The tendon of the sternocleidomastoid is precisely followed until the manubrium is reached. The palpating finger pads now point in a lateral direction.

The joint space is found directly underneath the finger pad when the finger palpates the medial end of the clavicle (▶ Fig. 2.42).

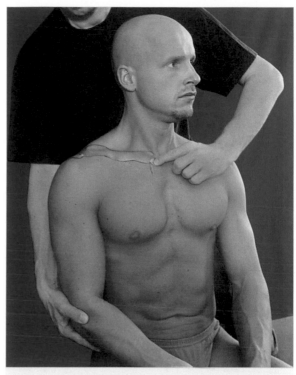

Fig. 2.43 Confirming palpation using shoulder girdle elevation.

Tip

Swelling of the capsule in patients with SC joint symptoms can make it significantly more difficult to find this joint. In this case, its position can be confirmed by moving the shoulder girdle. The best way to do this is through passive elevation of the shoulder by a push on the arm to proximal (▶ Fig. 2.43).

Jugular Notch

Starting at the medial end of the clavicle and the SC joint, the therapist palpates laterally along the inferior border of the clavicle. The muscular insertion of the clavicular part of the pectoralis major often makes exact identification of the inferior border more difficult. In addition, swelling of the costosternal transition, located directly caudal to the SC joint, can make palpation difficult. After approximately half of its course from medial to lateral, the anterior convexity of the clavicle becomes a posterior convexity.

2.6.4 Tips for Assessment and Treatment

Arthritis of the SC joint can cause local pain and pain projected to the shoulders as far as the jaw and the ear (Hasset and Barnsley, 2001). Moreover, capsular restriction can result in significant partial limitation of shoulder

girdle and arm elevation. A joint-specific test, for instance in the direction of traction, yields information about local mobility of the joint (▶ Fig. 2.44). In order to move the clavicle in the direction of traction, the therapist grasps the clavicle, supports the hand with the thenar laterally against its concavity and pulls it laterally, posteriorly, and slightly superiorly. Information about the extent of the separation in the SC joint is provided chiefly by touch, palpating the articular gap with the pad of a finger.

2.7 Local Palpation—Anterolateral

2.7.1 Overview of the Structures to be Palpated

- Coracoid process.
- Subscapularis tendon.
- Lesser tubercle of the humerus.
- Intertubercular sulcus.
- Greater tubercle of the humerus.
- Glenoid cavity.
- Supraspinatus—insertion.

2.7.2 Summary of the Palpatory Process

Further lateral, the clavicle forms the superior boundary of the infraclavicular fossa or clavipectoral triangle. The other boundaries are the clavicular portions of the deltoid

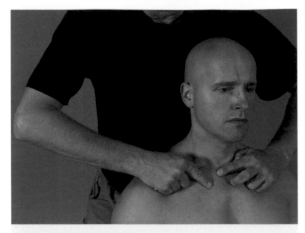

Fig. 2.44 Traction test of the SC joint.

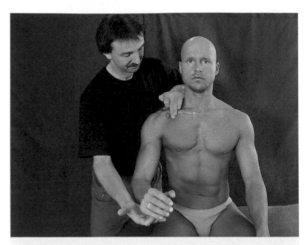

Fig. 2.45 Demonstrating the infraclavicular fossa.

and pectoralis muscle (see ▶ Fig. 2.39). These structures lie close together and it is occasionally quite difficult to differentiate between them; often this only succeeds with the help of movements by the other joint components.

The palpating hand moves systematically from medial to lateral and finds a new structure at almost every centimeter.

Access is obtained by locating the infraclavicular fossa and the coracoid process.

2.7.3 Palpation of Individual Structures
Coracoid Process
Starting Position

The patient sits on a chair or a treatment table. The arm is close to the body, the lower arm resting on the thigh. The therapist stands behind the patient. For the rest of the procedure, here depicted on the patient's right shoulder, the therapist's left hand palpates and the right hand guides the patient's arm in order to place the shoulder joint in the desired position or offer various degrees of resistance (▶ Fig. 2.45).

Alternative Starting Positions

Once the structures of the lateral shoulder region can be reliably found with these exercises, palpation should be tried from other, more difficult starting positions—for example, with the patient supine, arm raised.

Technique

As already described, the infraclavicular fossa is particularly easy to visualize with muscular activity in adduction. Its direct lateral, deep, bony boundary is the coracoid process. The following procedure is recommended for finding this prominent process.

With muscles tensed, the palpating finger (the middle finger is preferred here—▶ Fig. 2.46) is placed in the fossa and remains there, even when the arm is returned to the resting SP and relaxed. Now the pressure of the middle finger is increased laterally; the bony resistance of the medial boundary of the coracoid process is immediately felt.

When the index finger of the palpating hand is placed directly next to the middle finger, its pad is lying directly on the coracoid (▶ Fig. 2.47).

Palpation is continued in a lateral direction. The middle finger of the left hand remains in the infraclavicular fossa.

The index finger is moved laterally by approximately 1 finger width with moderate pressure. At this point, there is a distinctly palpable depression between the lateral edge of the coracoid and the lesser tubercle of the humerus (▶ Fig. 2.48).

In the following, it is possible to identify the borders of the tip of the coracoid process from all sides: from superior, inferior, and lateral (▶ Fig. 2.49). It becomes noticeable that the coracoid process is a remarkably large structure.

> **Tip**
>
> It is advisable to use care in applying pressure here during palpation, since pressure against the coracoid can often be uncomfortable.

As a reminder: four ligaments and three muscles that are part of the roof of the shoulder insert at the coracoid. This is a junction point for the forces that stabilize the shoulder joint and can pull the shoulder girdle in an anterior direction. The lower aspect of the coracoid plays an important part in visualizing the spatial orientation of the glenoid cavity.

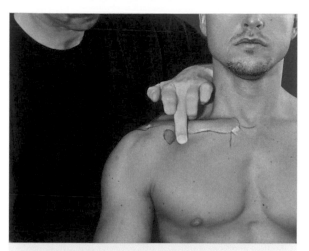
Fig. 2.46 Palpation of the infraclavicular fossa.

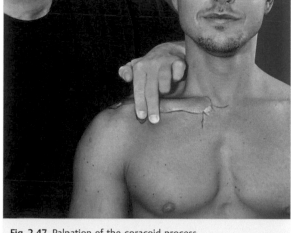
Fig. 2.47 Palpation of the coracoid process.

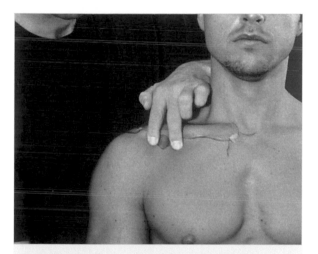
Fig. 2.48 Coracoid process—medial and lateral borders.

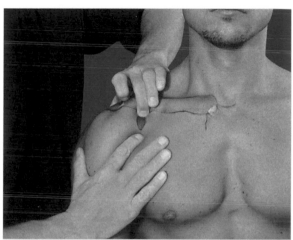
Fig. 2.49 Coracoid process—superior and inferior borders.

Comments and Exercises for the Coracoid Process

The coracoid process changes its position in relation to the clavicle during movement of the arm, especially during shoulder flexion. The following exercise is recommended to give the therapist an idea of the position of the coracoid process during this movement.

One finger of the right hand palpates the coracoid process between its superior border and the clavicle. The other hand facilitates passive flexion of the shoulder. It becomes obvious that the tip of the coracoid process moves closer to the clavicle during this movement as the scapula increasingly rotates. This is cross-checked by extending the shoulder, and it is observed that the coracoid process moves away from the clavicle. However, this cannot be felt as clearly, since the scapular movement associated with shoulder extension is significantly smaller than movement occurring with flexion of the shoulder. The fibers of the clavicular part of the deltoid also tense during this movement and hinder palpation.

Although the coracoclavicular ligaments are mainly viewed in connection with stabilization of the AC joint, their kinetic role now becomes clear. The facilitated passive movement of the shoulder tenses the soft tissue surrounding the shoulder joint and the scapula follows the movement. The scapula first moves on the clavicle at the AC joint until the joint's ligaments are placed under tension and the clavicle starts to rotate. The palpating finger on the coracoid process registers this short latency time.

When the arm is elevated, the coracoid process tilts in a posterosuperior direction and the conoid ligament is placed under tension, causing the clavicle to rotate posteriorly. During shoulder joint extension, selective tension in the trapezoid ligament assists anterior rotation. Preventing friction during movement of the coracoid in relation to the clavicle, there is often a bursa between the two structures, and in rare cases (< 1%, Faraj, 2003), a joint.

Spatial Orientation of the Glenoid Cavity

The therapist is now familiar with all structures needed to fully describe the alignment of the shoulder joint socket in space. Its position is a result of the scapula adapting to the shape of the thorax. The glenoid cavity usually opens laterally, anteriorly, and slightly superiorly, and is a direct extension of the spine of the scapula.

It is angled at approximately 20 to 30° anteriorly away from the frontal plane. This angle is very much dependent on the individual shape of the thorax. The glenoid cavity faces more lateral when the back is flat and more anterior when the thoracic spine is hyperkyphotic. This alignment may also change in the different SPs. When the patient lies prone, supine, or on the side, the position of the scapula on the thorax and the resulting spatial orientation of the glenoid cavity changes.

Hence, therapists need landmarks for reliable orientation to determine the exact alignment of the joint socket. This can only be defined using a connecting line. The ends of this line are located in the acromial angle and the inferior aspect of the coracoid process.

Technique

The right thumb is placed over the posterior angle of the acromion (acromial angle) and the index finger is placed on the inferior aspect of the coracoid process. The line connecting these points defines the alignment of the glenoid cavity.

This line travels from posterolateral to anteromedial when viewed from above (▶ Fig. 2.50) and travels anteriorly at a slight angle when viewed from the side (▶ Fig. 2.51).

This illustrates the angle of the glenoid cavity in the sagittal plane.

Alternative Starting Positions

If the therapist finds it easy to determine the alignment of the glenoid cavity when the shoulder is at rest, they should practice locating the connecting line with the patient in other SPs or the arm in other positions (e.g., full elevation). Each time they do this, they should attempt to visualize the position of the glenoid cavity in space.

Tips for Assessment and Treatment

It is extremely important that the manual therapist be able to exactly identify the plane of the glenoid cavity for the assessment of joint play and the application of manual therapeutic glides. A translational technique at the joint socket thus signifies a spatial adjustment to the anterior, medial, and somewhat inferior. If the therapist does not glide the humeral head exactly along this line, the test results will not be diagnostically conclusive.

In applying the translational technique to move the humerus to the posterior, the direction must be selected far enough to the lateral so that vulnerable structures, particularly the glenoid labrum, are not endangered by compression (▶ Fig. 2.52).

Subscapularis Tendon

An obvious depression marks the lateral edge of the coracoid process and can be felt underneath the index finger. The lesser tubercle of the humerus lies immediately lateral to this. Its location is confirmed by passively moving the hanging arm into medial and lateral rotations (▶ Fig. 2.53). Only the lesser tubercle moves underneath the index finger during this movement. Needless to say, no movement is observed at the coracoid process.

When the shoulder is positioned in end-range lateral rotation, the wide tendon of the subscapularis is placed under tension and pushes against the palpating finger so

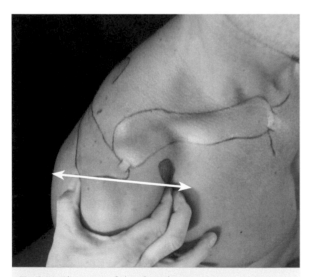

Fig. 2.50 Alignment of the glenoid cavity—near-cranial view.

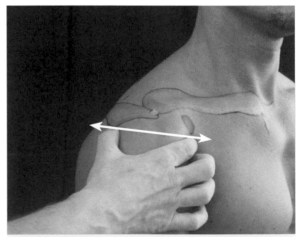

Fig. 2.51 Alignment of the glenoid cavity—lateral view.

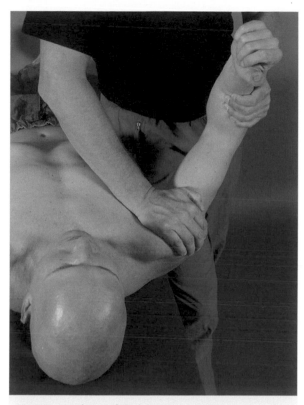

Fig. 2.52 Translation of the humerus to posterior.

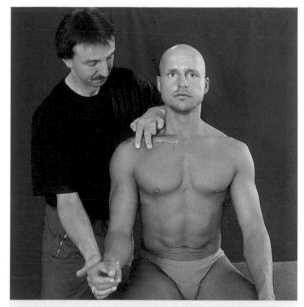

Fig. 2.53 Searching for the lesser tubercle of the humerus.

that it moves anteriorly onto the surface of the skin. When the palpating index finger applies more pressure to the tense tendon, the tendon responds with a very firm and somewhat elastic consistency.

Lesser Tubercle of the Humerus

The lesser tubercle is shaped like an upside-down tear-drop. Its tip becomes thinner more inferiorly and merges into a ridge of insertion, the crest of the lesser tubercle. The intertubercular sulcus forms its lateral boundary (▶ Fig. 2.54).

The insertion of the subscapularis occupies the entire surface of the lesser tubercle. Superficial fibers extend from here as a transverse ligament over the intertubercular sulcus and ensure that the long tendon of the biceps brachii remains in the groove. The latissimus dorsi and the teres major insert at the distal-running crest of the lesser tubercle.

The insertion of the subscapularis tendon can be painful and inflamed as a result of overloading. It can also be trapped underneath the roof of the shoulder, resulting in a painful arc when the arm is raised.

Deep portions of the tendon can be captured between the head of the humerus and the glenoid cavity in an internal impingement.

Intertubercular Sulcus

Technique

Method 1

The middle finger now takes over the position of the index finger. The sulcus can be palpated by moving the index finger further lateral across the lesser tubercle. By continuously passively rotating the arm medially and laterally, the therapist can confirm the position of the slender depression of the sulcus as it moves back and forth underneath the finger and can feel the edges of the sulcus (greater and lesser tubercles) (▶ Fig. 2.55 and ▶ Fig. 2.56). This method is more difficult when parts of the deltoid are well developed.

Method 2

If the sulcus cannot be found using the direct method described above, the therapist can resort to using an indirect method. When the shoulder is actively abducted in the scapular plane (scaption), the sulcus is found directly underneath a gap in the deltoid muscle.

The patient is instructed to hold the shoulder in abduction in the scapular plane so that the intermuscular gap between the acromial and clavicular parts of the deltoid becomes distinct. The palpating finger is positioned along the length of the intermuscular gap (▶ Fig. 2.57). The left index finger is used when the right side is being palpated. The sulcus is found directly underneath the intermuscular gap in this position. The index finger remains in the intermuscular gap while the arm is brought back to its SP (the neutral physiological position of the shoulder joint). The palpating finger is very probably lying over the sulcus

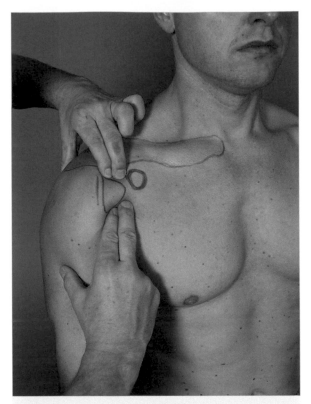

Fig. 2.54 Position and size of the lesser tubercle.

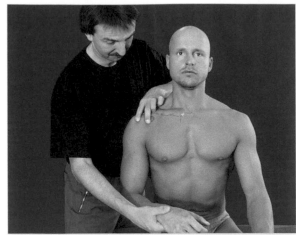

Fig. 2.55 SP Palpation—intertubercular sulcus.

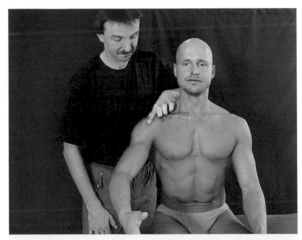

Fig. 2.57 Searching for the gap in the deltoid.

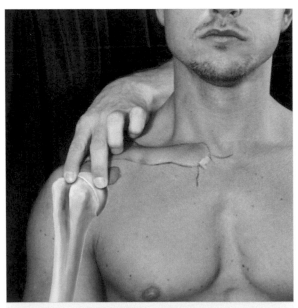

Fig. 2.56 Palpation of the intertubercular sulcus—detailed view.

being sought. The location of the intertubercular sulcus under the index finger is confirmed by repeated slight rotational movement of the arm in the shoulder joint.

Tips for Assessment and Treatment

The symptoms associated with tendon sheath disease at the long head of the biceps in the intertubercular sulcus are well known in soft-tissue disorders of the shoulder. Treatment usually involves the use of local physical therapy techniques, including Cyriax cross-frictions. Treatment is only successful when palpation is precise.

The location of the intertubercular sulcus should therefore be practiced with patients in other SPs.

Greater Tubercle of the Humerus

The instructions for locating the parts of the greater tubercle completes the description of the palpatory circle of the lateral structures of the shoulder. The greater tubercle offers three small surfaces (facets) for insertion of rotator cuff muscles:

• Anterior facet—supraspinatus, insertion field: 18 to 33 mm long, 12 to 21 mm wide

- Middle facet—infraspinatus, insertion field: 20 to 45 mm long, 12 to 27 mm wide
- Posterior facet—teres minor, insertion field: 20 to 40 mm long, 10 to 33 mm wide (Curtis et al., 2006).

The following palpation is intended to demonstrate the extent of the tubercle and to permit precise location of the three rotator cuff muscle insertions. Physical therapy techniques (e.g., transverse friction) can be applied in other starting positions, where clinically more problematic aspects are more easily accessed (see ▶ Fig. 2.18 and ▶ Fig. 2.62).

The previous palpation demonstrated the medial edge of the greater tubercle by finding the intertubercular sulcus. All three facets show a typical orientation of their position in relation to the humeral shaft (▶ Fig. 2.58):

- The anterior facet is perpendicular to the sulcus.
- The middle facet is angled approximately 45° posteroinferior to the sulcus.
- The posterior facet is at a 45° angle to this and thus is once more parallel to the shaft of the humerus and in the sagittal plane.

Technique

Anterior Facet

The extended index finger is supported by its radial side against the edge of the acromion and oriented at a right angle to the sulcus (▶ Fig. 2.59). Because of the intra- and interindividual difference in size of the acromion (Engelhardt et al. 2017), the accessible surface of this facet also varies. It is bordered at the front by the sulcus. The palpating finger feels this border and slips forward into the sulcus. The lateral boundary becomes distinct when the index finger slides off to the side.

Middle Facet

Palpating posteriorly from the sulcus past the approximately 2-cm-long anterior facet, the examiner arrives at the middle facet when the palpating finger slides over the 45° angle to the posteroinferior (▶ Fig. 2.60). To feel the facet as a surface, one can also palpate with the pad of the thumb. Palpation shows that this surface is bordered medially by the edge of the acromion and laterally by a roundish surface sliding down in an inferior direction.

Posterior Facet

In the same way, after approximately 2 cm, the thumb slips over an edge at a 45° angle in a posteroinferior direction and thus lands on the posterior facet of the

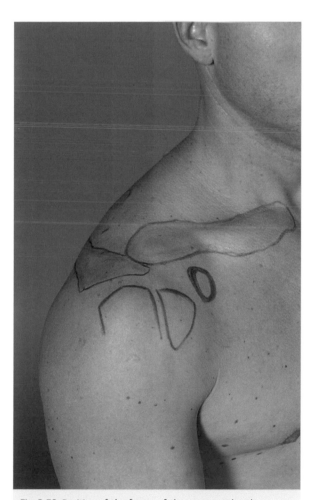

Fig. 2.58 Position of the facets of the greater tubercle.

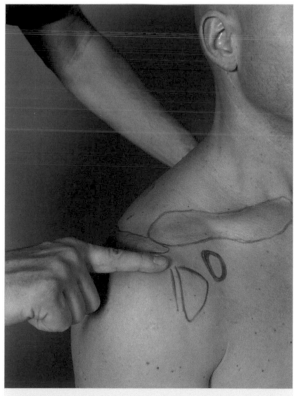

Fig. 2.59 Palpation of the anterior facet.

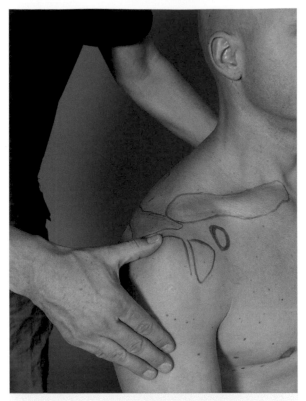

Fig. 2.60 Palpation of the middle facet.

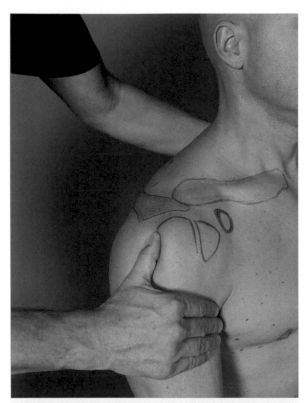

Fig. 2.61 Palpation of the posterior facet.

greater tubercle. The thumb is now parallel to the intertubercular sulcus (▶ Fig. 2.61).

Supraspinatus—Insertion

The outer sections of the greater tubercle can be palpated, in sitting position, lateral to the intertubercular sulcus (see also ▶ Fig. 2.58). These parts are of little clinical interest though. Important insertion areas of the supraspinatus and infraspinatus muscles are difficult to access below the acromion when the arms are set in the physiological null position.

Starting Position

For this test, the patient is positioned with the upper body at an angle (raised approximately 60° from the supine position), leaning against the foot section of the treatment table. To make the insertion of the supraspinatus accessible, the anterior facet of the greater tubercle must be brought forward. To do this, the patient's arm is brought into extension (approx. 30–40°) in slight abduction with end-range internal rotation (approx. 90°), so that the back of the hand is touching the lumbar spine (▶ Fig. 2.62). This position was already described by Cyriax in 1984 and confirmed in studies by Mattingly and Mackarey in 1996.

Now the clinically important point of insertion, measuring 1.5 to 2 cm², lies directly anterior and medial to the acromial spine, on a small bony horizontal plateau of the humerus(▶ Fig. 2.63 and ▶ Fig. 2.64).

Technique

To find the insertion, the therapist follows the edge of the acromion from the posterior angle to the anterior tip (see ▶ Fig. 2.24). The palpating index finger should now be positioned in such a way that the pad of the finger lies on the bony plateau, the fingernail is horizontal, and the edge of the index finger is pushing against the tip (▶ Fig. 2.65).

If the fingertip is brought from the tip of the acromion in an anterior direction to the anterior edge, one arrives at the end of the plateau, when the finger slips off in an inferior direction and the fingernail is parallel to the humeral shaft. The medial boundary of the anterior facet plateau is found when the finger slips off into the sulcus. If the palpating finger is moved laterally, the end of the plateau is found when the finger slips inferiorly by 45° onto the middle facet (compare also ▶ Fig. 2.55, ▶ Fig. 2.56, ▶ Fig. 2.57).

Tips for Assessment and Treatment

Cyriax cross-frictions are administered when this palpation is being used to provoke pain in the assessment and/

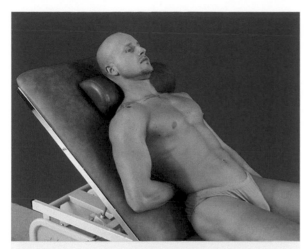

Fig. 2.62 SP—palpation of the site of insertion for the supraspinatus.

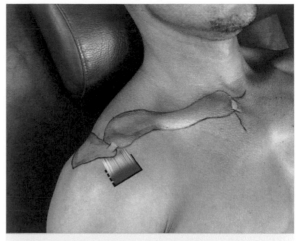

Fig. 2.63 Position of the supraspinatus—site of insertion.

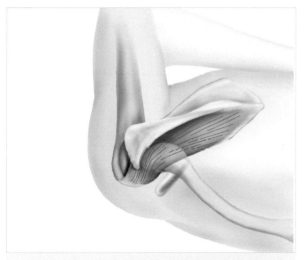

Fig. 2.64 Course of the supraspinatus with arm forward.

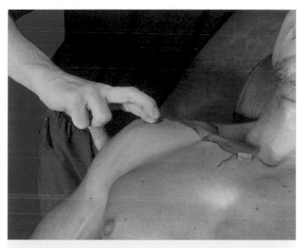

Fig. 2.65 Technique—transverse friction at the supraspinatus.

or treatment of insertion tendinopathy. The index finger is placed on the skin and moves medially for a short distance, applying only a minimal amount of pressure. Once on the plateau, the finger pushes deeper into the tissues and moves laterally without rubbing the skin (▶ Fig. 2.65 and ▶ Fig. 2.66). Increased pressure is applied to provoke pain; for treatment, the technique is applied sub-clinically in per-second increments.

The therapist should always be aware that the palpating finger can never make direct contact with the site of insertion. Deltoid muscle bundles and the subacromial/subdeltoid bursa lie superficial to the insertion. The bursa can also be inflamed and painful.

The therapist can only be certain that painful palpation of this region is due to a supraspinatus insertion tendinopathy by appropriately assessing the function of the shoulder joint.

If there is a tendinopathy present, resulting from an external impingement, it is more likely that the superficial portions of the tendons at the anterior edge of the plateau are affected.

Treatment for Tendinitis

The direction of the transverse friction in the pressure phase (medial or lateral) is largely not significant. Applying pressure in a lateral direction has proven ergonomically advantageous. The intensity is moderate if the objective is pain relief.

Treatment for Tendinosis

The transverse friction is applied with constant, considerable pressure in both directions.

To reach the deep portions of the tendons on the articular side, when treating an internal impingement,

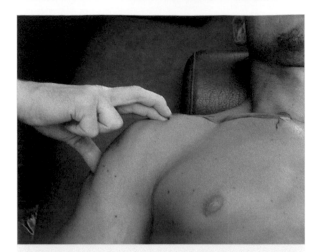

Fig. 2.66 Alternative view.

transverse friction is applied posteriorly, on the facet, directly before the acromial tip.

Tips

- It is sometimes difficult to find the tip of the acromion in the suggested starting position. The patient's SP is no longer upright-sitting and the therapist has to palpate through the stretched anterior sections of the deltoid muscle. In this case, it is advisable first to find this tip with the arm in resting position and then position the arm.
- To make the palpation ergonomical, it is also recommended that the treatment table is sufficiently elevated and that the therapist stands behind the patient's shoulder.

Bibliography

Colegate-Stone T, Allom R, Singh R, Elias DA, Standring S, Sinha J. Classification of the morphology of the acromioclavicular joint using cadaveric and radiological analysis. J Bone Joint Surg Br. 2010; 92(5):743–746

Curtis AS, Burbank KM, Tierney JJ, Scheller AD, Curran AR. The insertional footprint of the rotator cuff: an anatomic study. Arthroscopy. 2006; 22 (6):609.e1

Cyriax JH. Textbook of Orthopaedic Medicine, Vol. 2: Treatment by Manipulation Massage and Injektion. 11th ed. London, England: Bailliere Tindall; 1984

Depalma AF. Surgical Anatomy of Acromioclavicular and Sternoclavicular Joints. Surg Clin North Am. 1963; 43:1541–1550

Engelhardt C, Farron A, Becce F, Place N, Pioletti DP, Terrier A. Effects of glenoid inclination and acromion index on humeral head translation and glenoid articular cartilage strain. J Shoulder Elbow Surg. 2017; 26 (1):157–164

Faraj AA. Bilateral congenital coracoclavicular joint. Case report and review of the literature. Acta OrthopBelg. 2003; 69(6):552–554

Gokeler A, van Paridon-Edauw GH, DeClercq S, Matthijs O, Dijkstra PU. Quantitative analysis of traction in the glenohumeral joint. In vivo radiographic measurements. Man Ther. 2003; 8(2):97–102

Hassett G, Barnsley L. Pain referral from the sternoclavicular joint: a study in normal volunteers. Rheumatology (Oxford). 2001; 40(8):859–862

Kapandji IA. Funktionelle Anatomie der Gelenke. 4. Aufl. Stuttgart: Thieme; 2006

Mattingly GE, Mackarey PJ. Optimal methods for shoulder tendon palpation: a cadaver study. Phys Ther. 1996; 76(2):166–173

Saccomanno MF, DE Ieso C, Milano G. Acromioclavicular joint instability: anatomy, biomechanics and evaluation. Joints. 2014; 2(2):87–92

Sewell MD, Al-Hadithy N, Le Leu A, Lambert SM. Instability of the sternoclavicular joint: current concepts in classification, treatment and outcomes. Bone Joint J. 2013; 95-B(6):721–731

Thiel W. Photographischer Atlas der Praktischen Anatomie. 2. Aufl. Heidelberg: Springer; 2006

Tubbs RS, Shah NA, Sullivan BP, et al. The costoclavicular ligament revisited: a functional and anatomical study. Rom J MorpholEmbryol. 2009; 50 (3):475–479

Werner A, Mueller T, Boehm D, Gohlke F. The stabilizing sling for the long head of the biceps tendon in the rotator cuff interval. A histoanatomic study. Am J Sports Med. 2000; 28(1):28–31

Williams PL. Gray's anatomy. 40th ed. Edinburgh: Churchill Livingstone; 2009

Winkel D. Nichtoperative Orthopädie und Manualtherapie. Anatomie in vivo. 3. Aufl. München: Urban & Fischer bei Elsevier; 2004

Chapter 3

Elbow Complex

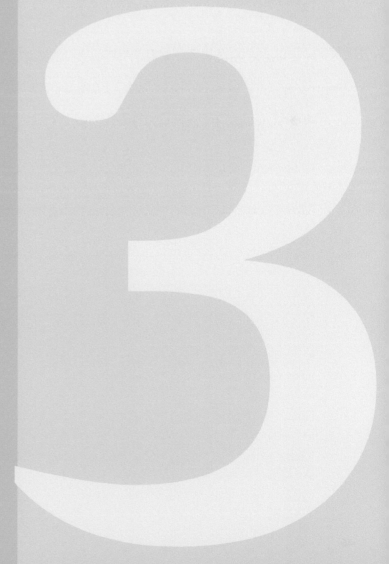

3 Elbow Complex

3.1 Introduction

3.1.1 Significance and Function of the Elbow Complex

The function of the middle joint of the upper limb (elbow joint) is to increase or decrease the distance between the hand and the body or face. Its second function is hand rotation, which occurs in the forearm. The fact that rotation of the distal portion of the extremity is not located exclusively in the middle joint is functionally and also anatomically the most significant difference between this joint and the middle joint of the lower extremity, the knee joint. Flexion and extension mainly take place in the humeroulnar joint (HUJ). The most important joint for controlling rotation of the hand is the proximal radioulnar joint (PRUJ). The humeroradial joint (HRJ) merely functions as an adapter between the center for flexion/extension in the HUJ and the rotational movements of pronation/supination in the PRUJ.

All three joints are found within a capsule that provides sufficient freedom of movement for the very large range of flexion/extension movements and lateral stability when the elbow is extended (collateral ligaments). Moreover, the annular ligament of the radius holds the radius to the ulna and thus directly assures the stability of the PRUJ.

Most bony structures can be reached laterally and posteriorly; only a few can be reached medially. Apart from a few exceptions, the joint space is usually hidden underneath well-developed soft tissue. It is therefore necessary to enlist the help of guiding muscles and spatial relationships to locate the joint. By way of example, when therapists want to reach the anterior radius, they must orient themselves on the medial edge of the brachioradialis, then palpate from this point deep into the tissues.

The accuracy of hand placement, for example, for manual therapeutic tests of joint play, depends on identification of the bony articular components and perception of how articular surfaces are spatially positioned.

In addition to the intricate bony structure, the elbow joint is also characterized by an arrangement of many, at times slender, muscles, which can be subdivided into one extensor (biceps brachii) and several flexors. It is particularly these that become symptomatic with stress syndromes of tendons and insertions (tennis or golfer's elbow) and make it necessary for the therapist to find the precise location of the lesion. These synergists originate on or near the epicondyles of the humerus.

3.1.2 Common Applications for Treatment in this Region

A wide variety of techniques are used to assess and treat the elbow joint, including blood-pressure measurement, testing reflexes in the biceps and triceps, electrotherapy and cryotherapy, as well as local transverse friction and manual therapeutic techniques applied to the individual parts of the joint.

3.1.3 Required Basic Anatomical and Biomechanical Knowledge

Precise palpation used to recognize and differentiate deep-lying structures is only valuable if the therapist can relate the findings to existing knowledge of topographical relationships. When searching for structures, therapists therefore need to have a good idea of how the bones of the elbow joint are spatially positioned. They must be able to visualize and identify the most important structures from different perspectives.

The cylindrical shaft of the humerus becomes wider and flatter. It forms edges (margins) and ridges (crests) that end in epicondyles and act as origins for a number of muscles.

The lower extremity of the humerus forms the proximal body of the elbow joint (condyle of the humerus) that is divided into the capitulum and the trochlea (▶ Fig. 3.1). Seen in the sagittal plane, the trochlea is convex from anterior to posterior. In the frontal plane, it is concave due to a longitudinal central groove.

Humeroulnar Joint (HUJ)

The HUJ is a hinge joint with an axis that varies in flexion and extension. This axis has a three-dimensional orientation so that the movement takes place in three anatomical directions. In extension, the ulna always moves in valgus. In flexion, its movement is variable, either in varus or in valgus (Matthijs et al., 2003). The ulna is considerably more massive proximally than distally and with the trochlear notch forms an articular surface with a deep

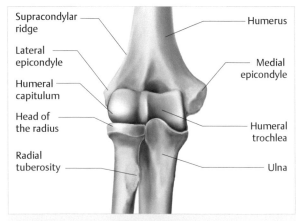

Fig. 3.1 Topography of the bones—anterior view.

socket that is inclined approximately 45° with reference to the ulnar shaft. The passive stability of the humeroulnar joint is produced chiefly by the shape of the articular surface; the deep trochlear notch surrounds the trochlea by about 180° (Milz et al., 1997). This type of stability is called form closure it occurs when both articulation surfaces have a small, almost identical radius of curvature (Matthijs et al., 2003).

The anatomy of the cartilaginous coating of the trochlear notch can vary. Many notches have no, or almost no cartilaginous coating (Milz et al., 1997). This means that in numerous humeroulnar joints there is no contact in the middle or that there is a certain incongruence between the notch and the trochlea.

Since 1993, Eckstein et al. have reported on this incongruence in several publications. According to them, the trochlea is often larger than the notch and in nonweight-bearing position is braced against the walls of the notch. With increasing load, the trochlea sinks deeper into the notch and the congruence increases (Eckstein et al., 1995).

Humeroradial Joint (HRJ)

The spherical shape of the capitulum has a very small radius and points in an anterodistal direction. Proximally, the radius is rather delicate in comparison to its distal end and with its head forms two articular surfaces that articulate simultaneously with the humerus and the ulna (▶ Fig. 3.2). The facet of the head forms a kind of trochoginglymus with the capitulum of the humerus. In contrast to the HUJ, the passive stability is not due to the bony construction of the articular surfaces but rather to the structure of the capsular ligaments, a so-called force closure. In this case, it is the capsule and the ligaments that, when they are stretched, create a force that maintains the physiological contact zones of the articular surfaces (Matthijs et al., 2003). As a result of the incongruence between the two articulating surfaces, the capsular folds (plicae) protrude into the articular space. In the HRJ, 60% of the axial load is transmitted from the lower arm to the

upper arm, and compression is increased even more by extension (with valgus) and pronation, as well as by the action of the hand extensors. Thus it is understandable that muscle action of the hand extensors can provoke pain from osteoarthritis or impingement of capsular folds. This complicates differentiation in investigation of lateral elbow pain in grasping movements, since, in addition, laxity and instability of the HRJ are also causes of lateral elbow pain (O'Driscoll et al., 1991).

Proximal Radioulnar Joint (PRUJ)

The PRUJ is formed by the radial circumference acting as articular head and the radial notch of the ulna with the annular ligament of the radius as the articular socket; it is a rotatory joint (▶ Fig. 3.2). The articular surface of the ulnar radial notch runs from anteromedial to posterolateral. In turning motions of the lower arm, the head of the radius is centered in an osteofibrous ring composed of the notch and the ligament. Although the entire circumference is lined with cartilage, one part never comes into contact with the ulnar articular surface but articulates exclusively with the annular ligament of the radius. The annular ligament of the radius lies directly on the circumference and therefore cannot contract. Thus, a laxity is to be expected as a pathologically altered mobility rather than capsule-determined hypomobility (Matthijs et al., 2003).

The head of the radius is oval. The longer diameter of the oval is approximately 28 mm and the shorter is 22 mm.

Due to a lateral overhang, the head of the radius is not exactly positioned as an extension of the radial shaft. The longer diameter of the oval is in the null position. In this position, the shaft moves further away from the ulna in a radial direction, which leaves room for the radial tuberosity (with the insertion of the long biceps tendon and an intervening bursa) to pass between the two lower arm bones. At the end of the pronation the radial tuberosity can be felt pressing out through the soft tissue in a lateral direction, thus becoming accessible for local therapeutic interventions. In complete supination, the radial tuberosity points forward and can be palpated in the depth of the cubital fossa.

Soft-tissue lesions are among the most frequent complaints seen in physical therapy practice in the area of the elbow joint. Knowing the names and position of muscles that arise at the humeral epicondyle is among the therapist's anatomical skills. The muscles to be palpated will be described in more detail in later sections of the chapter. For the moment, a few interesting aspects can be described.

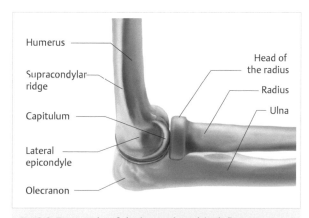

Fig. 3.2 Topography of the bones—lateral (radial) view.

Humerus

Supracondylar ridge

Capitulum

Lateral epicondyle

Olecranon

Head of the radius

Radius

Ulna

Muscle Origins at the Lateral Epicondyle of the Humerus

In 90° flexion, the lateral elbow muscles are almost parallel to each other (▶ Fig. 3.3). Clinically unremarkable, the

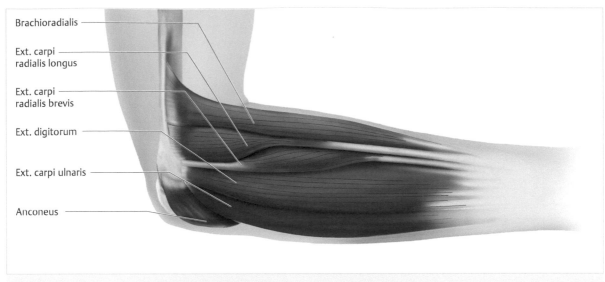

Brachioradialis

Ext. carpi
radialis longus

Ext. carpi
radialis brevis

Ext. digitorum

Ext. carpi ulnaris

Anconeus

Fig. 3.3 Topography of the muscles—lateral (radial) view.

brachioradialis (lateral margin of the humerus) and the extensor carpi radialis longus (medial supracondylar ridge) arise in a direct line. Several muscles arise directly on the lateral epicondyle; their tendons very often blend into each other and are in contact with the humeroradial capsule—extensor carpi radialis brevis and extensor digitorum, extensor carpi ulnaris and anconeus. Knowledge about the precise position of the origins comes from studies of preparations by Omer Matthijs at Texas Tech University in Lubbock. The short radial hand extensor is one of the structures that most commonly suffer from soft-tissue irritation such as insertion tendinopathy or tendinosis (tennis elbow). It is often therapeutically stretched. However, the stretched position used up to now (elbow extension and pronation and flexion and ulnar abduction of the wrist) was not the optimal position for the lengthening of its sarcomeres. In 1997, Lieber et al. described the fact that extension is not a stretching position and Ljung et al. stand by the idea that pronation does not contribute to the lengthening of the extensor carpi radialis brevis (Ljung et al., 1999). The pulling sensation in the usual stretching position could also be caused by stretching of the superficial ramus of the radial nerve. The extensor carpi ulnaris, anconeus, and supinator muscles also arise at the lateral epicondyle, but at the elbow they are clinically rather unremarkable.

Muscular Origins at the Medial Epicondyle of the Humerus

Some superficial muscles of the upper arm that contribute to flexion of the wrist originate with a common tendon (common head) at the distal tip of the medial epicondyle (▶ Fig. 3.4): flexor carpi radialis muscles, palmaris longus, flexor carpi ulnaris, and, deeper, the humeral head of the flexor digitorum superficialis. The common head, which is up to 1 cm long, can cause medial elbow pain (golfer's elbow). Only the pronator teres originates separately, from a plateau on the anterior side of the epicondyle. A few centimeters distal to the elbow joint, a tendinous, sharp-edged structure radiates from the biceps brachii to the fascia of the lower arm—the bicipital aponeurosis or lacertus fibrosus (see ▶ Fig. 3.12).

Neural Structures

In the therapeutic investigation of a joint, neural structures play a special role and are of great interest for differential diagnosis. Therefore, it is important to realize that all three main nerves for the innervation of the lower arm and hand (median, radial, and ulnar nerves) must pass by the elbow joint (▶ Fig. 3.5). In doing this, each one runs through at least one muscular passage that can develop into a bottleneck and exert pressure on the nerve. For this reason, peripheral nerve compression is an alternative to soft-tissue irritation that must be taken seriously, such as tennis or golfer's elbow.

The **radial nerve** travels posteriorly along the humerus in the radial groove, crosses over the elbow joint anteriorly, and passes through two sections of the supinator muscle.

In the radial tunnel (▶ Fig. 3.6), it passes through the sharp-edged tendon of the extensor carpi radialis brevis muscle and the sharp-edged arcade of the supinator muscle, where it can be affected by neurocontusion (Moradi et al., 2015), which is often misdiagnosed as tennis arm.

The groove for the **ulnar nerve** is the most well-known neural passage at the elbow. The ulnar nerve is the only large peripheral nerve of the arm that crosses over the

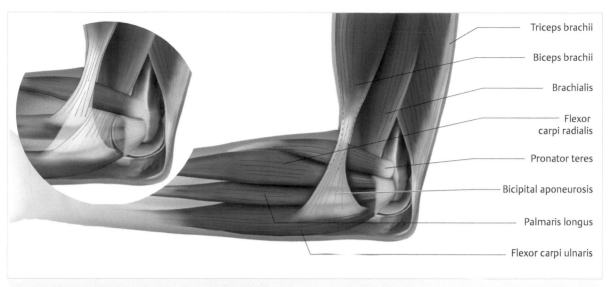

Fig. 3.4 Topography of the muscles—medial (ulnar) view.

Triceps brachii
Biceps brachii
Brachialis
Flexor carpi radialis
Pronator teres
Bicipital aponeurosis
Palmaris longus
Flexor carpi ulnaris

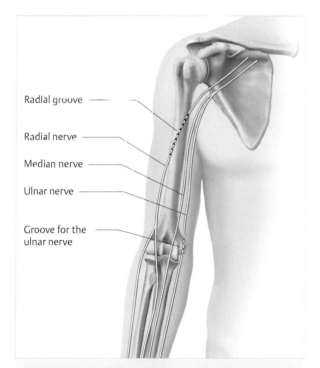

Radial groove
Radial nerve
Median nerve
Ulnar nerve
Groove for the ulnar nerve

Fig. 3.5 Pathways of the most important peripheral nerves of the arm.

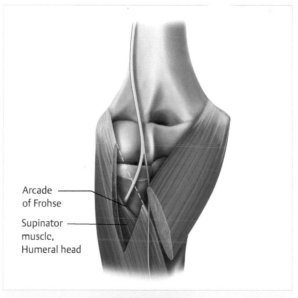

Arcade of Frohse
Supinator muscle, Humeral head

Fig. 3.6 Radial tunnel (after Omer Matthijs).

posterior side of the elbow (▶ Fig. 3.7). Largely unknown are possible nerve compressions on entry into the cubital tunnel (CT). Andreisek et al. (2006) write that cubital tunnel syndrome is the second most common nerve compression syndrome of the upper extremity. Even moderate compression of the CT, such as the physiological example of a vigorous flexion, causes a distinct decrease in volume. In his 2001 monograph, Grana

describes cubital tunnel syndrome, next to medial epicondylopathy, as a common cause of medial elbow pain in US throwing-event athletes. The pathology was known as long ago as 100 years but Feindel and Stratford first coined the name in 1958 (Robertson and Saratsiotis, 2005).

A very detailed description of the CT is given by O'Driscoll et al. in their publication (1991b). The basis is the bony groove for the ulnar nerve between the trochlea and the medial epicondyle. The floor of the tunnel is formed by the HUJ capsule and the ulnar collateral ligament that runs in it (Robertson and Saratsiotis, 2005). The roof is formed by the humeral and ulnar heads of the

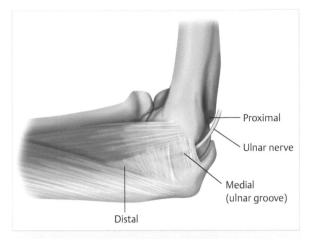

Fig. 3.7 Passage of the ulnar nerve in the cubital tunnel.

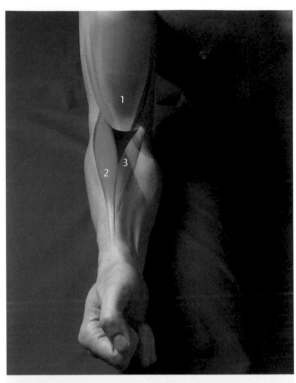

Fig. 3.8 Position and boundary of the cubital fossa.

flexor carpi ulnaris that arise from the lateral epicondyle and the olecranon respectively. They form a 3-cm-long triangle over which the deep aponeurosis of the muscle spreads and covers the tunnel. In 70% of O'Driscoll et al.'s preparations, the proximal boundary is formed by an approximately 4-mm-long ligament-like retinaculum (cubital tunnel retinaculum or Osborne ligament). It extends between the epicondyle and the olecranon. If the retinaculum is present, it can be palpated 90% of the time. With increasing flexion, it tightens itself and raises the pressure in the cubital tunnel by up to 20 times (Polatsch et al., 2007); in extension, it becomes lax. The presence of the retinaculum is associated with possible neural compression pathology; the absence is associated with a possible anterior dislocation of the ulnar nerve over the medial epicondyle and possible friction neuritis. Further proximal, the ulnar nerve may be compressed by the triceps brachii.

3.2 General Orientation—Anterior

3.2.1 Boundaries of the Cubital Fossa

The surface anatomy begins anteriorly at the crook of the elbow (cubital fossa). From here, palpation of the structures on the medial side, then the lateral elbow, and finally posterior structures is introduced. The cubital fossa has a triangular shape. The following structures form its boundaries (▶ Fig. 3.8):
- The muscle belly and the tendons of biceps brachii and brachialis proximally (1).
- Brachioradialis laterally (2).
- Pronator teres medially (3).

The brachial artery and the median nerve run together in the cubital fossa under the lacertus fibrosus to the middle of the lower arm (see ▶ Fig. 3.8 and ▶ Fig. 3.13). Further on, the rounded tendons of the biceps brachii and

brachialis insert at the corresponding tuberosities of the forearm bones.

3.3 Local Palpation—Anterior

3.3.1 Overview of the Structures to be Palpated

- Humerus—medial shaft.
- Biceps brachii.
- Neurovascular bundle:
  ○ Brachial artery.
  ○ Median nerve.
- Brachialis.
- Pronator teres.
- Brachioradialis.
- Proximal radioulnar joint (PRUJ).

3.3.2 Summary of the Palpatory Process

The various structures that make up the crook of the elbow are found by extensive palpation, beginning at the medial side of the humerus and ending at the structures of the cubital fossa.

The medial structures of the upper arm can be followed in two directions:

- The therapist first palpates inferiorly and anteriorly in the cubital fossa.
- Palpation in a distal direction and medially to the medial epicondyle is described later.

In particular, therapists search for a bundle of nerves and vessels located medially, which will guide them to the anterior aspect of the elbow joint.

Finally, the individual structures of the cubital fossa are differentiated from one another.

Starting Position

The following starting position (SP) is suitable when practicing (▶ Fig. 3.9). The patient sits on a stool at the side of the treatment table on which the therapist is seated. The elbow is supported on the therapist's thigh. The elbow joint is flexed and positioned mid-way between pronation and supination. The crook of the elbow should always be facing upward, indicating the neutral position of the upper arm.

This rather unusual SP has two main advantages when palpating the medial humerus and the cubital fossa:
- The areas to be palpated are freely accessible.
- It is easy to place the elbow joint in other positions.

The latter point is advantageous when the palpation is confirmed using joint movement or when certain muscles or nerves are initially elongated and placed under tension.

Alternative Starting Positions

Naturally, other positions can be used to reach the following structures. Nevertheless, care must always be taken to avoid squeezing soft tissue surrounding the elbow joint and to ensure that the position of the joint itself can be modified. Palpation on one's own upper arm is also possible if the elbow joint is stably supported and the second hand has free access to the medial upper arm and the crook of the elbow (▶ Fig. 3.10)

3.3.3 Palpation of Individual Structures

Humerus—Medial Shaft

Palpation of the anterior crook of the elbow begins quite far proximal in order to find reliable access to the boundaries of the cubital fossa. It is important for medial palpation of the upper arm that the triceps is hanging freely and the muscles are generally relaxed.

Technique

Large areas of the medial and lateral aspects of the humeral shaft can be accessed between the anterior elbow flexors and triceps brachii. This can be done on the medial side by lifting the flexor mass slightly with the flat hand and applying a slight, deep pressure with the finger pads (▶ Fig. 3.11).

This palpation technique locates the shaft of the humerus very quickly, and several thin structures can be observed running along the length of the shaft. Transverse palpation to the humerus is used here, that is, anterior-posterior. When palpating posteriorly, the therapist comes across the soft tissue of the triceps brachii, which is separated from the flexor side by a very firm intermuscular septum.

> **Tip**
>
> As nerves and vessels accompany these structures, the palpation should be very flat and applied with the appropriate amount of pressure. The humerus and the neurovascular bundle are easily accessible in almost every upper arm from the axilla to the distal forearm.

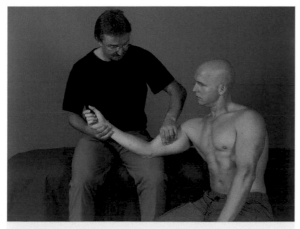

Fig. 3.9 SP for palpation of the anterior aspect.

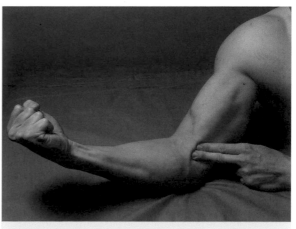

Fig. 3.10 Self-palpation of the arm—for practice purposes.

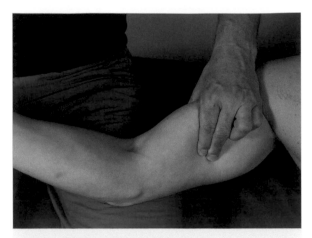

Fig. 3.11 Palpation of the medial humerus.

Biceps Brachii

Generally, the contours of the biceps can be felt very well when the muscles contract against a slight resistance. The medial edge guides therapists to the bundle of nerves and vessels as well as certain structures in the cubital fossa.

Technique
Bicipital Aponeurosis

The therapist looks for the muscle-tendon junction of the biceps brachii during continuous, slight muscle contraction. The muscle belly tapers distally and divides into two tendons that run in somewhat different directions. When hooked medially, it has very sharp edges, but when palpated anteriorly, the structure is flat and broad and presents as a coarse, collagenous plate (lacertus fibrosus or bicipital aponeurosis). It can be followed distally and medially but is then lost in the fascia of the forearm over the muscle belly of the pronator teres (▶ Fig. 3.4 and ▶ Fig. 3.10).

Biceps Tendon

The therapist can reach the main biceps tendon by hooking around the muscle-tendon junction from a lateral position. The tendon can be felt even better by adding isometric contraction and supination in the SP described above. If it is followed systematically with transverse palpation on the tendon distally, it leads the palpating finger to the distal end of the cubital fossa.

Radial Tuberosity

To reach the radial tuberosity, the biceps tendon must be followed deeply, with increasing pressure, as far as the floor of the cubital fossa. The tendon disappears when the patient pronates the forearm maintaining isometric flexion. It reappears when supinated in isometric flexion and is more easily palpable. On the other hand, the tuberosity itself can be reached without muscle activity. The

identification is confirmed by passive pronation and supination of the forearm. In supination, pressure is felt from the tuberosity against the palpating finger. The tendinous insertion is found here. During pronation, it wraps itself around the radius and penetrates between the two forearm bones to the posterior. There it can be felt to project at the same level (2 to 3 finger widths distal to the head of the radius during end-range pronation).

> **Tip**
>
> Palpation of tendon and insertion can be used as techniques for provocative diagnosis. Anterior pain in the crook of the elbow triggered by contraction indicates tendinopathy at the insertion. Passive pronation leads to the conclusion of a problematic passage of the tuberosity with attached soft tissue, usually because of a swollen bursa between the inserting tendon and the tuberosity (bicipitoradial bursa).

3.3.4 Neurovascular Bundle

Two important peripheral motor nerves supplying the forearm and hand, as well as two large blood vessels, travel through the medial region of the upper arm (▶ Fig. 3.13):
- Median nerve.
- Ulnar nerve.
- Brachial artery.
- Basilic vein.

The basilic vein, the deep brachial artery, and the median nerve form a neurovascular bundle that can be palpated over the entire length of the humerus. The ulnar nerve is also part of this bundle until the mid-upper arm. From there it travels separately and crosses the elbow joint posteromedially.

The other structures (median nerve and both blood vessels) run along the upper arm, first in the bicipital groove and then anteriorly and medially (through the cubital fossa) over the elbow joint to the forearm.

These are the longitudinal structures that were observed during the transverse palpation of the medial humerus.

Technique
Brachial Artery

The patient is instructed to maintain a moderately strong isometric elbow flexion and supination. The same transverse palpation technique is used as for the humerus (see ▶ Fig. 3.11). The bundle of nerves and blood vessels is found slightly posterior to the medial border of the biceps, where it lies in a soft-tissue groove, the bicipital

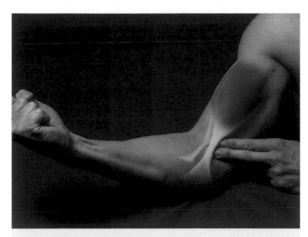

Fig. 3.12 Bicipital aponeurosis and the brachial artery—self-palpation.

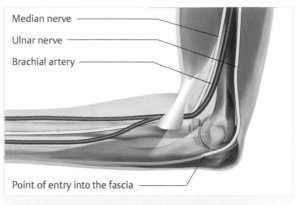

Median nerve

Ulnar nerve

Brachial artery

Point of entry into the fascia

Fig. 3.13 Nerves and blood vessels—medial (ulnar) view.

groove. This means that the palpating fingers have to be slightly flexed to enable the finger pads to reach these structures.

With the muscles now relaxed again, the pulsation of the brachial artery can be felt with moderate, flat pressure. It can be easily followed distally to the cubital fossa. The artery crosses underneath the bicipital aponeurosis and heads toward the middle of the cubital fossa (see ▶ Fig. 3.12). Then it divides into the radial artery and the ulnar artery, which cannot be found by palpation until they reach the distal forearm near the wrist.

Blood pressure is usually measured just before the artery crosses underneath the bicipital aponeurosis, with the aid of a blood-pressure cuff and a stethoscope.

Tip

If the therapist is not certain that the artery has been found, the palpation can be confirmed by finding the pulse at the wrist and then increasing the pressure applied to the point where the brachial artery is presumed to be. The pulse at the wrist will become weaker if the presumed location is correct. With the exception of severe vascular disease, there are no risks to the patient when pressure is applied for a short amount of time.

Median Nerve

The median nerve accompanies the artery until just before the cubital fossa. First it runs under the lacertus fibrosus, which, in rare cases, can irritate the nerve (Gregoli et al., 2013). Before it begins its median course in the forearm, the nerve runs through a passage between the ulnar and humeral heads of the pronator teres. Compression

neuropathies of the median nerve can arise when this muscle is very tense.

The nerve will roll back and forth underneath the transversely palpating fingers on the medial upper arm when slightly more pressure is applied to the humerus (see ▶ Fig. 3.10). This feeling is typical for the palpation of a neural structure.

Tip

It is relatively easy to differentiate the median nerve from the parallel blood vessel. It goes without saying that the nerve neither pulsates nor changes the quality of the radial pulse at the wrist. The location and pathway of a nerve can be confirmed by palpating the nerve as it is placed under alternating tension and relaxation. This procedure carries no risk for the patient as peripheral nerves can usually cope quite well with short, moderate pressure. Pressure occasionally causes formication in the periphery.

In this SP, the median nerve is placed under tension using elbow extension and, when necessary, wrist extension. The nerve becomes tauter underneath the palpating fingers.

Brachialis

First the therapist returns to the medial muscle-tendon transition of the biceps. Proceeding from anterior to medial along an imaginary line from the muscle-tendon transition to the medial epicondyle (see ▶ Fig. 3.23), one first reaches the brachial artery and the median nerve. Under these and on the line to medial, there is a portion of the brachial muscle belly that continues to the ulnar tuberosity, lying somewhat under the pronator teres. One or two finger pads are placed flat from anterior onto the assumed spot where they encounter the muscle-tendon transition of the biceps (not illustrated). The location is

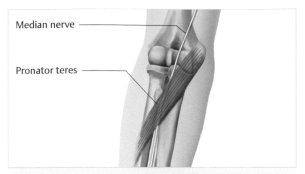

Median nerve

Pronator teres

Fig. 3.14 Position of the pronator teres—anterior view.

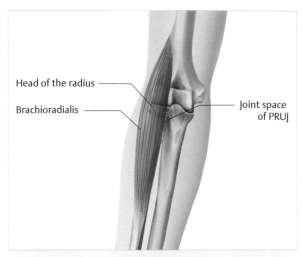

Head of the radius

Brachioradialis

Joint space of PRUJ

Fig. 3.15 Position of the joint space—proximal radioulnar joint (PRUJ).

confirmed by alternating contraction and relaxation of the flexed muscle.

Pronator Teres

The cubital fossa is formed medially by the lateral edge of the pronator teres. This muscle has already been encountered during palpation of the bicipital aponeurosis (see ▶ Fig. 3.14). It originates on the humerus proximal to the medial epicondyle and crosses over the proximal forearm onto the shaft of the radius (▶ Fig. 3.14).

Technique

Following the palpated muscle belly of the brachialis distally, the therapist encounters the lateral edge of the pronator teres. The identification is confirmed by end-range active pronation performed by the patient with some degree of pressure. The edge of the pronator teres can be followed distally to the end of the cubital fossa before it disappears under the muscle belly of the brachioradialis.

Brachioradialis

This muscle is the only flexor of the elbow joint innervated by the radialis nerve. Its slender muscle belly forms the lateral boundary of the cubital fossa (▶ Fig. 3.15). It becomes distinctly noticeable particularly with contraction against resistance in flexion, in a position that is neutral for pronation/supination.

Technique

If the medial edge of the constantly contracted muscle belly is followed proximally it leads the palpating finger to the distal third of the humerus on the lateral side, to the lateral margin of the humerus and to palpation of the radial nerve (see ▶ Fig. 3.36). With pronounced isometric tension, it pulls the soft tissue of the lateral upper arm flat and usually forms an easily recognized concavity at the level of the fleshy insertion.

3.3.5 Proximal Radioulnar Joint (PRUJ)

The medial border of the brachioradialis precisely marks the junction between the head of the radius and the ulna at the cubital fossa (▶ Fig. 3.15).

Technique

One palpating finger is placed in the middle of the cubital fossa, between the lateral biceps tendon and the medial edge of the brachioradialis. With marked deep pressure in the cubital fossa and somewhat laterally, the movement of the radial head can be felt when the forearm is turned over. The therapist now has an idea of where the PRUJ can be found: on the medial border of the brachioradialis at the height of the head of the radius.

3.3.6 Tips for Assessment and Treatment

- It is very important that all therapists be aware of the exact position of the neurovascular bundle on the medial side of the humerus. Colleagues who experience the position and size of these structures for the first time during courses on palpation are surprised at the ease with which these structures can be reached and, therefore, compressed.
- Whether applying classical massage therapy, underwater massage, or a manipulative technique in manual therapy, the therapist must protect the medial upper arm and the crook of the elbow from any permanent pressure or tension. Local and precise applications to well-defined areas are an exception.
- Familiarity with the course of the biceps brachii tendon is extremely helpful when confirming the presence of a tendinopathy or bursitis at the insertion.

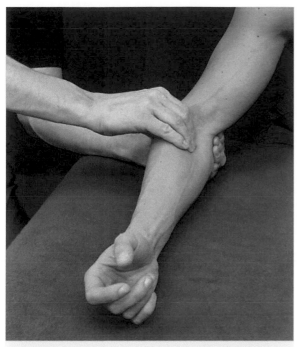

Fig. 3.16 Laxity test at the proximal radioulnar joint (PRUJ).

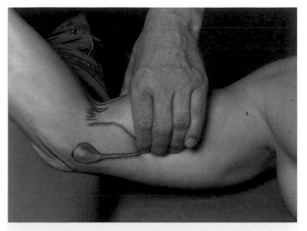

Fig. 3.17 Palpation of the medial shaft of the humerus.

• Translational movements of the radial head with respect to the ulna or the humerus for diagnostic or therapeutic purposes are part of every manual therapist's repertoire. Knowledge of how far to medial the head of the radius extends and its boundaries with the ulna ensures the use of the correct technique. These tests, together with fixation of the humerus in the HRJ, are used to confirm capsular hypomobility or laxity, and in the PRUJ (▶ Fig. 3.16), with fixation of the ulna, exclusively to confirm laxity.

3.4 Local Palpation—Medial

3.4.1 Overview of the Structures to be Palpated

• Humerus—medial border.
• Ulnar nerve.
• Groove for the ulnar nerve and the cubital tunnel.
• Medial supracondylar ridge and medial epicondyle of the humerus.
• Sites of insertion at the medial epicondyle, common head, pronator teres.
• Differentiation in the presence of epicondylitis.
• Quick orientation on the forearm.

3.4.2 Summary of the Palpatory Process

Local palpation begins again on the medial aspect of the shaft of the humerus. The previously sought neural structure in the neurovascular bundle is located and its pathway followed down onto the forearm.

Then come the bony and muscular structures. Finding their location and differentiation from other structures is of particular interest in the context of medial epicondylitis.

Hoppenfeld (1992) used a simple and helpful technique to visualize the position of the forearm muscles originating on the medial epicondyle. This will be presented at the end of this section (▶ Fig. 3.28).

Starting Position

It is recommended that the therapist uses either the practice SP or the alternative SPs from the anterior palpation (see ▶ Fig. 3.9). The therapist sits on a treatment table and the patient sits on a stool in front of the table. The elbow is resting on the therapist's thigh. The shoulder is flexed and slightly abducted. The elbow joint is flexed and placed in mid-position between pronation and supination.

3.4.3 Palpation of Individual Structures

Humerus—Medial Border

Local medial palpation begins by returning to the medial aspect of the shaft of the humerus (▶ Fig. 3.17).

Technique

The therapist attempts to feel the shaft beneath the small amount of soft tissue by using a flat, transverse technique. The grip has already been described in detail in the local palpation of the anterior aspect. It is advisable to just grasp the upper arm from below for some of the following techniques. For the sake of orientation, it is advisable to look for the structures of the medial neurovascular bundle, which has already been found by palpation, in the bicipital groove at the medial edge of the humerus (▶ Fig. 3.18).

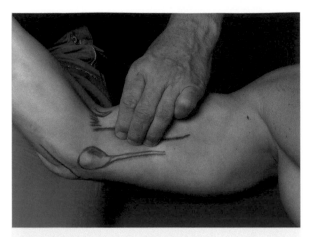

Fig. 3.18 Palpation in the bicipital groove.

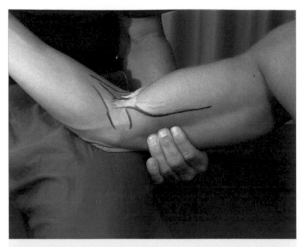

Fig. 3.19 Palpation of the ulnar nerve proximal to the groove.

Ulnar Nerve

About halfway down the upper arm the ulnar nerve separates itself from the other structures in the neurovascular bundle. It runs in a posterior direction, accompanies the triceps brachii, and passes through the medial intermuscular septum (▶ Fig. 3.19 and ▶ Fig. 3.21). This path is approximately 8 cm long (Grana, 2001). The ulnar nerve crosses the elbow joint posteriorly in the groove of the ulnar nerve (at the start of the cubital tunnel) and runs toward the ulna and between the flexor carpi ulnaris and the flexor digitorum profundus (Polatsch et al., 2007) in a distal direction to the forearm, only becoming palpable again at the distal forearm (see Chapter 4, Hand; in particular see ▶ Fig. 4.66).

Technique

The palpating fingers move from the medial humeral shaft in a posterior direction. The muscle belly of the triceps brachii uses the medial intermuscular septum as an expanded, membranous surface of origin. Both can be felt under slight isometric extension. The ulnar nerve is palpated from anterior against the septum and triceps. With transverse palpation directly on the nerve, there is a typical rolling feeling under the palpating finger. The nerve is followed distally and posteriorly, with transverse palpation, toward the medial epicondyle.

Tip

Only experienced therapists can be certain that they have found the ulnar nerve. It is often necessary to use the following measure to gain confidence. The ulnar nerve is placed under tension by passively flexing the elbow and, when necessary, extending the wrist. The nerve then becomes tauter when palpated and can be rolled back and forth underneath the fingertips with the typical feel of peripheral nerves.

Groove for the Ulnar Nerve and the Cubital Tunnel

The groove for the ulnar nerve can be felt on the posterior aspect of the distinct protrusion of the medial epicondyle. The ulnar nerve lies in this groove and is accompanied by a small artery.

Technique

The nerve can be felt best by using transverse palpation when the elbow is moderately flexed (approximately 40–70°). With greater flexion, the nerve is placed under tension and pushes the palpating finger out of the groove. It now becomes clear that only pointed objects can knock against the ulnar nerve especially when the elbow is flexed. Habitual and traumatic subluxation of the nerve can be occasionally observed at this site.

The nerve can be followed again more proximally up onto the medial humerus. Distally, it is no longer as easy to feel the ulnar nerve since, at the level of the epicondyle, it enters the cubital tunnel (▶ Fig. 3.20). In 70% of cases, the entry into the tunnel is marked by a ligamentous retinaculum that runs transverse to the course of the nerve from the epicondyle to the olecranon. With increasing flexion, it contracts and fixates the nerve in the groove; with extension, it relaxes. If a palpating finger is positioned between the epicondyle and the olecranon (humeroulnar groove), with the pad of the finger on the nerve and the fingertip pointing distally, it is possible to press against the retinaculum and feel its course. The best starting position for this is a flexion of 70 to 90%. Directly distal to the retinaculum the nerve is followed approximately 3 cm further along with transverse palpation, through the aponeurosis of the flexor carpi ulnaris, until it disappears downward between the muscle bellies of the flexor carpi ulnaris and flexor digitorum profundus muscles. Its further course on the ulnar side of the

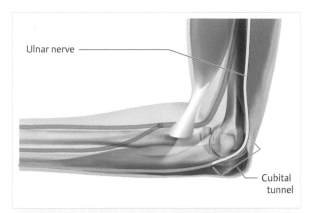

Fig. 3.20 Passage of the ulnar nerve in the groove and the cubital tunnel.

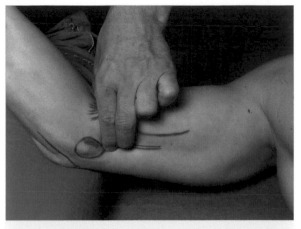

Fig. 3.21 Palpation of the medial intermuscular septum.

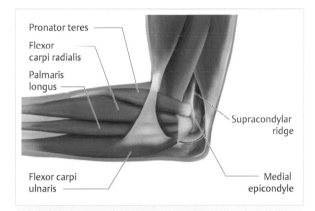

Fig. 3.22 Topography of the muscles—medial (ulnar) view.

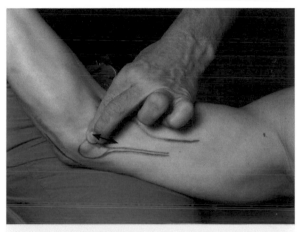

Fig. 3.23 Palpation of the origin of the pronator teres.

forearm as far as the pisiform bone is known from topographic anatomy. At this point it becomes palpable again.

The floor of the cubital tunnel can also be felt for part of its course. A finger is placed in the humeroulnar groove with the fingertip pointing laterally toward the ulna, past the ulnar nerve. The medial surface of the olecranon is followed proximally and distally. At the most anterior boundary of this surface is the capsule of the HUJ, which is often impinged (Boxer's elbow, Robinson et al., 2017).

Medial Supracondylar Ridge and Medial Epicondyle of the Humerus

Technique

Palpation begins again at the medial humeral shaft (see ► Fig. 3.11) and follows the bone systematically in a distal direction. It is clearly felt that the humerus becomes broader and acquires a sharp edge. The sharp-edged medial supracondylar ridge guides the palpation onto the tip of the well-developed medial epicondyle. This is the starting point for the palpation of all further muscle attachments in this region (► Fig. 3.22).

Sites of Insertion at the Medial Epicondyle (Pronator Teres, Common Head)

Two palpations of muscular insertions start at the tip of the medial epicondyle.

Technique

Pronator Teres

A bony plateau can be clearly felt when the therapist slides the fingers in an anterior direction down from the tip toward the cubital fossa. This is the insertion of the pronator teres (► Fig. 3.23). The therapist can be sure of having located the pronator teres correctly when active pronation pushes the palpating fingers away from the plateau. The pronator teres rarely causes epicondylitis (except in some throwing-event athletes; Grana, 2001). Long-term tension in the muscle belly can endanger the median nerve as it passes through the muscle.

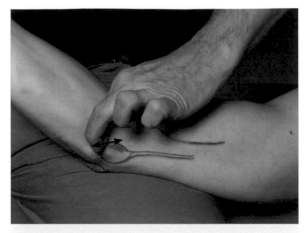

Fig. 3.24 Palpation of the distal tip of the epicondyle.

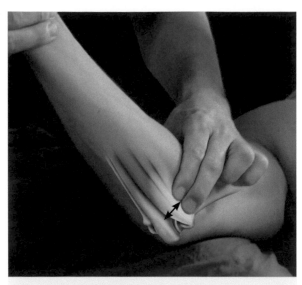

Fig. 3.25 Transverse palpation of the common head.

Common Head

When the therapist slides distally from the tip of the medial epicondyle toward the wrist, a taut, rounded structure of approximately 1 cm in width is felt (▶ Fig. 3.24). This structure turns into soft muscle tissue after only a short distance. The communal tendon of origin (common head) is formed by the convergence of three tendons onto the distal tip of the medial epicondyle: the radial and ulnar flexors of the hand and the tensor of the aponeurosis of the hand (▶ Fig. 3.22). The humeral head of the superficial finger flexors joins the common head deep in the tissues (not palpable).

Tip

Muscle activity confirms the correct location. When the patient flexes the wrist or fingers against resistance, tension in the tendon immediately results in counterpressure.

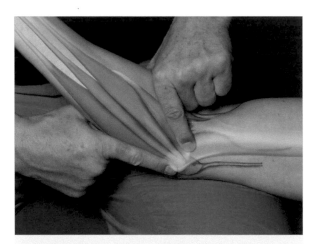

Fig. 3.26 Borders of the common head.

Other Techniques

Common Head

The dimensions of the common head can be visualized using two additional techniques.

The first technique involves the use of transverse palpation to determine the thickness of the tendon and the tendon-muscle junction (▶ Fig. 3.25). The patient's shoulder can be placed in a small amount of lateral rotation to allow better assessment of this region.

The second technique involves determining the length of the common head by placing the index fingers on either side of the tendon (▶ Fig. 3.26). Once again, a moderate amount of activity in the finger or wrist flexors can facilitate locating the tendon.

3.4.4 Differentiation in the Presence of Epicondylitis

The inserting muscular structures seen at the medial epicondyle are responsible for the symptoms associated with golfer's elbow syndrome. Winkel (2004) described three types of epicondylitis that mainly differ from one another by the location of the lesion along the above-described course. The techniques are used for diagnostic provocation in assessment or for treatment. The aim is to first find the most painful point and to then treat this area with appropriate physical therapy methods, including the possible use of cross-frictions according to Cyriax.

Types of Medial Epicondylitis

- Type I. common flexor origin on the distal tip of the medial epicondyle; pathology more likely to be inflammatory insertion tendinopathy.
- Type II. tendon of the common head; pathology tends to appear as tendinosis (most frequently occurring form of golfer's elbow).
- Type III. muscle-tendon junction; more of an inflammatory pathology.

Technique

Type I

To reach the insertion of the sturdy common head directly on the epicondyle, a technique is used where the finger pad points toward the distal tip of the epicondyle. In this case, the pad of the index finger of the more proximal hand is used.

The flexors are also approximated to relax the tendon and to provide free access to the insertion. This is achieved by passively moving the patient's hand into a flexed position.

The side of the index finger pushes down on the tendon and the finger pad points toward the epicondyle and applies pressure. If necessary, the middle finger is placed on top of the index finger for support. The index finger maintains this posture, increases the pressure, and moves from posterior to anterior (toward the cubital fossa). If epicondylitis is present at this location the patient will confirm this by reporting pain.

Types II and III

The therapist now turns the proximal forearm so that the pad of the index finger pushes down directly onto the approximately 1-cm-wide tendon (▶ Fig. 3.27). Direct pressure is applied onto the tendon during palpation; the direction of movement remains the same.

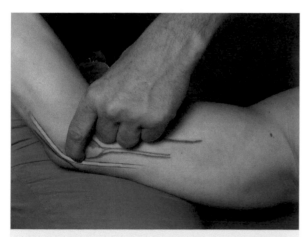

Fig. 3.27 Palpation of the ulnar nerve in the cubital tunnel.

If the therapist wishes to access the muscle-tendon junction, the palpating finger slides approximately 1 cm further distal.

The muscle-tendon junction (type III) can be differentiated from the tendon itself (type II) by its greater width and its softer consistency.

Quick Orientation on the Forearm

As already mentioned, the following muscles are found on the medial epicondyle:
- Flexor carpi ulnaris (travels along the ulna to the wrist).
- Palmaris longus (found in the middle, traveling superficially to the wrist).
- Humeroulnar head of the flexor digitorum superficialis (found in the middle, traveling deeper in the tissue to the wrist).
- Flexor carpi radialis (travels at an angle toward the radius and down to the wrist).
- Pronator teres (travels at an angle toward the radius).

Several of the tendons belonging to these muscles will be re-encountered when palpating the wrist. It is not possible to precisely differentiate the muscle bellies in the forearm from one another. It is only possible to distinguish the pronator from the common head of the hand and finger flexors.

Technique

The position of the muscles in the forearm and their alignment to the wrist can be visualized using a trick, and it is recommended that therapists try this out beforehand on their own arm.

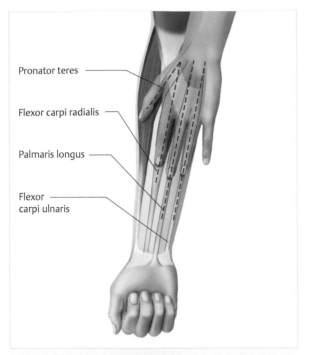

Fig. 3.28 Topography of the muscles in the forearm—anterior view.

Pronator teres

Flexor carpi radialis

Palmaris longus

Flexor carpi ulnaris

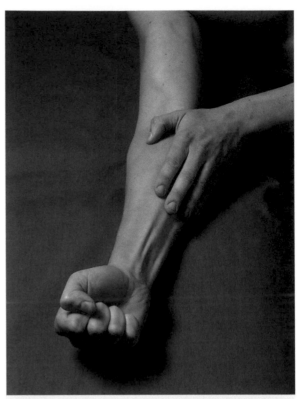

Fig. 3.29 Quick orientation on the forearm.

The forearm to be palpated is positioned so that the elbow joint is slightly flexed.

The left hand is positioned on the place on the medial epicondyle at which the thenar and hypothenar converge. The fingers are spread out slightly and rest on the forearm. Apart from the small finger, each finger represents the position and course of one of the muscles that originate from the epicondyle (▶ Fig. 3.28 and ▶ Fig. 3.29).

Tips

The actual position of the muscles can be confirmed using muscle contraction:
- The muscle belly of the pronator teres becomes distinct underneath the left thumb of the applied hand when the patient strongly pronates at end range.
- The index finger indicates the course of the flexor carpi radialis, and the tendon in the distal forearm becomes distinct with active wrist flexion and hand abduction.
- The ring finger is positioned over the ulnar flexor of the wrist. Wrist flexion combined with hand adduction activates this muscle.
- Not everyone possesses the palmaris longus. When present, this muscle is found in the middle of the anterior forearm, and the middle finger indicates its position. Further details can be found in Chapter 4, Hand.

3.4.5 Tips for Assessment and Treatment

Symptoms presenting on the medial side can be an indication for problems at the HUJ or the presence of soft-tissue lesions in the muscles inserting there. The therapist will quickly become aware of which type of pathological condition he or she is dealing with during the assessment. Structures are differentiated by assessing passive movement and testing against resistance.

Soft-tissue lesions, popularly known as golfer's elbow, can be easily confirmed by the action of finger and wrist flexors against the greatest resistance possible. The damaged structure can only be precisely identified by local palpation. It is always necessary to establish a differential diagnosis between a golfer's elbow and a cubital tunnel syndrome. In particular, in the presence of burning and distally radiating pain, the therapist should consider this possibility of neural irritation. Precise palpation shows the position of the nerve in comparison to the muscular structures. The predictive value of the flexion compression test (Beekman et al., 2009) for the presence of cubital tunnel syndrome is good. For the test, direct pressure is applied to the ulnar nerve with the elbow held in maximal flexion. Local and nonlocal pain can thus be provoked quickly.

3.5 Local Palpation—Lateral

3.5.1 Summary of the Palpatory Process

The humerus is once again the starting point when searching for specific, important structures.

The first part of the palpation on the lateral elbow is mainly directed toward the bony structures in the humeroradial joint (► Fig. 3.2). The muscular structures are then made accessible. The same applies as for the medial side: the exact location should be found that indicates the presence of epicondylitis.

Starting Position

It is recommended that the arm rests on a treatment table with the shoulder in abduction (between 45° and 90°). The elbow is flexed to about 90° and placed in mid-pronation/ supination. The therapist sits lateral to the patient (► Fig. 3.30).

3.5.2 Locating the Most Important Osseous Structures

Overview of the Structures to be Palpated

- Humerus—lateral border and lateral intermuscular septum.
- Lateral supracondylar ridge.
- Lateral epicondyle and the lateral condyle of the humerus.
- Capitulum humeri and anconeus.
- Humeroradial joint space (HJS).
- Head and neck of the radius.
- Brachioradialis and the radial nerve.
- Extensor carpi radialis longus.

- Extensor carpi radialis brevis.
- Extensor digitorum.
- Extensor carpi ulnaris.

Humerus—Lateral Border and Lateral Intermuscular Septum

As on the medial side, the increased width of the distal humerus can also be felt laterally. The therapist searches for the humerus in the inferior third of the upper arm between the flexor and extensor groups of muscles.

Technique

The finger pads are placed flat over the lateral side of the upper arm and palpate transversely (► Fig. 3.31). The aim is to find a hard structure with rounded contours (humeral shaft).

While searching for the humerus, the palpating fingers may slide over a layer that is solid but still yields elastically to pressure. This is the lateral intermuscular septum. As on the medial side, the triceps has a membranous enlargement of its surface of origin. The septum is especially pronounced when the patient tenses the triceps and the therapist attempts to palpate the muscle from anterior. The humerus can be palpated immediately anterior to the septum.

Lateral Supracondylar Ridge

Technique

As transverse palpation continues distally along the humerus, the rounded palpatory feel changes into a sharp edge. The palpating finger is now located over the lateral supracondylar ridge, which is found immediately proximal to the lateral epicondyle. This is the origin of the extensor carpi longus, with the brachioradialis directly proximal to it.

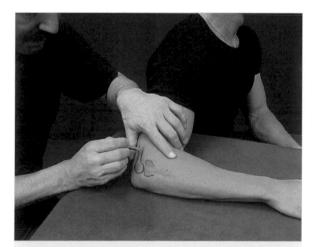
Fig. 3.30 Starting position for palpation of the lateral aspect.

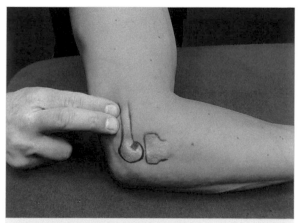
Fig. 3.31 Palpation of the lateral humerus.

Lateral Epicondyle of the Humerus

Technique

The following description is based on the most recent anatomical knowledge and corrects statements that have been made up to now about the morphology of the epicondyle and position of the muscular insertions. ► Fig. 3.32 was created by Omer Matthijs on the basis of numerous dissections of elbow preparations at the Texas Tech University Health Science Center performed by Dr. P. Sizer, Dr. M. Smith, and Dr. J.-M. Brismée. This drawing largely agrees with the description from MRI studies of preparations by Zoner et al. (2010) and was released for publication at the time.

The sharp edge of the supracondylar crest is followed further distally. It broadens into an almost-triangular structure with a lateral surface and three corners (► Fig. 3.32).

The superior edge (on the top in ► Fig. 3.32) is also a surface of origin for the extensor carpi radialis longus. The anterior flat edge is the surface of origin of the extensor carpi radialis brevis, extensor digitorum, extensor digiti minimi, and the extensor carpi ulnaris. The supinator uses a small area of the posterior edge as the point of origin. Directly above lies the largest mound of the small lateral surface, the actual lateral epicondyle. This rise, very shallow compared to its medial opposite number, is found by palpating with a rounded movement using one finger pad.

The significantly new information in this description is the changed position of the origin of the extensor carpi radialis brevis. It is now known to arise at the anterior and not, as previously assumed and often published, at the superior edge of the epicondyle. This has enormous consequences for the most important soft-tissue manipulation at the elbow in tennis elbow syndrome (see ► Fig. 3.44).

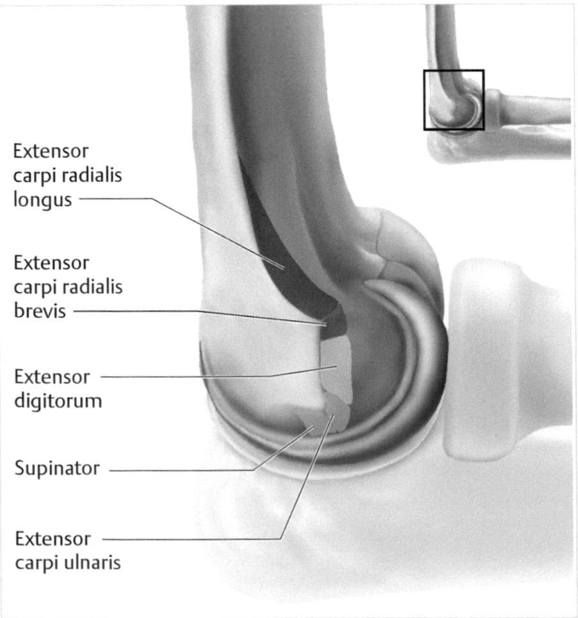

Tip

Correct definition of the contours of the lateral epicondyle depends decisively on systematically following the supracondylar crest with its two extensions in a distal direction. This can be done with transverse palpation over the respective ridges. The distal ridge is covered by the tendons that insert there and is clearly more difficult to feel.

Capitulum Humeri and Anconeus

Starting at the anterior ridge, the therapist palpates a short stretch anteriorly toward the crook of the elbow, using one fingertip and moderate pressure, and encounters a rounded convex structure, the anterior aspect of the capitulum humeri. Oriented in a distal direction, the ridge of the radial head offers direct bony resistance.

Starting at the rounded posterior end (► Fig. 3.33) palpation moves posteriorly from a convex structure and encounters the lateral surface of the olecranon. The rounded structure is the posterior portion of the capitulum humeri, the shape of which can only be felt when the elbow joint is flexed.

The whole lateral surface between the lateral epicondyle, lateral olecranon, and posterior side of the HRJ is covered by the muscle belly of the anconeus, whose contraction during extension can be well felt by direct flat palpation of the muscle belly (► Fig. 3.34).

Extensor carpi radialis longus

Extensor carpi radialis brevis

Extensor digitorum

Supinator

Extensor carpi ulnaris

Fig. 3.32 Detailed anatomy of the lateral epicondyle of the humerus (after Omer Matthijs).

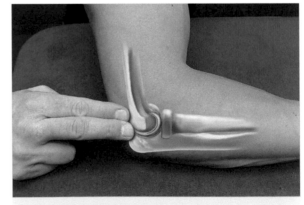

Fig. 3.33 Searching for the posterior capitulum of the humerus.

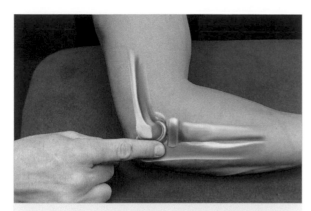

Fig. 3.34 Palpation of thehumeroradial joint (HRJ) space and the anconeus.

Humeroradial Joint Space (HJS)

The articular space of the HRJ can be reached in three ways:
- From the anterior aspect of the capitulum.
- From the posterior aspect of the capitulum.
- From the distal edge of the lateral surface with the lateral epicondyle always oriented distally.

The result of palpation should always be a narrow indentation and an adjacent ridge. The indentation is the articular space; the ridge is the head of the radius. There are several ways to confirm the correct location.

Tips

1. **Confirmation with movement:** the correct position of the palpating finger is determined by passively pronating and supinating the forearm. The joint space has been correctly located when movement is felt at the head of the radius.
2. **The simplest palpation access:** if the articular space of the HRJ is reached by moving distally from the distal edge of the lateral surface with the lateral epicondyle, palpation at this point is somewhat difficult because of the insertion tendons and it is difficult to feel the shape of the articular space. If the search is begun from the posterior aspect of the capitulum, the covering layer of extensor tendons is missing and the articular space between the rather straight radial head and the convex capitulum is wide open. This is the best point at which to find the articular space of the humeroradial joint (► Fig. 3.34).
3. **Palpation during movement:** the therapist can now understand how the joint space changes in a variety of elbow positions. The joint space can be best felt when the elbow is extended. With increasing flexion, the little radial head rocks and glides along the capitulum in an anterior direction and the capsule over the joint tenses, so that the capitulum is prominently palpable.

Head and Neck of the Radius

The contours of the proximal radius will become clear in the following section. When students feel this structure for the first time, they will be surprised by its position and particularly by the dimensions of the head of the radius.

Technique

Head of the Radius

The palpating finger starts at the joint space of the HRJ and slides distally for a short distance. The finger pads are now lying directly over the head of the radius and the more superficially located annular ligament of the radius. The expected height (proximal to distal length) is around 11 mm (Kuhn et al., 2012), which corresponds to about 1 finger width.

The therapist can feel the head of the radius rotating underneath the finger by rotating the forearm over a large range. As the head of the radius has a transverse elliptical form, the therapist can clearly feel the finger being pushed away when the forearm rotates from supination into pronation. The anterior boundary of the head of the radius is felt when the palpating finger consistently follows the head in an anterior direction. Now the index fingers can be used to grasp the boundary of the head of the radius that can be reached anteriorly and posteriorly and can be felt the entire length of the head (► Fig. 3.35). Most practitioners are surprised by the size, since it is much more prominent than the way it is depicted in anatomical illustrations or can be seen on anatomical models.

Tip

It is important that the therapist's finger remains on the head of the radius until soft tissue prevents further palpation. This soft tissue corresponds to the extensor carpi radialis longus and brachioradialis and will be highlighted later on.

As a reminder: the head of the radius is also accessible deep in the cubital fossa (see ► Fig. 3.15). Being able to recognize the entire dimensions of the head of the radius and its differentiation from the neck of the radius is the basis for manual therapy techniques at the HRJ and the PRUJ (see ► Fig. 3.16), as well as for locating important parts of the muscles.

Neck of the Radius

Further distal, the head tapers to the neck. If palpation follows the contours of the head with application of one finger pad, the finger normally slides deep, down to the neck. From this point, the radius can no longer be reached

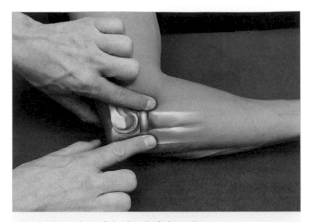

Fig. 3.35 Borders of the head of the radius.

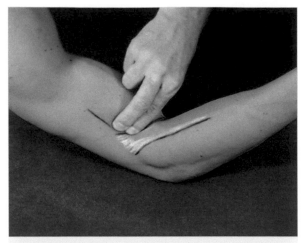

Fig. 3.36 Palpation of the radial nerve.

directly because there are muscles in the way of direct access. The next prominent structure in palpation further distal is the radial tuberosity whose convexity in end-range pronation can be felt through the belly of the flexor carpi ulnaris (usually the posterior part).

Brachioradialis and the Radial Nerve

The radial nerve crosses over the elbow joint laterally on the flexor side. The brachioradialis is the guiding structure for palpation.

Technique

Further palpation starts on the distal part of the upper arm. The muscle bulk of the brachioradialis is evident here, on the lateral border of the humerus. The slender muscle belly becomes prominent when it contracts against strong resistance opposing elbow flexion. The therapist can follow the muscle along its medial edge to its origin, where the active muscle pulls the soft tissue of the upper arm together and forms a shallow depression (▶ Fig. 3.36). Directly proximal to this, at the transition to the border of the biceps, the radial nerve can be felt with deep transverse palpation.

Tips

- The typical feeling of palpating peripheral nerves is felt with transverse palpation and slight posterior pressure against the bone: the nerve rolls back and forth under the finger.
- The brachioradialis is accompanied distally by its superficial ramus. Approximately a hand's breadth proximal to the wrist, this branch penetrates the fascia of the forearm, lies close to the surface, and can again be felt there.

3.5.3 Locating the Muscles and their Insertions

The muscle insertions of the posterior forearm in the region of the lateral epicondyle can be generators of lateral elbow pain, colloquially called tennis elbow. However, these are not the only pain generators. In establishing a differential diagnosis, arthritis of the HRJ or impingement of capsular plicae in the HR articular space should definitely be taken into account.

For successful location of soft-tissue irritations, it is necessary to know the following:
- The morphology of the lateral distal humerus.
- The inserting fibers of the extensor carpi radialis brevis and extensor digitorum merge into a common flat tendon so that here it is also possible to speak of a common head.
- These tendons are in contact with the deeper capsule of the humeroradial joint. This makes it difficult to determine with certainty whether lateral symptoms in the elbow joint involve soft tissue or the joint.

3.5.4 Locating the Lateral Insertion Tendinopathies

Position of the different types of tennis elbow (▶ Fig. 3.37):
- Tennis elbow, type I: insertion of the extensor carpi radialis longus.
- Tennis elbow, type II: insertion of the extensor carpi radialis brevis.
- Tennis elbow, type III: tendon of the extensor carpi radialis brevis.
- Tennis elbow, type IV: muscle-tendon junction of the extensor carpi radialis brevis.
- Tennis elbow, type V: insertion of the extensor digitorum.

Extensor Carpi Radialis Longus

The muscle bulk of the extensor carpi radialis longus is also evident on the supracondylar ridge. The therapist can observe the distinct, short, round, and usually noticeably prominent muscle belly when the wrist isometrically contracts while extended with hand abduction (▶ Fig. 3.38).

Technique

From the orientation point at the origin of the brachioradialis (lateral margin) palpation proceeds distally to the supracondylar crest.

In every case, muscle contraction pushes the palpating finger upward and away.

According to Winkel (2004), insertion tendinopathy is described as type I tennis elbow. Once the muscle is found, its borders can be visualized with continuous contraction (▶ Fig. 3.39).

Extensor Carpi Radialis Brevis

Using the SP described above, it is possible to locate a slender muscle belly of the short radial wrist extensors, which is the direct extension of the long radial hand extensors.

Technique

A shallow depression can be felt at the junction between the two muscle bellies when these muscles are contracted. This shallow indentation is located at the distal end of the belly of the long radial wrist extensor and at the proximal beginning of the belly of the short radial wrist extensor. Once the muscle has been located, the edges of the muscle belly can be followed (▶ Fig. 3.40). The brachioradialis forms its anterior boundary and the extensor digitorum its posterior boundary. The tendon of origin runs from the proximal beginning of the muscle belly to the distal edge of the lateral epicondyle. Three

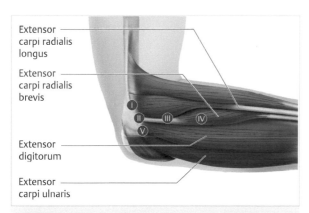

Fig. 3.37 Position of the different types of tennis elbow.

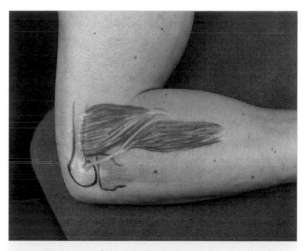

Fig. 3.38 Position of the lateral wrist extensors.

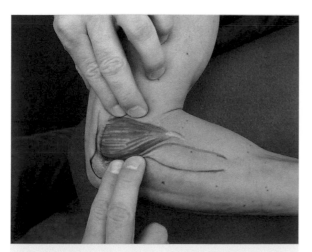

Fig. 3.39 Borders of the extensor carpi radialis longus.

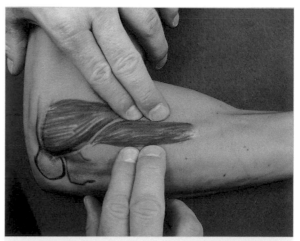

Fig. 3.40 Borders of the extensor carpi radialis brevis.

possible causes of a tennis elbow are ascribed to the extensor carpi radialis brevis (types II–IV, ▶ Fig. 3.41).

Tip

It is easy to locate the boundary between the two hand radial extensors and the brachioradialis. Its location can be confirmed by alternately actively flexing the elbow and extending the wrist. The posterior boundary to the neighboring extensor digitorum muscle is less distinct and is located with the aid of reciprocal inhibition, as will be described later in the text. The tendons of the longus and brevis muscles travel parallel to the radial side of the wrist joint, through the second tendon compartment.

The superficial part of the muscle belly of the extensor carpi radialis brevis is the only part that is accessible. The larger part of the muscle is found deeper in the tissues and is covered by neighboring muscles.

Extensor Digitorum

The extensor digitorum is noticeable on the anterior edge of the lateral epicondyle and the muscle belly is found between the extensor carpi radialis brevis and the extensor carpi ulnaris.

Technique

The muscle needs only to contract to differentiate it from the surrounding structures. The therapist resists wrist flexion by applying light pressure to the palm of the hand. This reciprocally inhibits all wrist extensors.

When combined with movement of the fingers (as if playing a piano), the medial and lateral borders of the muscle can be clearly differentiated from the wrist extensors (▶ Fig. 3.42).

Extensor Carpi Ulnaris

The medial hand extensors are also noticeable on the distal aspect of the anterior edge of the epicondyle and travel distally along the posterior border of the ulna.

Technique

The extensor carpi ulnaris can be differentiated from the ulna by feeling the differences in tissue consistency, that is, the resistance of the muscle to direct pressure of the palpating finger is rather soft and the resistance of the bone is distinctly hard.

Tip

In order to visualize the entire muscle, the therapist can ask the patient to alternate contraction in extension and ulnar abduction of the hand (▶ Fig. 3.43).

As has been described above, the lateral border of extensor carpi ulnaris is differentiated from extensor digitorum by reciprocally inhibiting the hand extensors and contracting the finger extensors.

Neither the origin, the tendon, nor the muscle-tendon junction are known to be associated with lateral elbow symptoms. This muscle appears to be insignificant for clinical practice.

3.5.5 Tips for Assessment and Treatment

Local Palpatory Techniques for Type II Tennis Elbow

Pain-provoking transverse friction techniques have been mentioned for the assessment and treatment of all types of tennis elbow. As type II tennis elbow (in combination

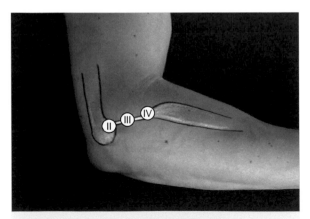

Fig. 3.41 Position of tennis elbow types II to IV.

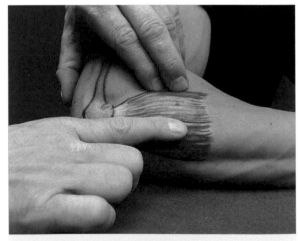

Fig. 3.42 Borders of the extensor digitorum.

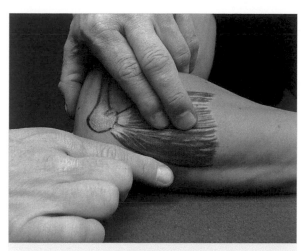

Fig. 3.43 Borders of the extensor carpi ulnaris.

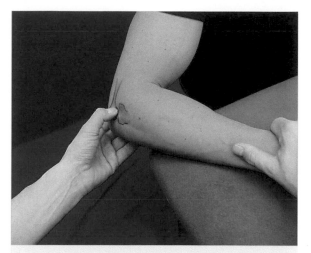

Fig. 3.44 Transverse frictions for the treatment of type II tennis elbow.

with type V) occurs most frequently, the technique for type II tennis elbow will be described in the following section.

Starting Position

There are two points of emphasis in this SP:
- The patient's arm should be resting on a treatment table with moderate shoulder abduction and elbow flexion.
- The elbow should protrude over the edge of the table to allow it to be easily reached from all sides.

The therapist uses one hand to conduct the technique and the free hand to stabilize the patient's arm on the treatment table.

Technique

The treatment hand grasps the elbow joint with the finger pads hooking onto the medial side. The finger pads stabilize the transverse frictions applied by the thumb (▶ Fig. 3.44).

The pad of the thumb touches the anterior edge of the lateral epicondyle.

With distinct pressure against the anterior edge, the thumb is pushed in a straight movement toward the crook of the elbow. The thumb is pulled back to the tip without pressure but maintaining skin contact. The tendinous origin of the extensor carpi radialis brevis cannot be palpated as an elevation since it attaches flat to the anterior edge.

This palpation is painful when tennis elbow symptoms are present. The therapist should therefore adjust the amount of pressure applied during treatment. Administration of treatment is governed by the rules of pain relief in inflammatory irritations: moderate intensity and therapeutic pressure in only one direction.

Tip

It can be quite strenuous for the therapist to apply this technique even for several minutes. An efficient technique should be used that does not require a great deal of strength. Therapists should not friction by moving the joints of the thumb. Instead, the unsupported arm should be positioned almost horizontally, and movement should be conducted using the wrist or the entire arm. An alternative hand position with a push from distal against the insertion, with movement in an anterior-posterior direction, is also possible.

3.5.6 Palpation in the Radial Tunnel

Although irritation of the radial nerve was already reported much earlier, it was Eversmann (1993) who described the notion of radial tunnel syndrome as compression of the radial nerve by the supinator muscle. The clinically relevant course of the radial nerve is limited by the supinator, extensor carpi radialis longus, and brevis muscles (Moradi et al., 2015) (▶ Fig. 3.45). At two different places in close proximity compression can often be exerted:
- At the level of the head of the radius; at the sharp-edged aponeurosis of the inferior extensor carpi radialis brevis muscle (Vergara-Amador and Ramírez, 2015).
- At the level of the neck of the radius; at the sharp-edged boundary of the superficial belly of the supinator muscle (arcade of Frohse; Moradi et al., 2015; Spinner, 1968) and the recurrent branches of the radial artery (leash of Henry, Ducic et al., 2012).

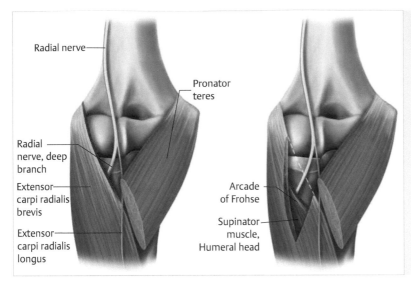

Fig. 3.45 Passages in the radial tunnel (after Omer Matthijs).

Radial nerve

Pronator teres

Radial nerve, deep branch

Extensor carpi radialis brevis

Extensor carpi radialis longus

Arcade of Frohse

Supinator muscle, Humeral head

Provocative Palpation of the Radial Nerve at the Level of the Head of the Radius

This palpation can be used to confirm the suspicion of a contusion of the radial nerve at the inferior extensor carpi radialis brevis muscle.

Starting Position

As suggested for palpation of the lateral side of the elbow, the shoulder is in moderate abduction and the elbow is flexed to 90°. Passive extension of the hand causes approximation of the hand extensors. Palpation is easier when the elbow joint is freely accessible. Each passage can be accessed in two positions of the forearm (pronation and supination). The results of provoked palpation of a passage are verified as negative only if the typical pain cannot be provoked in these two forearm positions. Otherwise, a pathological condition of the tendon of the extensor carpi radialis brevis muscle or of the humeroradial joint must be assumed.

Technique 1: Pronated Forearm Position

In this position, the radial nerve is sought between the tendon of the extensor carpi radialis brevis muscle and the muscle belly of the extensor carpi radialis longus muscle. The forearm is pronated and the hand is passively positioned in extension. The thumb, coming from the side and with the thumb joint strongly flexed, is positioned on the head of the radius so that the tip of the thumb presses against the bony ground. The thumb is guided along the head of the radius in an anterior direction until it presses against the muscle belly of the extensor carpi radialis longus. To confirm the location, the therapist has the patient isometrically contract the muscles in radial hand

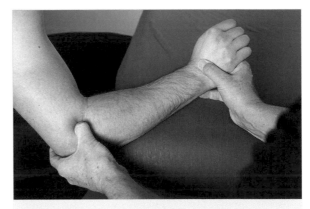

Fig. 3.46 Technique 1—in pronated forearm position.

extension and can thus palpate the edge of the muscle belly. Then pressure is applied sharply deep in the tissue and the patient is asked to describe the perceived sensation (▶ Fig. 3.46).

Technique 2: Supinated Forearm Position

In this position, the radial nerve is sought between muscle bellies of the extensor carpi radialis longus and brachioradialis muscles. The forearm is now supinated and the hand continues to be passively positioned in extension. Starting from the position used for palpation with technique 1, the thumb is guided over the belly of the extensor carpi radialis longus nearly without any pressure until the tip of the thumb feels the belly of the brachioradialis. With the patient isometrically contracting the muscles with the elbow flexed, the therapist confirms the correct location of edge of the muscle. Then pressure is applied sharply deep in the tissue and the patient is asked to describe the perceived sensation (not illustrated).

Provocative Palpation of the Radial Nerve at the Level of the Neck of the Radius

This palpation can be used to confirm the suspicion of a contusion of the radial nerve at the arcade of Frohse.

Starting Position

The position of the arm in flexion and of the hand in extension is the same as in the palpation of the head of the radius. Here too, each passage can be accessed in two positions of the forearm (pronation and supination). The results of provoked palpation of a passage are verified as negative only if the typical pain is not be provoked in these two forearm positions. Otherwise, a pathological condition of the transition between the muscle and tendon of the extensor carpi radialis brevis must be assumed.

Technique 1: Pronated Forearm Position

The palpation procedure, confirmation of the correct location between the extensor carpi radialis brevis muscle-tendon transition and the muscle belly of the extensor carpi radialis longus, provocation, and requesting the patient to describe the sensation are all the same as described above. The starting point for palpation is now the neck of the radius (not illustrated).

Technique 2: Supinated Forearm Position

Starting from the end position of technique 2 with the pronated forearm, the thumb is brought over the muscle belly of the extensor carpi radialis longus against the edge of the brachioradialis. Confirmation of the correct location between the extensor carpi radialis brevis muscle-tendon transition and the muscle belly of the extensor carpi radialis longus, provocation, and requesting the patient to describe the sensation are all the same as described above (▶ Fig. 3.47).

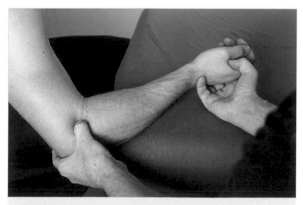

Fig. 3.47 Technique 2—in supinated forearm position.

3.6 General Orientation—Posterior Humerus

3.6.1 Summary of the Palpatory Process

Therapists orient themselves on the posterior aspect of the elbow joint to:
- palpate warmth and swelling;
- determine the relationship between the three bony elevations.

Starting Position

Although a special SP is not necessary, the posterior aspect of the elbow should be accessible. This is possible in a variety of arm positions, for example, with shoulder flexion or extension.

3.6.2 Palpating Warmth and Swelling

The posterior side of the elbow is the only area that is covered by very little soft tissue. It is easy for the therapist to recognize and palpate swelling of the capsule or the olecranon bursa. The presence of warmth in the inner joint space can only be ascertained on this side of the elbow.

Technique

Temperature is assessed using the back of the hand. The fingertips search for swelling. Capsular swelling is seen immediately medial or lateral to the olecranon. The therapist places the finger pads directly over the capsule and palpates using a gentle, slow technique (▶ Fig. 3.48).

A swollen bursa can be easily recognized with the naked eye. The fluid moves back and forth in the bursa when the fingers palpate the bursa directly (▶ Fig. 3.49).

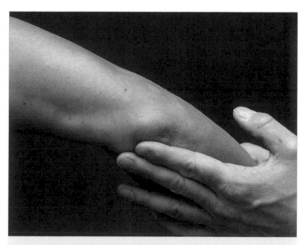

Fig. 3.48 Palpation of the elbow joint capsule.

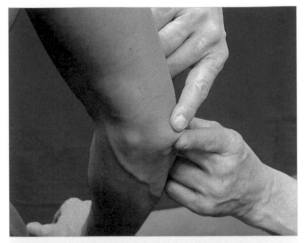

Fig. 3.49 Olecranon bursa—palpation technique.

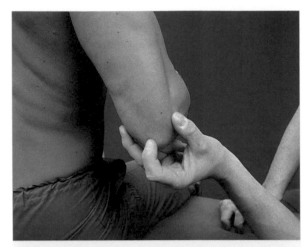

Fig. 3.50 Palpation of bony reference points.

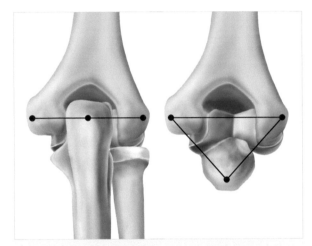

Fig. 3.51 Position of reference points during extension and flexion.

The Relationship between the Three Bony Elevations

The relationship between the palpable sections of bone in different joint positions will be described here. The clinical reference points consist of the tip of the olecranon and the two epicondyles of the humerus.

These landmarks should form an equilateral triangle when the elbow is flexed to 90° and form a line when the elbow is extended (▶ Fig. 3.50 and ▶ Fig. 3.51).

The relationship between these three points provides the therapist with a general overview of the position of these sections of bone. It is important to know whether the position of these bony landmarks is physiological when treating patients following trauma. If the therapist recognizes deviations from the norm, radiological clarification is recommended before mobilizing.

Bibliography

Andreisek G, Crook DW, Burg D, Marincek B, Weishaupt D. Peripheral neuropathies of the median, radial, and ulnar nerves: MR imaging features. Radiographics. 2006; 26(5):1267–1287

Beekman R, Schreuder AH, Rozeman CA, Koehler PJ, Uitdehaag BM. The diagnostic value of provocative clinical tests in ulnar neuropathy at the elbow is marginal. J Neurol Neurosurg Psychiatry. 2009; 80(12):1369–1374

Ducic I, Felder JM, III, Quadri HS. Common nerve decompressions of the upper extremity: reliable exposure using shorter incisions. Ann Plast Surg. 2012; 68(6):606–609

Eckstein F, Löhe F, Hillebrand S, et al. Morphomechanics of the humeroulnar joint: I. Joint space width and contact areas as a function of load and flexion angle. Anat Rec. 1995; 243(3):318–326

Eversmann WW. Entrapment and compression neuropathies. In: Green DP, Hotchkiss RN, eds. Operative Hand Surgery. 3rd ed. New York: Churchill Livingstone; 1993:1341–1385

Grana W. Medial epicondylitis and cubital tunnel syndrome in the throwing athlete. Clin Sports Med. 2001; 20(3):541–548

Gregoli B, Bortolotto C, Draghi F. Elbow nerves: normal sonographic anatomy and identification of the structures potentially associated with nerve compression. A short pictorial-video article. J Ultrasound. 2013; 16 (3):119–121

Kuhn S, Burkhart KJ, Schneider J, et al. The anatomy of the proximal radius: implications on fracture implant design. J Shoulder Elbow Surg. 2012; 21 (9):1247–1254

Lieber RL, Ljung BO, Fridén J. Sarcomere length in wrist extensor muscles. Changes may provide insights into the etiology of chronic lateral epicondylitis. Acta OrthopScand. 1997; 68(3):249–254

Ljung BO, Fridén J, Lieber RL. Sarcomere length varies with wrist ulnar deviation but not forearm pronation in the extensor carpi radialis brevis muscle. J Biomech. 1999; 32(2):199–202

Matthijs O, van Paridon-Edauw D, Winkel D. Manuelle Therapie der peripheren Gelenke. Bd. 2: Ellenbogen, Hand. München: Urban & Fischer bei Elsevier; 2003

Milz S, Eckstein F, Putz R. Thickness distribution of the subchondral mineralization zone of the trochlear notch and its correlation with the cartilage thickness: an expression of functional adaptation to mechanical stress acting on the humeroulnar joint? Anat Rec. 1997; 248(2):189–197

Moradi A, Ebrahimzadeh MH, Jupiter JB. Radial tunnel syndrome, diagnostic and treatment dilemma. Arch Bone Jt Surg. 2015; 3(3):156–162

O'Driscoll SW, Bell DF, Morrey BF. Posterolateral rotatory instability of the elbow. J Bone Joint Surg Am. 1991a; 73(3):440–446

O'Driscoll SW, Horii E, Carmichael SW, Morrey BF. The cubital tunnel and ulnar neuropathy. J Bone Joint Surg Br. 1991b; 73(4):613–617

Polatsch DB, Melone CP, Jr, Beldner S, Incorvaia A. Ulnar nerve anatomy. Hand Clin. 2007; 23(3):283–289

Robertson C, Saratsiotis J. A review of compressive ulnar neuropathy at the elbow. J Manipulative Physiol Ther. 2005; 28(5):345

Robinson PM, Loosemore M, Watts AC. Boxer's elbow: internal impingement of the coronoid and olecranon process. A report of seven cases. J Shoulder Elbow Surg. 2017; 26(3):376–381

Spinner M. The arcade of Frohse and its relationship to posterior interosseous nerve paralysis. J Bone Joint Surg Br. 1968; 50(4):809–812

Vergara-Amador E, Ramírez A. Anatomic study of the extensor carpi radialis brevis in its relation with the motor branch of the radial nerve. Orthop-Traumatol Surg Res. 2015; 101(8):909–912

Winkel D. Nichtoperative Orthopädie und Manualtherapie. Anatomie in vivo. 3. Aufl. München: Urban & Fischer bei Elsevier; 2004

Zoner CS, Buck FM, Cardoso FN, et al. Detailed MRI-anatomic study of the lateral epicondyle of the elbow and its tendinous and ligamentous attachments in cadavers. AJR Am J Roentgenol. 2010; 195(3):629–636

3

Chapter 4

Hand

4 Hand

4.1 Significance and Function of the Hand

The **osseous construction** of the hand and foot developed in the same manner during a long period of evolution. Even today, many similarities can be discovered between these two sections of the skeleton. It is well known that the acquisition of upright stance and bipedal locomotion differentiates the skeleton of the upper limb fully from the skeleton of the lower limb.

Hand function can be divided into three main areas: prehension, touch, and gesture/communication.

As the end organ of the upper limb, the hand is a well-developed working instrument with a **large variety of very fine functions.** Kapandji (2006) described the different types of grasp. These include power grips and precision handling, with pinching (bi-digital grasping using the thumb and index finger) being the most important function.

The precision with which the visually impaired are able to recognize different surfaces, materials, and consistencies is always impressive. The high density of mechanoreceptors in the skin of the hand and particularly of the fingertips provides humans with the extraordinary ability to perceive differences in the smallest of areas (ability to discriminate). The large sensory supply of the hand is mirrored in the hand's representation in the sensory cortex.

The hand naturally plays an important role in nonverbal communication, the interaction between gestures, mimic, and body posture. Everyone is familiar with typical, common, and international gestures and positions of the hand, such as connecting the thumb and the index finger into a circle (forming an "O") and holding the other fingers straight or relaxed in the air to indicate that everything is okay.

4.1.1 Causes of the Diversity of Functions in the Hand

A large number of joints in the wrist and the fingers, with some of these joints being very mobile. The amazing interaction between the bones of the wrist (carpal bones) is based on the three-dimensional movements seen in every bone during forward and backward movements of the palm (flexion and extension of the wrist) and sideways movements (ulnar and radial deviation of the wrist). With two joint lines (radio- and mediocarpal) in the hand, the carpus gives the hand the amazing mobility of a range of motion up to 180° for flexion and extension.

- **Opposition of the thumb and the finger.** The ability of the thumb bones to turn toward the other fingers (opposition) is shared by many primates. The particular spatial orientation of the trapezium in relation to the other bones of the carpus is the chief factor in this ability. Thus, at rest, the relaxed thumb hangs approximately 35° in a palmar direction, 15° in a radial direction (Zancolli et al.,1987). These two characteristics, combined with the special muscles acting on the thumb, enable opposition. Not only the thumb, but also the fingers are able to oppose. This becomes clear when therapists view the palmar aspect of the extended hand and flex each finger individually. In flexion, every fingertip points to the carpometacarpal joint.
  - Finger opposition can also be identified when the thumb touches the small finger. The finger pads of the thumb and fifth finger come into contact, not the sides of the fingers. Metacarpal V also has its own opponens muscle (▸ Fig. 4.1).
- A stable bony center as the foundation for grasp.
  - Mobility, expression, and functional diversity are impossible without a stable base. The different types of grasp and the development of strength are almost impossible without a central fixed point within the hand.
  - This stable center is located in the transition between the carpus (here the distal row of carpal bones) and the bases of metacarpals II to V (carpometacarpal joint line). This area is identified by the rigidity of the articular connections. All anatomical parameters, such as the jagged joint line, articular surfaces of complex structure, and a dense supply of ligaments, indicate stability, not mobility.
  - This carpal and the metacarpal junction also form a bony transverse arch that is comparable to the

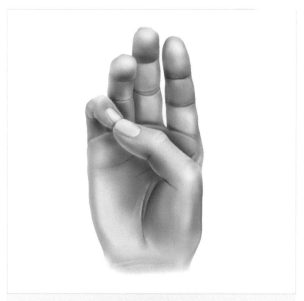

Fig. 4.1 Opposition of the thumb and the fifth finger.

transverse arch of the foot in its position, significance, and the point of its evolutionary development. It is the osseous foundation for the carpal tunnel (carpal groove).

- Pliancy of the palm.
  ○ The proximal ends of the metacarpals articulate firmly with each other and with the carpus. Distally, connected by syndesmoses, they move very freely against each other. The palm can therefore flatten itself out—important for power grips—as well as cupping the hand—which is of importance for precision handling using the fingers.
  ○ Moreover, the palm does not possess interfering muscle mass, in contrast to the short muscles in the sole of the foot.
  ○ Finally, the reinforced fascia of the hand (palmar aponeurosis) can be tightened by muscles designed especially for this purpose (palmaris longus).
- Selective muscular control.
  ○ The extraordinary presence of the hand in the primary motor center of the precentral gyrus (Williams, 2009) as well as the developmentally most recent tracts of the voluntary motor system, constitute the motor basis of the functional diversity. Just the functionally vital pincer grip requires finely tuned coordination based on small motor units (▶ Fig. 4.2).

4.1.2 Common Applications for Treatment in this Region

Hand symptoms constituting a therapeutic challenge are numerous and include almost the entire palette of postoperative, traumatic, and nontraumatic symptoms of the extremities.

The special feature of this section of the skeleton is the close proximity of clinically relevant structures in a tight area. The therapist searches for the source of most symptoms either in the carpus or its close proximity. Nontraumatic problems are rarely observed toward the

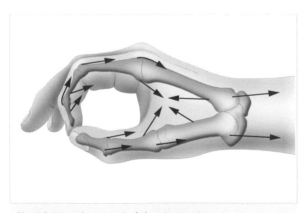

Fig. 4.2 Muscular control of the pincer grip.

forearm or the fingers. Therefore, the carpus region and the anatomical structures surrounding the carpus take up the largest proportion of the precise palpation of the hand.

Common Pathological Conditions in the Hand

- **Arthritis,** mainly caused by rheumatic disease or trauma. Joint inflammation is not only seen in the wrist area; it can also be observed in the distal radioulnar joint (DRUJ) and the first carpometacarpal joint, which must be kept in mind in differential diagnosis of radial or ulnar symptoms.
- **Restrictions in mobility,** mostly as a result of immobilization, for example, following fractures near the joint (Colles fracture). When presented with a hand with restricted mobility, the crucial issue for the therapist is to locate the point of restriction. Should the therapist start treating the radiocarpal joint, or should the local carpal bones be assessed first?
- **Instability in the hand region is a common cause of symptoms.** They can be present at various points:
  ○ Globally at the carpal joint lines: mid-carpal instability is located at the mediocarpal joint between the two rows of carpal bones (Lichtman, 2006). Palmar dislocations of the radiocarpal joint are typically encountered with rheumatoid arthritis.
  ○ Local, within the carpus: here, attention is on the lunate. It is held in position with intrinsic ligaments within the proximal row of scaphoid and triquetrum. If one of these ligaments ruptures as a result of a trauma, the lunate most often dislocates with a translational component in a palmar direction.
  ○ Further instabilities can be observed at the DRUJ and the carpometacarpal joint.
- Soft-tissue conditions.
  ○ The passage of tendons through compartments and the carpal tunnel, for example, and also the fixed points of the long muscles in the wrist provide sufficient opportunity for the development of overuse problems. The entire spectrum of possible pathological conditions can be observed here: tenosynovitis, myotenosynovitis, and insertion tendinopathy. On the dorsal side, the tendons travel in tendon compartments. On the palmar aspect, nine tendons and one nerve are bundled together in the carpal tunnel. Symptoms in this region can often be improved with precisely applied treatments.
  ○ The ulnar disk is the most important component of the triangular fibrocartilage (TFC) complex. Inflammation and trauma of the ulnar disk are common causes of local ulnar pain (Pang and Yao, 2017).
- **Nerve compression.** As in the elbow, all three large peripheral nerves can be compressed here too, in their tunnel at the wrist or in the immediate vicinity.

The median nerve can be compromised in the carpal tunnel. A variety of provocative tests for carpal tunnel syndrome are based on the careful location of the point of constriction. Cyclists occasionally compress the ulnar nerve in the Guyon canal ("handlebar palsy"). The radial nerve can be compressed as it passes through the fascia of the forearm into the superficial tissue.

- The therapist's challenge is to identify the causative laxity and thus the reason for the symptoms, using understanding of the local biomechanics and precision in locating the articulating bones. The necessary foundation for this task is knowledge of local surface anatomy based on good topographic and morphological knowledge.

It is an advantage of surface anatomy on the hand that patients are usually able to describe their symptoms exactly. With the exception of neural irritation, referred pain is not expected so far distally in the limb. In regard to diagnosis, this means that besides the assessment of function, the pain reported is of great importance to identify the affected structure.

4.1.3 Required Basic Anatomical and Biomechanical Knowledge

Students require a certain amount of important background information to understand the instructions for local palpation:

- The construction of the skeleton of the hand and fingers and, in particular, the name and position of the carpal bones and the longitudinal divisions of the hand.

- The names and positions of the tendons that cross over the wrist.
- The position and dimensions of the retinacula that keep the long tendons in the extensor compartments and the carpal tunnel.
- The position and construction of narrow passages for peripheral nerves in the hand, in particular the carpal tunnel.

4.1.4 Axial Divisions of the Skeleton of the Hand into Columns and Their Clinical Significance

There have been exact anatomical representations of the hand since Da Vinci and Vesalius. Since that time, there has been no change in the choice of the simpler, more transparent dorsal view for a description of the anatomy (Berger, 2010). In addition to the familiar horizontal anatomical divisions of the hand into the carpus, metacarpus, and phalanges (► Fig. 4.3), the skeleton of the hand can also be divided in an axial direction (► Fig. 4.4). The so-called columnar design was already described by Navarro in 1937 (Matthijs et al., 2003).

This classification is the result of experience when addressing clinical aspects. Each column consists of one or two "rays" (metacarpals plus phalanges) and the corresponding longitudinally positioned carpal bones:

- **Radial column**: this column comprises the first and second rays as well as the trapezium and scaphoid (distal pole). Experience shows that arthrotic changes are most frequently detected here. The scaphoid articulates with four neighboring carpal bones and the radius so that it controls the biomechanics of both capitate and

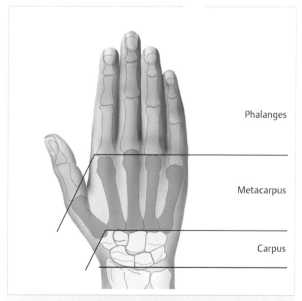

Fig. 4.3 Horizontal divisions of the skeleton of the hand.

Phalanges

Metacarpus

Carpus

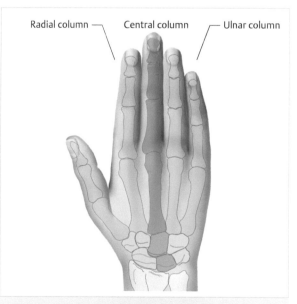

Radial column — Central column — Ulnar column

Fig. 4.4 Axial divisions of the skeleton of the hand (ray concept).

lunate. Hypomobility and fractures, particularly of the scaphoid, are encountered most frequently in the radial column. Within this column, the thumb column can be considered separately since the skeleton of the thumb is set apart from the rest of the carpus by the special orientation of the trapezium. This would then include the first ray, trapezium, and scaphoid (▶ Fig. 4.5).

- **Central column:** the principal ray of the hand (metacarpal III and middle finger) plus the capitate, scaphoid (proximal pole), and lunate form the central column. In addition to the location of hypomobilities, the clinical particularity of this column is the frequent occurrence of local instabilities, especially of the lunate, with possible dislocations fixed in a nonphysiological position and under stress. Finally, dislocation is promoted by the sagittal angling of the distal radius (volar tilt) and the arrangement of the deep palmar ligaments (▶ Fig. 4.6). Local mobility tests of the articular connections of the lunate to the neighboring articulation partners test the local stability if it is possible to determine precisely the location of the individual carpal bones.
- **Ulnar column:** the connections between the fourth and fifth rays, hamate, and triquetrum opposite the articular disk of the DRUJ are known to be hypermobile and can cause symptoms. The stability of the ulnar column depends to a large degree on the intact condition of the TFC complex.

4.1.5 The Carpus

The arrangement of eight carpal bones in two rows provides the basis for the anatomical structure of the carpus. In this arrangement in rows, the proximal row of carpal bones has a particular importance. With the exception of the flexor carpi ulnaris, no extrinsic muscle is directly attached to this row. The pisiform is indeed classified as a carpal bone, but biomechanically it is not part of the proximal row.

This independence from muscular influence marks the function of the proximal row as an intercalated segment that mediates between two rigid entities (distal forearm and distal carpal row of the metacarpals). The proximal row is able to perform this function through large, passive accompanying movements during planar movement (extension and flexion) and marginal movement (ulnar and radial abduction). The planar and marginal movements of the hand are assigned to two articular rows: radiocarpal and mediocarpal joints, where each carpal bone has its own degree of motion (De Lange et al., 1985). The mobility of the marginal movements depends on the position of the forearm. At complete supination, the forearm is pulled distally by contraction of certain fibers of the interosseous membrane of the forearm, and the degree of radial abduction is less than in full pronation. Scaphoid and lunate articulate with the corresponding articular groove at the radius (scaphoid fossa and lunate fossa), the triquetrum with the articular disk of the ulna. The radius has a total of two angles in relation to its longitudinal axis: an ulnar and a palmar tilt (see ▶ Fig. 4.18).

The distal row articulates with the proximal row in the mediocarpal joint; both rows have a generally convex form. It is only radially that the curvature between the scaphoid and the two trapezoid bones turns around. This makes it possible for the trapezoid and the trapezium to glide onto the scaphoid in extension (with radial abduction), which, in end-range motion, brings them into the direct vicinity of the distal radius. The mediocarpal joint is a hinge joint that permits radial extension and ulnar flexion around an oblique axis, known in the literature as a dart-throwing motion (Moritomo et al., 2007).

4.1.6 Kinematic and Kinetic Model of the Hand

The carpus is responsible for ensuring that the hand is optimally positioned in space for its various tasks. To achieve this, a high degree of mobility must be reached while ensuring stability (Ryu and Klin, 2010).

In terms of kinematics, the biomechanical model of the carpus consists of two rigid parts moving toward each other with an intercalated segment:

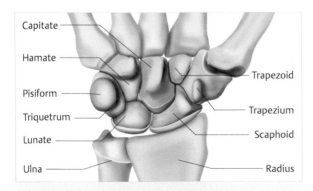

Fig. 4.5 Topography of the carpus—palmar view.

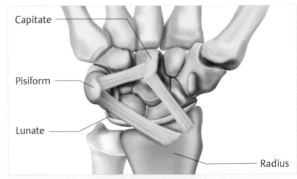

Fig. 4.6 Deep extrinsic palmar ligaments.

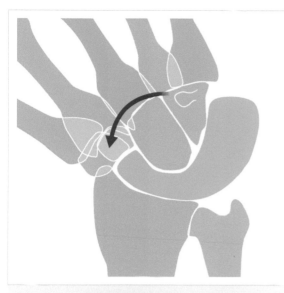

Fig. 4.7 Compensatory accompanying movements of the proximal row during radial abduction.

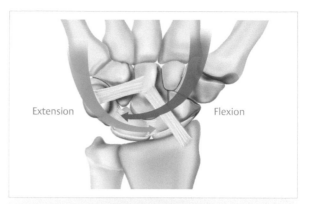

Fig. 4.8 Kinetic model of the hand during grasping movements.

- The rigid parts are the proximal radius and the metacarpal bones including the distal carpal row.
- The proximal carpal row is the intercalated segment, which in every position represents a stable socket toward distal and a head toward proximal. The proximal carpal row achieves this with compensatory movements between the individual members of this row (▶ Fig. 4.7).

Ryu refers to this as the "four-unit concept": distal carpal row plus the scaphoid, lunate, and triquetrum bones (Ryu and Klin, 2010).

The task of this model is to ensure a high degree of mobility under compressive forces in every position at the same time. The stability of the hand is ensured by the bony and, in particular, capsuloligamentous structures. With the exception of the flexor carpi ulnaris muscle, the carpus is completely traversed by the tendons of the extrinsic muscles. These tendons insert at the bases of the metacarpals and the finger skeleton.

In terms of kinematics, the greatest challenge involves ensuring the stability of the carpus while actively grasping objects. The maximum grasping force comes about when the hand is held in slight extension. This means that at the moment of grasping, the hand extensors, hand flexors, finger flexors, and thumb flexor are active and thus exert compression force on the carpus. In the middle position of the hand, of the total compression force transferred to the forearm, around 50% is transferred via the radial column, 30% via the central column, and 20% via the ulnar column (Hara et al., 1992).

At the moment of grasping, during the activity of the two radial hand extensors, the mediocarpal joint is in

slight radial extension. This results in two mechanisms (▶ Fig. 4.8):

- The compressive force on the radial side presses the distal pole of the scaphoid palmarly in the direction of flexion (Kobayashi et al., 1997). This flexion tendency transfers it over an intrinsic ligament (scapolunate ligament) to the lunate.
- The radial extension stretches a part of the deep extrinsic ligaments, that is, the arcuate or triquetral capitate ligament, in a palmar direction. This exerts an extensory force on the triquetrum that transfers this extension tendency to the lunate via an additional intrinsic ligament (triquetral lunate ligament).

Hence, the lunate takes on a flexion tendency from radial and an extension tendency from ulnar, and if the intrinsic ligaments are intact, it remains neutral for flexion and extension.

Different types of trauma to the ligament and carpal instabilities of the hand sustained during a fall on the hand can be explained by this model.

4.1.7 Triangular Fibrocartilage Complex (TFC)

The stability of the ulnar carpus and the distal radioulnar joint is controlled by the TFC complex (▶ Fig. 4.9).

Functions

- Stabilizes the carpus on the ulna and radius.
- Load bearing.
- Stabilizes the DRUJ.

Main Components

The main components are the articular disk of the DRUJ, the ulnar collateral ligament of the wrist joint, the deep ulnocarpal ligaments, and the synovial sheath of the extensor carpi ulnaris tendon. The disk extends between

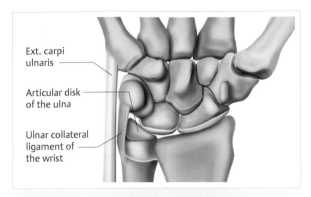

Fig. 4.9 Components of the TFC complex.

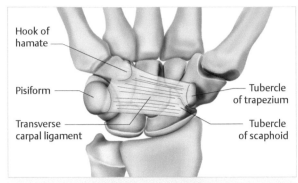

Fig. 4.10 Boundaries of the carpal tunnel.

the ulnar styloid process and the border of the radial articular surface for the DRUJ and is supported by ligaments.

The margins of the TFC complex have a vascular and nociceptive supply. Thus it can be the direct source of pain, a frequent cause for ulnar symptoms of the wrist.

4.1.8 Construction of the Carpal Tunnel

The two rows of carpal bones form a transverse arch, the carpal tunnel. The term "row" is actually quite confusing. The construction of the carpal arch becomes clear when the therapist examines the parts of bone that protrude palmarly (▶ Fig. 4.10):

- Radial: scaphoid tubercle and trapezium.
- Ulnar: pisiform and the hook of hamate.
- On the floor of the groove lie the lunate and capitate bones. The transverse carpal ligament encloses this carpal arch, forming the carpal tunnel.
- Schmidt and Lanz (2003) give the diameter of the tunnel as between 8 and 12 mm.

The following structures pass through the carpal tunnel:
- The four tendons of the flexor digitorum profundus (▶ Fig. 4.11).
- The four tendons of the flexor digitorum superficialis (▶ Fig. 4.12).
- The tendon of the flexor pollicis longus (▶ Fig. 4.13).
- Median nerve (▶ Fig. 4.13 and ▶ Fig. 4.14).

In the past, the flexor carpi radialis tendon was considered part of the carpal tunnel. Its course underneath the ligament is listed as a separate passage in topographical anatomy (Beckenbaugh in Cooney, 2010).

4.1.9 Extensor Tendons and their Compartments

The tendons of the long (extrinsic) muscles that move the hand and finger skeletons are held close to the radius and ulna in their palmar and dorsal aspects and at the sides of

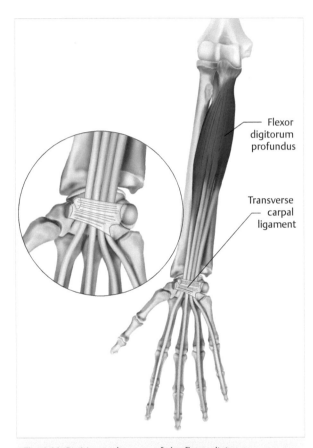

Fig. 4.11 Position and course of the flexor digitorum profundus.

the forearm by a deep thickening of the forearm fascia (flexor and extensor retinacula).

The retinacula maintain the position of all the tendons in relation to the forearm, even during large rotatory movements of the hand or the forearm. The extensor retinaculum extends between the radius and the tendon sheath of the flexor carpi ulnaris and is attached to the bones between the respective tendon compartments, so that small osteofibrous canals are formed for the passage

4

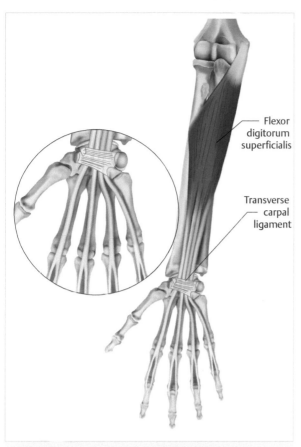

Fig. 4.12 Position and course of the flexor digitorum superficialis.

- Flexor digitorum superficialis
- Transverse carpal ligament

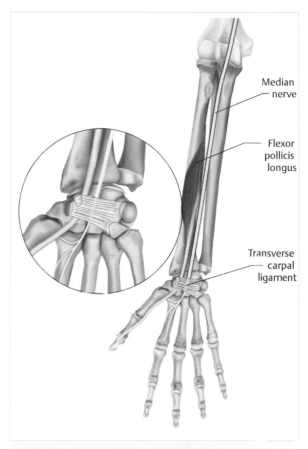

Fig. 4.13 Position and course of the flexor pollicis longus.

- Median nerve
- Flexor pollicis longus
- Transverse carpal ligament

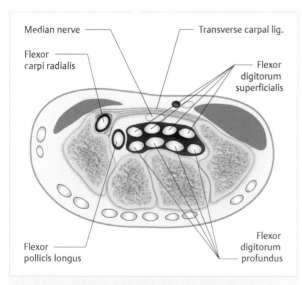

Fig. 4.14 Cross-section through the carpal tunnel.

- Median nerve
- Transverse carpal lig.
- Flexor carpi radialis
- Flexor digitorum superficialis
- Flexor pollicis longus
- Flexor digitorum profundus

of the tendons (▶ Fig. 4.16). Tendon sheaths protect the tendons at this point from frictioning during movement.

The six canals through which the tendons pass are named tendon compartments (▶ Fig. 4.15).

Tendon Compartments from Radial to Ulnar

- First compartment: abductor pollicis longus (APL) and extensor pollicis brevis (EPB).
- Second compartment: extensor carpi radialis longus (ECRL) and extensor carpi radialis brevis (ECRB).
- Third compartment: extensor pollicis longus (EPL).
- Fourth compartment: extensor digitorum (ED) and extensor indicis (EI).
- Fifth compartment: extensor digiti minimi (EDM).
- Sixth compartment: extensor carpi ulnaris (ECU).

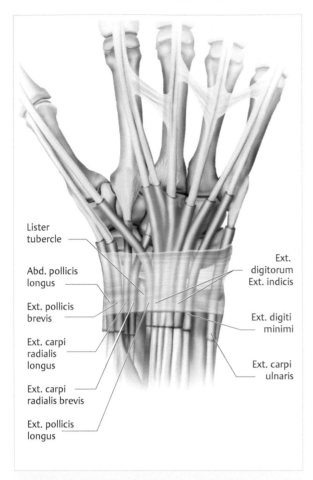

Lister tubercle

Abd. pollicis longus

Ext. pollicis brevis

Ext. carpi radialis longus

Ext. carpi radialis brevis

Ext. pollicis longus

Ext. digitorum
Ext. indicis

Ext. digiti minimi

Ext. carpi ulnaris

Fig. 4.15 Compartments for the wrist and finger extensor tendons.

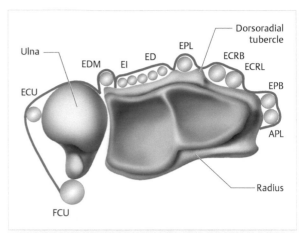

Fig. 4.16 Extensor tendons and retinaculum extensorum—distal view after Omer Matthijs). FCU: flexor carpi ulnaris. ECU: extensor carpi ulnaris. EDM: extensor digiti minimi. EI: extensor indicis. ED: extensor digitorum. EPL: extensor pollicis longus. ECRB: extensor carpi radialis brevis. ECRL: extensor carpi radialis longus. EPB: extensor pollicis brevis. APL: abductor pollicis longus.

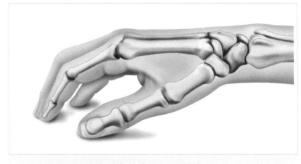

Fig. 4.17 Topography of the bones—radial view.

4.2 General Orientation—Dorsal

4.2.1 Summary of the Palpatory Process

The following instructions for finding the structures of the hand start on the dorsal aspect. The therapist first gains a general impression of the dimensions of the carpus and its proximal and distal boundaries so that precise information can be obtained on the size of the carpus and metacarpus. The therapist looks for distinct bony edges and points. This lays the groundwork for very local display of the extensor tendons in their tendon sheaths as well as of the individual carpal bones.

Starting Position

For the hand to be palpated, a relaxed position is selected that can be maintained without muscle activity. When palpating osseous structures, it is essential that all types of muscular contraction be avoided by placing the hand

and forearm on a level surface (▶ Fig. 4.17). If this is not done, the more superficially located tendons will be placed under tension and impede the specific search for deeper-lying structures. The therapist sits next to the ulnar side of the hand.

Tip

Directions will be described using the terms radial (toward the thumb), ulnar (toward the small finger), dorsal (toward the back of the hand), and palmar (toward the palm). This may take a while to get used to, but it enables the use of exact terminology and therefore understanding. For example, the joint space of the DRUJ is found radial to the head of the ulna.

4.2.2 Palpation of Individual Structures

Proximal Boundary of the Carpus (Radiocarpal Joint Line)

The boundary between the proximal row of carpal bones and the forearm marks the joint space for the radiocarpal joint. In particular, the joint line orients itself on the edges of the radius and ulna.

Technique

The palpating finger moves first from distal, so that the fingertip can meet the radius and the head of the ulna (transverse palpation, ▶ Fig. 4.18). It is most effective to start on the radial side of the hand in a depression at the carpus (radial fossa), which will be described in more detail below.

Transverse palpation at this point encounters a distinct, hard resistance when it reaches the edge of the radius. Moving a little more toward the palm, one can find the radial styloid process, the radial and right palmar boundary of the radius (▶ Fig. 4.19 and ▶ Fig. 4.20). Above the radial styloid are the tendons of extensor compartment I

and the V-shaped radial collateral ligament runs to the radial carpus (scaphoid and trapezium) from its tip.

The same technique is used to locate the boundaries of the carpus by palpating from radial to ulnar. The rounded tendons passing through their compartments in the wrist increasingly interfere with the palpation more ulnarly (▶ Fig. 4.21). When the palpating finger moves proximally from the second and third ray it feels, exactly when it reaches the radius at the level of the ulnar head, the drop-shaped dorsal tubercle of the radius, also known as the Lister tubercle (▶ Fig. 4.22). Directly distal to this is the edge of the radius. Further in the ulnar direction is the transition between radius and ulna. The level of the distal radioulnar articular space has been reached when the rather straight edge of the radius takes on a convex shape and the transition can be felt, on palpation, to be a small, V-shaped depression (▶ Fig. 4.23). The palpation ends distal to the ulnar head and the ulnar styloid process, located to the side (ulnar and dorsal) at the ulnar head (▶ Fig. 4.24).

4

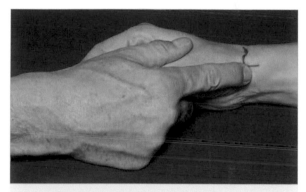

Fig. 4.19 Palpation of the radial styloid process.

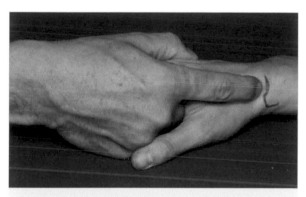

Fig. 4.18 Palpation of the radius from a distal position.

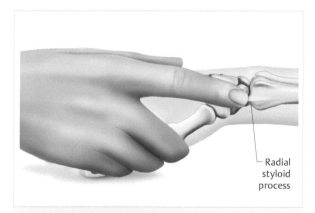

Radial styloid process

Fig. 4.20 Illustration of the palpation technique.

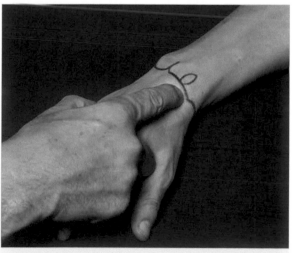

Fig. 4.21 Distal radial radius.

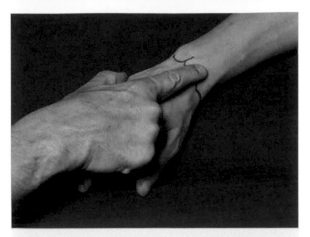

Fig. 4.22 Palpation of the dorsal tubercle of the radius.

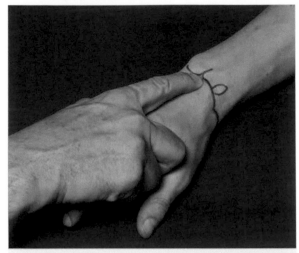

Fig. 4.23 Palpation of the distal radioulnar joint (DRUJ).

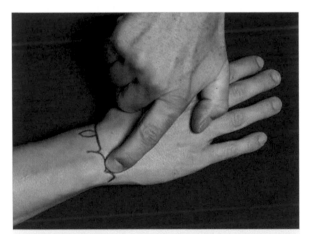

Fig. 4.24 Palpation of the distal head of the ulna and the ulnar styloid process.

Tip

If tendons hinder the palpation of the edge of the radius, the wrist is extended slightly and the hand relaxed. This causes the proximal row of bones to disappear in a palmar direction and relaxes the soft-tissue structures. The position of the extensor digiti minimi tendon at the level of the ulnar head confirms the position of the DRUJ space.

Alignment of the Radiocarpal Joint Space

For rapid location of the proximal boundary corresponding to the joint space of the radiocarpal joint, another structure must be found. Connecting the styloid process of the radius, the distal aspect of the dorsal radial tubercle, with the ulnar styloid process, easily yields a line that exactly reproduces the course and orientation of the radiocarpal joint space.

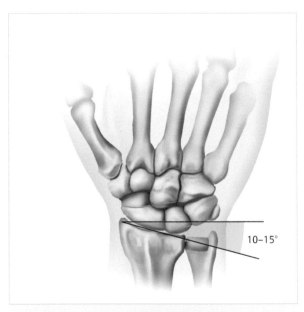

10–15°

Fig. 4.25 Alignment of the radiocarpal joint space.

It becomes clear that the orientation of the joint space is not exactly perpendicular to the forearm. In fact, seen from radial to ulnar, it runs obliquely proximal (▶ Fig. 4.25). Different angles are given in the literature. Taleisnik (1984) described the average value of this angle as 22° (12–30°), where the left–right differences, at an average of 1.5°, are very small (Hollevoet, 2000). Not depicted here, the joint surface of the distal radius in the sagittal plane, seen from the side, decreases from dorsal–distal to palmar–proximal. This palmar tilt measures an average of 11 to 15° (Taleisnik, 1984; Zanetti et al., 2001) and varies intraindividually by an average of 2.5° (Hollevoet, 2000). In addition, Zanetti reports changes in palmar tilt depending on the position of the forearm. In complete supination it is 29° but in complete pronation it is only 13°. This area is so precisely examined because there are so many global mobilization techniques available in manual therapy used to mobilize the whole hand at the radiocarpal joint. In using them, the therapist should have a spatial understanding of how the joint surfaces bend and vary.

Distal Boundary of the Carpus (Carpometacarpal Joint Line)

The distal boundary of the carpus is significantly more difficult to feel than the proximal boundary. The starting position is the same. The fingertips of the palpating hand still point in a proximal direction. First the joint line between the base of metacarpal III and the capitate or between metacarpal IV and the hamate is located. This can only be done centrally here, since further toward the radius, the joint line cannot be directly reached due to the protuberances on metacarpals II and III.

Technique

The palpating finger pad moves in a proximal direction directly on the shaft of the third or between the third and fourth metacarpals until it feels the base as an elevation (▶ Fig. 4.26). On top of this elevation is the very narrow joint space that is being sought. For this reason, the fingers must now be raised to their tips in order to feel the joint space as a narrow gap, very locally and with some pressure (▶ Fig. 4.27). This technique can be used for the joint space between metacarpal III and the capitate and for the joint space between metacarpal IV and hamate.

Tip

In our own experience, palpation is easier when it is initiated at metacarpal IV. The joint space felt there is somewhat wider and changes its size from radial to ulnar abduction.

At approximately the same level is the joint space between metacarpal V and the hamate. The base of metacarpal V offers another very helpful anatomical feature: a tuberosity for the insertion of the extensor carpi ulnaris (see ▶ Fig. 4.36). This can be easily felt perpendicularly from proximal.

The joint space to the radial, at metacarpal II, can be felt with the same technique. As already described, the ulnar aspect of metacarpal II and radial side of metacarpal III converge into a protuberance projecting proximally, a sort of styloid process. The extensor carpi radialis brevis inserts at this point (Rauber and Kopsch, 2003).

If the carpometacarpal joint line is drawn, this, together with the radiocarpal joint line, indicates the entire extent of the carpalia (▶ Fig. 4.28). The space between the two joint lines amounts to approximately two of the patient's finger widths. This is the basis for locating the individual bones of the carpus on the dorsal aspect of the hand.

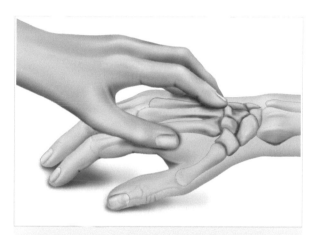

Fig. 4.26 Searching for the carpometacarpal joint line.

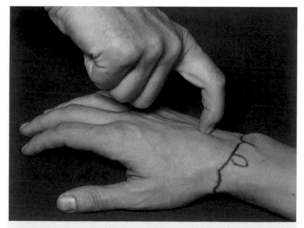

Fig. 4.27 Carpometacarpal technique.

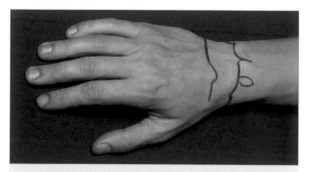

Fig. 4.28 Proximal and distal boundaries of the carpus.

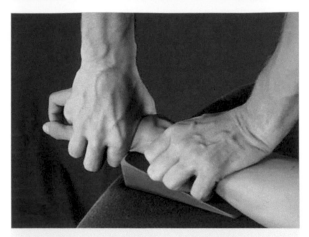

Fig. 4.29 Translational technique—carpus to palmar.

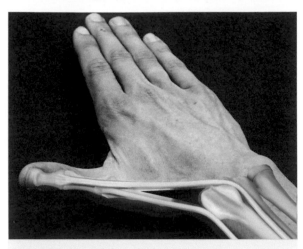

Fig. 4.30 Position of the radial fossa.

Tip

If it is difficult to find the joint space at the level of metacarpals III and IV with very sharp fingertip palpation, it can be more easily found if the patient moves the hand in radial abduction. No other kind of movement of this not very moveable joint line is helpful for confirmation.

4.2.3 Tips for Assessment and Treatment

Once found, the joint line of the radiocarpal joint is the definitive orientation point for several manual therapy techniques. The angle of the radioulnar joint line as well as of the dorsopalmar joint line (palmar tilt) must therefore be found and observed. The illustrated example (▶ Fig. 4.29) demonstrates a translational technique at the radiocarpal joint that is used for assessment and treatment. Here, the proximal row of the carpus is pushed toward the radius in a palmar direction. In this case, the therapist tries to compensate for the palmar tilt using a support under the forearm so that an almost perpendicular push on the distal hand, in a palmar direction, can succeed.

Evidently, the position of the forearm on the supportive surface and the handling itself require correct knowledge of the position and alignment of the joint space and the articular bones.

4.3 Local Palpation of the Dorsal Soft Tissues

4.3.1 Summary of the Palpatory Process

After the dimensions of the carpus and its boundaries have become clear, the soft tissue (tendons, vessels, and nerves) is at the mid-point of the local orientation on the dorsal surface of the hand. The palpation again begins radially, finishes ulnarly, and reveals the exact position of the extensor tendons.

Starting Position

The patient's hand and forearm are relaxed and rest on a supportive surface, which is as level as possible. The therapist generally sits to the side. The palm of the hand should face downward, enabling the dorsal and ulnar aspect of the wrist to be precisely palpated. If structures are being sought more on the radial side, the hand is positioned with the small finger downward.

4.3.2 Palpation of Individual Structures

Radial Fossa (Anatomical Snuffbox)

A triangular depression can be found in the radial region of the carpus that has already been used as a starting position for the palpation of the boundary of the carpus. This depression is called the radial fossa, or the "anatomical snuffbox" (▶ Fig. 4.30). Therapists can easily observe and palpate swelling here caused by inflammation in the wrist.

The following structures form the boundaries of the radial fossa:
- Proximal = distal radius.
- Dorsal = extensor pollicis longus tendon (tendon compartment III).
- Palmar = extensor pollicis brevis tendon (tendon compartment I).

Technique

Usually, the participating muscles must contract so that the position of the bordering tendons can be located and the radial fossa identified. The patient's hand is positioned with the small finger downward, and the patient is instructed to move the thumb upward toward the ceiling (extension of the thumb).

If the radial fossa is not yet obvious, the bordering extensor tendons of the thumb can be identified using a transverse palpation technique.

The two tendons of the thumb extensors come closer to each other more distally. The structures of the radial column are found in the floor of this depression (scaphoid and trapezium; see ▶ Fig. 4.42 and ▶ Fig. 4.43).

Extensor Tendons and their Compartments

The tendons of the long (extrinsic) muscles that move the hand and finger skeletons are held close to the radius and the ulna in their dorsal aspects at the side of the forearm by a thickening of the forearm fascia at the radius and ulna.

This extensor retinaculum maintains the position of all extensor tendons on the forearm skeleton, even during large rotary movements of the hand or forearm. The extensor retinaculum is attached to the bones between the respective tendon compartments, causing small osteofibrous canals to be formed for the passage of the tendons (▶ Fig. 4.15). Tendon sheaths protect the tendons from frictioning during movement.

The six canals through which the tendons pass are referred to as tendon compartments.

Technique

First Compartment

The ulnar side of the patient's hand is still positioned downward and the radial fossa is made distinct by moving the muscles of the thumb (▶ Fig. 4.31 and ▶ Fig. 4.32). The most palmar tendon bundle of the tendons shown here is located using transverse palpation. The patient then relaxes the thumb and the tendon bundle is followed proximally until the bony resistance of the radius is felt. This is the point where both tendons pass underneath the retinaculum through the first compartment. It lies directly over the radial styloid process.

The first compartment is one of the most common sites for tenosynovitis, and inflammation here is named de Quervain disease.

Technique

Second Compartment

The dorsal radial tuberculum is the starting point for further differentiation of compartments II and III.

From this point, the palpating finger points in a radial direction. With very slight, rhythmical extension and flexion of the hand and direct palpation with one finger pad, contractions of the tendons belonging to the extensor carpi radialis longus and brevis can again be felt. Both tendons together use the second tendon compartment. If they are followed further distal (approx. 2 cm) while the patient is working the muscle continuously, a V-shaped separation of the two tendons is found shortly before they cross under the tendon of the extensor pollicis longus. It can even be possible to follow both tendons to their insertions

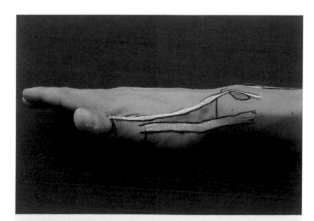

Fig. 4.31 Tendons of the first and third compartments.

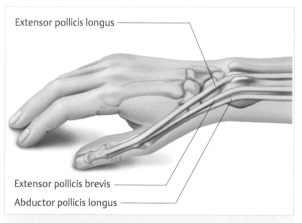

Extensor pollicis longus

Extensor pollicis brevis

Abductor pollicis longus

Fig. 4.32 Topography of the ulnar tendons (first and second compartments).

with the same palpation technique. The tendon of the extensor carpi radialis longus inserts more radially at the base of metacarpal II and the tendon of the brevis inserts between the bases II and III at the styloid protuberance of the carpometacarpal joint line (see ▶ Fig. 4.28)

Technique

Third Compartment

The dorsal tubercle of the radius serves as a pulley for the extensor pollicis longus tendon. Here, coming from the distal forearm, the tendon changes direction toward the distal phalanx of the thumb (▶ Fig. 4.33). If palpation is carried out directly ulnar to the tuberculum, with continuous extension movements of the thumb, the tension in the tendon can be felt.

Technique

Fourth Compartment

The tendons of the fourth compartment are found immediately ulnar to the extensor pollicis longus tendon. It is easy to palpate the extensor digitorum tendons. To do this, the patient lifts up the fingers one at a time, as if playing a piano. The palpating finger on what is believed to be the tendon compartment is immediately pushed away upward by the tendons. The tendon of the second muscle, the extensor indicis, which uses this tendon compartment, cannot be demonstrated in isolation.

Technique

Distal Radioulnar Joint Space and the Palpatory Technique for the Fifth Compartment

Further palpation of the dorsal soft tissue in the hand is directed toward the head of the ulna, with the forearm lying prone and relaxed.

The head of the ulna is flanked by two tendons. The tendon of the extensor digiti minimi can be felt radial to the ulnar head with slight, rhythmical contractions of the muscle and followed further proximally and distally (▶ Fig. 4.34). Its course directly radial to the ulnar head marks the position of the underlying joint space of the distal radioulnar joint (DRUJ). The tendon in compartment five is a guiding structure for location or confirmation of the joint space position (see ▶ Fig. 4.23).

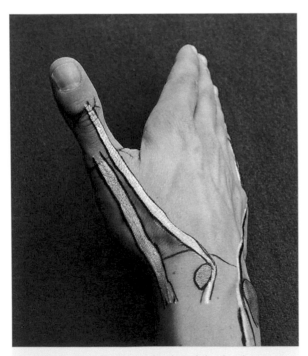

Fig. 4.33 Dorsal radial Lister tubercle and the thumb extensor tendons.

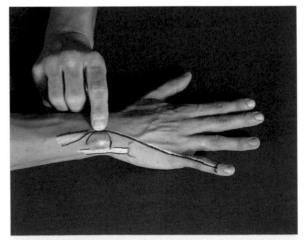

Fig. 4.34 Palpation of the extensor digiti minimi.

Technique

Sixth Compartment

The extensor carpi ulnaris tendon is found immediately ulnar to the head of the ulna. It can be distinctly felt at the level of the carpus if the muscle is rhythmically contracted (extension with ulnar abduction of the hand). It is easily followed distally down onto its insertion at the base of the fifth metacarpal and proximally as it passes by the head of the ulna. The tendon travels through the sixth compartment in a shallow osseous groove (▶ Fig. 4.36).

If two fingers are allowed to remain on the tendon in their position next to the ulnar head and the forearm is supinated, it seems that the ulnar head has turned under the tendon, which is now lying on the ulnar head dorsally. This impression is deceptive; the tendon in the groove remains where it is while the radius swings around. The ulnar head remains on the flexor side of the elbow. It is simply more visible and more accessible in pronation. In extreme supination and instability of the DRUJ, the ulnar edge of the radius can pinch and irritate the tendon sheath.

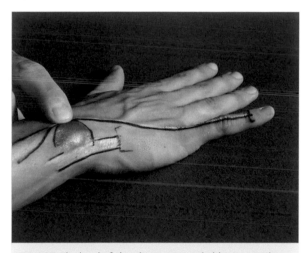

Fig. 4.35 The head of the ulna is surrounded by two tendons.

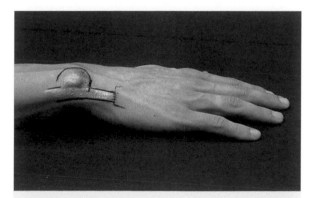

Fig. 4.36 Position of the tendon of the extensor carpi ulnaris.

4.3.3 Radial Nerve, Cephalic Vein, and Radial Artery

On average, approximately 8 cm proximal to the radial styloid process (Robson, 2008), the superficial branch of the radial nerve penetrates the forearm fascia passing through the gap between the tendons of the brachioradialis and extensor carpi radialis longus (Balakrishnan et al., 2009). This is the transition between the middle and distal thirds of the forearm, directly proximal and radial to the short muscle bellies of compartment I. It continues distally, directly under the skin, and can be felt next to the tendons of compartment II.

Technique

Radial Nerve

Initially, the contracted muscle bellies of the thumb extensors are located. The hand forms a fist (including the thumb) and is facilitated into ulnar deviation and extension of the wrist (Finkelstein maneuver). The radial nerve rolls underneath the transversely palpating fingertips immediately proximal and radial to the muscle bellies.

The nerve can be followed over its entire radial course (▶ Fig. 4.37):
- Penetrating the forearm fascia, it can be felt here for the first time.
- Then it crosses over the tendons of the first compartment.
- At the distal radius, it runs along tendon compartment II. Robson (2008) describes the distance to the radial tubercle as approximately 1.5 cm.
- The cephalic vein accompanies the radial nerve in radial fossa I, crossing over the groove superficially. This is an appropriate site for intravenous access as the vein is located just beneath the skin and is usually easy to reach. The weak pulsation of one branch of the radial artery can be felt when palpating deep in the fossa with a slight pressure against the osseous floor (scaphoid)

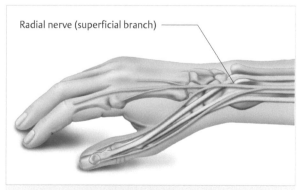

Fig. 4.37 Branches of the radial nerve—ulnar view.

Radial nerve (superficial branch)

4

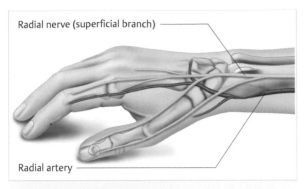

Fig. 4.38 Course of the radial artery.

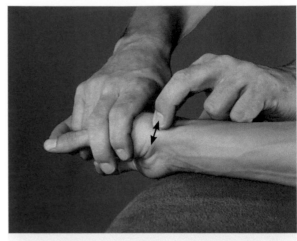

Fig. 4.39 Transverse frictions at the tendons of the sixth compartment.

(▶ Fig. 4.38). The radial artery accompanies the radial nerve for 72% of the way (Robson, 2008).
- Finally, the nerve and the vein can still be followed as they cross the tendon of the extensor pollicis longus; the nerve again rolls back and forth under the finger pad on transverse palpation with light pressure.

Tip

The tension in the radial nerve increases when the elbow is extended and the hand is flexed. The nerve's superficial position makes it susceptible to compression and friction, often caused by tight bracelets and heavy watches (so-called Wartenberg disease; Spies et al., 2016).

4.3.4 Tips for Assessment and Treatment

As already emphasized, the passages of tendons and their synovial sheaths through the extensor compartments are predestined for inflammatory processes. The first compartment is one of the most common sites for tenosynovitis. Tendosynovitisstenosans, known as de Quervain disease, is found at the level of the extensor retinaculum or proximal to the muscle-tendon transition.

Technique

Transverse Friction at the First Compartment

Transverse friction is used for provocative diagnosis or therapy of tenosynovitis. The patient's hand and thumb are first positioned without causing pain, in extension and with ulnar deviation. This places the tendon and synovial sheath under sufficient tension to ensure that they do not disappear deeper into the tissue or roll away from underneath the finger when pressure is applied during frictioning.

The free hand holds onto the back of the patient's hand and stabilizes the thumb. The index finger is placed over the affected site, and the middle finger is placed with light pressure over the index finger as a support. The frictions are conducted by applying pressure from palmar to dorsal exactly perpendicular to the fibers of the tendon (▶ Fig. 4.39). The fingers return to the starting position without applying pressure, but nevertheless maintaining skin contact. This technique is also to be applied 5 cm proximally at the muscle-tendon transition, if this is the location of the irritated spot.

Transverse Frictions for Insertion Tendinopathies in the Sixth Compartment

Another example of the application of local palpation of the hand is the application of transverse frictions onto the insertion for the extensor carpi ulnaris at the base of the fifth metacarpal.

As the tendon comes from a proximal position and inserts directly into the base, the therapist is faced with the challenge of even reaching the site of insertion.

This can be achieved when two aspects are taken into consideration:
- The tendon must be pushed deep into the tissues onto the carpal bones.
- The palpating finger pads come from a proximal position and rest against the base of the metacarpal.

Both are successful if the hand to be treated is arranged in a position that permits a passive approach to the tendon and the palpating hand is positioned with pronation of the forearm (▶ Fig. 4.40).

The actual transverse frictions are conducted by applying pressure from palmar to dorsal (▶ Fig. 4.40).

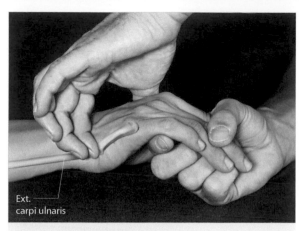

Fig. 4.40 Transverse frictions—radial view.

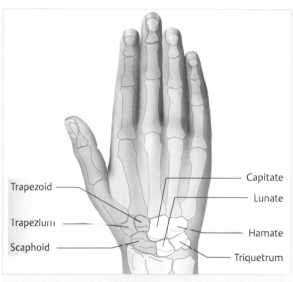

Fig. 4.41 Parts of the radial column.

If the therapist wishes to mainly treat the synovial sheath in the sixth compartment, the technique is used as for the first compartment:

- Tendon and synovial sheath are tightened by positioning the wrist in radial deviation and flexion (not illustrated).
- The technique is applied perpendicular to the tendon; pressure is applied during the movement from palmar to dorsal.

This fundamental procedure can be used for all other conditions of the synovial sheath.

4.4 Local Palpation of the Dorsal Aspect of the Carpal Bones

4.4.1 Summary of the Palpatory Process

The therapist now has a general idea of the dimensions of the carpus and metacarpus. The superficial soft-tissue structures on the back and edges of the hand have been located.

The next step involves palpating deep in the tissue to differentiate the individual wrist bones in the carpus from one another (▶ Fig. 4.41). Therefore, therapists orient themselves on the longitudinal divisions of the hand, the columns, consisting of rays (metacarpals and phalanges) and carpal bones. Palpation begins radially and finishes ulnarly.

Starting Position

The patient's hand and forearm relax again on a supportive surface, which is as level as possible. The therapist generally sits to the side. The palm of the hand should face downward to enable the dorsal and ulnar aspect of

the wrist to be precisely palpated. If more radial structures are being sought, the hand is placed with the small finger downward.

4.4.2 Carpal Bones in the Radial Column

Bones in the Radial Fossa

The radial fossa is formed when the thumb extends to the side. The therapist is familiar with its tendinous and bony borders. The carpal bones will now be palpated in the floor of the snuffbox.

Technique

Scaphoid

The index finger of the palpating hand comes from a distal position and strokes over the thumb in a proximal direction until the pad of the index finger is resting in the fossa. The tip of the index finger can now feel the edge of the radius very clearly, and the pad of the index finger is resting directly over the radial aspect of the scaphoid (▶ Fig. 4.42).

Tip

The palpation is confirmed using the pattern of scaphoid movement during passive radial and ulnar deviation of the hand. With the scaphoid in ulnar abduction, the pad of the index finger is pressed out of the fossa while with radial abduction it lies in a more pronounced depression.

Trapezium

To palpate the borders of the trapezium, the tip of the index finger must be turned so that it points distally toward the tip of the thumb by rotating the palpating hand 180°. The pad of the index finger rests again in the shallow depression of the radial fossa. The fingertip now comes into contact with the hard, bony resistance of the trapezium (▶ Fig. 4.43).

Tip

The correct location is confirmed through a small motion. The tip of the index finger should not feel any movement during small-range, passive extension of the thumb (▶ Fig. 4.44).

The scaphoid again disappears deep into the tissue during small-range radial deviation, and the distinct edge of the trapezium remains palpable.

First Carpometacarpal Joint

Since the carpometacarpal joint of the thumb is a possible cause of symptoms at the radius, both hypomobility and arthritis, its location is of great interest.

The index finger initially remains on the scaphoid with the fingertip resting on the trapezium. The palpating index finger now slides a few millimeters distally.

If the patient's thumb is now passively extended, it must be possible to feel movement. The base of metacarpal I now pushes against the palpating finger. This is the location of the joint space seen from radial.

With constant slight movement of the thumb, the entire extent of the base can be felt. Dorsal and palmar thumb movements (abduction, adduction) are useful if the therapist wishes to follow the base on the palm. Adduction of the thumb causes the base to protrude palmarly (▶ Fig. 4.45).

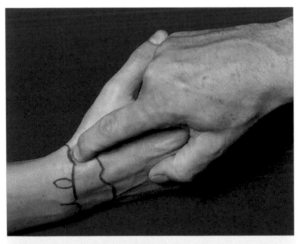

Fig. 4.42 Location of the scaphoid.

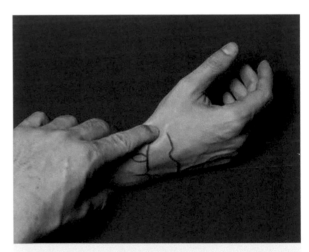

Fig. 4.43 Location of the trapezium.

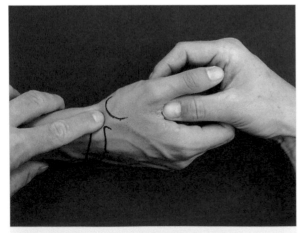

Fig. 4.44 Confirmation of the correct location of the trapezium using movement.

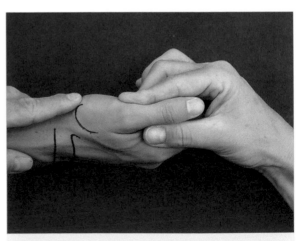

Fig. 4.45 Palmar palpation of the first carpometacarpal joint space.

During this movement, the base follows the rolling and gliding behavior according to the concave-convex rule of local biomechanics.

Tips for Assessment and Treatment

The following examples demonstrate possible uses for local palpation of the radial column.

- **Local mobility tests**
  - Once a carpal bone has been located, it is possible to move it specifically in the joints, to palmar and dorsal, together with its adjacent bones ("ballottement tests," Reagan et al., 1984). By comparing sides, information can be obtained on possible changes in mobility, that is, hypermobility or hypomobility. In particular, minor or end-range restrictions in wrist mobility can be identified.
  - An example is the isolated movement of the scaphoid on the radius (▶ Fig. 4.46). This is achieved by resting the ulnar side of the patient's hand against the body to stabilize the hand. One hand grasps around the radius to fixate it. The other holds onto the scaphoid on its dorsal and palmar aspects. Now the scaphoid is displaced to dorsal and palmar (taking into account the palmar tilt of the radius) and the range of the motion is compared to that in the other hand.
- Similar changes in mobility can also be found in the often-painful arthritic condition (acute basal joint arthritis) of the carpometacarpal joint of the thumb. One of the manual therapy techniques that can be used here is traction at the carpometacarpal joint (▶ Fig. 4.47), which assesses the current level of elasticity in the capsule by pulling on the first metacarpal. The advantage of accurate knowledge of local anatomy is demonstrated during the necessary precise stabilization of the trapezium.
- Transverse friction applied to the capsule of the first carpometacarpal joint has been proven effective in relieving pain. This is only possible if the therapist is able to find the joint space with palpation.

4.4.3 Carpal Bones in the Central Column

It is hardly possible to locate further carpalia dorsally by means of palpation. The structures can only be differentiated from each other by specific palpation from the ulnar aspect. For this reason, we need guiding lines and spatial relations on the back of the hand. The boundaries of the carpus must be drawn in.

Technique

Capitate

The palpation starts distally. The hand of the therapist is positioned along the extended axis of the patient's hand.

The capitate extends from the carpometacarpal line (end at the base of metacarpal III) by two-thirds of the distance to the radius on the back of the hand. The width of the capitate on each side is approximately 1 mm greater than the base of metacarpal III. The capitate is drawn in, including this widening, with a convex curve proximally (▶ Fig. 4.48).

Approximate Dorsal Location of the Lunate and Scaphoid

Landmarks for the further differentiation of the carpal bones are the dorsal radial tubercle and the space of the DRUJ. The scaphoid is halfway along the line connecting the capitate and the dorsal radial tubercle, and the lunate is halfway along the line from the capitate to the DRUJ. Another connecting line shows the boundary between lunate and scaphoid. To form this line, the dorsal radial tubercle is connected with the joint space of the DRUJ. Halfway along this line is the joint line between the two carpal bones.

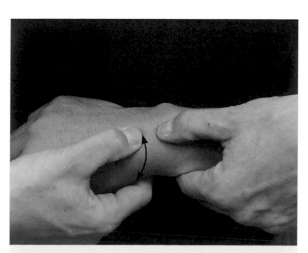

Fig. 4.46 Translational technique radius with respect to scaphoid.

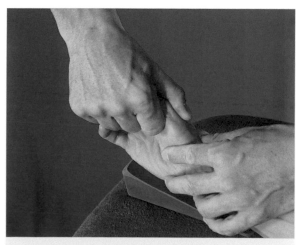

Fig. 4.47 Traction of the first carpometacarpal joint.

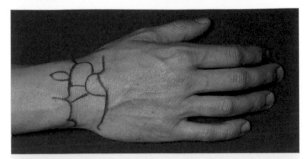

Fig. 4.48 Position of the capitate.

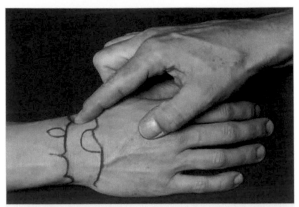

Fig. 4.49 Palpation of the dorsal surface of the scaphoid.

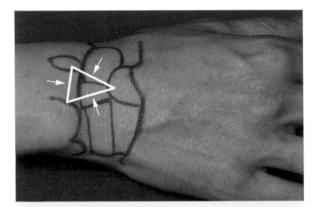

Fig. 4.50 Position of the scaphoid and the lunate.

Scaphoid and Trapezoid

The scaphoid was already found in the radial fossa. The boundary with the lunate is known. Finally, the extent of the distance to radial and distal must be found. The radial boundary of the dorsal view of the scaphoid is found by palpating from the known location (halfway from the capitate to the dorsal radial tubercle) with a slight amount of pressure, down to the radial edge of the carpus. The edge of the scaphoid has been reached when the palpating finger slips radially off the dorsal surface (▶ Fig. 4.49). This lies approximately between the base of metacarpal II and the dorsal radial tubercle. The boundary is drawn here; it extends distally for approximately two-thirds of the way from the edge of the radius to the base of metacarpal II (see ▶ Fig. 4.48).

From this boundary, the space between the scaphoid and the base of metacarpal II is filled out, in order to represent the position of the trapezoid. Distally, it has the same width as the base of metacarpal II. It hardly makes sense to describe the position of the trapezium in the dorsal view since it is tilted by approximately 35° to palmar in relation to the plane of the other carpal bones.

Lunate

The confirmed position of the lunate, halfway along the line connecting the capitate and the joint space of the

DRUJ has already been described. Now the position is definitively drawn in. The lunate extends from the scaphoid to the joint space of the DRUJ and from this point to the capitate (▶ Fig. 4.50).

The boundary of the correct location with respect to the edge of the radius is found by flexing and extending the hand. In direct palpation with one finger pad on the lunate, it becomes clear that when the hand is extended, the lunate disappears in a palmar direction and it becomes possible to feel the edge of the radius.

4.4.4 Tips for Assessment and Treatment

In particular, the assessment of lunate mobility on the capitate or the radius provides therapists with information on the presence of lunate instability within the central column.

Mobility is often restricted in the articulation between lunate and scaphoid and can interfere with mobility in both the proximal row of the carpal bones and movements in the wrist as a whole.

4.4.5 Carpal Bones in the Ulnar Column

The palpation begins proximal, on the forearm. The recommended position for the therapist is on the thumb side of the hand, allowing free access to the ulnar column (▶ Fig. 4.54).

Technique

Triquetrum

The first landmark is the ulnar head; from there, the ulnar styloid process is found again. The next bony structure distal to the ulnar head is the triquetrum. In the transition to the triquetrum, a depression is found that indicates the position of an articular disk. When the fingertip feels this depression as a narrow concavity (opposite ulna and triquetrum), the triquetrum is lying under the finger pad

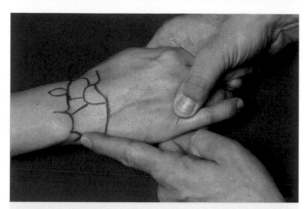

Fig. 4.51 Location of the triquetrum.

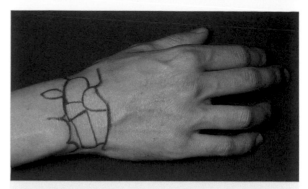

Fig. 4.52 Position of the triquetrum and the hamate.

(▶ Fig. 4.51). It is convex, curving toward the ulna. This convexity increases in radial abduction and decreases markedly in ulnar abduction. In this way, the correct location is confirmed by movement. The ulnar boundaries of this concavity are connected with the lunate and this describes the entire extent of the triquetrum. It becomes clear that a narrow gap between the proximal border of the triquetrum and the ulnar head remains. This is the location of the TFC complex, especially of the ulnar disk.

It is easy for the thumb and the index finger to hold onto the dorsal triquetrum and palmar pisiform and to move these bones, with the articular disk, opposite the head of the ulna in a dorsopalmar direction (▶ Fig. 4.52).

This movement is always extensive compared with the previously described movements within the carpus. The range of motion indicates the presence of a laxity and therefore the ability of the TFC complex to stabilize the ulnar column.

Tips

In principle, it is relatively easy to locate the triquetrum because it is the most prominent carpal bone distal to the head of the ulna. There are situations, however, that require additional reassurance. The following possibilities are used to confirm the location:
- The therapist palpates the dorsal aspect of the triquetrum and passively flexes and extends the wrist. The triquetrum protrudes dorsally during flexion and disappears in a palmar direction during extension.
- When conducting radial and ulnar deviation of the wrist, it becomes evident that the normal rolling and gliding movements are accompanied by rotation. The triquetrum becomes more prominent during radial deviation and disappears again in a palmar direction during ulnar deviation. This makes the large range of motion in the ulnar direction possible and permits the base of the fifth metacarpal to move closer to the ulna.

Hamate

The hamate is not very conspicuous ulnarly but becomes increasingly prominent radially toward the capitate. It mainly has a triangular form, with the wide section facing the capitate (▶ Fig. 4.56).

The hamate fills a gap between the triquetrum and the base of the fifth metacarpal and can also be felt in another concavity at the ulnar edge of the hand.

Tip

In summary, the contour of all the bones palpated from the ulnar aspect (▶ Fig. 4.53) is wave-shaped: the ulna is convex, the disk lies in a narrow concavity, the triquetrum is distinctly convex, the hamate feels concave, and the fifth metacarpal is distinctly convex.

If the therapist wishes to include the hamate in the local assessment of mobility or in mobilizing techniques, this is possible by locating the hamate directly proximal to the base of the fourth metacarpal (see ▶ Fig. 4.55).

4.4.6 Tips for Assessment and Treatment

The hypermobility stronghold in the hand is found here in the ulnar column. Physical therapists often have to support themselves on the ulnar side of the heel of the hand, where they are subject to local pressure. It is therefore not surprising that ulnar instability causes aggravation of symptoms during professional training. Often it is necessary to recommend the wearing of a special hand bandage that gives increased support to the ulnar column (Wrist restore, www.iaom.de, www.bernhardreichert.de).

In connection with local hypermobility of the ulnar column and/or of the distal radioulnar joint and as a result of axial pressure loads, inflammation or trauma of the TFC, especially of the articular disk of the ulna, can cause

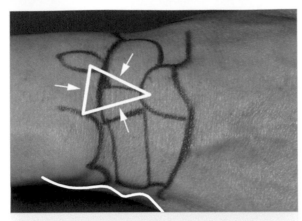

Fig. 4.53 Overview of the position of the carpals and ulnar wave shape.

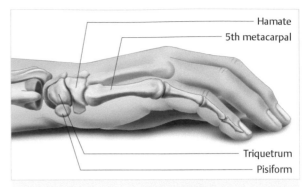

Fig. 4.54 Topography of the ulnar column.

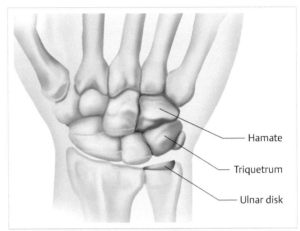

Fig. 4.56 Position of the hamate in the ulnar column.

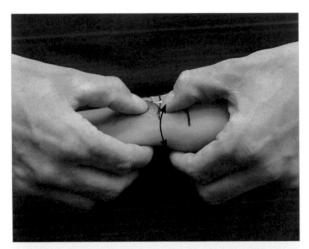

Fig. 4.55 Differentiating between the head of the ulna and triquetrum on the surface.

symptoms ulnarly, palmarly, or dorsally on the ulnar side of the wrist.

Diagnostically, pain should be provoked in end-range pronation or supination of the forearm (Vezeridis et al., 2010) or of the hand as well as through further loading through pulling or pressure with end-range movements of the hand toward ulnar or radial. Supporting oneself with an extended hand to get up from a sitting position ("press test," Lester et al., 1995) is highly sensitive with respect to ruptures of the disk. The "ulnar fovea sign" (Tay et al., 2007) is just as diagnostically valid for detecting trauma of the disk ligament as magnetic resonance imaging (MRI) (Schmauss et al., 2016). Tay described the manual provocation test as follows: The tip of the therapist's thumb presses against the more palmar side of the distal ulnar head into a space between the ulnar styloid process and the flexor carpi ulnaris tendon (▶ Fig. 4.57). The test is positive if the pain described by the patient can be reproduced. During testing, the patient's entire

arm is relaxed and the elbow is flexed approximately 90 to 110°. The forearm and wrist are in a neutral position.

4.5 General Orientation—Palmar

4.5.1 Summary of the Palpatory Process

The second large section in palmar palpation of the hand is specific identification of the carpal bones and visualization of the carpal tunnel. The transitional region between the distal forearm and the wrist will be covered in the following palpations.

The distal forearm generally appears to be a surface traversed by numerous tendons, blood vessels, and neural structures. The question is the location of the actual distal osseous boundary of the lower arm and identification of the soft-tissue structures that can be differentiated from each other by palpation.

Further distal is the region that is usually called the heel of the hand, the convergence of the thenar and hypothenar eminences. This is the osseous fixed point (origin) of numerous short, intrinsic muscles for the first and fifth fingers. This is the region of the carpal tunnel,

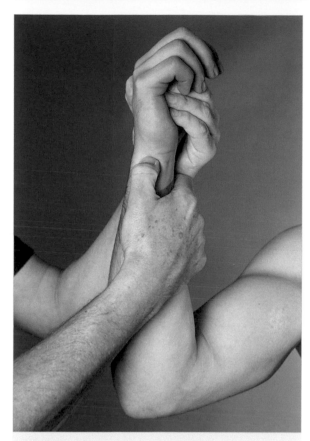

Fig. 4.57 Ulnar fovea sign (Tay et al., 2007).

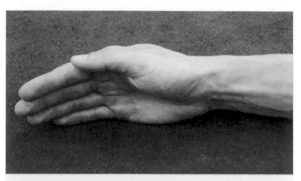

Fig. 4.58 SP for palmar orientation.

▶ Fig. 4.42) and followed over the tendons in a palmar direction, and over the radial styloid process. It is easy to access the radius immediately palmar to the tendons in the first compartment. The shape of its edge can also be well demonstrated at this point. The flexor tendons interfere greatly with palpation further toward the middle of the forearm and the ulna.

Tip

If the therapist wishes to palpate the edge of the radius further, the hand must be flexed significantly and, most importantly, moved into passive flexion. The therapist then positions the palpating finger vertically, palpates between the tendons, and attempts to hook around the edge of the radius. The line of the radiocarpal joint reveals itself if the palpation is successful. Comparable to the dorsal aspect, the joint line runs at a slight angle so that it is more proximal on the ulnar side and more distal on the radial side (▶ Fig. 4.59). Halfway between the radial styloid process and the DRUJ joint space is a small round prominence that represents the transition between the joint facets for the scaphoid and lunate of the joint surface of the radius. The carpal ligaments arise at this prominence.

known as the site of one of the most common peripheral compression neuropathies, carpal tunnel syndrome. Its position and extent can be precisely determined by palpation.

Starting Position

For the following palpations, it is recommended that the forearm rests on a level surface in a neutral or slightly supinated position (▶ Fig. 4.58). The therapist should be positioned next to the hand. In palpating one's own carpal bones, this starting position should be modified with the hand positioned vertically.

4.5.2 Edge of the Radius

Therapists require considerable skill and experience to feel the distal edge of the forearm. The boundary of the radius can be well accessed only at a few points. A large number of thick tendons prevent free access to the rest of the border. Therapists are only able to bypass the tendons with skill and by applying slightly more pressure.

Access is once more sought in the radial fossa. With perpendicular palpation, radially, the radius is found (see

It also becomes evident that in comparison to the dorsal line, the palmar line is displaced slightly proximally, demonstrating that the radius is a little longer on its dorsal than its palmar side (palmar tilt). This is important for the translational techniques of manual therapy, independent of whether it is a movement of the entire carpus or of individual carpal bones with respect to the radius.

The distal boundary of the carpus cannot be found by palpation. In the following sections, the accessible palmar eminences of the carpal bones are discussed. They give a relative orientation of the palmar carpometacarpal joint line.

4.6 Local Palpation of the Palmar Soft Tissues

4.6.1 Summary of the Palpatory Process

The patient is instructed to tighten the fist with the wrist flexed. The therapist then examines the tendons in the wrist area. Frequently, three tendons can already be observed in the middle of the wrist (flexor carpi radialis, palmaris longus, flexor digitorum superficialis).

These tendons and other soft-tissue structures crossing over the wrist will be differentiated from one another and identified. Once again, the palpation begins radially and ends on the ulnar side.

Netter (1992) labeled the structures in the radial section the **radial trio** (▶ Fig. 4.60). These are listed from radial to ulnar:

- Radial artery.
- Flexor carpi radialis tendon.
- Flexor pollicis longus tendon.

Netter (1992) labeled the ulnar area on the palmar side of the forearm the **ulnar trio** (▶ Fig. 4.61):

- Flexor carpi ulnaris tendon.
- Ulnar nerve.
- Ulnar artery.

4.6.2 Palpation of Individual Structures

Flexor Carpi Radialis and Tubercle of Scaphoid

The patient makes a fist and flexes it with minimal activity and constant contraction.

The palpation is conducted from radial to ulnar and locates the thick tendon of the flexor carpi radialis first. This is the most radial tendon. The tendon protrudes even further when wrist flexion is combined with radial deviation (▶ Fig. 4.62).

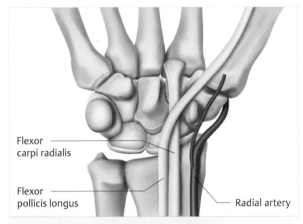

Fig. 4.60 "Radial trio" according to Netter.

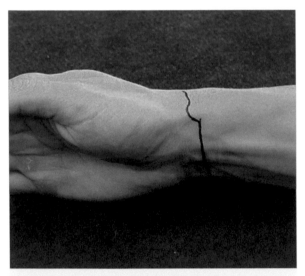

Fig. 4.59 Radiocarpal joint line—palmar view.

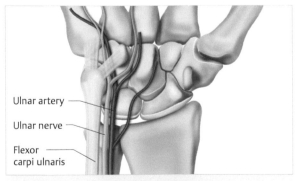

Fig. 4.61 "Ulnar trio" according to Netter.

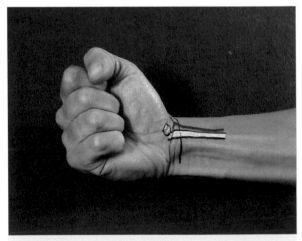

Fig. 4.62 Flexor carpi radialis tendon and tubercle of the scaphoid.

When the therapist follows the tendon more distally, the tendon guides the palpating fingers onto an important bony reference point: the tubercle of scaphoid. The tendon is not found on this tubercle, but rather passes ulnar to the tubercle, where it subsequently travels underneath the transverse carpal ligament via a compartment separate to the carpal tunnel, and inserts into the base of the second metacarpal.

Radial Artery

Feeling the pulsation of the radial artery is the most common method for determining heart rate by means of palpation. The artery is most clearly palpable immediately radial to the flexor carpi radialis on the flat plateau of the radius (▶ Fig. 4.63).

Therapists are familiar with its further course, which is only partially palpable, from their knowledge of topographical anatomy. In the wrist, it deviates dorsally, shortly proximal to the scaphoid tubercle, dips into the radial fossa between the tendons of the first compartment and the scaphoid, crosses under the extensor pollicis longus tendon, and continues in a dorsal direction between metacarpals II and III. It often accompanies the superficial branch of the radial nerve.

Flexor Pollicis Longus

The final radial triad structure is the tendon of the flexor pollicis longus. Similar to the radial artery, this tendon is also found directly radial to the tendon of the flexor carpi radialis but is located slightly deeper in the tissue beneath the artery. With repeated flexion of the thumb joint, it can be distinctly felt. Contraction of the muscle belly can be clearly felt a little more proximally. This tendon is one of the 10 structures that pass through the carpal tunnel.

Tip

If it is still difficult to differentiate the tendons from one another, the wrist should be actively extended to reciprocally inhibit and relax the carpal flexor.

4.6.3 Summary of all Radial Structures

The palpable structures on the radial side of the hand have the following order from dorsal to palmar:
- Tendon of the extensor pollicis longus (third compartment).
- Dorsal radial tubercle.
- Tendons of the extensor carpi radialis longus and brevis (second compartment).
- Superficial branch of the radial nerve, cephalic vein.
- Tendons of the extensor pollicis brevis and the abductor pollicis longus (first compartment).
- Radial artery.
- Tendon of the flexor pollicis longus.
- Tendon of the flexor carpi radialis.

Palmaris Longus

Three centrally located tendons are observed initially when the patient makes a fist. The middle tendon belongs to the palmaris longus. It runs through the carpal tunnel to the palmar aponeurosis. This tendon is more clearly visualized when the thumb and little finger are opposed (▶ Fig. 4.64). The tendon is a landmark structure for the course of the median nerve that lies directly below the tendon and runs through the carpal tunnel.

This muscle is the most variable muscle described in the anatomy of the motor apparatus. According to the literature, it is lacking in an average of 15% of cases (Mbaka and Ejiwunmi, 2009). Its tendon is preferred by surgeons as autologous substitute material (Bain et al., 2015).

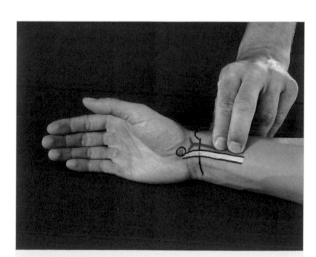

Fig. 4.63 Palpation of the radial artery.

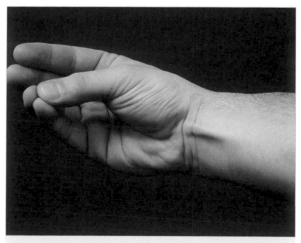

Fig. 4.64 Demonstration of the palmaris longus tendon.

Flexor Digitorum Superficialis

The patient is instructed to make a tight fist again. The therapist palpates further ulnarly and identifies another tendon that is especially easy to palpate when the patient additionally increases the pressure from the fourth and fifth fingers onto the palm of the hand. This is the tendon of the flexor digitorum superficialis. Both the superficial and the deep finger flexor, together with four tendons, run through the carpal tunnel.

Flexor Carpi Ulnaris and Pisiform

Another tendon can be felt with repeated contraction of the fist in flexion with ulnar abduction of the hand with distinct resistance or broad hand movement to ulnar (▶ Fig. 4.65). The flexor carpi ulnaris tendon lies very ulnarly and guides the palpating finger distally onto the pisiform.

Tip

The tendon is only very rarely visible as the fascia of the forearm is very soft at this point. Therefore, a large

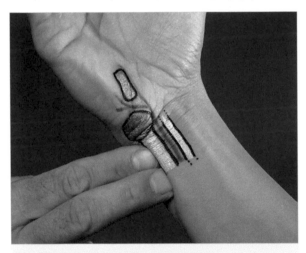

Fig. 4.65 Palpation of the flexor carpi ulnaris.

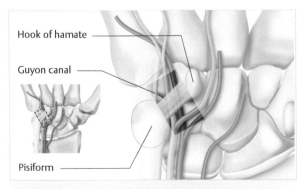

Hook of hamate

Guyon canal

Pisiform

Fig. 4.66 Topography of the ulnar trio and the Guyon canal.

amount of muscle activity and palpation immediately proximal to the pisiform is required to identify the tendon.

Ulnar Artery and Nerve

It is not as easy to feel this artery as on the radial side. For this reason, this palpation requires absolute relaxation of the tendons and muscles on the palmar side and some patience.

The pulse of the ulnar artery can be felt between the tendons of the flexor digitorum superficialis and flexor carpi ulnaris by positioning the finger pads over this area with a small amount of pressure. In its further course, the artery runs over the carpal tunnel and sends a branch into the Guyon canal. The main artery runs under the palmar aponeurosis in an arc, over the metacarpus (superficial palmar arch), where it gives off additional branches.

The ulnar nerve lies in the distal forearm, directly ulnar to the ulnar artery (▶ Fig. 4.66). The fingers are again positioned vertically between the tendons of the flexor carpi ulnaris and flexor digitorum superficialis for this palpation (▶ Fig. 4.67). The nerve can occasionally be confused with a relaxed tendon since it has approximately the same diameter. When the therapist palpates superficially and perpendicularly, the nerve will roll back and forth underneath the palpating finger and its position and consistency do not change during active finger flexion.

The artery and nerve can be followed for at least 3 to 4 finger widths proximally until they are covered by the tendons of the finger flexors. The nerve can also be followed further distally (▶ Fig. 4.68). It passes over the wrist here, directly radial to the pisiform, and divides into two branches. One branch disappears with the branch of the ulnar artery between the pisiform and the hamate in the Guyon canal; the other runs radial of the hamate to

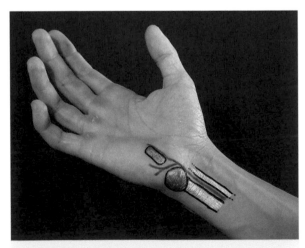

Fig. 4.67 Overview of the radial structures on the palmar aspect.

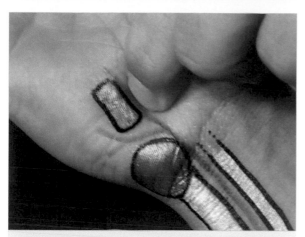

Fig. 4.68 Palpation of the ulnar nerve directly adjacent to the hook of hamate.

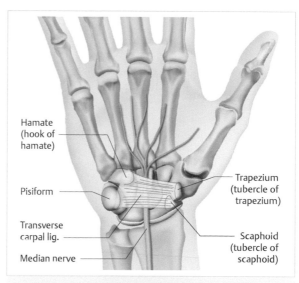

Fig. 4.69 Boundaries of the carpal tunnel and the median nerve.

the inner surface of the hand. Next to the hamate, the nerve is also palpable (▶ Fig. 4.68).

4.6.4 Summary of all Ulnar Structures

The palpable structures on the ulnar side of the distal forearm have the following order from dorsal to palmar:
- Extensor digiti minimi tendon (fifth compartment).
- Head of the ulna with the ulnar styloid process and TFC complex.
- Extensor carpi ulnaris tendon (sixth compartment).
- Flexor carpi ulnaris tendon.
- Ulnar nerve and artery.
- Flexor digitorum superficialis tendon.

4.6.5 Tips for Assessment and Treatment

The Guyon canal is formed by both of its neighboring osseous structures, pisiform and the hook of hamate, as well as the superficially situated pisohamate ligament. This ligament is one of the two extensions of the flexor carpi ulnaris tendon originating on the pisiform.

Compression neuropathies of the ulnar nerve in the canal are known as "handlebar palsy." These pressure lesions develop when weight is placed on the ulnar aspect of the hand, the wrist is positioned in extension, and the hand radially deviated.

4.7 Local Palpation of the Palmar Aspect of the Carpal Bones

4.7.1 Summary of the Palpatory Process

The chief objective of palpating carpal bones accessible from palmar is to demonstrate the position of the carpal

tunnel by finding the ulnar and radial bony landmarks (▶ Fig. 4.69). Then the osseous boundary points of the carpal tunnel are connected at the surface in order to clarify the extent of the tunnel.

First the radial and ulnar bony wall is found. Then the distal boundary of the forearm is once more palpated and defined and the position of the carpal bones on the floor of the tunnel (lunate and capitate) is determined by means of guiding lines and spatial orientation. Finally, the transverse carpal ligament is drawn in as the roof of the carpal tunnel.

Starting Position

The SP for the palpation of palmar soft tissue is also the standard SP here. To confirm some locations, motions are used with the hand positioned vertically. A well-relaxed hand is important at this point, so that palpation of the carpus is not disturbed by contracted tendons in the distal forearm or contracted thenar and hypothenar muscle bellies.

4.7.2 Palpation of Individual Structures

Pisiform

The therapist starts on the pisiform bone. It has already been discovered and palpated at the end of the flexor carpi ulnaris tendon (see ▶ Fig. 4.65). The pisiform can hardly be overlooked at the base of the hypothenar eminence. The therapist palpates around it with a vertically positioned fingertip. The result of palpating the edges is almost a circle. When the outer boundary is marked on the hand, the figure is surprisingly large. Here too, it is possible to see the difference compared to the depictions of established anatomical models.

The pisiform transfers the pull of the tendon onto the hook of hamate and the base of the fifth metacarpal. In this respect, it can be said that the pisiform is the only carpal bone on which the tendon of an extrinsic hand muscle inserts. Since the pisiform lies markedly above the level of the other carpal bones and the ulna, it functions like a sesamoid bone, contained within the flexor carpi ulnaris tendon. This tendon has no sheath, but it is also not exposed to friction exerted by the hand or forearm skeleton in any hand position.

Moreover, the pisiform is positioned in the middle of the hypothenar muscles and provides a bony fixed point, for example, for the abductor of the small finger. This becomes obvious when the patient is instructed to relax the hand and then rhythmically abduct and adduct the small finger extensively. Contraction of the abductor pulls the pisiform in a distal direction and, from this direction, tenses the flexor carpi ulnaris tendon.

The pisiform can be held by the thumb and index finger and moved sideways on the more dorsally positioned triquetrum when the hand is relaxed (▶ Fig. 4.70 and ▶ Fig. 4.71). On the other hand, with a broad extension of the hand, it is imprisoned between the flexor carpi ulnaris tendon and the pisometacarpal ligament. Therapists tend to use this situation to apply local pressure on the hand. But sometimes there are reports of pisotriquetral osteoarthritis.

Tip

The pisiform can be accessed from all sides. Its edge can even be palpated in the space between the pisiform and the hook of hamate (Guyon canal). Therefore, the palpating finger is positioned almost vertically, and the wrist relaxed in slight flexion (▶ Fig. 4.72). If local pressure in the canal should cause a tingling feeling in the patient's hypothenar eminence, the branch of the ulnar nerve has been touched.

Hook of Hamate

Another carpal bone accessible on the ulnar side of the palm is the hamate. It is recognized by its prominent process, the hook. It can be found quickly by using a trick described by Hoppenfeld (1992) that can also be used in palpation on one's own hand.

The therapist places the middle section of the thumb's interphalangeal joint fold over the pisiform (▶ Fig. 4.73). The tip of the thumb points toward the middle of the palm. From this point, the distance to the hamulus is approximately the length of the terminal phalanx of the thumb.

If the pad of the thumb applies light pressure, the bony resistance of the hook of hamate will be felt immediately (▶ Fig. 4.74).

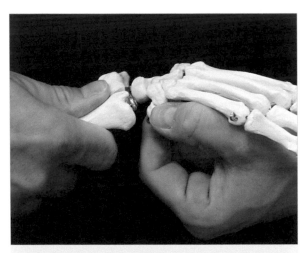

Fig. 4.70 Location of the pisiform on an anatomy model.

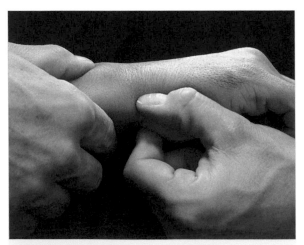

Fig. 4.71 Location of the pisiform on the surface.

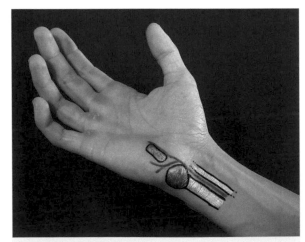

Fig. 4.72 Position of the pisiform and hook of hamate.

4

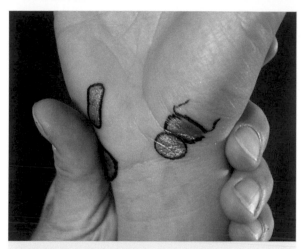

Fig. 4.73 Location of the hook of hamate—phase 1.

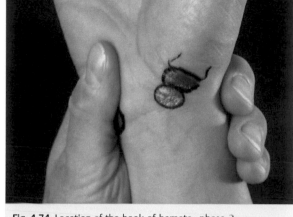

Fig. 4.74 Location of the hook of hamate—phase 2.

The therapist can attempt to locate the boundaries of the hook of hamate by applying the same technique used in the palpation of the edges of the pisiform.

The pisiform and the hook of hamate form the ulnar osseous boundary of the carpal tunnel.

Between the two is the Guyon canal, through which a branch of the ulnar nerve and the ulnar artery run. The Guyon canal can also be reached here, with vertical and transverse palpation techniques. Directly radial to the hamulus, the continuation of one branch of the ulnar nerve can be felt.

Scaphoid

The scaphoid and trapezium form the radial boundary of the carpal tunnel. Both bones have tubercles that can be very easily identified using palpation of the palmar aspect of the hand. The tubercle of the scaphoid has already been noticed during palpation of the palmar soft tissues. The flexor carpi radialis is the guiding structure here (▶ Fig. 4.75).

To locate the tuberculum precisely, the flexor carpi radialis is first displayed by making a fist in palmar flexion, emphasizing the tension on the radial side of the hand.

The radially prominent tendon guides the transverse palpation onto the distinctive bony landmark of the tubercle of the scaphoid. The precise position and extent becomes clear with palpation in a circle around the tuberculum.

The tuberculum is perceived as a rounded, bony point that becomes more prominent when the hand is in extension and radial abduction.

The therapist should keep in mind that the tendon is not present on the tubercle, but rather guides the palpation to this point. The flexor carpi radialis passes through its own canal adjacent to the carpal tunnel and onto the base of the second metacarpal (▶ Fig. 4.76).

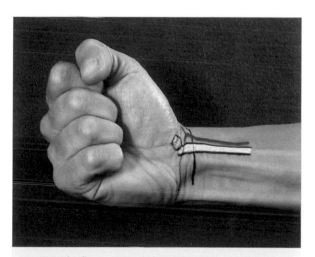

Fig. 4.75 The flexor carpi radialis tendon leads onto the tubercle of the scaphoid.

Trapezium

The tuberculum of the trapezium is next to the scaphoid, on the thumb side, and separated from it by a very small groove. The finger should be positioned almost vertically to palpate the groove. This groove feels similar to the anterior V in the AC joint and marks the joint space between the scaphoid and trapezium, as part of the mediocarpal joint line. The tubercle is again identified as a rounded, hard structure.

The pattern of movement in the two neighboring carpal bones can be used to confirm the location. It is based on the local arthrokinematic convex-concave rule as well as the associated rotation that each carpal bone conducts during movements of the wrist (DeLange, 1987).

The pad of the middle finger comes from a radial direction and is positioned over the scaphoid. The pad of the

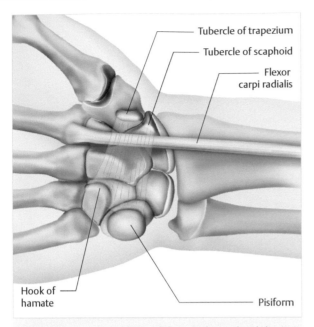

Fig. 4.76 Osseous boundaries of the carpal tunnel and the flexor carpi radialis tendon.

- Tubercle of trapezium
- Tubercle of scaphoid
- Flexor carpi radialis
- Hook of hamate
- Pisiform

index finger is positioned directly next to it on the trapezium (► Fig. 4.77).

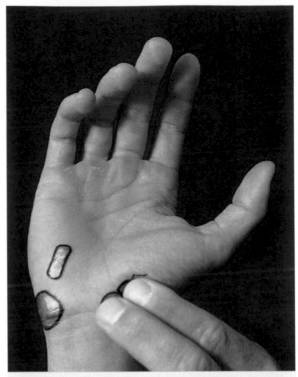

Fig. 4.77 Location of the scaphoid using radial deviation of the hand.

Tips

- The wrist is first actively or passively extended and flexed. The positioned finger pads follow the movement of the hand. The two carpal bones move against each other. During wrist extension, the scaphoid becomes more prominent and the trapezium less distinct. Flexion causes the trapezium to protrude, and the scaphoid disappears dorsally. The groove between the two bones now becomes even more prominent and it is possible to hook onto the trapezium from proximal.
- The finger pads remain on the tubercles and the hand is now moved into radial or ulnar deviation. The scaphoid becomes clearly more superficial during radial deviation and virtually pushes the middle finger away from the hand (► Fig. 4.77). The opposite pattern of movement is observed during ulnar deviation of the hand (► Fig. 4.78).

The joint space of the carpometacarpal joint lies as a direct extension of the tuberculum of the trapezius toward the bones of the thumb. The base of metacarpal I can be very easily visualized dorsally by adduction of the thumb. The base protrudes in a palmar direction during this movement (see ► Fig. 4.45).

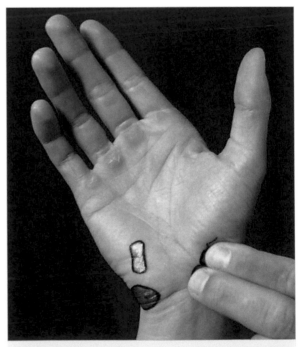

Fig. 4.78 Location of the trapezium using ulnar deviation of the hand.

Ulnar Head and Radiocarpal Joint Space

Now the osseous walls of the carpal tunnel are defined and the carpal bones forming the floor of the tunnel (central column) can be found.

To visualize the precise location, auxiliary lines and spatial orientation are needed, since the lunate and capitate, covered by soft tissue, cannot be directly palpated.

Display of the precise position of the radiocarpal joint space is the first visual aid. Finding the radial edge was already described in the section on overall palmar orientation. Now the palpating finger is oriented at the ulnar aspect of this line, directly proximal to the pisiform (▶ Fig. 4.79). The ulnar head is sought by means of circular palpation. Once more, the DRUJ lies at the radial boundary; the distal boundary forms a portion of the radiocarpal joint space. Now all the requirements for finding the lunate have been completed (▶ Fig. 4.80).

Lunate and Capitate

The proximal boundary of the lunate is the radiocarpal joint space formed by the connection of the radial styloid process with the distal aspect of the DRUJ space. Approximately in the middle of the connection, using vertical

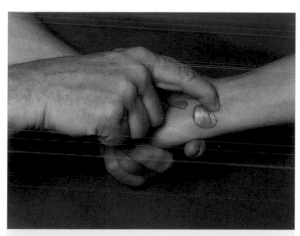

Fig. 4.79 Palpation of the palmar head of the ulna.

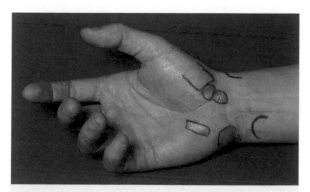

Fig. 4.80 Overview of structures accessible from palmar.

palpation, moderate pressure, and a little patience, the boundary between the joint facet of the radius for the scaphoid (scaphoid fossa) and the joint facet for the lunate (lunate fossa) can be felt as a slight eminence. It lies directly ulnar to the tendons of the flexor carpi radialis. This defines the extent of the lunate in the radial direction. As with the dorsal location, the joint space of the DRUJ is the radial boundary. The distal extent is visualized by a connecting line between the radial styloid process and the middle of the pisiform bone (▶ Fig. 4.81).

The capitate lies directly distal to it. It is reached indirectly halfway along a line between the pisiform and the tuberculum of the trapezium (▶ Fig. 4.81).

Transverse Carpal Ligament and the Carpal Tunnel

Since the osseous walls and the carpal bones of the floor have been found, the transverse carpal ligament that covers the carpal arch to form a tunnel is added. Because direct palpation cannot be exact, auxiliary lines are again used to arrive at a precise visualization. The area can be reliably distinguished from the hard carpal bones or the soft structures of the palm by its tough elastic consistency. And yet, it is not possible to establish a clear boundary by palpation. Beckenbaugh (2010) describes the start of the carpal tunnel at the distal aspect of the lunate bone. For reliable visualization of the tunnel, one concludes that the ligament must be situated between the visualized carpal bones, and this is supported by the literature.

The dimensions of the ligament become clear when the therapist draws lines between the ulnarly positioned pisiform and hook of hamate and the tubercles of the scaphoid and trapezium on the radial side.

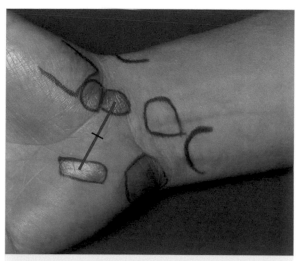

Fig. 4.81 Position of the lunate.

4

Two facts in particular stand out when examining the drawing on the skin:
- The ligament is quite large.
- The ligament is not square, but rather resembles a trapezoid with a wide ulnar edge.

Despite this, the large dimensions of the drawing of the ligament should not mislead the therapist; the distance between the bony walls of the carpal tunnel is the width of a small finger.

Median Nerve

In addition to the nine tendons that pass through this narrow carpal tunnel, the median nerve also travels through the tunnel with a very superficial pathway (▶ Fig. 4.82). Its course cannot be followed by palpation, and guide structures as well as information from topographical anatomy are needed. The palmaris longus marks its position in the distal forearm. The nerve lies directly below the tendon and runs superficially through the carpal tunnel and then chiefly supplies the motor innervation of the hypothenar.

The nerve position in the carpal tunnel is not constant. It shifts with movements of the fingers, the hand, even proximal and distal movements of the elbow and shoulder. Sixty degree extensions of the hand change its position by an average of 19.6 mm to distal and 10.4 mm to proximal after 65° flexion. Finger movements from maximal extension to maximal flexion cause an excursion of the nerve of a total of 9.7 mm. Even 90° elbow flexion and shoulder abduction and adduction can move the nerve in the carpal tunnel by another 2.5 to 2.9 mm (Wright et al., 1996).

4.7.3 Tips for Assessment and Treatment

The advantages of locating the carpal bones on the palmar aspect of the wrist fall into two groups:
- **Exact location of the carpal bones.** This is especially useful when individual bones have to be accurately differentiated from one another for local tests and treatment at the wrist joint. Using the example of dorsal and palmar location of the scaphoid, it becomes apparent that the palmarly and dorsally positioned fingers are not found directly opposite one another. The scaphoid runs significantly further to distal than in its dorsal aspect. The therapist cannot avoid having to precisely locate the bony landmarks, as tests would otherwise prove inconclusive.
- **Provocation of compression neuropathies.** The presence of nerve compression syndromes in the hand can be proven by using local pressure on the narrowing passage to provoke symptoms. This applies to the carpal tunnel syndrome and the compression of the ulnar nerve in the Guyon canal. Knowledge of local surface anatomy is useful in the carpal tunnel area when Tinel and Tetro tests are being used:

In the Tinel test, percussion is applied to the carpal tunnel to provoke the patient's symptoms (▶ Fig. 4.83).

In 1998, Tetro et al. described a new carpal compression test with continuous local compression of the carpal tunnel with the hand flexed (▶ Fig. 4.84). The arm lies with the elbow extended and the forearm supinated. With the hand flexed by 60°, pressure is exerted on the carpal tunnel with two thumbs. The test is positive if symptoms set in within 30 seconds. With a sensitivity of

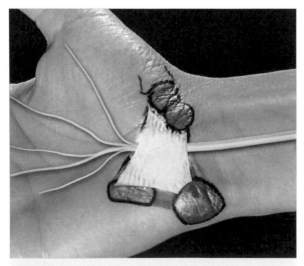

Fig. 4.82 Projection of the transverse carpal ligament and the median nerve.

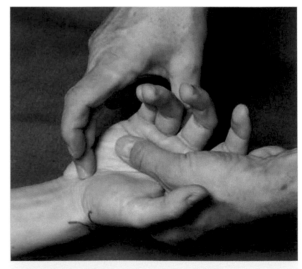

Fig. 4.83 Tinel test.

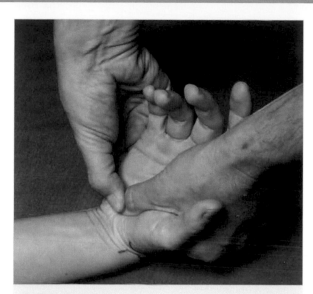

Fig. 4.84 Tetro test.

85% and a specificity of 95%, the test is one of the most reliable in clinical diagnostics.

Bibliography

Bain GI, Eng K, Lee YC, Mcguire D, Zumstein M. Reconstruction of chronic foveal TFCC tears with an autologous tendon graft. J Wrist Surg. 2015; 4(1):9–14

Balakrishnan C, Bachusz RC, Balakrishnan A, Elliot D, Careaga D. Intraneural lipoma of the radial nerve presenting as Wartenberg syndrome: a case report and review of literature. Can J Plast Surg. 2009; 17(4):e39–e41

Beckenbaugh RD. The Carpal Tunnel Syndrome. In: Cooney WP, ed. The Wrist: Diagnosis and Operative Treatment. 2nd ed. Philadelpia: Lippincott Williams & Wilkins; 2010:1105

Berger RA. Anatomy of the Wrist. In: Weinzweig J, ed. Plastic Surgery – Secrets Plus. 2nd ed. St. Louis: Mosby; 2010:939–945

De Lange ALH, Kauer JMG, Huiskes R. A kinematical study of the human wrist joint [Doctoral Thesis]. Nijmegen, NL: Universität Nijmegen; 1987

Die International Academy of Orthopedic Medicine.https://www.iaom.de

Hara T, Horii E, An KN, Cooney WP, Linscheid RL, Chao EY. Force distribution across wrist joint: application of pressure-sensitive conductive rubber. J Hand Surg Am. 1992; 17(2):339–347

Hollevoet N, Van Maele G, Van Seymortier P, Verdonk R. Comparison of palmar tilt, radial inclination and ulnar variance in left and right wrists. J Hand Surg [Br]. 2000; 25(5):431–433

Hoppenfeld S. Klinische Untersuchung der Wirbelsäule und Extremitäten. 2. Aufl. Stuttgart: Fischer; 1992

Ihle JEW, van Kampen PN. Vergleichende Anatomie der Wirbeltiere. 2nd ed. Heidelberg: Springer; 2011

Kapandji IA. Funktionelle Anatomie der Gelenke. 4. Aufl. Stuttgart: Thieme; 2006

Kobayashi M, Garcia-Elias M, Nagy L, et al. Axial loading induces rotation of the proximal carpal row bones around unique screw-displacement axes. J Biomech. 1997; 30(11–12):1165–1167

Kuhn S, Burkhart KJ, Schneider J, et al. The anatomy of the proximal radius: implications on fracture implant design. J Shoulder Elbow Surg. 2012; 21(9):1247–1254

Lester B, Halbrecht J, Levy IM, Gaudinez R. "Press test" for office diagnosis of triangular fibrocartilage complex tears of the wrist. Ann Plast Surg. 1995; 35(1):41–45

Lichtman DM, Wroten ES. Understanding midcarpal instability. J Hand Surg Am. 2006; 31(3):491–498

Matthijs O, van Paridon-Edauw, D, Winkel D. Manuelle Therapie der peripheren Gelenke, Bd. 2: Ellenbogen, Hand. München: Urban & Fischer bei Elsevier; 2003

Mbaka GO, Ejiwunmi AB. Prevalence of palmaris longus absence–a study in the Yoruba population. Ulster Med J. 2009; 78(2):90–93

Moritomo H, Apergis EP, Herzberg G, Werner FW, Wolfe SW, Garcia-Elias M. 2007 IFSSH committee report of wrist biomechanics committee: biomechanics of the so-called dart-throwing motion of the wrist. J Hand Surg Am. 2007; 32(9):1447–1453

Netter FH. Farbatlanten der Medizin, Bd. 7: Bewegungsapparat I. Stuttgart: Thieme; 1992

Pang EQ, Yao J. Ulnar-sided wrist pain in the athlete (TFCC/DRUJ/ECU). Curr Rev Musculoskelet Med. 2017; 10(1):53–61

Rauber A, Kopsch F. Anatomie des Menschen. Bd. 1 Bewegungsapparat. 3. Aufl. Stuttgart: Thieme; 2003

Rauber A, Leonhardt H, Eds. Anatomie des Menschen: Lehrbuch und Atlas. Bd. 1, Bewegungsapparat. Stuttgart: Thieme; 1987

Reagan DS, Linscheid RL, Dobyns JH. Lunotriquetral sprains. J Hand Surg Am. 1984; 9(4):502–514

Robson AJ, See MS, Ellis H. Applied anatomy of the superficial branch of the radial nerve. Clin Anat. 2008; 21(1):38–45

Ryu J, Klin J. Biomechanics of the Wrist. In: Weinzweig J. Plastic Surgery – Secrets Plus. 2nd ed. St. Louis: Mosby; 2010: 961–963

Schmauss D, Pöhlmann S, Lohmeyer JA, Germann G, Bickert B, Megerle K. Clinical tests and magnetic resonance imaging have limited diagnostic value for triangular fibrocartilaginous complex lesions. Arch Orthop Trauma Surg. 2016; 136(6):873–880

Schmidt HM, Lanz U. Chirurgische Anatomie der Hand. 2. Aufl. Stuttgart: Thieme; 2003

Spies CK, Müller LP, Oppermann J, Neiss WF, Hahn P, Unglaub F. Die operative Dekompression des Ramus superficialis des Nervus radialis: Das Wartenberg-Syndrom. Oper Orthop Traumatol. 2016; 28(2):145–152

Taleisnik J, Watson HK. Midcarpal instability caused by malunited fractures of the distal radius. J Hand Surg Am. 1984; 9(3):350–357

Tay SC, Tomita K, Berger RA. The "ulnar fovea sign" for defining ulnar wrist pain: an analysis of sensitivity and specificity. J Hand Surg Am. 2007; 32(4):438–444

Vezeridis PS, Yoshioka H, Han R, Blazar P. Ulnar-sided wrist pain. Part I: anatomy and physical examination. Skeletal Radiol. 2010; 39(8):733–745

Williams PL. Gray's anatomy. 40th ed. Edinburgh: Churchill Livingstone; 2009

Wright TW, Glowczewskie F, Wheeler D, Miller G, Cowin D. Excursion and strain of the median nerve. J Bone Joint Surg Am. 1996; 78(12):1897–1903

Zancolli EA, Ziadenberg C, Zancolli E, Jr. Biomechanics of the trapeziometacarpal joint. Clin OrthopRelat Res. 1987(220):14–26

Zanetti M, Gilula LA, Jacob HA, et al. Palmar tilt of the distal radius: influence of off-lateral projection initial observations. Radiology. 2001; 220:594–600

Zanetti M, Hodler J, Gilula LA. Assessment of dorsal or ventral intercalated segmental instability configurations of the wrist: reliability of sagittal MR images. Radiology. 1998; 206(2):339–345

4

Chapter 5

Hip and Groin Region

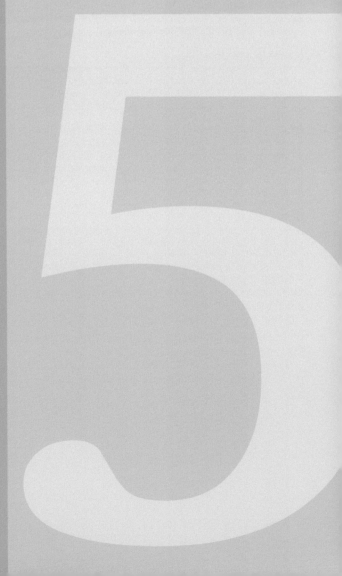

5 Hip and Groin Region

5.1 Introduction

5.1.1 Lumbar-Pelvic-Hip Region

The lumbopelvic-hip (LPH) region is a functional unit composed of the hip joints, pelvic connections, and the lumbar spine. As this book addresses the precise palpation of the joints of the limbs, the lateral and anterior hip complex will be selected and discussed in detail. The posterior hip and pelvic region is discussed in Chapter 9.

5.1.2 Functional Significance of the Pelvis and Hip Joint

The LPH region is subject to the principles of bipedal locomotion, as is the case for the entire construction of the lower limb. Support and locomotion are the most important aspects of these principles.

With this in mind, the first role of the LPH region is to form a connection between the lower limbs and the trunk. The sacroiliac (SI) joints are very large and rigid in comparison to the more delicate sternoclavicular joint that forms the junction between the upper limb and the trunk. The very steep articular surfaces and the tilted position of the sacrum make the construction and ligamental stability in the SI joint complicated in many respects.

The small movements observed in the SI joints and the pubic symphysis are especially necessary to cushion the transmission of loading, that is, for shock absorption. The principle of shock absorption is not only seen in the pelvis, but is also demonstrated in all sections of the lower limbs.

The complex connection between the lower limbs and the vertebral column also results in movement of the hip joint being transmitted directly onto the vertebral column. Movements of the pelvis and more superior movements acting on the pelvis also affect the other components of the LPH region. This becomes clear when looking at the example of hip extension. The normal range of hip extension is 10 to 15°. This movement is transmitted very quickly onto the articulations of the pelvis (SI joints and symphysis) and from there immediately onto the inferior segments of the lumbar spine.

While sitting, the pelvis transfers the load of the body to the surface on which the individual is seated or standing, and not to the legs.

Especially thick parts of the ilium transfer the load of the body from the SI joint to the acetabulum when the individual is upright.

5.1.3 Pathology and Common Applications for Treatment in this Region

The hip symptoms encountered in daily practice are numerous and very varied. If pain in the buttocks and groin is reported, functional differentiation of the pain generators is a diagnostic challenge that often requires considerable time and effort. The pain can originate in the lumbar spine, the pelvic connections, or the hip joints. The pain generators in pelvis and hip can be a variety of tissues: capsules, subchondral bones, labrum of the acetabulum, muscular insertions, tendons, bursae, peripheral nerves. An additional complication is the fact that pain generators close to the trunk can transmit symptoms as referred pain or pain projected to the legs, and this can extend the area in which pain is perceived (Lampert, 2009). For this reason, it is advisable when examining the LPH region to include in the diagnosis all components of the motor apparatus that could be possible causes of the symptoms.

Common Pathological Conditions in the Hip

- **Lateral hip symptoms:** Soft-tissue conditions over the greater trochanter (tendinosis, trochanteric bursitis) and referred pain in the hip joint.
- **Local posterior hip symptoms:** Insertion tendinopathy of the ischiocrural muscles, piriform syndrome, hamstring syndrome, femoroacetabular impingement, lesions of the acetabular labrum.
- **Groin pain:** Insertion tendinopathy (e.g., of the adductors), irritation of the pubic symphysis, referred pain originating in the lumbar spine or the SI joint, and naturally, problems in the hip joint (arthrosis, arthritis, labrum lesion, femoroacetabular impingement), compression neuropathy.

This selection is just a partial listing of all the hip and groin symptoms that are commonly met in a physical therapist's practice. Symptoms that occur on the dorsal aspect of the pelvis often originate in a pain generator in the spinal column or the sacroiliac joint.

Most hip and groin symptoms can be differentiated from one another by using special tests during assessment. Precise palpation is nevertheless required when tests do not help the therapist and when the exact position of the lesion needs to be identified and confirmed.

5.1.4 Required Basic Anatomical and Biomechanical Knowledge

To understand instructions for local palpation, the student needs some essential background information:
- The bony construction of the pelvis, especially the accessible elevated areas of bone.
- The geometry of the proximal femur, especially the femoral neck anteversion (FNA) angle.
- The names and positions of the muscles that cross over the hip joint with special emphasis on the extensors and adductors.

Bone Anatomy

Pelvis

The remarkable aspect of the bony pelvis is the three-dimensional construction of the large bones that form a ring. It is very difficult to illustrate this in the two-dimensional illustrations that are available to therapists. Therefore, it is important for the therapist to develop the ability to visualize the structure of the ring from different perspectives.

The bony landmarks of the pelvis, whose precise location will be discussed in this section, mainly lie on the anterior aspect (▶ Fig. 5.1).

These are consolidated into the anteriorly accessible sections of the ilium and pubis.

The local anatomy of the deep structures in the posterior pelvis will also be addressed in this section on palpation of the hip region (▶ Fig. 5.2).

The ischial tuberosity is the only posterior reference point that will be sought. All other structures will be discussed in Chapter 9.

Pubic Symphysis

The symphysis, an important component of the pelvic ring, exerts significant control of the hip bones and strongly influences the SI joints. This means that the symphysis offers the greatest resistance to the effects of movement on the pelvic ring.

It is very long, at 4 to 5 cm, but this is not apparent because it is tilted approximately 45° from anterocranial to dorsocaudal (▶ Fig. 5.8). In the middle, between the two symphyseal rami of the pubic bone, is a fibrocartilaginous disk. This interpubic disk varies in thickness and develops, from the age of 10, an increasingly wide articular cavity, which, from the age of 30, develops a synovial membrane. The symphysis is stabilized by the superior interpubic ligament and the arcuate ligament of the pubis. The arcuate ligament is the most important stabilizer. It consists of thick fibers running in an arc, which insert directly medial to the insertions (origin) of the gracilis on the rami of the pubic bone. Large shear forces can lead to irritations at this point; these shear forces arise with loading on a single foot. In walking, there is a vertical and ventral translation of 2.2 and 1.3 mm respectively (Meissner, 1996).

Through its highly differentiated innervation (ilioinguinal and genitofemoral nerves, T12-L2, as well as the pudendal nerve, S2-S4), the symphysis is a potential pain generator with a uni- or bilateral pain perception area in the lower abdomen, anal, and genital areas and toward the medial thigh. Arthropathies of the symphysis are divided into four stages and are often associated with instability (increased translation). Palpation to locate an irritated muscular structure in adductor problems should always include the possibility of symphyseal irritation.

Hip Joint

The geometry of the bones in the joint can predispose the hip joint for certain pathologies: femoroacetabular impingement with/without lesions of the acetabular labrum, as well as coxarthrosis. The hip joint undergoes multiple changes during development, and individual variations of the spatial relation between femoral head and acetabulum are the rule.

The variations in size given for the caput-collumdiaphyseal (CCD) angle are well known. This angle

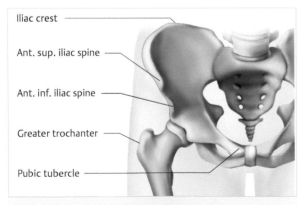

Fig. 5.1 Pelvic structures—anterior view.

Iliac crest

Ant. sup. iliac spine

Ant. inf. iliac spine

Greater trochanter

Pubic tubercle

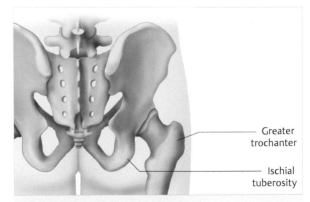

Fig. 5.2 Osseous structures—posterior view.

Greater trochanter

Ischial tuberosity

describes the superomedial orientation of the femoral head with respect to the shaft; at birth it is approximately 150°. Reduction of the angle with advancing age to approximately 133° at the age of 15, and even lower in adults, varies inter- and intraindividually. Overall, there is agreement in the literature that a coxa vara exists from approximately 120° and less. This can favor the occurrence of a femoroacetabular impingement between the collum femoris and the border of the acetabulum. A CCD angle of over 135°, a coxa valga, is a predisposing factor for early coxarthrosis but also involves the danger of overloading the labrum at the superior edge of the acetabulum (Matthijs et al., 2003).

The antetorsion angle (ATA) is one of the determinants of the hip joint's degree of rotation. The greater it is, the greater is the inward rotation capacity of the hip joint in normally elastic soft tissue (capsule and muscles). The ATA determines the degree of anterior twisting of the femoral neck with respect to the shaft. In drawings, the position of the shaft is usually represented as a transverse connection through the condyles at the distal femur (▶ Fig. 5.3).

Children have a large ATA (Rudorff 2007) and can therefore often achieve remarkable inward rotation. As the skeleton grows, the ATA is reduced to an average of 14 to 15° (von Lanz and Wachsmuth, 2004) as variously reported in the literature. Reduction of the 35° ATA of early childhood (Matthijs et al., 2003) results in inter- and especially intraindividual differences.

Determination of the ATA is of interest when it is found that there is a difference in rotational capability of the hip joints between one side and the other. The degree of inward plus outward rotation should always be the same. The ATA determines the distribution in favor of inward or outward rotation. However, this widespread opinion of teachers in the field of physical therapy was challenged by Tavares Canto et al. (2005). In his study, he found no significant correlation between the ATA and the degree of rotation, so the conclusion must be drawn that additional parameters, such as the geometry of the acetabulum, influence hip rotation.

Manual determination of the ATA by palpation of the lateral major trochanter has special importance in preoperative diagnosis of children with cerebral palsy, before derotation osteotomy. There are also validation studies from authors (Ruwe et al., 1992; Chung et al., 2010) that confirm the accuracy of this test.

The greater trochanter is especially easy to access on the **femur.** The remaining structures are either hidden by thick layers of soft tissue or can only be identified using guiding structures.

The size of the greater trochanter in living subjects is astonishing. For example, the posterior area between the trochanter and the lateral border of the ischial tuberosity amounts to only approximately 2 to 3 finger widths.

Once again, illustrations and common anatomical models cause confusion as the trochanter is too small in these examples and the spatial relationship to the pelvis too large.

In recent years, the geometry of the acetabulum coxae has also been substantiated. It is angled in all three planes. In the frontal plane, the angle is approximately 60° in children and approximately 45° to the transverse in adults (▶ Fig. 5.4). In the transverse plane, the acetabulum is often not uniformly inclined laterally out of the sagittal plane. The upper portion describes an approximately 20° angle, the lower a 45° angle, which creates a distinct torsion of the acetabulum. In the sagittal plane, the acetabulum is tipped backward by approximately 30°, which causes the notch in the acetabular edge to point down and forward.

Relevant Anterior Soft Tissues

The position of the anterior muscles is usually divided into the following:
- The lateral femoral triangle (▶ Fig. 5.5).
- The medial femoral triangle (▶ Fig. 5.6)

This topographical classification aids orientation on the anterior aspect.

The **lateral femoral triangle** is bordered by the following:
- The tensor fasciae latae (medial edge of the muscle belly).
- The sartorius (lateral edge of the muscle belly).

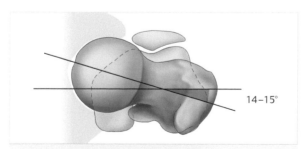

Fig. 5.3 The femoral neck anteversion angle.

14–15°

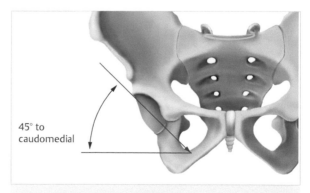

45° to caudomedial

Fig. 5.4 Angling of the acetabulum.

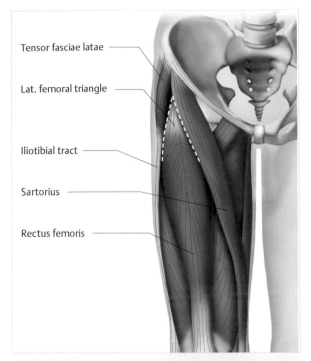

Fig. 5.5 Lateral femoral triangle.

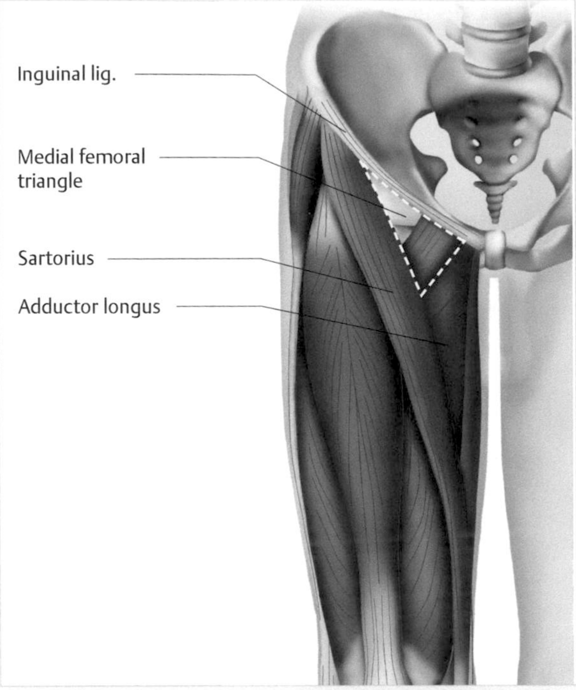

Inguinal lig.

Medial femoral triangle

Sartorius

Adductor longus

Fig. 5.6 Medial femoral triangle.

This area is actually not a triangle, but is instead shaped like an arrowhead with its tip pointing upward. The triangle does not have a third border. The two participating muscles are in contact with the anterior superior iliac spine (ASIS). This is the most important osseous orientation point on the anterior pelvis.

The anterior inferior iliac spine (AIIS) and rectus femoris are found deep in this triangle.

The **medial femoral triangle** is the actual trigonum femorale (femoral triangle) and was first described by the Italian anatomist Antonio Scarpa (1752–1832). It is a proper triangle and is formed by the following:
• The sartorius (medial edge of the muscle belly).
• The adductor longus (medial edge of the muscle belly).
• The ligament of the groin (inguinal ligament).

In addition to the previously mentioned ASIS, the pubic tubercle is also another important bony point for orientation.

Knowledge of this triangle helps the therapist to locate lesions in the clinically important flexor and adductor muscle groups. Furthermore, the position of the large neurovascular bundle directly anterior to the hip joint can be identified.

The following are the structures (from lateral to medial) (▶ Fig. 5.7):
• The femoral nerve.
• The femoral artery.
• The femoral vein.

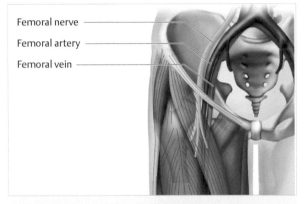

Femoral nerve
Femoral artery
Femoral vein

Fig. 5.7 Neurovascular bundle in the groin.

The vessels leave the pelvic space together and cross under the inguinal ligament in the vascular lacuna, while the nerve accompanies the iliopsoas muscle passing through the lacuna musculorum. The inguinal ligament is a gathering of fasciae of the anterolateral muscles, thus not a real ligament in the usual sense. It extends between the ASIS and the pubic tubercle, another important osseous landmark. Lateral to the ASIS, the inguinal ligament is very flat and tapers visibly along its spiral course to medial. The groin (sulcus inguinalis) only coincides with the inguinal ligament in thin individuals. With an even slightly increased proportion of body fat, the groin falls below the level of the ligament. The superficial inguinal lymph nodes lie in the groin; they will not be discussed further here. The inguinal area cranial to the inguinal ligament is explained in Chapter 11.

Pubic Symphysis

The symphysis, an important component of the pelvic ring, exerts significant control of the hip bones and strongly influences the SI joints. This means that the symphysis offers the greatest resistance to the effects of movement on the pelvic ring.

It is very long, at 4 to 5 cm, but this is not apparent because it is tilted approximately 45° (Mens et al., 1999) from anterocranial to dorsocaudal (▶ Fig. 5.8). In the middle, between the two symphyseal rami of the pubic bone, is a fibrocartilaginous disk. This interpubic disk varies in thickness and develops, from the age of 10, an increasingly wide articular cavity, which, from the age of 30, develops a synovial membrane. The symphysis is stabilized by the superior interpubic ligament and the arcuate ligament of the pubis. The arcuate ligament is the most important stabilizer. It consists of thick fibers running in an arc, which insert directly medial to the insertions (origin) of the gracilis on the rami of the pubic bone. Large shear forces can lead to irritations at this point; these shear forces arise with loading on a single foot. In walking, there is a vertical and ventral translation of 2.2 and 1.3 mm respectively (Meissner, 1996).

Through its highly differentiated innervation (ilioinguinal and genitofemoral nerves, T12-L2, as well as the pudendal nerve, S2-S4), the symphysis is a potential pain generator with a uni- or bilateral pain perception area in the lower abdomen, anal, and genital areas and toward the medial thigh. Arthropathies of the symphysis are divided into four stages and are often associated with

instability (increased translation). Palpation to locate an irritated muscular structure in adductor problems should always include the possibility of symphyseal irritation.

Relevant Posterior Soft Tissues

The hamstring muscles and the insertion of their common head onto the ischial tuberosity are the soft-tissue structures posterior to the hip joint that are important for palpation (▶ Fig. 5.9).

The muscle bellies of the biceps femoris, semimembranosus, and semitendinosus converge proximally and form a common tendon of origin.

Contrary to common belief, the muscle bellies are not aligned along the middle of the proximal femur, but are rather angled in a medial direction. The reason for this angled course is seen in the more medial position of the tuberosity.

Fibers from the tendon of origin (especially the segments of the biceps femoris muscle) sometimes even merge further into the sacrotuberous ligament (Mercer et al., 2005) and can therefore, theoretically, directly influence the SI joint (Woodley, 2005).

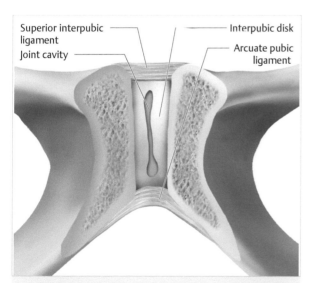

Fig. 5.8 Structure of the pubic symphysis.

Superior interpubic ligament
Joint cavity
Interpubic disk
Arcuate pubic ligament

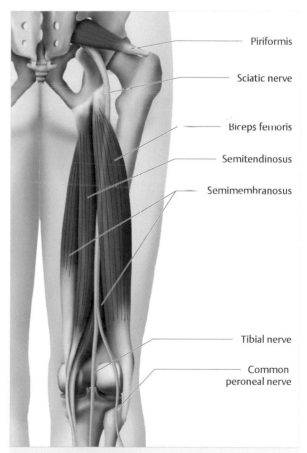

Fig. 5.9 Important posterior soft-tissue structures.

Piriformis
Sciatic nerve
Biceps femoris
Semitendinosus
Semimembranosus
Tibial nerve
Common peroneal nerve

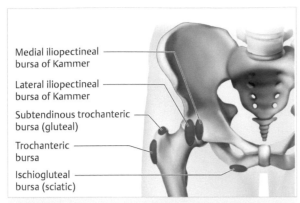

Fig. 5.10 Bursae of the hip region (after Omer Matthijs).

Labels in figure:
Medial iliopectineal bursa of Kammer
Lateral iliopectineal bursa of Kammer
Subtendinous trochanteric bursa (gluteal)
Trochanteric bursa
Ischiogluteal bursa (sciatic)

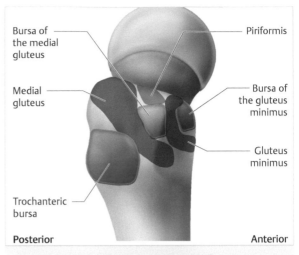

Fig. 5.11 Bursae at the greater trochanter (after Omer Matthijs).

Labels in figure:
Bursa of the medial gluteus
Medial gluteus
Trochanteric bursa
Posterior
Piriformis
Bursa of the gluteus minimus
Gluteus minimus
Anterior

The functional importance of this muscle group is viewed far beyond its concentric-dynamic actions (extension of the hip joint, flexion of the knee joint). Proximally, the hamstrings assist other muscles to help control the pelvis in the sagittal plane and prevent the pelvis from tilting down anteriorly. Toward the knee joint, the hamstrings develop their strongest contraction at the end of the swing phase. The muscles decelerate the anterior swing of the leg just before heel strike to prevent excessive loading on the passive structures in the joint.

In hip flexion and extension, the sciatic nerve moves in its course along the lateral tuberosity and the common head. Especially in adduction, it is compressed against neighboring structures. As a result of scar formation after muscle injuries, long periods of sitting, fast running, or exaggerated stretching exercises of the ischiocrural muscles, the nerve can become irritated through friction or stretching (hamstring syndrome; Puranen and Orava, 1991).

Bursae

The course of muscles along bony eminences and edges as well as insertions involves a large number of bursae in a variety of locations. ▶ Fig. 5.10 gives an overview of those that could be of clinical interest in the case of bursitis and are often indirectly palpable. These are the following:

- The **iliopectineal bursa,** lodged between the underside of the iliopsoas nerve and the iliopubic ramus, which protects the muscle against friction where it passes under the inguinal ligament.
- **Bursae of the greater trochanter**—here, under the insertion of the gluteus minimus and medius muscles, there is a subtendinous bursa under each. On the lateral surface, on the boundary with the iliotibial tract, is the trochanteric bursa (Pfirrmann et al., 2001).
- The **sciatic bursa of the gluteus maximus,** located at the inferomedial aspect of the sciatic tuberosity, which reduces friction between the muscle and the tuberosity.

Relevant Lateral Soft Tissues

Tendinosis and bursitis at the greater trochanter are known sources of lateral hip pain (Barratt et al., 2017). The study by Pfirrmann et al. (2001) clarifies the position of the gluteal insertions and bursae (▶ Fig. 5.11).

Seen from posterior to anterior, there is a continuous alternation between bursae and insertions. Each insertion of the gluteus minimus has its own bursa to protect it from friction. The largest bursa covers the posterior facet of the greater trochanter, the distal and lateral portions of the gluteus medius tendon, and the proximal portion of the vastus lateralis origin (Pfirrmann et al., 2001).

5.2 Local Palpation—Lateral

5.2.1 Overview of the Structures to be Palpated

- Greater trochanter.
- Femoral neck anteversion angle (FNA).
- Insertions and bursae at the greater trochanter.

5.2.2 Summary of the Palpatory Process

This palpation involves finding easily accessible structures. It starts by locating and palpating the entire surface of the greater trochanter. The greater trochanter is palpated to provoke pain in locally inflamed soft tissues and to identify one of the most important aspects in the geometry of the proximal femur: the FNA angle.

Starting Position

The patient is in prone position, the arms rest next to the body, and a foot roll can be positioned underneath the ankles. This prone position only needs to be modified for patients suffering from hip joint or lumbar spine symptoms.

To locate boundaries and surfaces of the greater trochanter and to determine the ATA, the knee must be bent for rotational movement of the hip joint. The therapist stands on the contralateral side.

5.2.3 Palpation of Individual Structures

Greater Trochanter

As almost the only directly accessible section of the proximal femur, the greater trochanter acts as an important orientation point in the lateral region of the hip. It is the site of insertion for several small muscles coming from the pelvis, lengthens the lever for the small gluteal muscles, and its palpation allows conclusions regarding the geometry of the femur.

The greater trochanter is naturally found laterally, at around the same level as the tip of the sacrum approximately at the start of the post-anal furrow (see ▸ Fig. 9.32). The trochanter is located approximately 1 hand width inferior to the iliac crest.

Technique

The trochanter is found and recognized in the region described by palpating the area, applying moderate deep pressure, and feeling a hard resistance. With perpendicular palpation, its superior and anterior and posterior borders can be distinctly felt (▸ Fig. 5.12). If the anterior and posterior borders are grasped between thumb and index finger, the width of the trochanter becomes clear (▸ Fig. 5.13). Directly lateral, in the same plane, a large surface of the trochanter can be felt, on which the small gluteus muscles insert, protected by a few bursae.

> ### Tip
>
> As this region is often obese, palpation may be difficult and it may be necessary to confirm the location using the following aid.
>
> The therapist flexes the ipsilateral knee and uses the leg as a lever to alternately medially and laterally rotate the hip joint. The trochanter then rolls back and forth underneath the palpating finger so that both its lateral surface and its superior aspect can be easily palpated.
>
> This is the starting point of the dorsal palpation that will follow.

Femoral Neck Anteversion Angle

The FNA angle helps determine the amount of medial rotation at the hip joint. The larger the angle is, the greater the ability of the hip joint to medially rotate—providing the soft tissues (capsule and muscles) have normal elasticity.

In children with cerebral palsy, the angle is determined before derotation osteotomy. Rapid manual determination of the FNA (also known as the ATA "Antetorsion Angle") goes back to Drehmann (1909) (Tönnis and Legal, 1984) and is based on estimation or goniometric measurement of the angle at the moment when the most lateral forward curve of the trochanter is palpated (Ruwe et al., 1992). The exactitude of this rapid determination is amazingly high. Ruwe et al. (1992) describe the average difference between the trochanteric eminence angle test and intraoperative measurements to be approximately 4° with an intratester error of 5°. The excellent validity and reliability of this test was confirmed again by Chung et al. (2010).

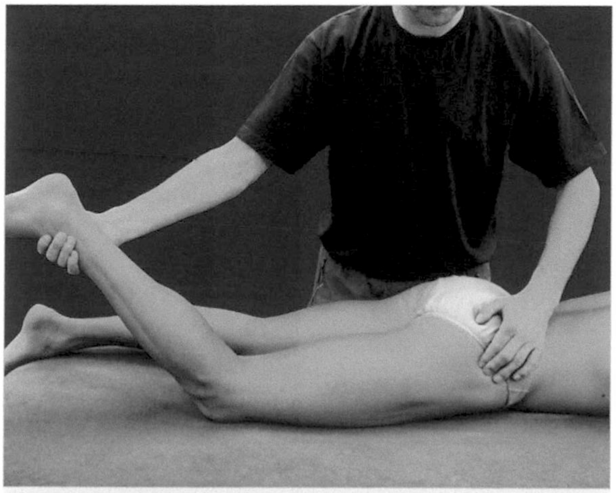

Fig. 5.12 Palpation of the tip of the trochanter.

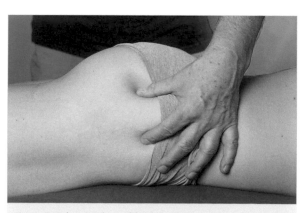

Fig. 5.13 Palpating the width of the trochanter.

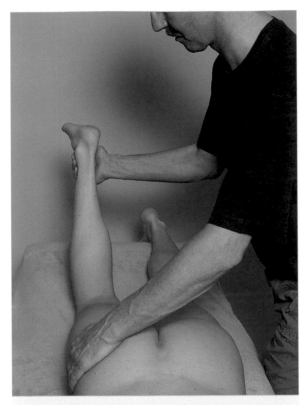

Fig. 5.14 Demonstrating the FNA angle—phase 1.

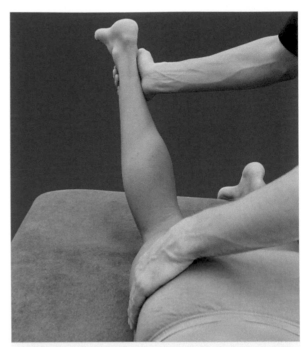

Fig. 5.15 Demonstrating the FNA angle—phase 2.

Technique

The therapist positions the hip in neutral rotation and flexes the knee. The flat hand palpates laterally over the trochanter (▶ Fig. 5.14).

The hip is placed in medial rotation by moving the leg laterally away from the sagittal plane. The therapist should now be able to visualize the greater trochanter moving in a large arc around the head of the femur during the medial rotation movement.

While continuing to palpate, the medial rotation movement is stopped at the position where the trochanter is felt to be most lateral (▶ Fig. 5.15).

Now the femoral neck is in the frontal plane and the angle of antetorsion can be determined (estimated in angular degrees or measured with a goniometer). The expected average is approximately 10 to 16° (Schneider et al., 1997). The values depend in part on imaging procedures and vary intraindividually (approx. 5°; Schneider et al., 1997) and interindividually.

Palpation of the Insertions and Bursae at the Lateral Greater Trochanter

The site of insertion of the pelvitrochanteric muscles and of the gluteus minimus muscles can be palpated for tenderness.

Starting Position

The patient is in side-lying position with the side to be palpated on top. The patient slides on the treatment table somewhat more to the side of the therapist. The hip and knee joints are slightly flexed. The knee joints are on top of each other with a soft cushion placed between them if desired. First, the accessible edges of the greater trochanter are demonstrated with perpendicular palpation and the border is marked on the surface (▶ Fig. 5.11).

Tip

If it is not possible to palpate the edges of the greater trochanter well, the correct location can always be confirmed easily by rotating the leg and moving the bone below the hand while doing the palpation.

A line is then drawn from anterior to posterior, dividing the demonstrated area into a proximal and a distal half. Perpendicular to this line, another line is drawn that divides this area into an anterior and a posterior half, forming quadrants.

- The anterior-proximal quadrant is marked with a marking on its anterior and its posterior third for the bursae of the gluteus minimus and medius muscles.
- The posterior-distal quadrant is filled in with a marking for the trochanteric bursa (▶ Fig. 5.11).
- The insertion of the tendon of the gluteus minimus extends from the anterior border of the anterior-distal

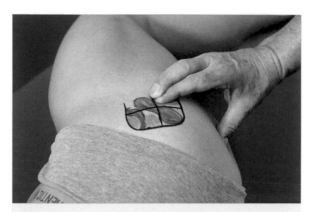

Fig. 5.16 Palpation of the trochanteric bursa.

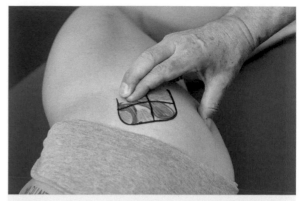

Fig. 5.17 Palpation of the insertions at the trochanter.

quadrant to the center third of the anterior-proximal quadrant.
- The insertion of the tendon of the gluteus medius extends from the posterior two-thirds of the anterior-distal quadrant to the upper half of the posterior-proximal quadrant (▶ Fig. 5.11).

Trochanteric Bursa

In addition to muscular or tendo-osseous complaints, bursitis in the region of the trochanter can be the source of local pain in the lateral buttocks. Inflammation of the trochanteric bursa of the gluteus maximus is most common. The technique described above can be used to palpate the side of the trochanter and the area medial to the gluteal tuberosity for pain sensitivity (▶ Fig. 5.16).

Tips for Treatment

As with any other prominent site with a bursa, it will not be felt as a structure. Only if the patient has bursitis will the patient respond to pain provocation and may possibly report the feeling of fluctuant synovial fluid in the swollen bursa during palpation.

Trochanteric bursitis has long been a known source of lateral hip pain. Detailed understanding of the morphology of the peritrochanteric bursae is important for confirming the diagnosis through palpation and for treatment, for example, with local infiltration. Dunn et al. (2003) studied the morphological connections and positions of the different peritrochanteric bursae in 21 cadavers. They located 121 bursae at 10 different sites. In addition to the many variations, a bursa between the greater trochanter and the gluteus maximus or the iliotibial tract was always observed. In most cases, a bursa with the gluteus minimus was also discovered.

Bursitis can be easily confirmed by applying direct pressure against the trochanter, especially with the patient in side-lying position. On the basis of its findings, the International Academy of Orthopedic Medicine differentiates insertion tendinopathies from bursitis by means

of direct provocative palpation in various positions of the hip joint. The starting point is with the patients lying on their side (not illustrated).
- The painful place on the trochanter is found with palpation.
- The palpation is repeated with active abduction.

If the intensity of the pain remains constant with abduction, the disorder is a tendinopathy. If pain decreases, it is a trochanteric bursitis.

Insertion tendinopathy can be treated with transverse frictioning on the trochanter using flat fingers (▶ Fig. 5.17).

Patients often report pain in the lateral buttocks. However, this does not necessarily mean that the pain originates in this region. In many cases, the pain is a result of referred or projected pain with the pain generators located further proximal. In addition to thorough functional testing, local palpation to provoke pain is very helpful for precisely locating the pain origin.

5.3 Local Palpation—Dorsal

5.3.1 Overview of the Structures to be Palpated

- Pelvitrochanteric fossa.
- Ischial tuberosity.
- Ischiocrural muscles and tendon of origin.

5.3.2 Summary of the Palpatory Process

In the following we turn to another bony structure that is easy to find, the ischial tuberosity (also tuberosity of the ischium). This is an important fixed point for thick ligaments that contribute to securing the sacroiliac joint (sacrotuberous ligament) and for strong extensors (ischiocrural muscles). The tendinous portions of these muscles converge at the tuberosity and can be felt as a large, common tendon.

Starting Position

The patient is prone, that is, the arms are close to the body and the ankles can be supported by a foot roll. The prone position may only be modified for patients with hip joint or lumbar spine symptoms.

In palpating the tendon at the ischiocrural origin, it can be advantageous to have the patient lie on their side with flexed hip joints.

5.3.3 Palpation of Individual Structures

Width of the Pelvitrochanteric Fossa

The fossa between the greater trochanter and the ischial tuberosity is depicted much too large in both anatomy textbooks and the usual models. In a leg in rotationally neutral position it is only 2 to 3 fingers wide. During external rotation, the fossa is considerably narrowed. As already discussed, the pelvitrochanteric muscles and the approximately thumb-wide sciatic nerve are located here (▶ Fig. 5.18).

Technique

Starting from the last technique, one hand is rotated and two fingers are pressed into the soft tissues on the posterior side of the greater trochanter, exerting a great deal of pressure. Now a consistency assessment is used to confirm the correct location and the proximity to the bony structures. The therapist presses one finger against the edge of the trochanter and the other finger in the direction of the tuberosity. In both cases, a hard, bony response is expected.

Ischial Tuberosity

The apophyseal enlargement on the posterior side of the ischium between its body and its ramus is called the ischial tuberosity. Overall, it is so far posterior that it only transmits weight onto the seat when an individual

is sprawling in a chair. When the pelvis is vertical, the long axis of the tuberosity is oriented from inferomedial to superolateral. Medially, its entire edge serves as the insertion of the sacrotuberous ligament and its lateral edge lies at the origin of the quadratus femoris muscle. The distribution of the insertions of the tendons and the position of the sciatic bursa are highly varied. Portions of the tendons can also transition directly into the sacrotuberous ligament without insertions into the tuberosity. The adductor magnus muscle mainly inserts at the ischiopubic ramus connecting ventrally (Windisch et al., 2017).

Technique

Method 1

From the back of the greater trochanter, the palpating finger falls into a pelvitrochanteric fossa that is approximately 2 fingers wide, bounded medially by the lateral edge of the tuberosity (see Chapter 9). In this gap are the quadratus femoris nerve and the sciatic nerve that run close by the edge of the tuberosity, which may undergo pathological friction there.

Method 2

With a fork grasp (thumb medial) the therapist follows the transverse fold of the buttocks in a medial direction until the thumb meets the tuberosity (▶ Fig. 5.19). The principal relevant feature for the palpation is the peak of the tuberosity.

Palpation for Muscle Activity in the Pelvic Floor

It is possible to palpate the muscle activity in the pelvic floor from the accessible caudal portions of the tuberosity without coming too close to the anal area.

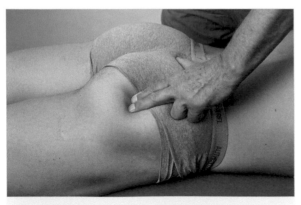

Fig. 5.18 Demonstration of the pelvitrochanteric fossa.

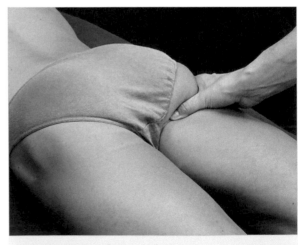

Fig. 5.19 Palpation of the ischial tuberosity.

Technique

To palpate the activity on the right side, the therapist stands next to the right side of the patient's body. Using flat fingers and palpating with the fingertips are recommended.

Starting from the tuberosity, move the fingertips in a medial direction and follow the bony contours. When the finger pads encounter firm elastic resistance, the pelvic floor has been reached. This is confirmed by relevant activity. If the muscles (levator ani muscle) are contracted, the finger pads are pushed out in a posterior direction.

Tips for Treatment

This palpation is suitable as a feedback method when instructing patients to stimulate or strengthen their pelvic floor muscles. Patients can also use this tactile feedback when doing exercises on their own.

Ischiocrural Muscle Bellies and Tendon of Origin

The aim is to palpate the borders of the muscles and their insertions. The bellies of the muscles become distinct when the muscles contract into knee flexion against resistance (► Fig. 5.20).

Technique—Muscle Bellies

The borders can be easily palpated by holding the contraction or rhythmically contracting and relaxing. It is noticeable that the muscles on the posterior thigh do not follow the axis of the leg, but have an angled course. They travel proximally and medially toward the ischial tuberosity.

Tip

As the muscles are approximated proximally in the prone position, the knee should not be flexed extensively and the therapist should not let the patient contract the muscle too strongly, to avoid the risk of muscle cramping. If the objective is to provoke tendinopathies or insertion tendinopathies by significant activity, an effective starting position is with the patient in prone position with the legs hanging over the treatment table. Here the knee can be flexed with a flexed hip. In this way, the ischiocrural muscles are proximally prestretched, easier to provoke, and not as likely to cramp.

The vastus lateralis of the quadriceps femoris forms the lateral boundary to the hamstrings, in particular the biceps femoris. This is all the more surprising because the vastus lateralis is expected to be found more anteriorly on the thigh than posteriorly. The quadriceps actually lies not only anteriorly and laterally beneath the iliotibial tract, but also quite posteriorly.

Technique—Tendon of Origin

The edges of the muscle can be easily followed more proximally. The muscles merge together into a common head and can therefore no longer be differentiated from one another. The common tendon of origin is found more on the lateral side of the tuberosity. The tendon itself can be differentiated from the surrounding softer tissues by palpating with the thumb and index finger (method 1, ► Fig. 5.21) or by using both hands (method 2, ► Fig. 5.22).

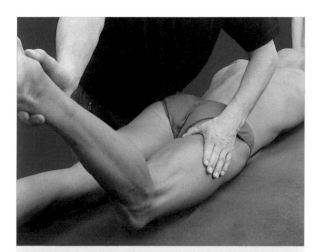

Fig. 5.20 Demonstration of the muscle bellies of the ischiocrural muscles.

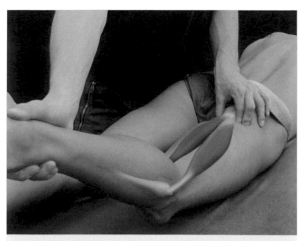

Fig. 5.21 Palpation of the common head—method 1.

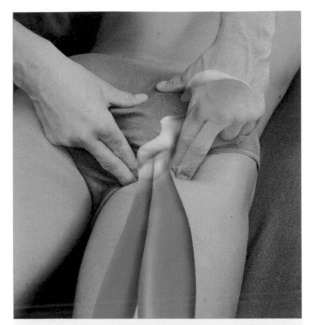

Fig. 5.22 Palpation of the common head—method 2.

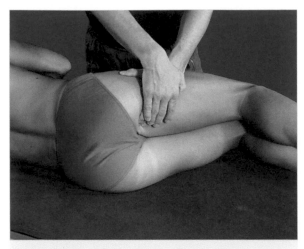

Fig. 5.23 Transverse frictions at the common head.

Tip

If contraction of the gluteus maximus impedes palpation, this muscle can be reciprocally inhibited by asking the patient to push the knee down into the treatment table.

Tips for Assessment and Treatment

Especially in athletes with muscle injuries, insertion tendinopathies or tendinopathies near an insertion, the ischiocrural muscles can exhibit local pain. Local palpation ensures accurate location of the injured structure.

Transverse friction, for provocation or treatment, is preferably performed with the patient lying on their side. In 2007, Askling and Thorstensson were able to show that ischiocrural injuries vary in type depending on the patient's sport and that the level of the injury influences the duration of rehabilitation: higher injuries (1–3 cm below the tubercle in dancers) required longer rehabilitation than lower injuries (7–10 cm below the tubercle in sprinters). According to them, palpation of the injury level can provide information about the duration of rehabilitation.

Technique

The therapist selects a starting position (SP) where the hips are clearly flexed so that the tendon of origin is placed under slight tension and remains still during frictioning. If necessary, the knees can be extended a little further.

The hand palpates distal to the ischial tuberosity and applies transverse friction. More pressure is applied during the movement from medial to lateral.

It is recommended that the other hand assists in the application of pressure to make this technique less tiring (▶ Fig. 5.23).

5.4 Local Palpation—Anterior

5.4.1 Overview of the Structures to be Palpated

The region is divided into two triangles to aid orientation. The borders of these triangles, as well as their contents, are the structures to be found.

- Lateral femoral triangle (borders and contents):
  - Sartorius.
  - Tensor fasciae latae.
  - Rectus femoris.
  - Anterior inferior iliac spine.
- Medial femoral triangle (borders):
  - Sartorius.
  - Adductor longus.
  - inguinal ligament.

5.4.2 Summary of the Palpatory Process

Local palpation of the anterior hip region in particular aims to locate the soft-tissue structures, that is, muscle bellies and their insertions, that are of particular clinical importance.

Palpation begins on the lateral triangle of the thigh (▶ Fig. 5.24). The bordering muscles and their edges will be precisely identified. The structures deep in the tissues

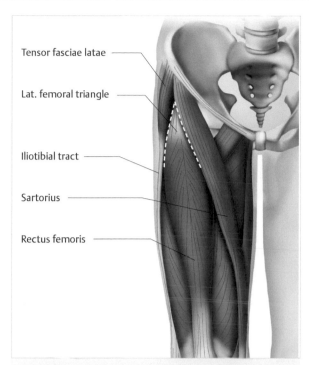

Fig. 5.24 Lateral femoral triangle.

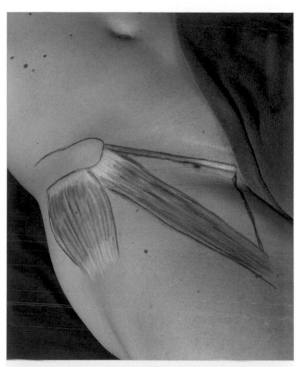

Fig. 5.25 Drawing of the lateral femoral triangle structures.

will be located with the aid of guiding structures and muscle contraction.

This is followed by the palpation of the medial triangle of the thigh. Its boundaries will also be located first, followed by the palpation of the structures (for instance, a nerve and vessel bundle) inside the triangle.

Starting Position

The patient is in a neutral side-lying position. A supportive roll is placed underneath the knees; the arms are relaxed and lie next to the body. The patient should remove sufficient clothing to allow access to the groin region. To confirm some locations, it will be necessary to flex or rotate the hip joint actively or passively.

5.4.3 Palpation of Individual Structures

Lateral Femoral Triangle

The following structures form the boundaries of the lateral triangle of the thigh:
• Lateral edge of the sartorius.
• Anterior edge of the tensor fasciae latae.

This area is actually not a triangle, but is instead shaped like an arrowhead with its tip pointing superiorly (▸ Fig. 5.25). The triangle does not have a third border. The ASIS is the most important osseous structure, lying at the head of the arrow.

Sartorius

The sartorius is the central muscle used for orientation. Its diagonal course over the thigh separates the lateral triangle from the medial triangle. It is rarely possible to recognize the edges of these muscles without muscular activity. For this reason, to visualize the muscle boundaries—and for the sartorius that reaches to about the middle of the thigh—contraction of the appropriate muscles is required.

The sartorius and tensor fasciae latae are hip joint flexors. Their position can be illustrated by actively flexing the hip. To do this, the patient is instructed to slightly raise the leg from the neutral hip position, during which the knee may be flexed slightly.

The sartorius becomes prominent when the hip joint additionally rotates laterally. The muscle belly can very frequently be observed along its course up to the middle of the thigh. Its position in the distal half of the thigh is visible only in very slender patients (▸ Fig. 5.26).

Its medial edge forms the border of the medial femoral triangle and its lateral edge the border of the lateral femoral triangle (▸ Fig. 5.27).

The lateral edge of the sartorius is now followed more proximally until the palpating finger encounters soft-elastic resistance on the lateral aspect. This is the anterior edge of the tensor fasciae latae (▸ Fig. 5.28).

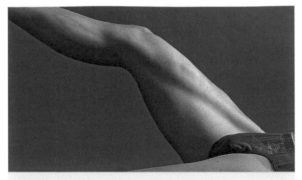

Fig. 5.26 Sartorius—entire course.

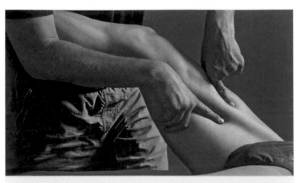

Fig. 5.27 Sartorius—palpation of the edges of the muscle.

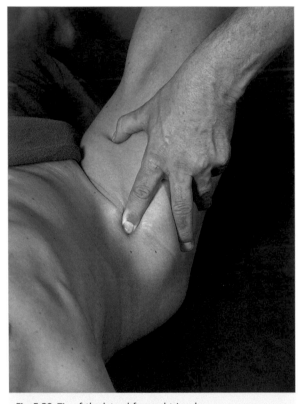

Fig. 5.28 Tip of the lateral femoral triangle.

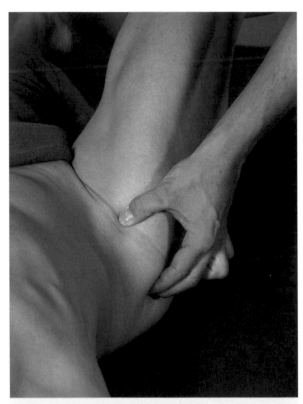

Fig. 5.29 Edges of the tensor fasciae latae.

Tensor Fasciae Latae

The tensor fasciae latae becomes particularly distinct when the patient moves the flexed leg from lateral rotation into medial rotation.

The anterior edge of the tensor fasciae latae can be palpated quite well, while the posterior edge usually merges into the fascia of the thigh (▶ Fig. 5.29).

The muscle belly is followed up onto its muscular origin. It becomes obvious that this involves not only the ASIS, as is often specified in anatomy books, but also a wide section of the iliac crest.

Rectus Femoris and Anterior Inferior Iliac Spine

The muscular edges of the tensor fasciae latae and sartorius meet superiorly and form an inverted V shape like an arrowhead. The tip is found immediately inferior to the ASIS somewhat below the sartorius. The rectus femoris forms the floor of this incomplete triangle of the thigh (▶ Fig. 5.30).

Where the muscular edges of the tensor fasciae latae and sartorius meet, the rectus femoris tendon of origin disappears deep into the tissue as it heads toward the AIIS.

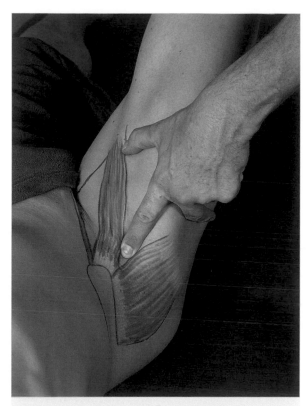

Fig. 5.30 Position of the rectus femoris tendon.

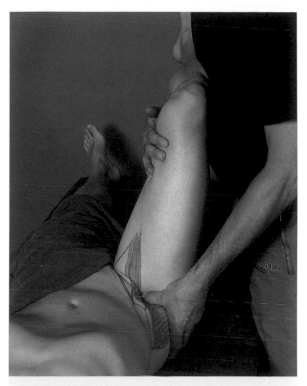

Fig. 5.31 Palpation of the tendon of origin for the rectus femoris.

To reach this insertion, the leg to be palpated is passively moved into approximately 90° hip flexion and the leg held in a horizontal position (▶ Fig. 5.31).

The patient must fully relax the leg during this part of the procedure. Using the thumb of the free hand, the therapist transversely palpates the deep tissue at the tip of the triangle, applying moderate pressure. An attempt is then made to locate the rectus femoris tendon. This tendon is somewhat firmer than the surrounding tissues. The start of palpation on the rectus is approximately a hand's breadth distal to the ASIS. Approximately 5 to 6 cm distal to the spine, the rectus dips under the sartorius and inserts at the inferior spine approximately 4 cm distal and medial to the ASIS (▶ Fig. 5.32).

Tip

The tendon can be immediately located when the patient rhythmically extends and flexes the knee slightly as if kicking a ball toward the ceiling. The surrounding hip flexors remain relaxed during this movement and the rectus femoris is the only muscle that is active.

Once the tendon has been found, the therapist follows the tendon to the AIIS. This structure has been reached when an osseous structure is felt. With flattened fingers but significant pressure against the spine, the entire pelvis should move a bit.

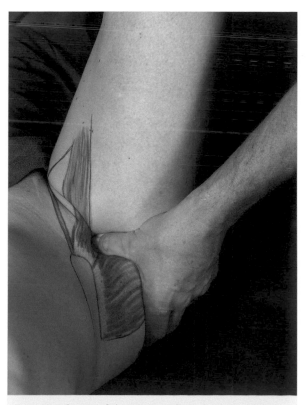

Fig. 5.32 Palpation of the anterior inferior iliac spine (AIIS).

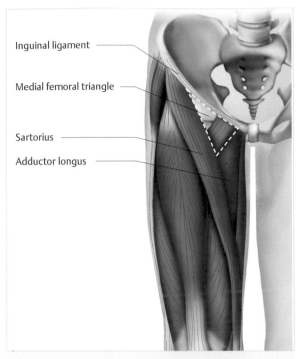

Fig. 5.33 Medial femoral triangle.

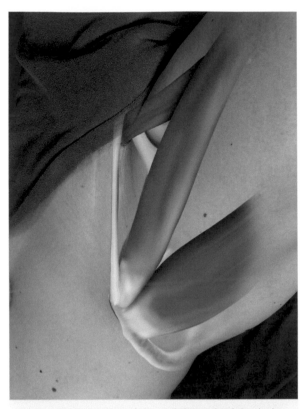

Fig. 5.34 Demonstration of the medial triangle of the thigh.

Medial Femoral Triangle

Overview of the Structures to be Palpated

(See ▶ Fig. 5.33 and ▶ Fig. 5.34):
- Sartorius.
- Adductor longus.
- Anterior superior iliac spine (ASIS).
- Inguinal ligament.
- Lateral cutaneous nerve of the thigh.
- Femoral nerve, artery, and vein.
- Iliopsoas muscle and iliopectineal bursa.
- Pectineus.
- Pubic tuberosity.
- Gracilis.

Sartorius

The sartorius is once again a crucial structure needed for orientation at the medial triangle of the thigh (▶ Fig. 5.27). The muscle is identified using the technique described above. Its medial edges are followed distally as far as possible until at least the middle of the thigh has been reached.

Adductor Longus

The patient moderately flexes the thigh then lowers it, abducting the hip to around 45°. All adductors work isometrically when the patient holds the leg in this position.

The adductor longus is the most prominent adductor of this muscle group (▶ Fig. 5.35). The anterior edge of the adductor longus is the definitive boundary of the medial femoral triangle.

> **Tip**
>
> If this activity is not enough to make the belly of the muscle visible or palpable, the therapist can position their hand on the medial knee joint and instruct the patient to push against the hand in an isometric contraction. This should suffice to make the entire length of the muscle distinct.

Anterior Superior Iliac Spine, Inguinal Ligament, and Lateral Cutaneous Nerve of the Thigh

The course of the groin ligament (inguinal ligament), the last bordering structure of the triangle, will now be clarified. This ligament extends from the ASIS to the pubic tubercle, the structure found immediately superolateral to the symphysis. This ligament of the groin is a fusion of several layers of fascia so that when perpendicular palpation is attempted, there is no clear edge to the structure.

The ASIS is differentiated from the ligament by assessing consistency.

Palpation can be performed with a finger or, as shown here, the pad of the thumb. The therapist begins in known territory—the iliac crest—and follows it with transverse palpation to distal and medial. As long as the thumb remains on the crest or the spine, the feeling is of a rounded structure, bone-hard on direct pressure (▶ Fig. 5.36 and ▶ Fig. 5.37). When the thumb slides down from the spine, the feeling on direct pressure is of a flat, elastic surface. Now it is possible to hook into the ASIS from distal and identify the inguinal ligament (▶ Fig. 5.38 and ▶ Fig. 5.39).

Directly medial to the ASIS and inferior to the inguinal ligament, the cutaneous femoris lateralis nerve can be transversely palpated in its course toward the thigh as a

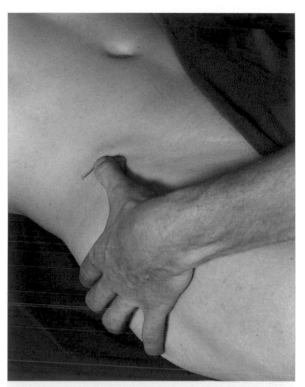

Fig. 5.36 Palpation of the superior anterior iliac spine.

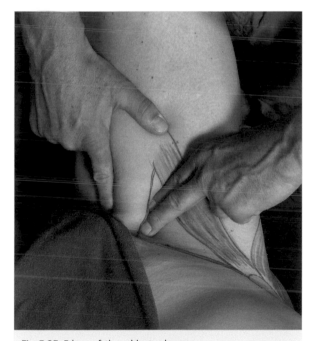

Fig. 5.35 Edges of the adductor longus.

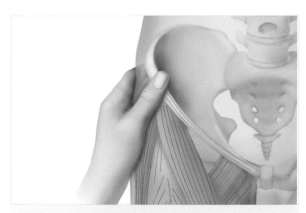

Fig. 5.37 Surface palpation of the ASIS.

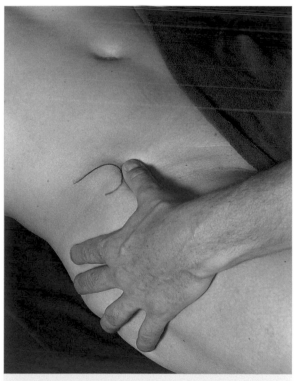

Fig. 5.38 Surface palpation of the inguinal ligament.

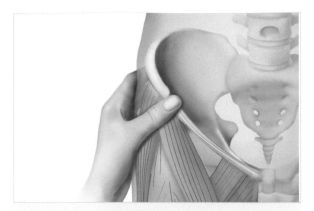

Fig. 5.39 Palpation of the inguinal ligament.

thin strand (approximately 3 mm in diameter). Its position in relation to bony landmarks is given in the literature as approximately 0.7 to 1.6 cm from the ASIS (Dias Filho et al., 2003; Doklamyai et al., 2008) and 5 to 6 cm from the femoral artery.

Once it has been found, it rolls back and forth under the fingertip with transverse palpation. It accompanies the iliacus muscle and crosses under the inguinal ligament very far to lateral. At the ASIS it angles to the lateral thigh, to which it provides sensory innervation over an area the width of a hand (Trepel, 2004). However, the course and branchings of the nerve are very variable (Doklamyai et al., 2008), so that it is possible that the nerve cannot be found, or that it will be located at a slightly different spot. A long period of compression in the lateral inguinal area can lead to repeated irritation (meralgia paresthetica).

The special structures listed above are found in the floor of the triangle. The process of locating them will now be described.

Femoral Nerve, Artery, and Vein

The femoral artery is a suitable landmark for further orientation in the medial femoral triangle. From this structure, other portions of the nerve-vessel bundle can be found, as well as other muscles (▶ Fig. 5.40).

Its course within the femoral triangle extends from the middle of the inguinal ligament to the tip of the medial femoral triangle. It provides the therapist with an idea of the location of the femoral head. The medial side of the hip joint lies directly under the vessel. The center of the femoral head lies between 15 and 24 mm lateral to the artery (Sawant et al., 2004).

For palpation, one or more finger pads are placed flat, with a small amount of pressure, on the middle of the inguinal ligament (▶ Fig. 5.41).

One of the finger pads feels the rhythmical pulse of the artery within a very short time. Topographical anatomy dictates that the nerve must be lying immediately lateral to the artery and the femoral vein immediately medial.

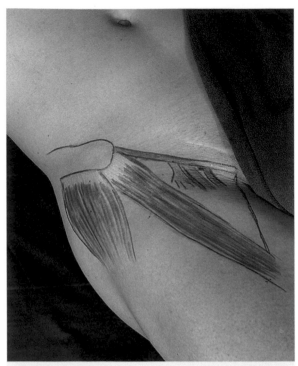

Fig. 5.40 Femoral artery, vein, and nerve in the medial femoral triangle.

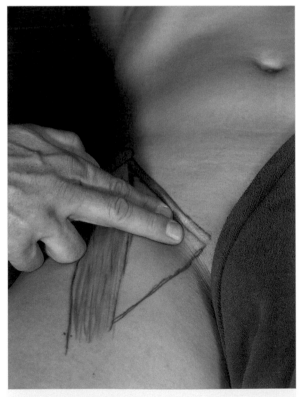

Fig. 5.41 Palpation of the femoral artery.

Iliopsoas Muscle and Iliopectineal Bursa

A portion of the iliopsoas muscle can be reached lateral to the nerve-vessel bundle, in the lateral superior angle of the medial thigh. The angle is determined by the inguinal ligament and the medial edge of the sartorius. The palpating thumb is placed at this point. Hip flexion brings the lesser trochanter and the muscle belly of the psoas major forward, making the muscle accessible. Usually, a flexion of 45° is sufficient, the foot can be supported on the bench and the thigh is passively stabilized. With these parameters, the technique is comparable to accessibility of the iliopsoas(▶ Fig. 5.42). Directly under this is the iliopectineal bursa, lying on the iliopectineal eminence or protuberance, which with deep pressure can only be indirectly located. In bursitis, this point is painful on pressure. Under the bursa is the capsule of the hip joint.

Proximal Insertion of the Pectineus

The insertion of the pectineus can be palpated on the sharp edge of the pectineal line immediately medial to the femoral artery and vein. The therapist pronates the forearm for this palpation and points the palpating finger pads toward the superior ramus of the pubis. The direction of pressure is roughly toward the patient's contralateral ASIS. The technique is optimal when the finger is positioned parallel to the inguinal ligament. The therapist applies frictions from medial to lateral during this palpation (▶ Fig. 5.43).

> **Tip**
>
> As the pressure of palpation is often quite uncomfortable, the therapist should apply pressure with care when conducting the technique. As with the palpation of all muscles presented in this book, this technique can be used to provoke pain and also to treat tendinitis.

Proximal Insertion of the Pubic Tuberosity, Adductor Longus, and Brevis

The adductor longus can be irritated at the proximal insertion, at the tendon, and also at the muscle-tendon transition. First the proximal insertion of the adductor longus at the pubic tuberosity is found. To do this, the palpating finger is brought somewhat to medial from the pectineal line (▶ Fig. 5.44). The pubic tuberosity lies at the cranial boundary of the pubic symphysis. Its shape, a large, distinct projection, allows it to be recognized from every direction. The adductor tendon has its proximal fixation at the lower edge of the tubercle. The insertion is accessible when the muscles are relaxed. The palpating finger is moved toward the tuberculum with the lower arm pronated and a certain amount of pressure (toward the ASIS lying opposite). In transverse friction, the

5

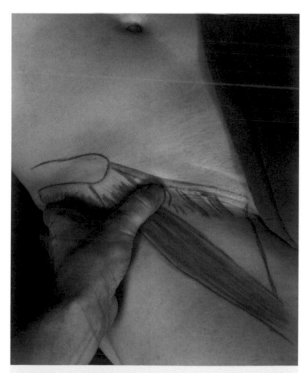

Fig. 5.42 Accessibility of the iliopsoas.

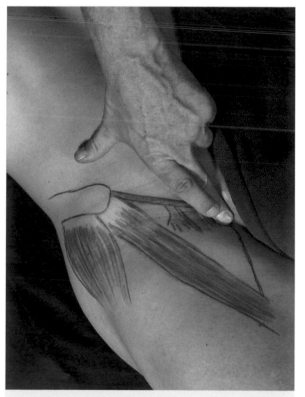

Fig. 5.43 Palpation of the pectineus.

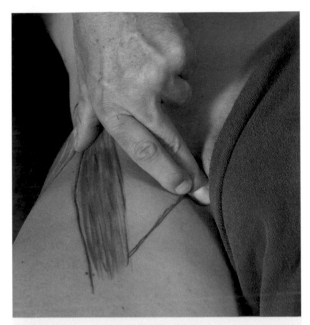

Fig. 5.44 Palpation of the pubic tubercle.

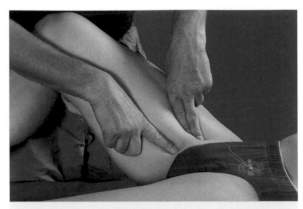

Fig. 5.45 Edges of the adductor longus.

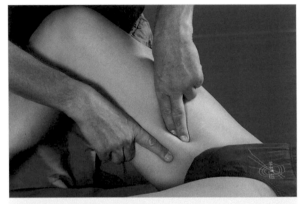

Fig. 5.46 Edges of the gracilis.

pressure is to superomedial and movement is from posterior to anterior. Muscle contraction is used to confirm that the location is correct. When the muscle contracts, the finger is pushed away from the insertion. If the insertion tendon is not directly found as a roundish structure, it is also possible to demonstrate the adductor longus muscle belly with the technique described above (▶ Fig. 5.45) and to follow it proximally to the insertion.

The tendon of insertion is subject to variation and may be divided into two tendons. The tendon(s) and the muscle-tendon junction can be easily differentiated from one another. The consistency of the muscle-tendon junction is considerably softer than the tendon. The tendon is a taut collagenous structure and is significantly firmer. The therapist is already familiar with the position of the muscle belly from the previously described boundaries of the medial femoral triangle.

The adductor brevis can be reached in the fossa posterior to the adductor longus muscle by using deep pressure (not illustrated). From this point, it can be followed to its insertion, somewhat anterior to the insertion of the longus.

Gracilis

To differentiate the position and course of the gracilis from that of the adductor longus, the muscle belly of the adductor longus must be displayed.

The patient holds the flexed leg as it falls to the side with an isometric contraction. The edges of the adductor longus muscle belly can be easily differentiated again from the surrounding soft tissues.

The patient is then instructed to push the heel into the treatment table (and toward the buttocks). The gracilis should tense here as it is a flexor of the knee (▶ Fig. 5.46). Its muscle belly is now prominent and can, in turn, be followed onto its insertion at the lower edge of the symphysis as far as the inferior ramus. Transverse friction at the insertion of the gracilis is performed with the same technique as for the adductor longus (over a larger surface).

Tip

If the gracilis cannot be clearly located using this method, the therapist uses the reciprocal inhibition principle again. The hip and knee are slightly flexed and the patient is instructed to let the knee fall to the side. The therapist then applies light resistance to the lateral knee. The patient must now contract the abductors, which reciprocally inhibits all of the adductors.

The patient is then instructed to contract the knee flexors again (now using its second action in the neighboring knee joint). At this point, the muscle belly of the gracilis protrudes clearly in relation to its surroundings.

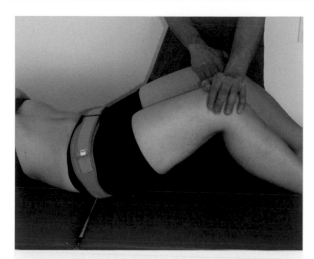

Fig. 5.47 Differentiation test for symphysis pathology.

Tip for Topographic Anatomy

The rami of the pubic bone serve as the origin of the adductors, arranged in the form of a horseshoe. A good mnemonic for the position of their proximal insertions is the word "PELOGRAM." PE stands for the pectineus, LO for the adductor longus, GRA for gracilis and M for adductor magnus. Only the adductor brevis is not included here.

Tips for Assessment and Treatment

The palpation of all muscle bellies and their insertions can be used to differentiate structures during assessment after an adduction resistance test indicates that these muscles can be considered as pain generators. These techniques may also be used as Cyriax cross-friction to treat certain pathological conditions in the soft tissues (e.g., insertion tendinopathy).

The therapist should nevertheless first consider the presence of a tendinopathy or insertion tendinopathy when involvement of the pubic symphysis has been excluded. The pain perception area for an irritation of the pubic symphysis can extend beyond the symphysis to the lower abdomen, the genital and anal area, as well as the adductors.

If resisted hip adduction in a neutral or flexed hip position is positive, it is recommended that the test is repeated with a seat belt positioned around the pelvis (► Fig. 5.47). The fixating seat belts commonly used in manual therapy are suitable for this. The resistance test that resulted in groin pain or adductor pain and was positive without the use of a seat belt is repeated with the seat belt in position.

If the repeated test causes significantly less pain, it is highly likely that the presumption is correct and the pubic symphysis or the SI joints are causing symptoms.

Bibliography

Askling C, Thorstensson A. Acute harmstrings strains involving the proximal free tendon attachement to the ischial tuberosity are associated with prolonged rehabilatation time. Barcelona 6th Interdisciplinary Word Congress on Low Back & Pelvic Pain; 2007

Barratt PA, Brookes N, Newson A. Conservative treatments for greater trochanteric pain syndrome: a systematic review. Br J Sports Med. 2017; 51(2):97–104

Chung CY, Lee KM, Park MS, Lee SH, Choi IH, Cho TJ. Validity and reliability of measuring femoral anteversion and neck-shaft angle in patients with cerebral palsy. J Bone Joint Surg Am. 2010; 92(5):1195–1205

Dias Filho LC, Valença MM, Guimarães Filho FA, et al. Lateral femoral cutaneous neuralgia: an anatomical insight. Clin Anat. 2003; 16(4):309–316

Doklamyai P, Agthong S, Chentanez V, et al. Anatomy of the lateral femoral cutaneous nerve related to inguinal ligament, adjacent bony landmarks, and femoral artery. Clin Anat. 2008; 21(8):769–774

Dunn T, Heller CA, McCarthy SW, Dos Remedios C. Anatomical study of the "trochanteric bursa." Clin Anat. 2003; 16(3):233–240

Lampert C. Läsionen des Lig. capitis femoris: Pathologie und Therapie. Arthroskopie. 2009; 22:293–298

Lanz T von, Wachsmuth W. Praktische Anatomie, Rücken. Berlin: Springer; 2004

Matthijs O, van Paridon-Edauw D, Winkel D. Manuelle Therapie der peripheren Gelenke, Bd. 3: Hüfte, Knie, Sprunggelenk, Fuß und Knorpelgewebe. München: Urban & Fischer bei Elsevier; 2003

Meissner A. Biomechanical investigation of the pubic symphysis. Unfallchirurg. 1996; 6:415–421

Mens JM, Vleeming A, Snijders CJ, Stam HJ, Ginai AZ. The active straight leg raising test and mobility of the pelvic joints. Eur Spine J. 1999; 8(6):468–473

Mercer SR, Woodley SJ, Kennedy E. Anatomy in practice: the sacrotuberous ligament. NZ J Physiother. 2005; 33:91–94

Pfirrmann CW, Chung CB, Theumann NH, Trudell DJ, Resnick D. Greater trochanter of the hip: attachment of the abductor mechanism and a complex of three bursae–MR imaging and MR bursography in cadavers and MR imaging in asymptomatic volunteers Radiology. 2001; 221(2):469–477

Puranen J, Orava S. The hamstring syndrome–a new gluteal sciatica. Ann Chir Gynaecol. 1991; 80(2):212–214

Rudorff von KD. Orthopädie für Physiotherapeuten. Steinfurt: Internationale Medizinische Akademie Steinfurt (IMAS) e.V.; 2007

Ruwe PA, Gage JR, Ozonoff MB, DeLuca PA. Clinical determination of femoral anteversion. A comparison with established techniques. J Bone Joint Surg Am. 1992; 74(6):820–830

Sawant MR, Murty A, Ireland J. A clinical method for locating the femoral head centre during total knee arthroplasty. Knee. 2004; 11(3):209–212

Schneider B, Laubenberger J, Jemlich S, Groene K, Weber HM, Langer M. Measurement of femoral antetorsion and tibial torsion by magnetic resonance imaging. Br J Radiol. 1997; 70(834):575–579

Spomedial. Belastung und Beanspruchung des Stütz- und Bewegungsapparates im Fußball. 2009. http://vmrz0100.vm.ruhr-uni-bochum.de/spomedial/content/e866/e2442/e12729/e12752/e12754/e12788/index_ger.html; Accessed: 16.10.2017

Tavares Canto de RS, Filho GS, Magalhaes L, et al. Femoral neck anteversion: aclinical vs radiological evaluation. Acta Ortop Bras. 2005; 13:171–174

Tönnis D, Legal H. Die angeborene Hüftdysplasie und Hüftluxation im Kindes- und Erwachsenenalter: Grundlagen, Diagnostik, konservative und operative Behandlung. Heidelberg: Springer; 1984

Trepel M. Neuroanatomie. Struktur und Funtion. München: Urban & Fischer Verlag bei Elsevier; 2004

Windisch G, Dolcet C, Auer B, et al. Anatomy of the ischial tuberosity [unpublished]. Graz: Institut für makroskopische und klinische Anatomie der Universität Graz; 2017

5

Chapter 6

Knee Joint

6 Knee Joint

6.1 Introduction

The knee joint is not only the largest joint of the body; it is also the joint with the most complicated biomechanics. It connects the longest bones to each other, has the largest articular cavity, has the largest sesamoid bone (the patella), and has the largest capsule (Matthijs et al., 2006). Therapists frequently have to deal with this joint in their daily work. Post-traumatic and postoperative treatment of the joint is part of the work of almost every rehabilitation clinic or physical therapy practice.

Comparatively, the large number of knee operations is extraordinary. The common indications for surgical intervention are arthritic changes in articular surfaces and injury to the complex ligamentous construction and the menisci. In the USA, more than 966,000 total knee arthroplasties were carried out in 2017 (HCPUnet, iData Research, 2018). According to estimates by Maradit Kremers et al. (2015) around 7 million Americans are living with a hip or knee replacement. In Germany, approximately 108,000 knee replacements were implanted in women alone in 2015. This makes this knee procedure the eleventh most common surgical procedure in women in Germany (German Federal Statistical Office, 2017). In addition to appropriate postoperative treatment, which has become quite sophisticated, the therapist also encounters traumatic and nontraumatic joint symptoms that at first seem difficult to classify and that require a systematic and technically precise examination procedure. Target-oriented palpation, combined with systematic interrogation and diagnosis, play a central role in identifying the location and cause of the symptoms.

6.2 Significance and Function of the Knee Joint

One of the basic principles of joint function in the lower limbs will also become obvious in the knee joint. It must be possible to lock the lower extremity into a stable weight-bearing pillar that also has remarkable mobility.

This **knee joint mobility** calls for a great deal of flexion that decreases the distance between the foot and the body. In such ordinary situations as squatting, climbing stairs with high risers, or getting into a car, it becomes clear why a high degree of flexion is necessary.

The second form of mobility is the **rotation of the knee joint.** This movement is linked to the angle of knee joint flexion and is only possible between approximately 20 and 130°. Between 20° flexion and maximal extension the knee joint is locked in terminal rotation. When the leg is loaded and in end-range extension, the femur rotates inward and the tibia, in open chain, turns in end-range outward rotation. If active rotation in end-range extension were possible, it would presumably be at the cost of stability, which is of particular importance in the extended position.

The **ability of the foot to rotate** is mainly anchored in the knee joint. The remaining rotation takes place in the motor complex consisting of the talotarsal joint and the transverse tarsal joints.

This capacity for rotation of the tibia in the knee joint places specific demands on the construction of the articulating bones at the knee joint. Axial rotation of the leg at the knee joint requires a central rotary column (primarily the posterior cruciate ligament), a flat rotary plate (proximal end of the tibia), and articular surfaces with almost only one single point of contact.

This flat rotary plate causes a high degree of **incongruence between the articular surfaces.** The knee would be unable to rotate as well if the tibial articular surface were more curved. Although incongruence facilitates rotation, stability and the transfer of load suffer. The menisci complement this joint, forming a mobile articular socket to balance the pointlike contact between the articular surfaces and to lubricate the joint.

As **stability** can no longer be provided by the bones, internal and external ligamentous structures (cruciate and collateral ligaments) as well as sections of muscle that radiate into the capsule (dynamization) fulfill this function. All these ligaments give each other functional support (Matthijs et al., 2006).

The cruciate ligaments are responsible for the primary security of the joint in the sagittal plane. This function can also be assessed using a test conducted in the sagittal plane, the drawer test, and the Lachman test. These ligaments also modulate tension to control the arthrokinematics during flexion and restrict the amount of medial rotation.

Knee joint stabilization in the frontal plane is the function of both the collateral ligaments and the posterior capsule.

The dynamization of different collagenous structures at a joint is not peculiar to the knee joint. However, it is quite distinct in this region. Dynamization in this context means that muscles, and sometimes their tendons, are attached to the capsule or menisci. Different sections of the capsule are placed under tension and strengthened when these muscles contract. During active movement of the knee, the femoral condyles not only roll over the menisci on the tibia in an anterior or posterior direction, the contraction of muscles also pulls on the menisci and causes movement.

6.3 Pathological Conditions and Common Applications for Treatment

6.3.1 A Selection of Possible Pathologies

It is beyond the scope and objectives of this book to list all types of disease and injuries seen in the knee joint. Therefore, only the most important groups are listed below:
• Capsular and noncapsular restrictions in movement.
• Laxity or instability.
• Traumatic and degenerative meniscus pathology, impingement of the meniscal horns.
• Injuries to ligaments or ligamental overuse syndromes.
• Injuries to the muscles or muscular overuse syndromes (including tendons and insertions).
• Disease of the femorotibial articular cartilage (for instance, osteoarthritis or osteochondrosis dissecans).
• Patellofemoral pathologies (for instance, chondromalacia patellae or patellofemoral pain syndrome, "young girl's knee syndrome").

6.3.2 Common Assessment and Treatment Techniques

• Assessment and mobilization of existing restrictions in mobility.
• Improvement of muscular tracking of the joint in cases of instability.
• Treatment of injuries in ligaments and muscles or the symptoms associated with overloading.

The high prevalence of irritation or injury to ligaments, tendons, and bursae shows in the established use of independent terms such as runner's knee (iliotibial band friction syndrome), jumper's knee (insertion tendinopathy of the patellar ligament at the apex of the patella), and housemaid's knee (prepatellar bursitis).

6.4 Required Basic Anatomical and Biomechanical Knowledge

Therapists must have a good basic knowledge of anatomy to locate specific important structures in the knee joint and its surroundings. Therapists are familiar with most bony and ligamentous structures through their training/studies and professional experience. It is important to develop a good spatial sense so that the construction of the joint can be considered from different perspectives. Presenting the structural complexity of the knee joint is beyond the scope of this book. Therefore, in what follows, only basic concepts will be discussed.

The knee joint is subdivided into the femorotibial joint and the patellofemoral joint.

6.4.1 Construction of the Femorotibial Joint

Embryologically, the knee joint develops from two structures, the medial and lateral compartments. The original synovial dividing wall gradually disappears in the course of development and only remains as the synovial plica. This original division can, however, be retained for anatomical and functional reasons. It is always true that the lateral compartment is more mobile. The slightly convex shape of the lateral tibial condyle and the more mobile, lateral meniscus, O-shaped and more deformable, back this up. In the frontal view, the knee joint can be divided into three levels (Matthijs et al., 2006):
• *Femorotibial joint:* selective, direct contact between femoral condyles and tibial condyles.
• *Meniscofemoral joint:* contact between the femoral condyles and the menisci.
• *Meniscotibial joint:* contact between the tibial condyles and the menisci.

The associated capsular portions are described in the same way, for example, meniscofemoral capsular portions.

The femur widens at the distal end and has two condyles (▶ Fig. 6.1). This may lead to classifying the knee joint as a condylar joint. Nevertheless, with its movements in flexion, extension, and inward and outward rotation, it must be classified as a trochoginglymus joint. The medial femoral condyle is longer than the lateral, to compensate for the oblique position of the femur. In contrast, the lateral condyle stands out somewhat further to anterior and acts as a lateral resistance to the patella.

The femoral condyles, together, form a grooved patellar face as a component of the patellofemoral joint. Distally and posteriorly, the condyles diverge and form the

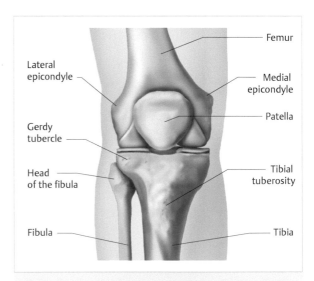

Fig. 6.1 Topography of the osseous reference points—anterior view.

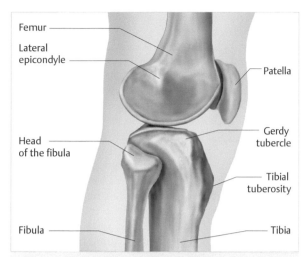

Femur

Lateral
epicondyle

Patella

Gerdy
tubercle

Head
of the fibula

Tibial
tuberosity

Fibula

Tibia

Fig. 6.2 Topography of the osseous reference points—lateral view.

intercondylar fossa, which is approximately 20 to 22 mm wide (Wirth et al., 2005), the resting place of the cruciate ligaments. Both femoral condyles are convex. In the sagittal plane, their curvature increases posteriorly (▶ Fig. 6.2), more distinctly in the lateral condyle. Accordingly, the articular surfaces of the condyles with the tibial condyles are smaller in flexion than in extension. The femoral condyles have an impression line, the sulcus terminalis, which in end-range extension points to the tibia and the anterior horns of the meniscus. In loaded position, pressure on the meniscus and tibia laterally initiates terminal rotation—with the medial condyle sliding to posterior with a longer gliding movement—and thus forces the femur to rotate inward. Proximal to the articular body, the femur has a medial and a lateral epicondyle, attachment points of the collateral ligaments.

The club-shaped enlargement of the **proximal tibia** (see ▶ Fig. 6.1) forms two cartilage-covered facets (tibial condyles) and an intercondylar area with the intercondylar eminence. These are the points of attachment for both menisci and both cruciate ligaments. Seen frontally, both tibial joint surfaces are slightly concave. Sagitally, the medial joint surface remains concave. In contrast, the lateral joint surface is slightly convex, which facilitates the arthrokinetic roll components in the lateral compartment. Further, seen in the sagittal plane, the tibial plateau falls off from the level of the tibial longitudinal axis by approximately 10° (Matthijs et al., 2006). In the embryo, this angle is 45° and regresses to varying degrees intraindividually. For this reason, it is very variable. On the proximal tibia, there are two large rough areas for the insertion of strong ligaments: the tibial tuberosity for the patellar ligament and the Gerdy tubercle for the principal insertion of the iliotibial tract. The two rough areas and the head of the fibula form an equilateral triangle.

Occasionally an additional sesamoid bone can be found in the knee joint. The fabella is embedded in the tendon of the lateral head of the gastrocnemius muscle at the level of the lateral femoral condyle. Reported figures for the frequency of occurrence of a fabella as a bone vary from 8 to 20% (Petersen and Zantop, 2009). If the fabella is not present as a bone, it can occur as a fibrous or fibrocartilaginous structure. It is in contact with important ligaments of the posterior capsule (oblique popliteal, arcuate popliteal, and fabellofibular ligaments).

The menisci, movable cups, equilibrate the incongruence between the femoral condyles and the tibia, bear weight when the joint is under load, and press synovia against the articular cartilage of the articulating condyles during movement, thus building a foundation for cartilage nutrition.

As central pillars or intracapsular ligaments, the **cruciate ligaments** control the arthrokinematics of the knee joint, ensure the integrity of the joint in the sagittal plane, and limit inward rotation. They usually run from the femoral intercondylar fossa to the tibial intercondylar area. They consist of several bundles of high tensile strength, helical type I collagen, encased in a synovial membrane. Strictly speaking, they are thus situated within the fibrous capsule (intra-articular) but without direct contact with the synovia (extrasynovial). Some parts of the cruciate ligaments are isometric and remain tensed in every joint position (companion bundles). Other portions are increasingly recruited in end-range movements (safety bundles; Fuss, 1989).

The **capsule** can be subdivided in various ways. Superficial and deep portions can be distinguished, or distinctions can be made according to direction. Thus, a distinction is made among the following:

- Medial capsule portions with the reinforcing medial collateral ligament (except at the level of the joint capsule).
- Lateral portions without direct reinforcement by the lateral collateral ligament.
- An anterior capsule with the patellar ligament, longitudinal and transverse retinacula, and the patellomeniscal ligaments. The anterior capsule forms a suprapatellar recess that inserts at the posterior half of the patellar base and displaces the patella downward by up to 8 cm under increasing flexion.
- Strengthening of the posterior capsule, for instance laterally, by the arcuate popliteal ligament and medially by the oblique popliteal ligament.

Protection in the frontal plane is provided by the **collateral ligaments** and the posterior capsule. The tension of all components increases with extension. The posterior capsule primarily protects in complete extension, whereas the collateral ligaments provide the primary stability against varus and valgus stress beginning with

6

slight flexion. The two collaterals differ morphologically and work synergistically in limiting outward rotation.

The medial collateral ligament has its femoral origin at the medial femoral epicondyle and the adductor tubercle and becomes significantly wider (3–4 cm) at the level of the articular space. According to Liu et al. (2010), it runs for a further approximately 6.2 cm from the articular space to the medial surface of the tibia, below the superficial pes anserinus. It has a superficial (anterior) and a deep (posterior) portion. The superficial portion twists during knee flexion and is therefore palpable as a convexity over the articular space. The posterior portion is in close contact with the base of the medial meniscus.

The lateral collateral ligament is comparatively short (approximately 5 cm), rounded, and thin. It has no capsular or meniscal contact. Its points of fixation are the lateral femoral epicondyle and the head of the fibula.

6.4.2 Construction of the Patellofemoral Joint

When seen from the front, the patella, the largest sesamoid bone in the human body, is basically triangular (▶ Fig. 6.3). The rounded base of the patella is about 1.5 cm thick and functions posteriorly as the point of insertion of the suprapatellar bursa and anteriorly as the point of insertion of the largest part of the quadriceps femoris. At 90° the base of the patella is flat and parallel to the shaft of the femur. For this reason, the anterior edge of the base is very simple and the posterior edge very difficult to palpate. The base is bounded laterally by projecting corners: the medial and lateral poles of the patella. From this point, the patella narrows to its apex, which is generally located at the level of the femorotibial articular space. The distal third is the point of insertion of the patellar ligament, both at the edges and to a lesser extent at the anterior and posterior surfaces. At the middle of the posterior surface of the patella is a longitudinal ridge, from which medial and lateral facets extend. These together make up the articular surface of the patella. The longitudinal eminence articulates with the groove of the femoral patellar surface, which, in extension, is the articulating partner. With increasing flexion, the lateral surfaces of the patella glide over the femoral condyles. During an extensive flexion, the patella describes movements that can be classified as:

- inferior glide, up to 8 cm;
- shift, lateral movements to medial and then to lateral;
- tilt, tipping about its longitudinal axis;
- rotation of the patellar apex to medial, in line with the terminal inward rotation of the tibia.

6.4.3 Proximal Tibiofibular Joint

In contrast to the elbow joint, only one bone in the medial joint of the lower extremity, the tibia, articulates with the bone of the proximal section of the extremity, the femur. The fibula forms an amphiarthrosis with the posterolateral head of the tibia; its articular space is oriented at approximately 45° from anterolateral to posteromedial (see ▶ Fig. 6.2). In some cases, the joint cavity communicates with the cavity of the femorotibial joint and must then be considered as a part of the knee joint. Functionally, the proximal tibiofibular joint (TFJ) is part of the tibiotarsal motor complex and moves in accompaniment with foot extension and flexion and all associated movements, especially in an anteroposterior direction. It is protected by ligaments that provide force closure and acts as point of insertion for several muscles, the most important being the biceps femoris. The biceps has a basically dislocating effect on the proximal TFJ.

6.4.4 Muscles of the Knee Joint

The **quadriceps femoris** muscle is the most important in extension of the knee joint (▶ Fig. 6.4). Its fibers insert in part at the anterior base of the patella and also run anterior via the patella and parapatellar as longitudinal retinacula, to the tibia. The vastus medialis, arising in part from the tendon of the adductor magnus (Scharf et al.,

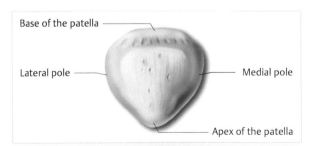

Fig. 6.3 Sections of the patella—anterior view.

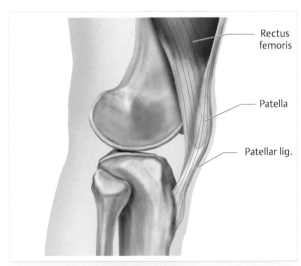

Fig. 6.4 Rectus femoris, patella, and ligament during knee extension.

1985) offers active resistance to the tendency for lateral movement, since it inserts at the chief medial stabilizer of the patella, the medial patellofemoral ligament (Panagio-topoulos et al., 2006). Probably the largest individual muscle in the body, the vastus lateralis inserts with a 5-cm-long tendon at the lateral aspect of the patellar base. The thickening of the muscle belly in contraction spans the iliotibial tract from the interior outward. Below the rectus femoris, as a branch of the vastus intermedius, is the articularis genus muscle. Its fibers radiate in the popliteal recess and, in active knee extension, span the recess and prevent femoropatellar impingement.

The **flexors of the knee joint** are more distinctly differentiated; they are the group of inward and outward rotators (▶ Fig. 6.5). The ischiocrural muscles (hamstrings) can be considered as agonists, while the further portions of the pes anserinus (sartorius and gracilis muscles) as well as the heads of the gastrocnemius and popliteal muscles act synergistically. The distribution of the

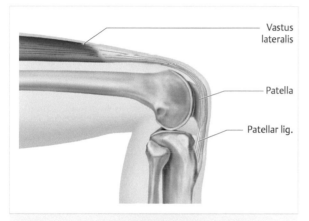

Fig. 6.5 Rectus femoris, patella, and ligament during knee flexion.

ischiocrural muscles on the distal thigh forms the proximal half of the rhomboid popliteal fossa.

The principal outward rotator, the biceps femoris, has a very variable distribution of its insertion tendon. It inserts chiefly at the head of the fibula (▶ Fig. 6.6), at the crural fascia and the tibia (Tubbs et al., 2006). Its fibers embrace the lateral collateral ligament. Some fibers radiate into the arcuate ligament of the knee and the tendon of the popliteal muscle (ibid.). Radiation into the posterior horn of the lateral meniscus is also described.

Another important structure is found lateral to the iliotibial tract. The tract, dynamized by the tensor fasciae latae, gluteus maximus, and vastus lateralis, functions as reinforcement of the lateral thigh fascia, which is located close to the lateral intermuscular septum. Directly proximal, it receives ligamentary radiations from the femur (Kaplan fibers). Its distal insertion is chiefly on the Gerdy tubercle, anterolateral on the tibial head. Other radiations are the fasciae of the foot extensors and the proximal and anterior patella (iliopatellar ligament), which can also create a tendency to move the patella to one side. At approximately 30 to 40° flexion of the knee joint, the tract is located directly over the lateral epicondyle. With increasing extension, it has an extensor effect; with increasing flexion, it acts as a flexor synergist. In addition, it has an external rotatory effect on the knee joint.

Medially, the pes anserinus muscles are the dominant anatomical feature (▶ Fig. 6.7). It is well known that fibers of the sartorius, gracilis, and semitendinosus muscles end in the superficial pes anserinus. These can be well differentiated proximal to the joint. Distal to the articular space, they run together in a broad insertion tendon that inserts at the medial tibial surface. They cross the knee joint behind the flexion/extension axis and thus act as flexors and inward rotators. A series of small bursae protects the insertion plate against friction from the medial collateral ligament and the tibial periosteum. The deep

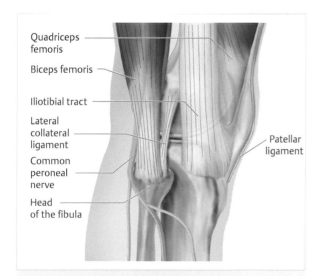

Fig. 6.6 Relevant lateral soft tissues.

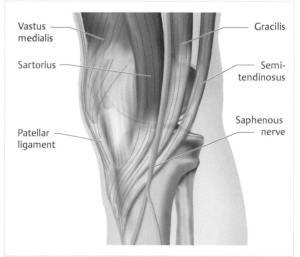

Fig. 6.7 Relevant medial soft tissues.

pes anserinus is formed by the tendon of the semitendinosus muscle that divides into five insertion bands. In addition to two insertions at the tibia, there are the radiations into the fascia of the popliteal muscle, the posterior horn of the medial meniscus, and the posteromedial capsule (oblique popliteal ligament). Its tendon is clearly prominent in the posterior thigh during flexion.

To posterior, the gastrocnemius is dominant at the surface; it forms the distal half of the rhomboid popliteal fossa with the division of its two bellies. Deep portions of the tendon radiate into the posterior capsule. The popliteal muscle is fleshy at its origin on the posterior proximal tibia. Its muscle belly is anterior to the medial gastrocnemius head and is therefore not directly palpable. The tendon that runs upward to proximal and lateral divides into three portions that insert at the medial meniscus and radiate into the posterolateral capsule. The actual insertion tendon crosses the articular space between the lateral collateral ligament and the joint components femorotibially and inserts approximately 0.5 cm distal and anterior to the lateral epicondyle.

From the introduction to the muscles of the knee joint presented so far it becomes clear that in addition to motor functions, the radiations into capsules, fasciae, or menisci are an important anatomical fact. The effect is the tensing of these structures with muscle contraction, which is called dynamization. At other joints, such as the shoulder joint, dynamization is also known. However, the difference in contact of muscles to articular structures is particularly pronounced here, at the knee joint. ▶ Table 6.1 provides a summary of all dynamizations.

6.4.5 Neural Structures

The most important neural structures pass along the back of the knee. Only a large branch of the femoral nerve, the saphenous nerve, crosses the joint medially (see ▶ Fig. 6.7). Its position is very variable. Usually it comes to the surface between the sartorius and gracilis muscles and runs subcutaneously in a distal direction (von Lanz and Wachsmuth, 2003).

Approximately 1 hand width proximal and posterior to the knee joint, the sciatic nerve separates into its two divisions. The tibial nerve runs through the middle of the popliteal fossa. Its expected size lies between the diameter of a pencil and that of a little finger. After branching from the tibial nerve, the peroneal nerve runs laterally and accompanies the biceps tendon to the head of the fibula. Distal to the fibular head, it crosses to anterolateral and branches again. At the level of the biceps tendon, the nerve is shifted approximately 1 cm to medial.

6.5 Palpation for Warmth and Swelling

6.5.1 Palpating an Increase in Temperature

An increase in temperature may be a sign of capsule irritation. The therapist can decide if this is the case by comparing sides and by also comparing the knee with the proximal and distal soft tissues. Obviously, both knees should have the same temperature when normal (▶ Fig. 6.8). However, examination of the joint in relation to its surroundings is of interest. The therapist can assume that a nonpathological joint feels colder than its surroundings, that is, compared with the soft tissues proximally and distally/laterally.

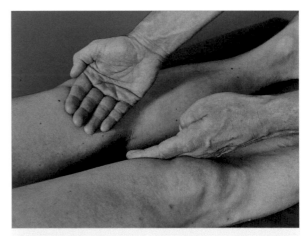

Fig. 6.8 Test for heat.

Table 6.1 Muscular attachments and dynamized structures

Quadriceps femoris	Anterior capsule (patellar ligament and a variety of retinacula), menisci (via the patellomeniscal ligaments)
Adductor longus	Medial collateral ligament
Biceps femoris	Lateral collateral ligament and the lateral meniscus
Popliteus	Posterior capsule (arcuate ligament of the knee) and the lateral meniscus
Semimembranosus	Posterior capsule (oblique popliteal ligament), medial meniscus, medial collateral ligament
Gastrocnemius	Posterior capsule

6.5.2 Palpating Edema

Summary of the Palpation Process

Swelling appears in various joint diseases and injuries involving, for instance, capsular ligaments, menisci, and cruciate ligaments. If it occurs within one hour after a trauma, the swelling is very probably a hemarthrosis. Slowly emerging articular effusions are most likely synovial in nature. Nontraumatic swelling that occurs immediately after stress is a sign of a cartilaginous lesion. On the other hand, gradually developing swelling after stress more probably indicates degenerative meniscopathy. In any case, swelling is a sign of joint disease. A detailed diagnosis, if necessary with additional joint-challenging tests designed to test stability and provoke pain, can in itself cause or intensify effusion and increased warmth around the joint.

Techniques will be described that identify the presence of edema in the joint in terms of:
- large effusions, evidence of severe swelling,
- medium-sized effusions, evidence of moderate swelling,
- minimal effusions, evidence of minor swelling.

Starting Position

The patient is either lying prone or sitting with their legs stretched out on a treatment table. The affected knee joint is extended as far as possible without aggravating pain. However, the knee must be fully extended to identify a small effusion, otherwise the test will most likely result in a false negative.

Large Effusions

It is not difficult to recognize a large joint swelling by visual inspection and palpation. In extension, the capsule is tight, posteriorly and laterally. In an intra-articular effusion, the fluid collects anteriorly, under the patella, and sometimes raises it.

Technique

This test aims to collect the synovial fluid underneath the patella and to identify the extent of the edema by applying pressure to the patella.

The thumbs of both hands are abducted here. The distal hand is positioned over the joint space of the knee. It prevents the synovial fluid from spreading distal and lateral to the patella (► Fig. 6.9).

The proximal hand starts stroking widely over the thigh approximately 10 cm superior to the patella so that the synovial fluid is milked out of the suprapatellar pouch and accumulates underneath the patella. This raises the patella. One finger of the proximal hand is then placed on the patella. Pressure is exerted in a posterior direction

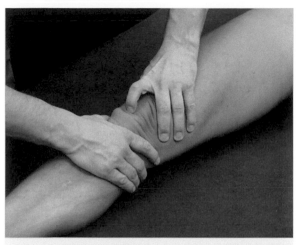

Fig. 6.9 Test for large effusions.

until the patella is once more in contact with its femoral glide.

The criterion for comparing swelling on the two sides is the time required for the patella to come in contact with the femur. The intra-articular effusion is then pressed against the palpating finger in a medial and lateral direction. The sign of a dancing patella is not present if extra-articular swelling is present (Strobel and Stedtfeld, 2013).

> **Tip**
>
> This test is also called the "dancing patella" test, "ballotable patella" test, or "patella ballottement" test, or the "patella tap" test. Execution of the test varies significantly. All forms are permissible providing the following details are observed: the fluid is gathered under the patella and held there while direct pressure to posterior is exerted on the patella.

Medium-sized Effusions

The "dancing patella test" is quite common; the test to identify medium-sized effusions is used less often.

Technique

The proximal hand again strokes distally. The distal hand forms a tight V between thumb and index finger. This V is supported from distal against the lateral borders of the patella and the finger pads are placed on the articular space (► Fig. 6.10).

During stroking, the synovial fluid is pushed distally underneath the patella. The V-formed hand feels an increase in pressure as the synovial fluid spreads out.

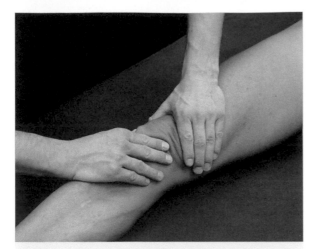

Fig. 6.10 Test for medium-sized effusions.

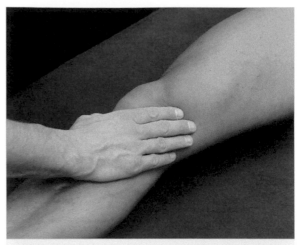

Fig. 6.11 Test for minimal effusions—phase 1.

The criterion for this test is the possibly different magnitude of this pressure on the two sides.

Minimal Effusions

It is very simple to identify a moderate- or large-sized edema in the knee joint. Recognition of a minimal effusion requires a special technique. The starting position must be full extension, held passively.

Technique—Phase 1

The therapist broadly strokes the medial side of the knee joint to proximal-lateral, at least three times (▶ Fig. 6.11). In this way, the synovial fluid is shifted to other parts of the joint.

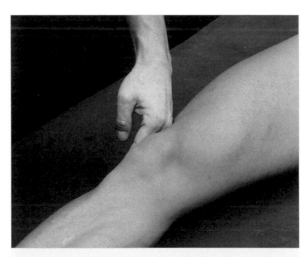

Fig. 6.12 Test for minimal effusions—phase 2.

Technique—Phase 2

Immediately thereafter, the lateral aspect of the knee joint is widely stroked once in a proximal direction, which pushes the synovial fluid into the joint cavity and to medial (▶ Fig. 6.12). The therapist simultaneously observes the medial joint space adjacent to the patella, which usually takes on a slightly concave shape. In a normal joint, there is a slight concavity here that remains concave if the effusion test is negative. When a small joint effusion is present, a small "bulge" is produced in the medial concavity while stroking the lateral side of the knee.

6.6 Local Palpation—Anterior

6.6.1 Summary of the Palpatory Process

Anterior palpation locates the boundaries of the patella and their connection to the tibia (▶ Fig. 6.13).

Starting Position

The patient sits in an elevated position, for example, on the edge of a treatment table. The therapist either sits in front of the patient or a little to the side (▶ Fig. 6.14).

When possible, the leg should hang freely over the couch and be able to flex freely when the therapist's hand facilitates movement.

This starting position (SP) ensures that the palpable structures on the anterior, medial, and lateral sides of the knee joint are freely accessible. This SP should only be considerably altered when palpating the posterior aspect of the knee. The patient exerts no static effort to retain this starting position and all muscles are relaxed. The patellar ligament is moderately tensed, and the entire base of the patella is accessible.

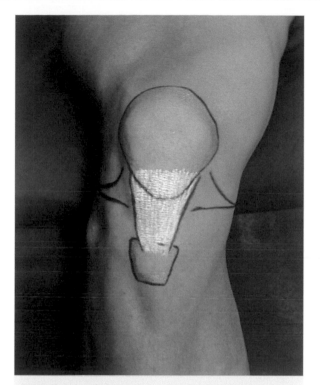

Fig. 6.13 Accessible structures on the anterior aspect.

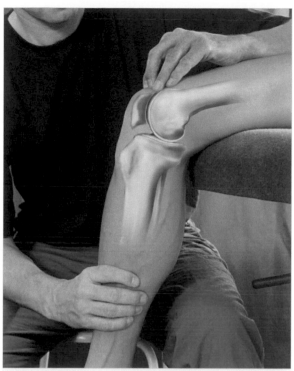

Fig. 6.14 Palpation of the base of the patella.

Alternative Starting Positions

The SPs described above are mainly used when practicing. Other SPs may be necessary in the everyday assessment and treatment of the knee joint. In these cases, the therapist may have to approach the knee from a different angle and position the knee with a different amount of flexion.

When the following palpation has been correctly applied to study partners or patients, it should be repeated in its modified forms:

• Full extension.
• Increasing amount of flexion.
• Patient in side-lying position.
• Without visual control.
• On arthritic and/or swollen joints.

When the knee is fully extended it is easier to palpate the base and the poles and more difficult to palpate the apex of the patella and the ligament through the laterally protruding infrapatellar Hoffa fat pad.

With increasing flexion due to increasing contraction of the anterior structures, all contours will be more difficult to find. Arthritis-related edema and bony deformation alter the expected consistency and contours of the respective structure.

6.6.2 Palpation of Individual Structures

Base of the Patella

The search for the borders of the patella begins at its base. As already mentioned in the topographic introduction to the knee joint, the base of the patella is very thick and has a front and back boundary.

When the knee is extended, only the anterior edge of the patellar base can be easily reached. It connects both poles in a curved line. Pressure on the apex can be used to tip the base upward and make the posterior edge accessible.

The posterior edge is the most important border in the flexed position. The palpation aims to identify this edge and differentiate it from the femur and the surrounding soft tissues. When the knee joint is flexed, the patellar base is parallel to the thigh and follows the shape of the patellar surface of the femur. Therefore, its boundaries can only be palpated during slight passive extension/flexion movement of the knee joint (▶ Fig. 6.14).

Tip

The facilitated movement of the lower leg should be minimal and completely passive! Any activity of the quadriceps makes locating the base of the patella extremely difficult.

Technique

The therapist places several fingertips on the thigh approximately 3 to 4 cm proximal to a line connecting the medial and lateral poles of the patella. They point to distal for transverse palpation of the edges (see ▶ Fig. 6.13). The second hand moves the joint in small, passive motions. This causes the patella to also describe small motions to proximal and to push its posterior edge against the fingertips of the palpating hand, and thus be located. The posterior edge can be followed to medial and lateral to both poles. This line tapers off somewhat in the center and thus represents the extension of the posterior groin, which separates the medial from the lateral facet. The anterior surface is not as wide as the posterior surface, so that an incline to the palpated edge drops off from the anterior surface to each side. To record the length of this anterior surface, a line can be drawn outlining it, starting from where the incline begins. Ultimately, two outlines of the patella are created.

Edges of the Patella

The borders of the patella are now defined by following the contours with transverse palpation, past both poles to the apex (▶ Fig. 6.15).

Technique

Compared with the medial side, it is relatively difficult to identify the exact border of the lateral pole of the patella. The lateral femoral condyle projects further to anterior

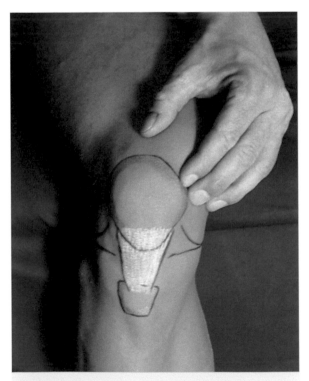

Fig. 6.15 Palpation of the medial pole of the patella.

than the medial condyle; its outline is similar to the shape of the patella. The knee joint must be moved occasionally to differentiate the patella from the lateral femoral condyle. The previously described perpendicular technique is used for palpation.

Apex of the Patella

The patellar ligament uses the distal third of the patella, including the apex, as proximal area of attachment. This distal border of the patella can therefore only be reached via the ligament.

Technique

The palpating hand approaches the apex using a perpendicular technique once more. Firm pressure is initially applied to the patellar ligament, which responds with a pronounced firm consistency. While maintaining the pressure on the ligament, the palpating fingertips attempt to make contact with the more proximal apex. The consistency of the apex is expected to be hard and the edge distinct (▶ Fig. 6.16). The edges of the patella in the area of the ligament's insertion can easily be located with the same technique.

Several soft-tissue pathologies of the patellar ligament (tendinosis, jumper's knee) can be located here. Therefore, precise pinpointing techniques are of great advantage. The treatment of these conditions will be discussed later in the text.

> **Tip**
>
> The ligament is reasonably tensed in the flexed position. Thus, firm pressure should be applied to the ligament. If it is not possible to differentiate the apex from the ligament, a further attempt is made with the knee in extension.

Patellar Ligament, Differentiation

The patellar ligament must be differentiated from the bony fixed points at its origin (patellar apex) and insertion (tibial tuberosity). Furthermore, the lateral contours can be discerned. Two techniques for this purpose will be described below:

▶ **Method 1.** Starting at the apex, the therapist palpates slightly more distally so that the fingers are directly on top of the ligament. The side borders are then sought from this position.

▶ **Method 2.** Two shallow indentations are found at the level of the patellar apex in knee joints, which are neither swollen nor arthritic. The anterior knee joint space can be accessed here. Starting at these indentations, the therapist

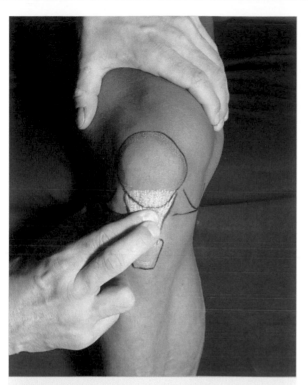

Fig. 6.16 Palpation of the apex of the patella.

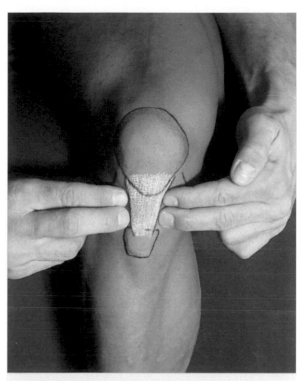

Fig. 6.17 Edges of the patellar ligament.

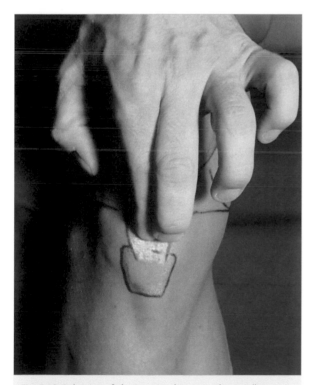

Fig. 6.18 Palpation of the junction between the patellar ligament and the tibial tuberosity.

palpates anteriorly and encounters the firm yet somewhat elastic consistency of the patellar ligament.

The edges of the ligament can be followed from the patella onto the tibial tuberosity (▶ Fig. 6.17). The palpation reveals that:

• the ligament is very wide;
• it converges and slightly tapers down into the tibial tuberosity.

Tibial Tuberosity

The tuberosity tapers off distally and merges into the anterior border of the tibia. This border can be easily palpated along the entire length of the leg. On its medial aspect, the tibia possesses a surface with a boundary posterior to the medial border of the tibia. A rough area is found on the lateral and proximal aspects of the tuberosity at the insertion of the iliotibial tract (Gerdy tubercle).

Technique

The patellar ligament is differentiated from the tibial tuberosity using the same technique (perception of differences in consistency) as for the apex.

With direct pressure on the ligament, a firm but elastic consistency is felt (▶ Fig. 6.18). If palpation is continued in a distal direction, the tuberosity is located as a distinctly hard resistance. The transition from elastic to hard consistency marks the proximal boundary of the tuberosity. Its greater size can be perceived by circular palpation with a flat fingertip. This is particularly successful in the case of a shape distorted by aseptic osteonecrosis (Osgood-Schlatter disease).

Tip

Insertion tendinopathies at the distal insertion of the ligament are well known but relatively rare. Now and then this region is painful to pressure because of bursitis, where the movement of fluid in the inflamed deep infrapatellar bursa (under the inserting ligament) or subcutaneous bursa of the tibial tuberosity (directly on the tuberosity) can be felt.

6.6.3 Tips for Assessment and Treatment

The palpation techniques used for the anterior region of the knee are used in two common assessment and treatment techniques:
- The assessment of mobility of the patellofemoral joint.
- Transverse frictions at the patellar ligament and the apex of the patella.

Techniques at the Patellofemoral Joint

Examining or restoring mobility of the patella on its femoral glide is important in postoperative treatment, for maintenance or restoration of knee flexion.

In the very early phases of postoperative treatment, this is possible when the knee is almost fully extended. It is easiest to move the patella in all directions in this position as the surrounding structures are most relaxed.

Treatment aims to preserve the elasticity of the capsule and the suprapatellar pouch in particular. Therefore, it is most important to maintain patellar mobility in a distal direction.

If necessary, stretching is used to restore mobility at a later stage of postoperative treatment. This only makes sense when the knee is positioned at maximum flexion. The knee is therefore assessed starting in this position and, when necessary, mobilized.

Surface anatomy techniques help therapists to locate the base of the patella precisely and to apply treatment effectively, even in joints that are still swollen. In this process, either the fingertips of the distal hand or the base of the proximal hand is placed on the base of the patella to exert a push to distal (▶ Fig. 6.19).

Transverse Frictions at the Patellar Ligament

Tendinopathies (especially tendinosis) of the patellar ligament are frequently occurring soft-tissue lesions in the

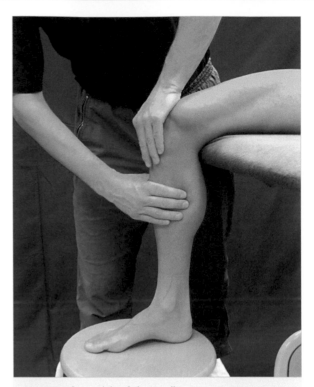

Fig. 6.19 Inferior glide of the patella.

knee joint. They are especially frequent in jumping sports with explosive extension or eccentric knee flexion (Tan and Chan, 2008). In their review, Van der Worp et al. (2011) report a frequency of up to 45% in competitive volleyball.

Transverse frictions are used to precisely locate and treat the affected part of this large structure.

If the technique targets the ligament itself, the joint should be positioned so that the ligament does not give way to the pressure of the fingers applying transverse frictions. The therapist should therefore choose to position the knee in flexion to initially place the ligament under tension (▶ Fig. 6.20).

The middle finger is placed on top of the index finger, with the index finger being used again to conduct the technique. The friction technique obtains its stability from the laterally supported thumb that exerts pressure transverse to the grain of the muscle fibers.

Tip

If this technique is being used during assessment to provoke symptoms, the therapist often has to be patient and palpate several points before they can find the (most-) affected part of the ligament. The therapist should stand a little proximal to the knee joint to prevent the body obstructing the palpating hand.

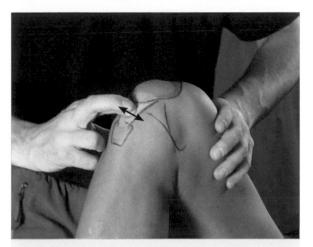

Fig. 6.20 Transverse frictions at the patellar ligament.

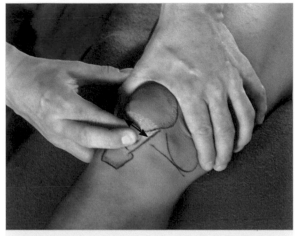

Fig. 6.21 Transverse frictions at the apex of the patella.

Transverse Frictions at the Apex of the Patella

It is not easy to palpate the junction between the ligament and the apex of the patella. If the therapist wishes to reach the edge of the bone, the ligament must first be pushed deeper into the tissues. This is only partially possible when the joint is flexed.

It is therefore recommended that the knee be almost fully extended, but not so much that excessive extension causes Hoffa fat pad to bulge and interfere with the technique. The finger pad applying the transverse frictions now points toward the apex. Sustained pressure is applied to the ligament and several points on the apex and the side edges of the patella are palpated (▶ Fig. 6.21).

The other hand stabilizes the patella proximally to prevent it moving to the side. It is also possible to apply slightly more pressure to the base of the patella so that the apex tilts to anterior and is easier to access.

6.7 Local Palpation—Medial

6.7.1 Summary of the Palpatory Process

Now that the therapist has finished palpating the anterior aspect of the knee, the side regions of the knee joint will be discussed next. A reliable point will be sought on the medial side to access the joint space. The articulating bones will be followed, if possible, from the anterior side of the knee to the posterior side. Essential bony reference points on the medial side:
• Boundaries of the medial joint space.
• Tip of the adductor tubercle.
• Medial epicondyle.
• Gastrocnemius tubercle.

Essential soft tissues that must be located:
• Medial patellotibial ligament.
• Meniscofemoral ligament.
• Mediopatellar synovial fold.
• Superficial medial collateral ligament.
• Insertions at the superficial pes anserinus.

Starting Position

The patient sits in an elevated position, for example on the edge of a treatment table. The therapist sits a little to the side, in front of the patient (▶ Fig. 6.22).

When possible, the leg should hang freely over the table and be able to flex sufficiently when the therapist's hand facilitates movement. This SP guarantees free access to the palpable structures on the medial side of the knee joint.

Alternative Starting Positions

The SP described above is mainly used when practicing. Other SPs may be necessary in the everyday assessment and treatment of the knee joint. In these cases, therapists may have to approach the knee from a different angle and position the knee with a different amount of flexion.

6.7.2 Boundaries of the Joint Space

The medial femoral condyle and the medial tibial plateau form the boundaries for the joint space. With some practice, it is possible to follow the joint space posteriorly for quite a distance until reaching the soft tissues of the pes anserinus muscles.

The edge of the tibial plateau is generally used to describe the spatial alignment of the femorotibial joint space.

Two dimples, or at least two areas, that are soft to touch are always found medially and laterally at the level of the apex of the patella. They are the most reliable approaches to making the contours of the joint components visible.

6

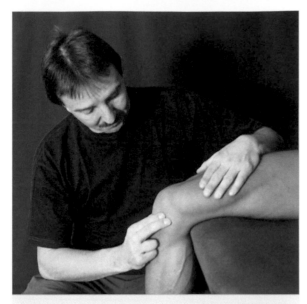

Fig. 6.22 Starting position for palpation of the medial aspect.

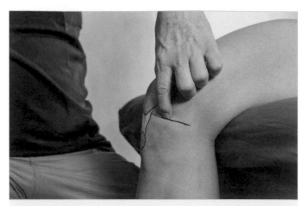

Fig. 6.23 Palpation of the edge of the tibia.

It is only at end-range extension that the infrapatellar Hoffa fat pad (corpus adiposuminfrapatellare) protrudes medially and laterally to the patellar tendon, making the finding of structures more difficult.

Technique—Tibial Plateau

If the therapist wishes to precisely palpate the edge of the tibial plateau, one hand comes from a proximal direction and palpates using a perpendicular technique while the other hand controls the leg.

The palpating finger pads are placed in the dimple medial to the apex of the patella. The fingertip pushes distally against the hard resistance of the edge of the tibia (▶ Fig. 6.23).

The tibial plateau can be followed posteriorly from this point onward for quite a distance when using this technique.

This tibial slope differs somewhat medially and laterally and can generally be expected between 4 and 10° (Nunley et al., 2014).

Tip

It will become harder to discern the edge of the tibia when palpating more posteriorly due to the presence of the medial collateral ligament. To increase confidence, the palpation can be confirmed by moving the leg. This is achieved more anteriorly on the tibia by passively extending the knee slightly so that the tibia pushes against the palpating fingertip. Extensive rotation is suitable to confirm the palpation further posteriorly.

Technique—Medial Condyle of the Femur

The palpating hand now comes from a distal position and is again positioned in the depression medial to the apex of the patella (▶ Fig. 6.24). The fingertip pushes down into the depression and attempts to reach the superior bony structure. The hard resistance felt is the cartilage coating of the articular surface of the medial femoral condyle. If the palpating fingers slip further proximal from this point, they come to a rubbery edge, the cartilage-bone boundary of the condyle, which is distinctly raised in arthritic knee joints as the result of increased pull on the capsule. Starting at the first point of hard contact, the femoral condyle is palpated further posteriorly (▶ Fig. 6.25). The palpation must follow the shape of the femoral condyle, which is expected to form a convex line (▶ Fig. 6.26).

As was the case when palpating the edge of the tibial plateau, it is hard to discern the edge of the femur for approximately 3 to 4 cm. The medial collateral ligament again hinders direct access here.

Tip

Occasionally it seems more appropriate to position the finger perpendicular to the surface of the knee and use the fingernail to palpate. The bony edge is then more distinct.

The finger encounters several soft structures further posteriorly. These are the muscles that are attached proximally to the pes anserinus.

The joint space can be followed further posteriorly when the therapist lifts the leg so that the thigh muscles hang down. The palpating finger can reach the femoral condyle more easily again on the posterior aspect.

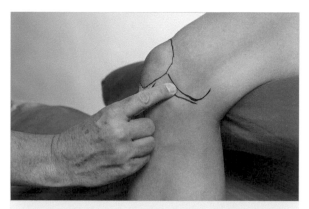

Fig. 6.24 Palpation of the medial condyle of the femur.

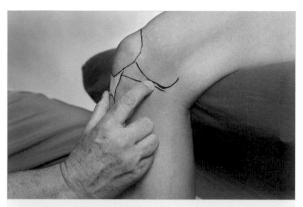

Fig. 6.25 Following the edge of the femoral condyle posteriorly.

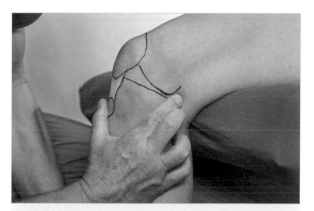

Fig. 6.26 Palpation of the posterior aspect of the femoral condyle.

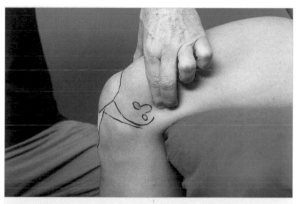

Fig. 6.27 Palpation of the adductor magnus tendon.

Adductor Tubercle and the Tendon of Adductor Magnus

The medial femoral condyle has three raised bony structures to be located: the adductor tubercle, the medial epicondyle, and the gastrocnemius tubercle. Important soft tissue parts are in contact with these raised structures. The descriptions follow an anatomical study by LaPrade et al. (2007) (▶ Fig. 6.29).

The most proximal raised structure is the adductor tubercle, which concludes with an apex in a proximal direction. At this site, the medial supracondylar crest ends and the tendon of the posterior part of the adductor magnus inserts. The especially strong elevation of the apex and the insertion can be palpated very well (▶ Fig. 6.27, ▶ Fig. 6.28).

To find the apex, the therapist uses the flat hand to stroke the medial thigh from the center to distal applying moderate pressure. The first bony structure encountered is the apex of the adductor tubercle. The dimensions of the apex can be precisely registered by using a local palpation technique with circular motion.

The round, taut tendon lies directly proximally to the apex and can be distinctly felt using transverse palpation with moderate pressure (▶ Fig. 6.27).

Tip

Sitting on the edge of the treatment table presses the posterior soft tissues of the thigh anterolaterally. If the pes anserinus muscles impede palpation of the tendon, the thigh can be lifted so that the muscles hang down (▶ Fig. 6.28). This allows reliable access to the tendon.

The entire adductor tubercle is quite large. This is where the medial patellar reticulum originates, which belongs to the transverse ligamentary apparatus of the patella (von Lanz and Wachsmuth, 2003).

For the location of additional structures, the therapist begins palpation:
- at the highest point of the tubercle—additional bony reference points.
- from the apex of the tubercle—origins of the portions of the medial collateral ligament.

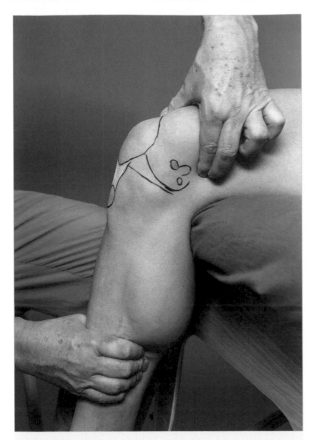

Fig. 6.28 Palpation after raising the thigh.

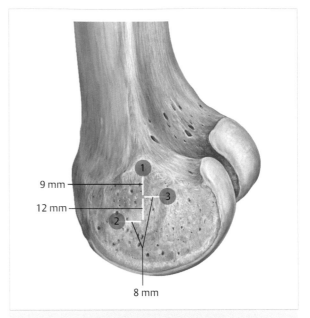

Fig. 6.29 Bony protuberances on the medial epicondyle. 1 = Highest point of the adductor tubercle, 2 = Medial femoral epicondyle, 3 = Gastrocnemius tubercle.

6.7.3 Medial Epicondyle of the Femur

LaPrade et al. (2007) describe the medial epicondyle of the femur as the most anterior and distal osseous prominence over the medial epicondyle.

The adductor tubercle is around 12 mm (9 to 15 mm) distal and around 8 mm (6 to 12 mm) posterior to the medial epicondyle. The therapist must keep this in mind in the sitting SP of the patient in which the spatial dimensions of distal and anterior are encountered (▶ Fig. 6.29).

6.7.4 Medial Gastrocnemius Tubercle

LaPrade et al. (2007) reported that the gastrocnemius tubercle was around 9 mm (7 to 11 mm) distal and around 8 mm (6 to 12 mm) posterior to the medial epicondyle (▶ Fig. 6.29).

6.7.5 Anteromedial and Medial Soft Tissues

Triangular Medial Articular Space

More soft-tissue structures can be palpated in the almost triangular articular space directly medial to the patella.

With moderate pressure and vertical fingertip and small medial to lateral movements, it is possible to feel the narrow medial patellotibial ligament that is part of the middle layer of the anterior capsule (▶ Fig. 6.30). With slight isometric contraction in extension, the ligament becomes taut.

Further to proximal on the medial femoral condyle, directly next to the edge of the patella, is the mediopatellar synovial fold (▶ Fig. 6.31). Individual folds vary in size, with a minimal width of 5 mm. In some cases, a fold can become inflamed as a result of impingement at the medial patellar edge, become thicker, and cause anterior knee pain. Pain can be provoked with pressure against the medial patellar edge when the knee is in 30° flexion.

The meniscotibial connections of the deep capsular layer can be reached in the triangular medial articular space, with pressure against the edge of the tibia. They cannot be recognized as structures but when inflamed, they can be provoked for pain. This is particularly successful when the knee joint is in 90° flexion and pronounced outward rotation, with significant pressure from proximal against the edge of the tibia (see ▶ Fig. 6.45).

Medial Collateral Ligament

During visualization of the bony structures, the collateral ligament made it more difficult to follow the edges. At the level of the knee joint space, it is approximately 3 to 4 cm wide. Now the ligament is to be visualized as completely as possible. The fixed point on the femur, the medial epicondyle, has already been found. The description below is based on the anatomical studies conducted

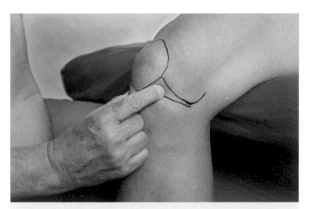

Fig. 6.30 Palpation of the medial patellotibial ligament.

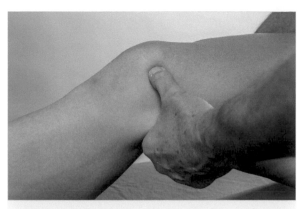

Fig. 6.31 Technique: Mediopatellar synovial fold.

6

by Liu et al. (2010), LaPrade et al. (2007), and Saigo et al. (2017).

Femoral Insertion Areas

The results of studies by Liu et al. (2010) and Saigo et al. (2017) coincide, reporting that in the femoral insertion area:

- The superficial medial collateral ligament originates 1 to 2 cm directly from the medial epicondyle. Only LaPrade et al. (2007) report the location as posterior to the medial epicondyle. From here, the superficial medial collateral ligament runs around 3 cm up to the joint line (Liu et al., 2010), where it can also be palpated.
- The oblique posterior part originates at an area between the medial epicondyle and the medial gastrocnemius tubercle. This can be visualized around 2 cm in direct distal line to the apex of the adductor tubercle (Saigo et al., 2017).

The significance of this very detailed anatomical knowledge will be explained later in the section on treatment tips.

Palpation Over the Articular Space

The palpating finger pads apply significant pressure to the depression medial to the apex of the patella. The fingertip is now positioned horizontally, aligned with the joint space (▶ Fig. 6.32).

When the therapist palpates along the edge of the tibia in a posterior direction, the palpating finger is soon pushed out of the tissues by a flat structure that is very firm and occasionally possesses a sharp edge. This structure makes it difficult to palpate the borders of the joint space.

This edge corresponds to the anterior border of the superficial medial collateral ligament. In principle, as long as the articular space cannot be distinctly felt, the collateral ligament reinforces the capsule and does not permit direct palpation of the bony structures.

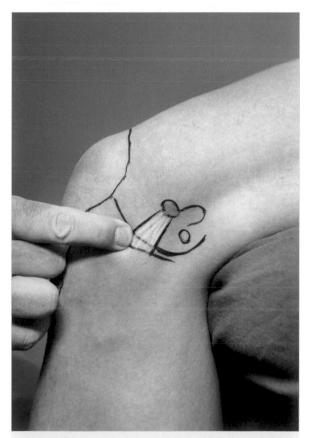

Fig. 6.32 Palpation of the medial collateral ligament, anterior edge.

The superficial portion is palpable as a distinct structure. With transverse anterior-posterior palpation on this portion, a convex eminence is felt, particularly distinctly in flexed position and poorly in extended position. The posterior boundary of this convex eminence, marking the superficial bundle, represents the transition to the posterior (or deep) portion of the collateral ligament.

The therapist can palpate the shift of the superficial part of the medial collateral ligament back when the joint is moved from extension to flexion. The therapist marks the anterior border of the ligament with the joint in extension. If the finger is kept at the palpated site and the knee is then moved into flexion; the pressure against the finger will ease when the ligament glides in a posterior direction.

Palpation continues on the posterior portion of the lateral ligament. The posterior boundary of the medial collateral ligament has been reached when the articular space can again be more clearly felt (▶ Fig. 6.33). The ligament has its closest connection to the medial meniscus in this area.

The posterior border can only be located by concluding that the ligament is no longer present when the articulating femur and tibia can be felt without interference from another structure. To palpate the

joint space, the therapist should push on the leg so that the thigh is slightly raised from the treatment table and the muscles are able to hang down (▶ Fig. 6.34).

Tibial Insertion

To identify the entire dimensions of this ligament, the therapist draws a line between its borders at the level of the joint space and the medial epicondyle. To visualize the further course to distal, the therapist can imagine that the ligament runs from the articular space for an average of another 6.2 cm (Liu et al., 2010) to distal and then somewhat anteriorly. At the anterior half of the medial tibial surface, it runs under the superficial pes anserinus and into the periosteum (▶ Fig. 6.35). Taking into account the ligament's total course running down to distal and anterior and the mass of collagen with which the ligament reinforces the capsule, it is understandable that the ligament is the primary brake for valgus stress and outward rotation of the joint.

Pes Anserinus Muscle Group

We now identify the structures that have interfered with finding, from posterior, structures close to the joint. This incorporates the group of muscles attached to the pes

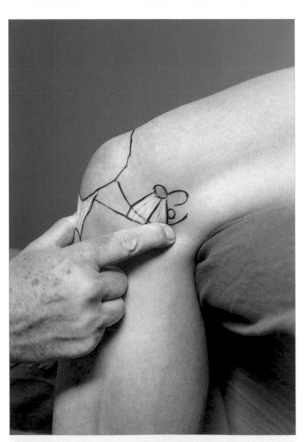

Fig. 6.33 Palpation of the posterior border.

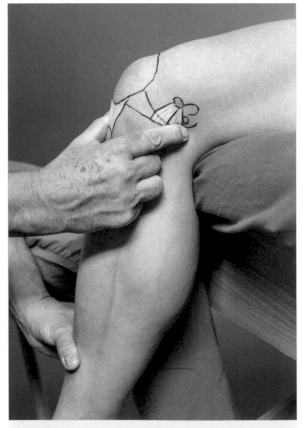

Fig. 6.34 Palpation of the posterior border after raising the thigh.

anserinus. The individual muscles are listed here from anterior to posterior:

- Sartorius.
- Gracilis.
- Semitendinosus.

Helfenstein and Kuromoto (2010) give the position of the insertion as 5 cm distal to the articular space. Symptoms (bursitis and tendinitis) are reported mainly by long distance runners.

Technique—Area of Insertion

It is impossible to differentiate the tendons from one another in the area of the pes anserinus when palpating locally and when examining anatomical specimens. The therapist can only identify the inferior border of the area of insertion (▶ Fig. 6.37).

The palpating hand is positioned flat over the medial aspect of the leg; the thumb is on the anterior edge of the tibia. When the therapist strokes over the leg from distal to proximal, the finger will first feel the more convex form of the gastrocnemius followed by a shallow concavity. The distal border of the superficial pes anserinus has been found once the finger feels a slightly convex area again (▶ Fig. 6.36).

Technique—Differentiation of Muscles

The individual muscles can be differentiated from one another proximal to the knee joint; this is best achieved posterior to the vastus medialis (▶ Fig. 6.38). Knee flexion causes the muscles to contract as a group. If necessary, medial rotation of the knee can also be used. The tendon that stands out the most distinctly with isometric contraction in flexion is the tendon of the semitendinosus.

Tip

The individual muscles can be located by using their selective actions at the other joint, the hip joint. The therapist can then locate:
- the sartorius using additional active hip flexion;
- the gracilis using additional active hip adduction;
- the semitendinosus using additional active hip extension.

Saphenous Nerve

The most important neural structures pass over the posterior side of the knee. Only one large branch of the femoral nerve traverses the joint medially: the saphenous nerve.

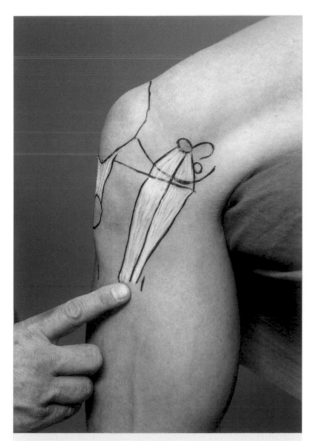

Fig. 6.35 Demonstration of the distal insertion of the medial collateral ligament.

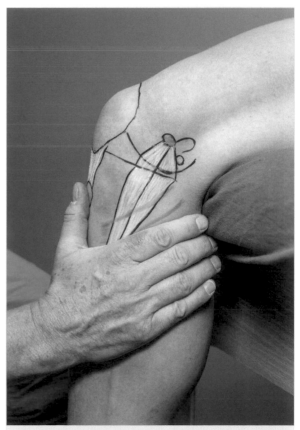

Fig. 6.36 Demonstration of the insertion area of the superficial pes anserinus muscles.

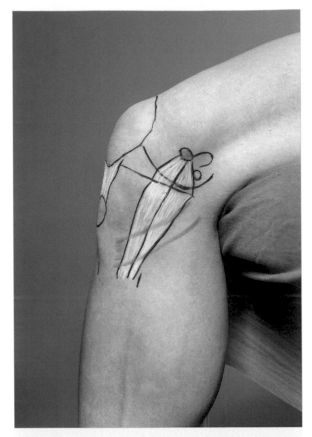

Fig. 6.37 Position of the superficial pes anserinus muscles.

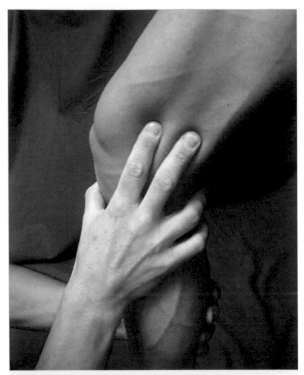

Fig. 6.38 Differentiation proximal to the knee joint.

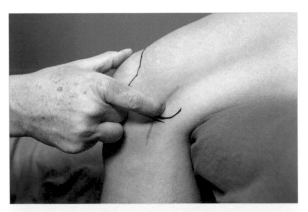

Fig. 6.39 Palpation of the saphenous nerve.

Its position varies widely (personal communication, Dos Winkel, 1992). The position depicted here is therefore only an example of individual situation.

Technique

A very specific technique is required when using palpation to locate neural structures. To palpate the movement of a peripheral nerve and/or its branch, the therapist hooks around the nerve with vertical finger pads and plucks it like a loose guitar string. Using anterior-posterior movements on the medial condyle or over the medial articular space, the therapist first attempts to find a thin structure, first with flat fingertips and then with vertical fingers. Locating the saphenous nerve is extremely difficult (▶ Fig. 6.39).

6.7.6 Tips for Treatment

Why Do Therapists Need to Locate the Joint Space?

As already mentioned, the edge of the tibial plateau is used to determine the spatial alignment of the joint space. This is very important for orientation when using translational manual therapy techniques. The joint space is not completely perpendicular to the longitudinal axis of the tibia. Instead, it tilts down distally by approximately 10°.

The illustrated examples demonstrate why identification of the joint space is necessary to glide the tibia posteriorly. This technique is used to produce the necessary back and forth femorotibial glide to allow the knee to flex freely.

Regardless of whether the joint is positioned in approximately 100° flexion (▶ Fig. 6.40) or at end of range (▶ Fig. 6.41), the therapist must pay attention to the exact spatial alignment of the joint in order to apply a parallel force.

Anteromedial Structures in the Articular Space

The menisci move posteriorly on the tibial plateau during knee flexion and anteriorly during knee extension. The anterior horns of the meniscus can be palpated in the joint space next to the apex of the patella when the knee is fully extended.

The Steinman II test is a provocative test for pain in the anterior horn of the meniscus. To conduct this test, the knee joint is first positioned in complete extension. The thumb of the testing hand applies significant pressure to the joint space adjacent to the apex of the patella (▶ Fig. 6.42). This pressure is painful in lesions of the anterior meniscal horn.

The knee joint is then slowly moved out of complete extension into flexion (▶ Fig. 6.43 and ▶ Fig. 6.44). At the same time, the meniscus glides to posterior on the tibia and moves away from the pressure of the thumb. Fading of the pain caused by pressure confirms the lesion in the anterior horn of the meniscus.

Transverse Friction of the Femoral Insertions of the Medial Collateral Ligament

In their anatomical study, Luyckx et al. (2016) describe the particular strain placed on the superficial medial collateral ligament at the femoral insertion site. This part of the medial collateral ligament retains its length throughout the whole range of motion and is therefore isometric. Deformation of the knee is observed in three planes during

6

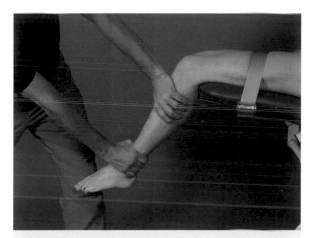

Fig. 6.40 Anterior-posterior gliding of the tibia on the femur.

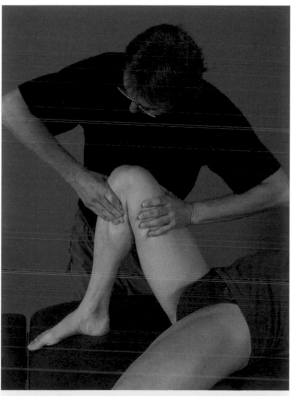

Fig. 6.41 Gliding with the knee prepositioned at end of range.

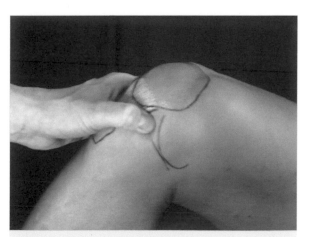

Fig. 6.42 Palpation of the joint space.

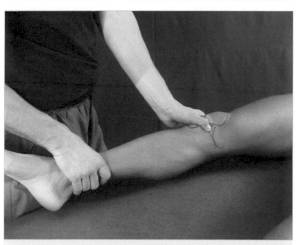

Fig. 6.43 Steinman II test, phase 1.

the movement from extension to flexion. Proximal to the joint line it rotates. As it does so, the anterior edge shifts its position noticeably toward posterior. von Lanz and Wachsmuth (2003) describe a bursa of the medial collateral ligament directly distal to the epicondyle that reduces friction of the ligament during knee movements against the femoral condyle. The rotation of the ligament brings about increased tension on the femoral insertion site. As a result, trauma of the medial collateral ligament can occur not only at the level of the articular space, but also at the proximal (and also distal) insertion. Luyckx et al. (2016) call for surgeons to also include the proximal insertion areas during reconstruction of a ruptured medial collateral ligament. Therapists should therefore use detailed palpation to precisely locate the site(s) of an injury.

Transverse Friction of the Meniscotibial Ligaments

The indentation adjacent to the apex of the patella is not only the starting point for locating the articulating surfa-

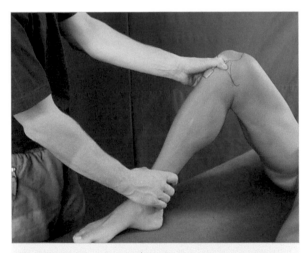

Fig. 6.44 Steinman II test, phase 2.

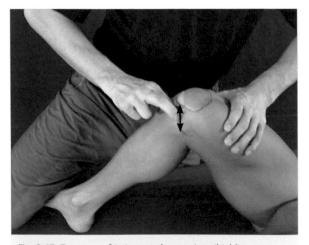

Fig. 6.45 Transverse frictions at the meniscotibial ligaments.

ces of the femur and tibia, it is also the starting point for the palpation of the meniscotibial ligaments. The coronary ligaments often cause symptoms in the anteromedial knee, especially in traumatic meniscal lesions. They insert a few millimeters distal to the articular space (Bikkina et al., 2005).

These ligaments are reached using a transverse friction technique. The palpating index finger is placed over the familiar indentation next to the apex of the patella so that the finger pad faces distally toward the tibial plateau (▶ Fig. 6.45). To facilitate access to the tibial plateau, the knee is positioned in lateral rotation so that the plateau protrudes more.

Transverse friction from posterior to anterior as far as the patellar apex is performed with pressure against the tibia. This technique can be used for both the provocation of pain in affected structures as well as for treatment.

Transverse Frictions at the Medial Collateral Ligament

The medial ligament is frequently injured. Experience shows that most of the lesions along the 9-cm-long ligament occur at the level of the joint space (Liu et al., 2010).

The therapist uses the previously described technique to locate the anterior edge of the ligament to precisely identify the affected part of the ligament (▶ Fig. 6.46). This ensures that the therapist is palpating at the level of the joint space. Next, the therapist applies posteroanterior transverse friction to the ligament with movements that cover the entire width of the ligament, in 5 mm segments, to posterior.

Joint Line Tenderness Test

This test is used, particularly in patients with arthritic knees, to differentiate between sensitivity caused by arthritis and a degenerative pathological condition of the meniscus. The test is conducted with the patient in the supine SP with the knee in 90° flexion. It can be used for the medial and lateral joint line (▶ Fig. 6.47). During medial rotation of the knee joint, the medial meniscus is distinctly palpable, while the lateral meniscus can be

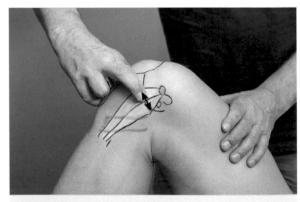

Fig. 6.46 Transverse frictions at the medial collateral ligament.

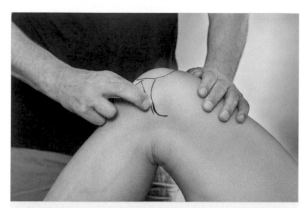

Fig. 6.47 Joint line tenderness test.

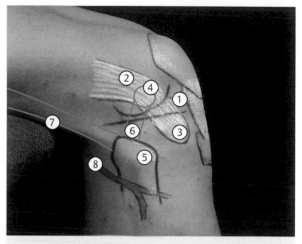

Fig. 6.48 Structures on the lateral aspect of the knee joint.
(1) Boundaries of the joint space.
(2) Iliotibial tract.
(3) Gerdy tubercle.
(4) Lateral epicondyle of the femur.
(5) Head of the fibula.
(6) Lateral collateral ligament.
(7) Biceps femoris.
(8) Common peroneal nerve.

distinctly palpated during lateral rotation (Malanga et al., 2003). When diagnosing a pathological condition of the meniscus, it should be combined with other tests (e.g., McMurray test). The scientific reliability of the joint line tenderness test is assessed differently in the literature with an average sensitivity of 0.72 and a specificity of 0.75 reported (Berberich, 2017).

Palpation starts at the anterior edge of the superficial medial collateral ligament with the therapist exerting heavy pressure with a small anterior-posterior movement. The movement is continued centimeter by centimeter in a posterior direction until the patient reports the typical pain. Then while the therapist continues to locate the sensitive site, the patient flexes the knee, increasing and decreasing range of motion. If the position of the sensitive site now changes, this indicates a meniscal lesion. If the position remains unchanged, the tenderness is caused by degenerative changes to the joint.

6.8 Local Palpation—Lateral

6.8.1 Summary of the Palpatory Process

Most of the procedure is identical to the one on the medial side. Initially, a reliable point will be sought on the lateral side to access the joint space. The articulating bones are followed from the anterior side of the joint onto the posterior side. Structures that cross over the joint space will be identified and named (▶ Fig. 6.48).

Starting Position

A starting position (SP) is again selected with the patient sitting high up, for example, on the edge of a treatment table. The therapist sits a little to the medial side, but still in front of the patient.

When possible, the leg should hang freely over the table and be able to flex extensively when the therapist's hand facilitates movement (▶ Fig. 6.49). This SP

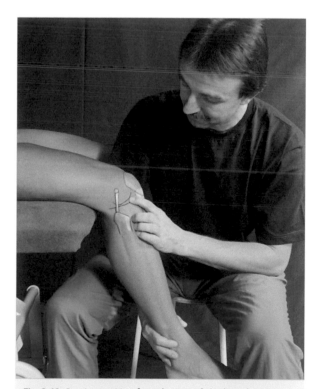

Fig. 6.49 Starting position for palpation of the lateral aspect.

guarantees free access to the palpable structures on the lateral side of the knee joint.

Alternative Starting Positions

The SP described above is mainly used when practicing. Assessment and treatment techniques often force therapists to use other angles of knee flexion in their everyday work with the lateral side of the knee joint. For this reason, to increase palpation skill, palpation should be repeated using the usual, everyday patient starting positions.

6.8.2 Palpation of Individual Structures

Boundaries of the Joint Space

The procedure and techniques applied here correspond to those in medial palpation. Therapists need to reorient themselves on the apex of the patella to easily reach the joint space. This is bordered by the lateral femoral condyle and the lateral side of the tibial plateau.

Technique—Tibial Plateau

The hand coming from the proximal direction uses a perpendicular technique to palpate the edge of the tibia precisely. The other hand is used to control the leg.

The palpating finger pads are placed in the dimple medial to the apex of the patella. The fingertip pushes distally against the firm resistance of the edge of the tibial plateau (▶ Fig. 6.50).

From here, the tibial plateau can be followed posteriorly for quite a distance using this technique. Again, the palpation is expected to follow a straight line and tilt down in a slightly inferior direction at the posterior side of the knee.

> **Tip**
>
> It will not be easy to discern the edge of the tibial plateau more posteriorly due to the presence of two soft-tissue structures. To improve the reliability of the palpation, the therapist can confirm the location by

moving the leg. Slight passive extension and extensive rotation of the joint are ideal for this.

Technique—Lateral Femoral Condyle and Lateral Patellotibial Ligament

The palpating hand now comes from a distal position and is again placed in the depression lateral to the apex of the patella. The fingertip pushes down into the depression and attempts to reach the proximal bony structure (▶ Fig. 6.51 and ▶ Fig. 6.52). The firm resistance felt is the cartilage coating of the articular surface of the lateral condyle. If the therapist slides slightly more proximally, another edge will be reached that corresponds to the boundary between the cartilage and the bone of the condyle.

Like the medial patellotibial ligament, the lateral ligament runs in the groove medial to the apex, steeply downward and almost parallel to the patellar ligament, to the tibia. It should be possible to feel it with deep pressure and transverse medial-lateral finger movement, but this is not always the case (not illustrated).

Starting at the first point of hard contact, the femoral condyle is palpated further posteriorly (▶ Fig. 6.53). The palpation must follow the shape of the femoral condyle and is expected to take the form of a convex line with a smaller radius than to medial.

It is generally easier to feel the bony borders of the joint space on the lateral side than on the medial side. If lateral palpation is still difficult, a vertical fingernail can be used. This makes it easier to feel the edge of the bone.

Soft tissues do not obstruct palpation of the posterior section of the joint space on the lateral side. Therefore, it is not necessary to raise the leg to allow the muscles to hang down.

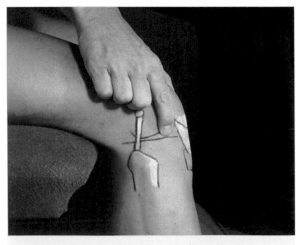

Fig. 6.50 Palpation of the edge of the tibia.

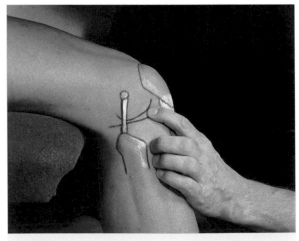

Fig. 6.51 Palpation of the anterior aspect of the femoral condyle.

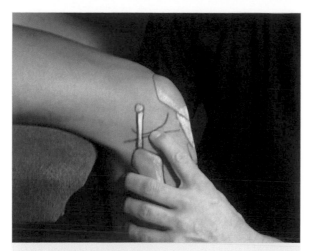

Fig. 6.52 Palpation of the lateral femoral condyle.

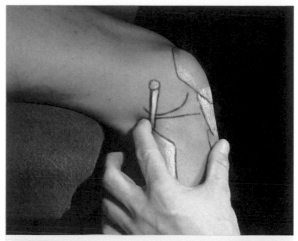

Fig. 6.53 Palpation of the posterior aspect of the femoral condyle.

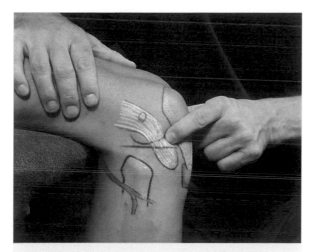

Fig. 6.54 Palpation of the iliotibial tract—anterior edge.

Iliotibial Tract

The iliotibial tract (see ▶ Fig. 6.6) is a flat, wide, firm-elastic structure when it crosses over the knee joint. It inserts immediately distal to the joint space on a roughened area (Gerdy tubercle) (▶ Fig. 6.2).

Overall, the tract does not seem as wide and firm as the superficial portion of the medial collateral ligament that crosses the articular space at a comparable point medially. The anterior edge of the tract is also not as sharp as in the medial collateral ligament.

Technique—At the Joint Space

The palpating finger pads apply firm pressure to the depression lateral to the apex of the patella. The fingertip is now aligned with the joint space.

When the therapist palpates laterally over the femoral and tibial condyles, the fingers are soon pushed superficially out of the joint space again (▶ Fig. 6.54). This marks the anterior boundary of the tract. The joint components are less clearly felt while the tract is crossing the articular space. The posterior boundary of the tract can also be determined in this way.

Technique—Proximal to the Knee Joint

The entire width of the tract can be located when this collagenous structure is tensed by the strong contraction of muscles. The muscles involved are the vastus lateralis (with knee extension) and tensor fasciae latae (with flexion and inward rotation).

The edges of the tract can be visualized closely proximal to the base of the patella with transverse palpation (▶ Fig. 6.55). A considerable number of the tract fibers run from the frontal aspect of the tract to the proximal edge of the patella and insert somewhat distal to the lateral vastus tendon. In flexion, these fibers (iliopatellar ligament) can be made to tense by isometric contraction in flexed position, which differentiates them clearly from the vastus fibers.

Gerdy Tubercle

The principal insertion of the tractus on the tibia has several possible names: Gerdy tubercle, lateral tibial tubercle, tubercle of the iliotibial tract.

Technique

It is usually easy to locate this area of roughness and its borders by again using several flattened fingers to stroke over the anterolateral side of the tibia slightly inferior to the joint space (▶ Fig. 6.56). This elevation is palpated as a semicircular structure directly inferior to the edge of the tibial plateau. Together with the tibial tubercle and the fibular head, it forms an equilateral triangle.

6

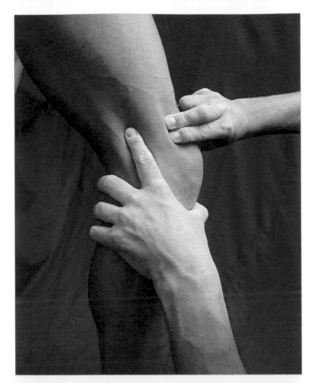

Fig. 6.55 Palpation proximal to the knee joint.

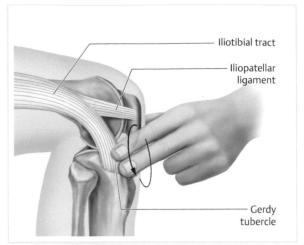

Fig. 6.56 Palpation of the Gerdy tubercle.

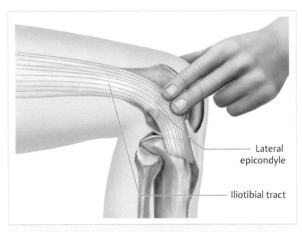

Fig. 6.57 Palpation of the lateral epicondyle of the femur.

Lateral Epicondyle of the Femur and Insertion of the Popliteal Tendon

This epicondyle is far less prominent than its medial counterpart; it can be found and felt by the same technique. It serves as a possible landmark when seeking the lateral collateral ligament.

Technique—Epicondyle

The same palpatory procedure is used here as for the medial side. The region is palpated with several flat fingertips and a small amount of pressure (▶ Fig. 6.57). The most prominent elevation is the lateral epicondyle. In some cases, a true tip of the epicondyle cannot be palpated due to the very flat curvature (Takeda et al., 2015).

Technique—Popliteal Tendon

The tendinous insertion of the popliteus can be felt from the epicondyle by palpating approximately 0.5 cm distal to the tip of the epicondyle and then 0.5 cm anterior. The insertion of the tendon, which runs between the collateral ligament and the capsule, can rarely be palpated as a distinct structure. Correct location is therefore confirmed by instructing the patient to rhythmically flex and extend the knee slightly. A contraction is felt underneath the palpating finger. However, this location process can be categorized as rather difficult (not illustrated).

Head of the Fibula

The next stage of the palpation of the lateral knee joint encompasses the entire dimensions of the head of the fibula. It is of interest because it serves as the point of insertion of the lateral collateral ligament and the biceps femoris, as well as being a component of the tibiofibular joint.

Technique

The location of the posterolateral tibial plateau can usually be determined without problems by initially using the flattened finger pads for palpation. The anterior, proximal, and posterior contours of the head of the fibula are identified next. Again, a perpendicular palpation technique is used.

When the fibular head is first found, its size is astonishing (▶ Fig. 6.58). It also becomes apparent that the head of the fibula has a tip that varies greatly between individuals and marks the lateral collateral ligament as well as the large portion of the biceps tendon.

If it is still difficult to locate this structure and palpate it in its entirety, the prominent tendon of the biceps femoris can be followed distally as far as the tip of the head of the fibula.

Lateral Collateral Ligament

The therapist can mark the course and dimensions of the lateral collateral ligament by drawing a line between the lateral epicondyle and the head of the fibula.

Technique

Since in the starting position for lateral knee joint palpation already described the ligament remains relatively

relaxed, direct location by transverse palpation is not always successful (▶ Fig. 6.59).

Two methods exist to make the ligament more distinct:
- The SP is altered to confirm the location. One finger remains in contact with the region where the ligament is presumed to be. The leg is placed in the "Patrick test position" (or "Figure Four test") by placing the leg to be palpated on top of the other leg so that this hip is positioned in flexion, abduction, and lateral rotation (▶ Fig. 6.60).
  - When the knee hangs down passively, the joint is subject to varus loading that produces tension in the collateral ligament.
  - The ligament can now be palpated as a short, thick, and rounded structure. The finger remains on the ligament while the leg is brought back into the original starting position.
- It takes a lot less effort to confirm the location of this ligament when the joint is moved passively into extensive lateral rotation. As the ligament extends inferiorly in a posterior direction, this position places the ligament under tension, making it easier to locate (not illustrated).

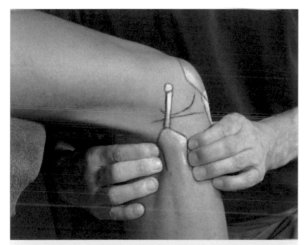

Fig. 6.58 Borders of the head of the fibula.

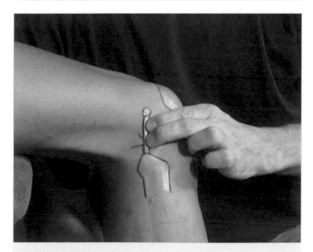

Fig. 6.59 Palpation of the lateral collateral ligament.

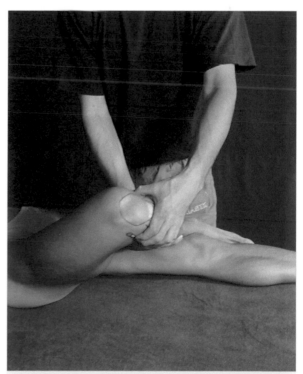

Fig. 6.60 Palpation with the aid of the Patrick test position.

Biceps Femoris

The biceps femoris is the only effective flexor *and* lateral rotator of the knee joint.

Its tendon is visible especially when the muscle isometrically contracts (▶ Fig. 6.61). Several of its fibers are evident on the lateral meniscus or hug the lateral collateral ligament. The largest part of the tendon inserts onto the head of the fibula.

Technique

The boundaries of the wide, prominent tendon can be found by transverse palpation on the anterior and posterior sides (▶ Fig. 6.62). The next anterior structure is the iliotibial tract and the next posterior structure the common peroneal nerve. The tendon can be easily followed to its insertion on the head of the fibula.

Common Peroneal Nerve

This nerve is one of the large peripheral nerves that cross over the knee joint. Therapists are familiar with its pathway from topographical anatomy. The nerve separates itself from the tibial nerve approximately 1 handwidth proximal to the joint (see ▶ Fig. 6.63). It then accompanies the biceps femoris tendon and crosses over the fibula inferior to its head before dividing into its deep and superficial branches.

Technique

A vertical fingertip slides to distal on the head of the fibula until the head is no longer felt as a bony thickening and only soft tissue can be felt. The nerve can be palpated slightly more posterior to this position and is "plucked" using a small transverse movement (proximal-distal) (▶ Fig. 6.63). The thickness of the nerve is surprising when it is first found.

6.8.3 Tips for Assessment and Treatment

Joint Space

The palpation of the lateral joint space is also used laterally when applying manual therapy glide techniques. In these techniques, the angle of glide has to be accurate to the degree (see ▶ Fig. 6.39).

Lateral Meniscus

The Steinman II test can also be used in the same manner to provoke symptoms in the anterior horn of the lateral meniscus.

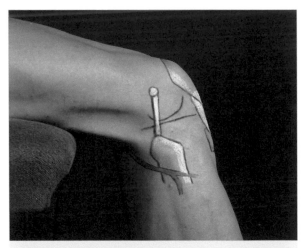

Fig. 6.61 Contraction of the biceps femoris.

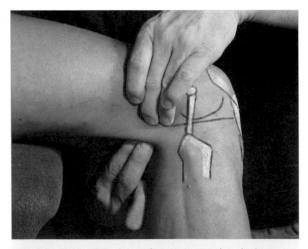

Fig. 6.62 Edges of the biceps femoris proximal to the knee joint.

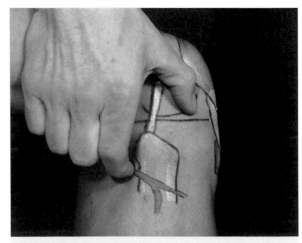

Fig. 6.63 Palpation of the common peroneal nerve.

Treatment of the Lateral Collateral Ligament

As was the case medially, transverse frictions can be used to confirm or treat painful lesions of the lateral collateral ligament.

Three possible methods are available to find the ligament:
- Transverse palpation along the joint space.
- Palpating from the ligament's bony attachments (epicondyle and head of the fibula).
- Moving the leg into the Patrick test position.

Experience has shown that approximately 90° knee flexion in prone lying is a suitable SP for the patient. The ligament can be placed under slightly more tension by laterally rotating the knee minimally to ensure that the ligament does not slide away as easily from underneath the finger that applies the frictions. Other SPs are also possible (▶ Fig. 6.64).

The therapist stands on the opposite side of the patient. One hand is used to stabilize the leg position while the other hand applies the frictions. The middle finger is placed on top of the index finger applying the frictions, and the thumb rests on the medial side of the knee to stabilize the hand.

After the ligament has been found, transverse friction is used for precise location of the damaged spot (▶ Fig. 6.65). The tendon is assessed in several small sections. The same technique is used with appropriate pressure to ease pain.

Iliotibial Band Friction Syndrome

There are a large number of causes for lateral knee pain. Symptoms are all too often ascribed to the femorotibial joint or the lateral meniscus. Therefore, we must point out two pathological possibilities that have nothing to do with joint pathology. Knowledge of surface anatomy is the indispensable prerequisite for recognizing and naming the cause of the symptoms.

Athletes who flex and extend the knee very often during movement can develop "runner's knee," otherwise known as the iliotibial band friction syndrome. This is caused by repeated rubbing of the iliotibial tract (also known as iliotibial band) over the lateral epicondyle during flexion and extension. In most cases, additional pathogenic factors, such as abnormal varus joint statics, also play a role.

The benefits of surface anatomy are demonstrated when therapists are able to confirm the presence of friction at the iliotibial tract or the bursa between the tract and epicondyle. Reaching the conclusion that these problems are due to a (more easily treatable) periarticular problem is important in setting the course for further assessment and treatment of the affected knee.

Arthritis of the Proximal Tibiofibular Joint

Another set of symptoms involves pain on the anterolateral aspect of the knee region and is related to arthritis in the joint between the head of the fibula and the posterolateral tibia. The fact that this does not usually involve the femorotibial joint is also of great importance.

The tibiofibular joint functionally belongs to the kinematic chain associated with the important joints of the foot (tibiotarsal complex). The fibula, in particular, moves during flexion and extension of the foot. Of course, this also occurs proximally. Trauma associated with "twisting the ankle" can damage the ligaments of the ankle and often results in the fibula changing its position with posterior laxity and sometimes dislocation in the proximal tibiofibular joint. Both of these conditions manifest themselves as anterolateral pain when present over a long period and is associated with irritation of the capsule.

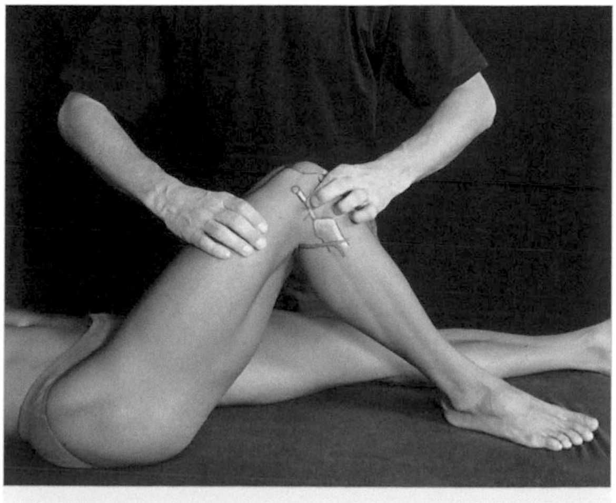

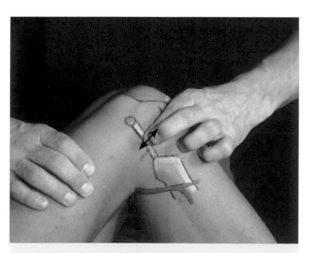

Fig. 6.64 Starting position for transverse friction at the lateral collateral ligament.

Fig. 6.65 Detailed view of the transverse friction.

Aside from this particular injury, the pain cannot be easily linked to any other precipitating factors.

Only local palpation of the anterior aspect of the joint or a well-conducted test of joint play at the tibiofibular joint can confirm the source of these symptoms (▶ Fig. 6.66).

6.9 Local Palpation—Posterior

6.9.1 Summary of the Palpatory Process

The hollow of the knee (popliteal fossa) characterizes the topographical anatomy and palpation of the posterior aspect of the knee joint. It is a diamond-shaped depression with muscles forming its boundaries.

The aim of surface palpation is to make the borders of the popliteal fossa and its contents accessible. For orientation in the popliteal fossa, it is advisable to induce tension in the soft-tissue structures (muscles and nerves) so that their contours become distinct.

Starting Position

The patient lies prone. The therapist places the leg in a position very similar to that for a straight leg raise test, although the sequence of positions deviates slightly (▶ Fig. 6.67).

The following combination is recommended for practice: a generous degree of flexion of the hip joint with extension of the knee joint (for this patient, it is approximately 50° flexion) as well as moderate extension of the foot.

The advantage of this SP is the unobstructed view of the hollow of the knee, the free access for the palpating hand, as well as the initial tension in the soft-tissue structures.

One hand stabilizes the position of the leg. Handling should permit the facilitation of additional ankle dorsiflexion to tighten other muscular and neural structures. The other hand is free to search for the structure being sought.

Alternative Starting Positions

This SP is not particularly comfortable for patients and is only recommended when practicing. Once therapists are able to reliably locate the described structure, they should therefore practice the palpation in other, more comfortable SPs. The position of the muscular structures is then confirmed using selective contraction of the muscles.

6.9.2 Palpation of Individual Structures

Neural Structures in the Popliteal Fossa

The following neural and vascular structures pass though the popliteal fossa (▶ Fig. 6.68):
- Tibial nerve.
- Common peroneal nerve.
- Popliteal artery and vein.

The neural structures in the popliteal fossa can be easily identified when the therapist uses the above-described SP and places the ankle in additional dorsiflexion. End-range hip flexion and extension of the knee have already

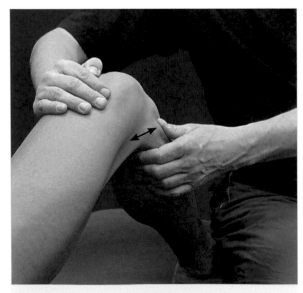

Fig. 6.66 Test of tibiofibular joint play.

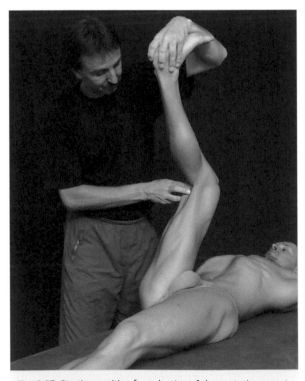

Fig. 6.67 Starting position for palpation of the posterior aspect.

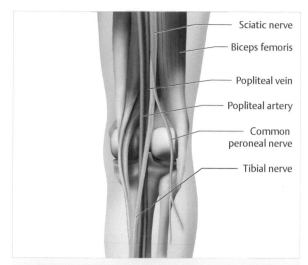

Fig. 6.68 Topography of the neurovascular bundle on the posterior aspect.

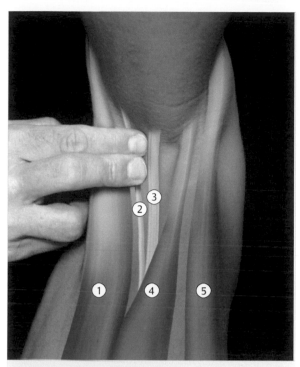

Fig. 6.69 Palpation of the tibial nerve.
(1) Biceps femoris.
(2) Common peroneal nerve.
(3) Tibial nerve.
(4) Semitendinosus.
(5) Gracilis.

almost stretched these peripheral nerves. The positioning of the foot causes them to be maximally tensed.

Technique—Tibial Nerve

The sciatic nerve divides into its two branches approximately 1 handwidth proximal to the knee joint. The tibial nerve is observed directly in the middle of the popliteal fossa. The stretched nerve feels very firm and elastic when palpated directly (▶ Fig. 6.69). The expected diameter of the structure can be described as varying from the thickness of a pencil to that of a small finger.

Tip

If the position of the leg does not stretch the nerve sufficiently to identify it as a firm structure, the therapist can additionally move the hip into adduction and medial rotation. This increases the passive tension in the nerve.

Technique: Common Peroneal Nerve—Posterior

After branching out from the tibial nerve, the common peroneal nerve passes laterally and accompanies the biceps tendon to the head of the fibula. It crosses further anterolaterally, distal to the head of the fibula, and then branches out.

The nerve is approximately 1 cm wide and found more medially at the level of the biceps tendon. The tension in the nerve makes it easy to clearly differentiate it from the tendon (▶ Fig. 6.70).

Tip

If the nerve does not feel like a firm structure because it is not stretched sufficiently, the therapist can additionally alter the position of the foot to increase tension. Adduction and supination are ideal for this. In theory, plantar flexion also increases tension, but its use is not as appropriate here because it causes the neighboring gastrocnemius to relax and makes it more difficult to differentiate the nerve from its surroundings.

Tendon of the Biceps Femoris

The biceps tendon forms the lateral border of the popliteal fossa. The tendon is stretched so much and is so prominent in this SP that it cannot be missed. Palpation of the tendon in a distal direction leads the therapist onto the head of the fibula again. Proximally, the disappearance of the distinct contour of the tendon marks the start of the muscle belly of the short head.

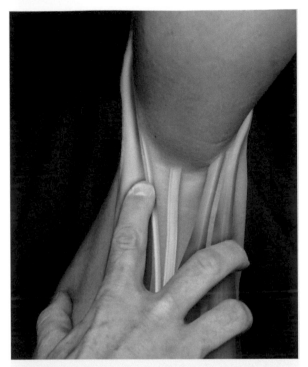

Fig. 6.70 Palpation of the common peroneal nerve.

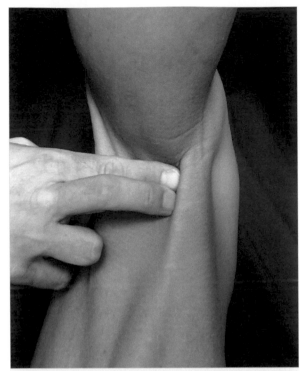

Fig. 6.71 Palpation of the tendon of the semitendinosus.

Tendons of the Pes Anserinus Muscles

It is significantly more challenging to differentiate the muscles forming the medial border of the popliteal fossa.

Technique—Tendon of the Semitendinosus

The semitendinosus has the most prominent tendon in this muscle group. It is easily found by moving medial from the middle of the hollow of the knee and hooking with the fingertips (▶ Fig. 6.71). The tendon can be followed a little distally. Its contours disappear into the collagenous plate of the superficial pes anserinus on the inner side of the knee.

> **Tip**
>
> If tissue conditions make precise location of the tendon difficult, the therapist can confirm the location by instructing the patient to actively extend the hip, which causes the tendon to clearly protrude.

Technique—Tendon of the Gracilis

The tendon of the gracilis can be palpated directly medial to the semitendinosus tendon, which is best achieved when the patient adducts the hip (▶ Fig. 6.72). These tendons are separated by a small gap.

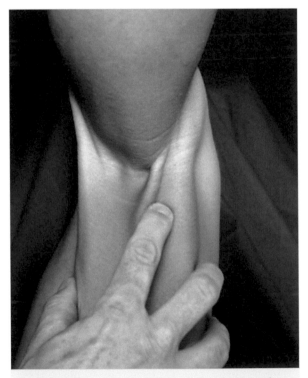

Fig. 6.72 Differentiation between the semitendinosus and gracilis.

Technique—Tendon of the Sartorius

The palpating finger can locate the more flattened structure of the sartorius further medially after passing another small gap in the muscles.

Precise differentiation of this muscle from the gracilis tendon is achieved by flexing the hip against resistance. This causes the gracilis to relax again and the sartorius becomes more distinct (no illustration).

6.9.3 Tips for Assessment and Treatment

Popliteal Fossa

Caution

Knowing how easy it is to reach very sensitive structures in the hollow of the knee, such as the peripheral nerves or their neighboring blood vessels, should prevent therapists from applying excessive pressure to the popliteal fossa. This area is at risk when applying underwater pressure massage and local friction techniques, for example, to the popliteus, or during mobilization when pressure is applied to the calf near the knee joint.

Transverse frictions should be applied very accurately to the biceps tendon or the muscle-tendon junction. It is very important that these structures be differentiated from the common peroneal nerve when conducting these techniques. Knowledge of the correct anatomy of living subjects provides therapists with the necessary basic skills.

Bibliography

Alvarez-Nemegyei J. Risk factors for pes anserinus tendinitis/bursitis syndrome: a case control study. J Clin Rheumatol. 2007; 13(2):63–65

Berberich K. Diagnostische Genauigkeit und Reabilität manueller Tests zur Untersuchung der unteren Extremität: Ein Umbrella Review [Bachelorarbeit]. Dresden: Dresden International University (DIU), Studiengang Bachelor of Science in Präventions-, Therapie- und Rehabilitationswissenschaften; 2017

Bikkina RS, Tujo CA, Schraner AB, Major NM. The "floating" meniscus: MRI in knee trauma and implications for surgery. AJR Am J Roentgenol. 2005; 184(1):200–204

Fuss FK. Anatomy of the cruciate ligaments and their function in extension and flexion of the human knee joint. Am J Anat. 1989; 184(2):165–176

HCPUnet, Healthcare Cost and Utilization Project. Agency for Healthcare Research and Quality. http://hcupnet.ahrq.gov (Accessed on December 20, 2012)

Helfenstein M, Jr, Kuromoto J. Anserine syndrome. Rev Bras Reumatol. 2010; 50(3):313–327

iData Research.2018. Total Knee Replacement Statistics 2017; https://idata-research.com/total-knee-replacement-statistics-2017-younger-patients-driving-growth/; last access 19 Oct 2019

Lanz T von, Wachsmuth W. Praktische Anatomie, Bein und Statik. 2. Aufl. Berlin: Springer; 2003

LaPrade RF, Engebretsen AH, Ly TV, Johansen S, Wentorf FA, Engebretsen L. The anatomy of the medial part of the knee. J Bone Joint Surg Am. 2007; 89(9):2000–2010

Liu F, Yue B, Gadikota HR, et al. Morphology of the medial collateral ligament of the knee. J Orthop Surg Res. 2010; 5:69

Luyckx T, Verstraete M, De Roo K, Van Der Straeten C, Victor J. High strains near femoral insertion site of the superficial medial collateral ligament of the Knee can explain the clinical failure pattern. J Orthop Res. 2016; 34(11):2016–2024

Malanga GA, Andrus S, Nadler SF, McLean J. Physical examination of the knee: a review of the original test description and scientific validity of common orthopedic tests. Arch Phys Med Rehabil. 2003; 84(4):592–603

Maradit Kremers H, Larson DR, Crowson CS, et al. Prevalence of Total Hip and Knee Replacement in the United States. J Bone Joint Surg Am. 2015; 97(17):1386–1397

Matthijs O, van Paridon-Edauw D, Winkel D. Manuelle Therapie der peripheren Gelenke, Bd. 3: Hüfte, Knie, Sprunggelenk, Fuß und Knorpelgewebe. München: Urban & Fischer bei Elsevier; 2003

Matthijs O, van Paridon-Edauw D, Winkel D. Manuelle Therapie der peripheren Gelenke, Bd. 3: Hüfte, Knie, Sprunggelenk, Fuß und Knorpelgewebe. München: Urban & Fischer bei Elsevier; 2006

Nunley RM, Nam D, Johnson SR, Barnes CL. Extreme variability in posterior slope of the proximal tibia: measurements on 2395 CT scans of patients undergoing UKA? J Arthroplasty. 2014; 29(8):1677–1680

Panagiotopoulos E, Strzelczyk P, Herrmann M, Scuderi G. Cadaveric study on static medial patellar stabilizers: the dynamizing role of the vastus medialis obliquus on medial patellofemoral ligament. Knee Surg Sports TraumatolArthrosc. 2006; 14(1):7–12

Petersen W, Zantop T. Das vordere Kreuzband: Grundlagen und aktuelle Praxis der operativen Therapie. Deutscher Ärzte-Verlag; 2009

Saigo T, Tajima G, Kikuchi S, et al. Morphology of the insertions of the superficial medial collateral ligament and posterior oblique ligament using 3-dimensional computed tomography: a cadaveric study. Arthroscopy. 2017; 33(2):400–407

Scharf W, Weinstabl R, Orthner E. Anatomische Unterscheidung und klinische Bedeutung zweier verschiedener Anteile des Musculus vastus medialis. Acta Anat (Basel). 1985; 123(2):108–111

Shamus J, Shamus E. The management of iliotibial band syndrome with a multifaceted approach: a double case report. Int J Sports Phys Ther. 2015; 10(3):378–390

Statistisches Bundesamt (Destatis). Gesundheitsberichterstattung des Bundes. http://www.gbe-bund.de (Accessed on October 4, 2017)

Strobel M, Stedtfeld H-W. Diagnostik des Kniegelenkes. 3. Aufl. Heidelberg: Springer; 2013

Takeda S, Tajima G, Fujino K, et al. Morphology of the femoral insertion of the lateral collateral ligament and popliteus tendon. Knee Surg Sports TraumatolArthrosc. 2015; 23(10):3049–3054

Tan SC, Chan O. Achilles and patellar tendinopathy: current understanding of pathophysiology and management. DisabilRehabil. 2008; 30(20–22):1608–1615

Tubbs RS, Caycedo FJ, Oakes WJ, Salter EG. Descriptive anatomy of the insertion of the biceps femoris muscle. Clin Anat. 2006; 19(6):517–521

van der Worp H, van Ark M, Roerink S, Pepping GJ, van den Akker-Scheek I, Zwerver J. Risk factors for patellar tendinopathy: a systematic review of the literature. Br J Sports Med. 2011; 45(5):446–452

Wirth CJ, Zichner L, Kohn D. Orthopädie und Orthopädische Chirurgie – Knie. Stuttgart: Thieme; 2005

Chapter 7

Foot

7

7 Foot

7.1 Introduction

7.1.1 Significance and Function of the Foot

Function

- **Transmission of body weight onto the underlying surface:** during the gait cycle and bipedal stand the construction of the foot absorbs shock and cushions the transfer of body load onto the underlying surface. The sole of the foot, a double angle lever, is perpendicular to the axis of the leg at rest and can distribute the weight of the body over a large surface.
- **Shock absorption:** this basic principle spans the entire lower limb and vertebral column. Shock absorption is achieved in the foot by:
  - calcaneal fat pad (Dhillon, 2013);
  - the bony construction, more similar to a cushioning sheet than an inflexible arch;
  - the astonishing range of motion within the tarsal joints.
- **Locomotion:** the gait cycle is the most complicated pattern of movement in the musculoskeletal system, followed by full elevation of the arm and the biomechanics of the upper cervical spine. The foot's function in the lower limb is to establish contact, support the weight of the body, adapt to uneven terrain, provide a stable supportive surface, and exercise propulsion. There are two different patterns in this activity:
  - In the landing phase (loading response) the foot performs a complete eversion movement (total pronation). The calcaneus moves into valgus and the forefoot (transverse tarsal joints) goes into extension, abduction, and pronation. The accompanying inward rotation of the talus then forces the tibia and later also the femur into accompanying inward rotation. This chain reaction begins at the calcaneus and ends approximately at T8.
  - Preparation for a chain reaction to introduce the push-off phase (total supination) begins proximally. The swing forward of the other leg causes a brief inward rotation of the hip joint in the stance leg that is transformed into outward rotation of the femur after absorption of the tension in the pelvitrochanteric muscles and the joint capsule. Finally, this femoral rotation pulls along the tibia and talus and the calcaneus responds with varus and inward rotation. The subsequent twisting makes the forefoot rigid and prepares it for load transfer as the calcaneus leaves the ground.
- **Sensory function:** information from the many mechanoreceptors in joints, ligaments, and the sole of the foot contributes to the coordination of standing and walking as well as to the creation of equilibrium. Injuries to structures such as the deep intrinsic ligaments between talus and calcaneus in the tarsal sinus, resulting from inversion trauma, can lead to chronic pain and in particular to feelings of instability during heel contact (Helgeson, 2009; Karlsson et al., 1997).

7.1.2 Special Characteristics of the Bony Construction

Hand and foot skeletons have many parallel aspects in phylogenetic development. Thus, the transverse articulation in hand and foot—root, middle, and terminal elements—can be comparably described (Starck, 1978). In comparison to the construction of the skeleton of the hand, the tarsal bones stand out from their surroundings with their noticeable increase in bony mass and their reduced mobility.

The skeletal arches, also recognizable in the structure of the hand, are universally recognized to be more pronounced in the foot as longitudinal and transverse arches, with the median arch higher than the lateral. Phylogenetically, the calcaneus has developed from a flat position and has pulled the talus along with it into a vertical position. This created the longitudinal arches that transmit the weight of the body to the underlying surface not rigidly but with great elasticity. Through the plantar aponeurosis, the plantar ligaments (plantaris longus ligament), and the short foot muscles, the longitudinal arches are secured as with a tension band.

It is noteworthy that in the evolution of the metatarsal area, the first ray together with the ray of the great toe has rearticulated with the remaining metatarsal bones. This development improved the ability of the foot to both support the body and partake in heel-toe gait, but was at the cost of grasp, with enormous losses being made here in comparison to the feet of primates.

The angle between the skeleton of the foot and the axis of the leg in two directions is almost perpendicular and is labeled the "double-angled lever construction." This enables locomotion on the soles of the feet and provides a long lever for the long muscles originating in the leg.

The talus has exceptional status. No muscles insert on it. All extrinsic tendons run past it, and no intrinsic tendons have their origin there. In a load-carrying situation, the talus distributes the body weight to the forefoot and heel. It functions as an adaptive intercalated segment (Landsmeer, 1961), comparable to the functioning of the carpal bones of the hand. In addition to contributing significantly to the extension and flexion capacity of the foot, the talus mediates rotation of the leg on the foot and vice versa.

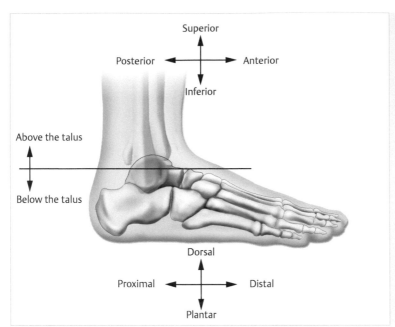

Fig. 7.1 Special nomenclature for the foot.

7.1.3 Features of the Nomenclature

The almost perpendicular relationship of the foot skeleton to the leg requires modification of the nomenclature for precise description of position and orientation of structures. As a result, a suggestion is offered for the following designations of position, so that the particular construction of the foot can be taken into account. The terms used above the talus are the usual ones; downward from the talus, the usual terminology is replaced by foot-specific terms. ▶ Fig. 7.1 indicates the boundary between the two terminologies with a transverse line through the talus.

7.1.4 Special Biomechanical Characteristics

An outstanding biomechanical characteristic in the foot is the formation of the kinematic complex consisting of the talocrural joint, the subtalar complex, and the transverse tarsal (TT) joint. This articular complex must always be viewed as a functional unit. The articular components always act together, especially during movement in a closed kinematic chain.

The transverse tarsal joint and its biomechanical connection to the ankle and talocalcaneonavicular (TCN) joints play another important role in the mobility and flexibility of the foot. Disorders within the kinematic chain—all of which lie along the Chopart (or TT) joint line—can only be identified using tests of joint play at the respective articulation.

The alignment of the subtalar complex during heel contact is decisive for the chain reaction from distal to proximal during the landing phase. The position and freedom

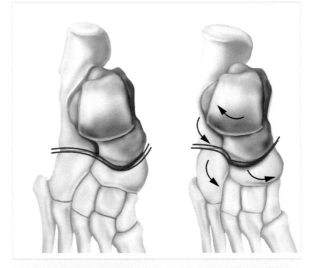

Fig. 7.2 Subtalar biomechanics.

of movement of the calcaneus determine further progress. For this reason, the subtalar complex is also known as a key joint.

The talus and calcaneus move in contrary motion, while the transverse tarsal joint always follows the movement of the calcaneus. In the landing phase, the calcaneus tips to the side in valgus position. Its distal end swings to lateral in abduction. At the same time, the talar head turns to medial, which is termed inward rotation or adduction. In inversion of the calcaneus in the push-off phase, the pattern of movement is the reverse for both; they press the distal tarsalia into a rigid position, which prepares them to take over the weight as the heel is lifted (▶ Fig. 7.2). The rotations of the talus and the lateral movements of the distal end of the calcaneus are often unrecognized and undervalued movement components that are essential for frictionless movement. In particular, the outward rotation of the talus is a decisive component that arises in association with most loaded flexion and extension positions of the talocrural joint (Van Langelaan, 1983; Huson, 1987, 2000; Lundberg, 1989).

The individual components of the motor complex influence each other and are always to be viewed, assessed, and, if necessary, treated as a unit when mobility is affected. Sites of hypomobility and hypermobility are often found adjacent to one another. Hence, all joints should be assessed individually in cases of abnormal mobility. Accurate knowledge of the position of the joint space is required to locate the respective joint.

7.1.5 Common Symptoms in the Foot

Any dysfunction of sensation, mobility, and motor control in the foot affects the more superior sections of the lower limbs, the pelvis, and vertebral column. Therefore, particular attention should always be paid to symptoms of the foot.

▶ **Arthritis.** arthritis primarily has traumatic or rheumatic origins. Traumatic arthritis mainly develops following the common twisting the ankle trauma. The anterior talofibular ligament reinforcing the anterolateral aspect of the ankle joint capsule is one of the most commonly injured structures in the musculoskeletal system. Therapeutic management of this ligament injury requires:
- monitoring signs of post-traumatic inflammation;
- detecting and treating the many possible complications;
- healing the ligament in physiological position to avoid posterior decentering of the loaded leg onto the talus.

Surface anatomy is a basis for local pain relief caused by injury and detection of certain complications, such as overstretching of peroneal tendon sheaths or the bifurcate ligament.

▶ **Restricted mobility.** hypomobility in the ankle joint, usually resulting from immobilization or arthritis, is very common. The other aspects of the motor complex must be included in the examination of limited movement. The examination is based on things such as precise knowledge about the position and orientation of the articular space of the transverse tarsal joints.

▶ **Laxities and instability.** post-traumatic ligamentary tendon laxity in the talocrural joint is well known. The anterior ligaments of the ankle have the task of holding the tibia on the talus during weight-bearing. This can no longer be upheld in cases of extreme laxity, so that the tibia is no longer positioned to posterior over the center

of the talus (Hintermann, 1999). During dorsiflexion in weight-bearing, dysfunctional arthrokinematics of the ankle can be confused with a restriction in mobility at the joint.

Other laxities may be hidden in the remaining components of the ankle, TCN, and TT (Chopart) joints' kinematic complex. Traumatic injuries of the interosseous ligaments between talus and calcaneus can lead to tarsal sinus syndrome, in which patients report symptoms such as a feeling of instability in the hindfoot (Akiyama et al., 1999) especially on heel contact. Ligamentary laxity in the transverse tarsal joints stops the movement of the foot in the landing phase (total pronation) too late and causes hyperpronation of the foot in the middle of the stance phase.

▶ **Pathological conditions in the soft tissues**
- **Tenosynovitis**
  In addition to ligamental injuries, inflammation of the Achilles tendon and synovial sheaths of the extrinsic (long) muscles of the foot is particularly painful. This can occur on both sides of the foot at the point where the extrinsic tendons change directions:
  ○ Lateral—peroneal muscles.
  ○ Anterior—ankle dorsiflexors, toe extensors.
  ○ Medial—deep ankle plantarflexors and toe flexors in the tarsal tunnel.
- Strain and traumatic overstretching as well as bleeding cause tenosynovitis.
- **Tendinopathy**
  Insertion tendinopathy is observed:
  ○ Medial: Tibialis posterior at the tuberosity of the navicular bone.
  ○ Lateral: Peroneus brevis at the base of metatarsal V.
  ○ Posterior: Insertion of the triceps surae at the Achilles tendon (calcaneal tuberosity).
- Painful or nonpainful tendonitis (which often leads to spontaneous ruptures) occurs at the tendons of the triceps surae (center portion) and the tibialis posterior (Yao et al., 2015).
- **Local plantar pain**
  Can be classified as follows:
  ○ Muscular insertion tendinopathy (e.g., flexor digitorum brevis and abductor hallucis) andneurocontusions (plantar branches of the tibial nerve).
  ○ Fasciosis or pain at the insertion of the plantar fascia: Plantar fascia pain is often associated with a bony growth at the insertion of the calcaneus ("heel spur") (Johal and Milner, 2012).

It is also possible for neural structures to be compressed or overstretched in the foot. Two peripheral nerves are most commonly affected:
- **The tibial nerve in the tarsal tunnel (posterior to the medial malleolus)**
  Narrowing of the tarsal tunnel, through which the flexor hallucis longus, flexor digitorum longus, and

tibialis posterior also travel, mainly compresses the neural structure (Hudes, 2010). The tibial nerve divides into two plantar nerves after it exits the tunnel.

- **The intermediate branch of the superficial peroneal nerve**
This nerve branch lies very close to the surface, anterolaterally and distally, on the leg. It crosses the talocrural joint medial to the malleolus fibularis. A possible injury can arise from overstretching in a sprain, from iatrogenic injury (Blair and Botte, 1994), or from irritation after carelessly executed transverse friction of the talofibular ligament.
The same distinguishing characteristics always indicate a nerve irritation: burning pain and sensory disorders in the nerve's area of supply.

7.1.6 Required Basic Anatomical and Biomechanical Knowledge

Therapists should have sound knowledge of topographical anatomy when palpating the foot. The following comments are intended to be a motivation for further study of the topography:

- **Bony Structures**
Therapists should also be familiar with the bony construction of the foot and its individual sections, the joint lines, as well as the names of the individual tarsal bones and their mobile connections (▶ Fig. 7.3). Transverse subdivision of the foot skeleton into phalanges, metatarsus, and tarsus is certainly well known. The Lisfranc line, with its rather rigid joints, divides the metatarsus and the

tarsus. The joints of the Chopart articular line (between talus and navicular bone medially and between the calcaneus and the cuboid laterally) are parts of the transverse tarsal articulations.

To emphasize the significance of the functional relationships in loaded foot movements, the participating joints are combined into the tibiotarsal complex (Padovani, 1975). This motor complex includes the talocrural joint, the subtalar complex (talocalcaneal joint) with two articular cavities, and the transverse tarsal joints. Functionally, the distal syndesmoses and the proximal tibiofibular joint are part of this complex.

- **Muscular Structures**
These include the tendons and tendon sheaths of the long (extrinsic) foot muscles, especially as they pass by the tibiotarsal complex and their insertions. ▶ Fig. 7.4 shows the course to medial and plantar in the tarsal tunnel. This space provides a passageway for three tendons, two blood vessels, and the tibial nerve. It is covered by the retinaculum flexorum to become a tunnel. ▶ Fig. 7.5 depicts the particular course of the peroneal muscles with a frequently changing course of tendons behind the lateral malleolus, the peroneal trochlea, and at the cuboid bone (peroneus longus). The foot and toe extensors pass by the talocrural joint dorsally (▶ Fig. 7.6). The position of their tendons explains the secondary functions: the tibialis anterior and extensor hallucis longus adduct and supinate the foot, while the extensor digitorum longus with its branch (peroneus tertius), the only evertor of the foot, also abducts and pronates. All tendons of extrinsic muscles (except for the Achilles tendon) are held against the skeleton of the foot with retinacula, and for protection against friction require tendon sheaths that are several centimeters long.

- **Ligamentous Structures**
The functionally and clinically important ligamentous apparatus of the foot is found extending laterally and medially from the malleoli (▶ Fig. 7.7 and ▶ Fig. 7.8). The talofibular ligaments control the position of the talar mortise, while the calcaneofibular tendon lies over the

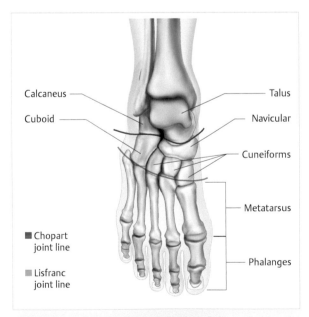

Calcaneus

Cuboid

Talus

Navicular

Cuneiforms

Metatarsus

■ Chopart joint line

■ Lisfranc joint line

Phalanges

Fig. 7.3 Topography of the skeleton of the foot.

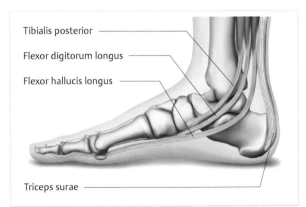

Tibialis posterior

Flexor digitorum longus

Flexor hallucis longus

Triceps surae

Fig. 7.4 Extrinsic muscles—medial aspect.

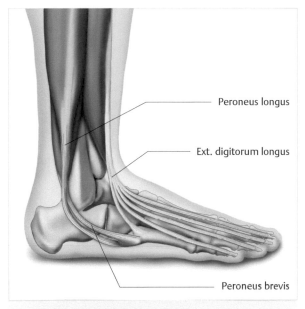

Fig. 7.5 Extrinsic muscles—lateral aspect.

- Peroneus longus
- Ext. digitorum longus
- Peroneus brevis

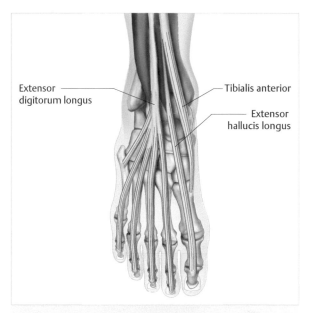

Fig. 7.6 Extrinsic muscles—dorsal aspect.

- Extensor digitorum longus
- Tibialis anterior
- Extensor hallucis longus

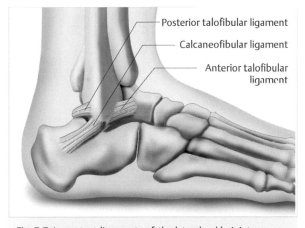

Fig. 7.7 Important ligaments of the lateral ankle joint.

- Posterior talofibular ligament
- Calcaneofibular ligament
- Anterior talofibular ligament

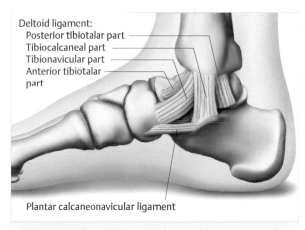

Fig. 7.8 Important ligaments of the medial ankle and TT joints.

Deltoid ligament:
- Posterior tibiotalar part
- Tibiocalcaneal part
- Tibionavicular part
- Anterior tibiotalar part

Plantar calcaneonavicular ligament

7

subtalar joints. The deltoid ligament is a coarse collagenous plate extending from the medial malleolus to the talus, calcaneus, and navicular bones. It is possible to see four separate ligaments in an anatomical preparation. This ligamentary complex appears much thicker and more stable than on the lateral aspect. The medial malleolus does not extend as far to plantar and, in addition, the ligamentary complex functions as a brake to pronation during the landing phase. The calcaneonavicular ligament closes the plantar articular space between talus, calcaneus, and navicular bones (calcaneonavicular ligament, spring ligament) and, together with other plantar ligaments and the short, intrinsic muscles, contributes to securing the medial longitudinal arch.

• Neural Structures

The tibial nerve passes on the medial side of the tarsal tunnel, divides into the medial and lateral plantar nerves and innervates the plantar intrinsic muscles. The possibility of compression neuropathy in the tunnel has already been noted. The deep and superficial peroneal (or fibular) nerves run dorsally on the foot. Whereas the deep branch innervates the dorsal intrinsic muscles, the superficial branches of the peroneal nerve are entirely sensory. They first emerge approximately 10 cm proximal to the talocrural joint under the fascia of the leg, divide into different branches, and run to the dorsum of the foot. The specific course of the cutaneus dorsalis intermedius will be described in chapter 7.4.

7.2 Local Palpation of the Medial Border of the Foot

7.2.1 Summary of the Palpatory Process

All relevant structures in the area of the ankle will first be located. Both the bony reference points and the clinically important soft-tissue structures are of interest.

This is followed by the palpation of all joint spaces on the medial side and extends down onto the first metatarsophalangeal joint (▶ Fig. 7.9). It is advisable to review the directional terms for the leg and foot as given in ▶ Fig. 7.1 before beginning.

Starting Position

The patient sits in an elevated position, for example, on the edge of a treatment table. The therapist sits on a stool on the lateral side of the foot. The patient's distal leg is placed on the therapist's thigh to stabilize the leg while the foot itself is unsupported and can move freely (▶ Fig. 7.10).

This starting position (SP) is not mandatory when practicing palpation. The therapist can also choose to position the patient differently. The starting position described places the patient in a comfortable sitting position and gives the therapist the best possible access with both hands to the freely moving and almost neutrally positioned foot.

7.2.2 Overview of the Structures to be Palpated

- Medial malleolus.
- Sustentaculum tali.
- Head and neck of the talus.
- Posterior process of the talus (medial tubercle).
- Tendon of the tibialis posterior.
- Navicular tuberosity.
- Position of the medial ligaments.
- Tendon of the flexor digitorum longus.
- Tendon of the flexor hallucis longus.
- Tibial artery and tibial nerve.
- Joint spaces on the medial border of the foot.

Medial Malleolus

The palpation starts by circling around the medial malleolus. The perpendicular palpation technique is used to locate the bony structures on the edge of the malleolus.

Technique

The posterior (facing the Achilles tendon) and plantar boundary of the medial malleolus should be palpated with the index finger from proximal and the anterior boundary and the transition to the articular space of the talocrural joint should be palpated with the index finger coming from distal (▶ Fig. 7.11).

In general, the boundaries are easy to access and can be marked clearly with transverse palpation. There is only one tendon that crosses a part of the edge and could somewhat impede palpation. The transition of the anterior edge to the talocrural articular space is not simple, since the tendon of the tibialis anterior hinders access to the tibialis anterior.

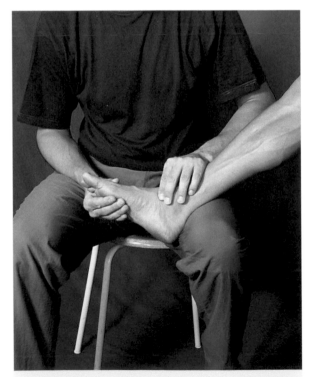

Fig. 7.10 Starting position for palpation of the medial aspect.

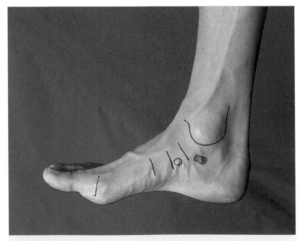

Fig. 7.9 Several structures drawn on the medial aspect of the foot.

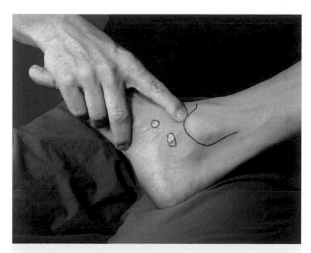

Fig. 7.11 Circling around the medial malleolus.

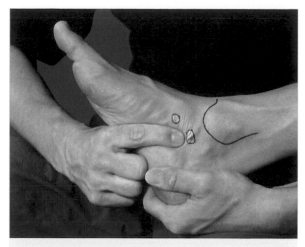

Fig. 7.12 Palpation of the sustentaculum tali.

Once the palpation has circled the medial malleolus, the therapist can identify where the most posterior, inferior, and anterior parts of the malleolus can be found.

The point that protrudes the most:

- distal will be later described as the anterior tip of the malleolus;
- inferior will be later described as the inferior tip of the malleolus;
- proximal will be later described as the posterior tip of the malleolus.

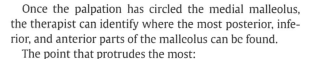

Tip

The therapist should avoid excessive prestretching of the medial soft tissues because the soft tissues can prevent free access to the bony edge of the medial malleolus if stretched. Checking the foot in mid-position of the joint is best done by using the hand coming from distal. When the edge of the medial malleolus is carefully followed, a little notch can be felt on the distal tip. This V-shaped notch separates the anterior portion of the medial malleolus (anterior colliculus) from the posterior portion (posterior colliculus) (Weigel and Nerlich, 2004).

Sustentaculum Tali

The next bony structure is found approximately 1 cm inferior to the plantar tip of the malleolus: the sustentaculum tali. This is a bony eminence on the calcaneus that protrudes in a medial direction. The sustentaculum tali is quite interesting in terms of its topography and functional anatomy:

- It bears a balconylike prominence medial to the head of the talus.

- The tarsal tunnel separates the two chambers of the talocalcaneal joint; it ends at the proximal boundary of the sustentaculum. The tendon of flexor hallucis longus crosses beneath it.
- Two ligaments insert at the sustentaculum tali: a section of the deltoid ligament and the calcaneonavicular ligament, also known as the spring ligament.
- The talus can be directly palpated on the medial aspect between the sustentaculum tali and the malleolus.

Technique

The sustentaculum tali can be clearly identified from an inferior direction. It is very difficult to identify its junction with the talus.

The therapist can access the inferior boundary by palpating the soft tissue from the sole of the foot toward the malleolus. The sustentaculum tali is the first osseous structure to be palpated that has a correspondingly hard feel (▶ Fig. 7.12).

The therapist gently places one finger between the inferior tip of the malleolus and the sustentaculum tali (that is, on the talus located underneath) to locate the rounded dorsal boundary and tilts the calcaneus medially (varus) and laterally (valgus) using small movements. In this way, it is possible to differentiate the sustentaculum tali, which is moveable, from the immovable talus.

The changes palpated during the valgus and varus movements represent the alternating tension and relaxation in the superficially located soft tissues (retinacula and deltoid ligament).

The posterior and anterior boundaries of the sustentaculum tali are also identified. This structure appears to be approximately 1 cm wide and approximately 2 cm long in total (Olexa et al., 2000). Distally, the head of the talus,

7

and proximally, the medial tubercle of the posterior talar process, articulate with it (▶ Fig. 7.14).

Head and Neck of the Talus

Palpating from the sustentaculum to distal, two bony eminences are encountered in rapid succession: the head of the talus and the tuberosity of the navicular bone. The head of the talus projects to medial directly next to the sustentaculum. If the tip of the palpating finger lies on the presumably correct spot, movement confirms the accurate location. For this purpose, the heel is tilted to medial and, if the subtalar biomechanics are normal, the head of the talus immediately turns away to lateral. Moving the calcaneus back to its former position allows the head to project to medial again.

Tip

If the therapist tilts the head of the talus by inverting the heel away to lateral, the distal boundary of the sustentaculum (palpation toward proximal) and the navicular tuberosity (still distinct) is reached in palpation toward distal.

Sections of the talus can be accessed from the anterior and posterior tips of the medial malleolus (▶ Fig. 7.13). Moving further distal from the anterior tip, the palpating finger immediately encounters the neck of the talus. The anterior-most portion of the deltoid ligament, the anterior tibiotalar ligament, inserts here. The posterior articular surfaces directly proximal to the malleolus are less distinctly felt. They lie directly above the posterior process of the posterior talar process.

Posterior Process of the Talus (Medial Tubercle)

Another bony reference point is found proximal and plantar to the medial malleolus. The medial tubercle of the posterior talar process thus lies in direct contact proximally with the sustentaculum.

Technique

The palpating finger applies moderate pressure to the posterior tip of the medial malleolus and gradually moves posterior and slightly inferior. Palpating to proximal from the sustentaculum is also a successful way of finding the tubercle. With circular palpation, the tubercle is found as another bony eminence (see ▶ Fig. 7.14). Another section of the deltoid ligament inserts here—the posterior tibiotalar part.

Tip

Movement is used to confirm the definite identity of this structure. The free hand facilitates alternating ankle dorsiflexion and plantar flexion. The posterior process of the talus increasingly pushes against the palpating finger during dorsiflexion and disappears into the tissues during plantar flexion. This results from the rolling and gliding motion of the talus during this movement and the associated changes in spatial position.

Tendon of the Tibialis Posterior

This is the most prominent tendon on the medial side. It is one of the tendons held on the foot and the skeleton of the leg by the flexor retinaculum. The extraordinary feature of its course is its position in a deep, separate groove (sulcus tendinis of the posterior tibial muscle) (von Lanz

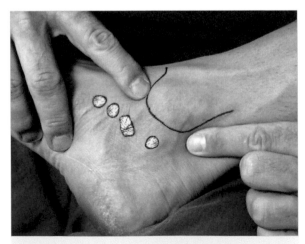

Fig. 7.13 Locating the neck and posterior process of the talus.

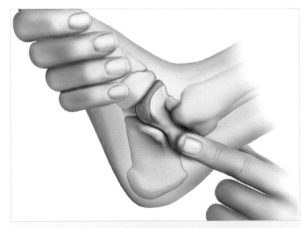

Fig. 7.14 Palpation of the posterior talar process.

and Wachsmuth, 2003) on the medial malleolus, just under the flexion-extension axis of the talocrural joint.

This tendon is used to guide the therapist onto the navicular, which is the last important bony reference point on the medial aspect of the foot.

Technique

Theoretically, the tendon can be found using a flat, transverse palpation technique, even when it is relaxed, over the malleolus. Practically, this often proves difficult (▶ Fig. 7.15).

The tendon is made more distinct for palpation by isometrically or rhythmically contracting the muscle with inversion of the foot (plantar flexion, adduction, and supination). This allows the tendon to be traced over its entire length, from the distal leg to its primary insertion on the navicular tuberosity.

Navicular Tuberosity

Following the tendon of the posterior tibial muscle systematically to distal, one reaches a bony eminence, the tuberosity of the navicular bone, whose size can be observed with rounded, circular palpation. To locate this structure precisely, the muscle should be relaxed and the tendon free of tension. The tuberosity presents as a distinct, rounded elevation. It feels hard when pressure is applied. In contrast, the tendon reacts with slightly more elasticity. To differentiate it from the head of the talus, which is also projecting in the close vicinity, the heel is tipped to medial, causing the head of the talus to swing to lateral and emphasize the proximal boundary of the navicular. The talonavicular articular space is found at this point. The extent of the tuberosity can be felt at the medial edge of the foot and also on the sole, by means of circular palpation.

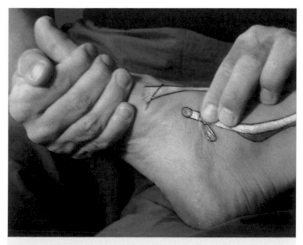

Fig. 7.15 Palpation of the tibialis posterior tendon.

7.2.3 Position of the Medial Ligaments

The sections of the deltoid ligament and the plantar calcaneonavicular ligament are the most important ligaments on the medial side of the foot (see ▶ Fig. 7.8).

By locating the bony reference points in the immediate vicinity of the medial malleolus, all reference points have been identified that are needed to establish the position of the deltoid ligament.

The deltoid ligament can be divided into several anatomical sections. Naming of the ligaments is based on the bony fixed points.

They include—according to their position from anterior (distal) to posterior (proximal)—the following:

- Anterior tibiotalar ligament: anterior tip of the medial malleolus—neck of the talus.
- Tibionavicular ligament: anterior tip of the medial malleolus—navicular tuberosity.
- Tibiocalcaneal ligament: plantar tip of the medial malleolus—sustentaculum tali.
- Posterior tibiotalar ligament: posterior tip of the medial malleolus—posterior process of the talus.

Technique
Deltoid Ligament

The individual ligaments of the deltoid ligament cannot be located by palpation. Their fibers flow together and there are too many other soft-tissue elements lying above them to permit direct contact (retinaculum flexorum and various tendons).

Only the dimensions of the ligaments can be identified, by drawing a line between the respective bony fixed points on the skin.

The advantages of this procedure are the production of a three-dimensional conception and comprehension of the tension in the different structures in a variety of joint positions.

For example, the therapist comprehends that the posterior tibiotalar ligament is placed under more tension as dorsiflexion of the ankle increases (▶ Fig. 7.16). The medial tubercle of the posterior process of the talus projects proximal and plantar and moves away from the medial malleolus. This tightens the ligament and supports the approximation of the articulating bones in the ankle.

For Further Practice

The following movements place the respective parts of the deltoid ligament under tension:
- Anterior tibiotalar ligament: by plantar flexion, abduction, and pronation.
- Tibionavicular ligament: by plantar flexion, abduction, and pronation.
- Tibiocalcaneal ligament: by valgus (tilting the calcaneus laterally).

- Posterior tibiotalar ligament: by dorsiflexion (with abduction and pronation).

lateral tilt of the heel causes the head of the talus to project to medial, thus tightening the ligament.

Plantar Calcaneonavicular Ligament

The plantar calcaneonavicular ligament passes underneath the head of the talus between the sustentaculum tali and the navicular tuberosity. It is palpable as a thick, rounded structure and converges with the tibialis posterior tendon onto the tuberosity.

The boundary with the neighboring bony fixed points is confirmed by moving the heel (with forefoot). The pad of the finger lies on the medially accessible aspect of the talar head between the sustentaculum and the navicular tuberosity. The fingertip points to plantar (▶ Fig. 7.17). When the heel is tilted to medial, the head disappears to lateral. Distally and proximally, the neighboring bony features become distinctly palpable. With pressure to lateral, the fingertip can hit the spring ligament. A pronounced

Tendon of the Flexor Digitorum Longus

This is the second tendon that, together with its tendon sheath, passes through the tarsal tunnel under the deep lamina of the retinaculum flexorum. Like the tendon described below, it can only be distinctly detected proximal to the talus and calcaneus.

The therapist first locates the tendon of tibialis posterior and follows it proximally until a point approximately 2 to 3 finger widths superior to the malleolus.

From the tendon, the therapist palpates posteriorly toward the Achilles tendon. The next bulging elevation felt is the tendon of the flexor digitorum longus (▶ Fig. 7.18 and ▶ Fig. 7.19).

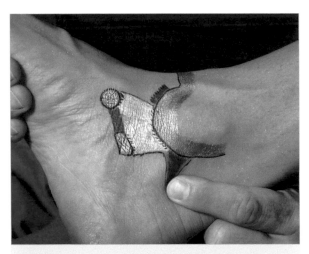

Fig. 7.16 Demonstration of the course of the posterior tibiotalar part.

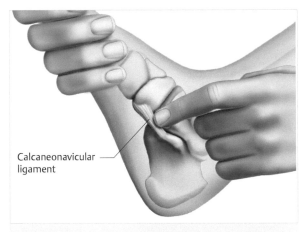

Fig. 7.17 Palpation of the plantar calcaneonavicular ligament.

Calcaneonavicular ligament

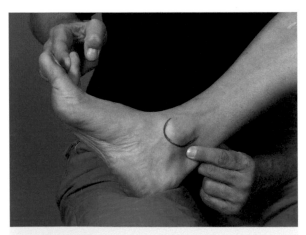

Fig. 7.18 Palpation of the flexor digitorum longus tendon.

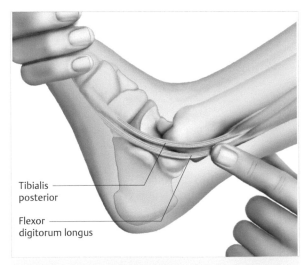

Tibialis posterior

Flexor digitorum longus

Fig. 7.19 Palpation of the flexor digitorum longus tendon.

Tip

As this area is often filled with fatty tissue, it is unlikely that the tendon can be located using transverse palpation alone. The therapist therefore uses active and rhythmical toe flexion to confirm the correct location. Now, the increase and decrease in tension in the tendon is rather distinct. If this is not successful, the tension in the tendon can also be increased, in order to feel it more clearly, by passive extension of the toes.

Tendon of the Flexor Hallucis Longus

The next tendon and its synovial sheath are palpated using the same method. This tendon is found immediately posterior to the above-described tendons and is the third tendon held on the skeleton of the leg and foot by the flexor retinaculum. To plantar, the tendon continues

in its own tibial groove and further on, between the two tubercles of the posterior talar process.

Starting at the tendon of flexor digitorum longus, palpation again moves slightly more posteriorly toward the Achilles tendon (▶ Fig. 7.20 and ▶ Fig. 7.21). The tendon of the flexor hallucis longus is palpated as the last firm and elastic structure before the Achilles tendon. The location is confirmed here using rhythmical active flexion of the first toe. Passive extension of the great toe also produces the desired tension of the tendon, which allows it to be more easily found. By transverse palpation, it is possible to follow the tendon in a plantar direction as far as directly proximal to the medial tubercle.

Additional Structures of the Tarsal Tunnel

In addition to the three tendons and synovial sheaths described above, three structures pass between the deep and superficial laminae of the retinaculum flexorum (von Lanz and Wachsmuth, 2003) behind the medial malleolus to the sole of the foot (▶ Fig. 7.22):

- Tibial vein.
- Posterior tibial artery.
- Tibial nerve.

The artery can be reliably palpated, as can the nerve, with a little more difficulty.

Technique—Posterior Tibial Artery

The posterior process of the talus is located first. From this point palpation moves somewhat proximal and the therapist applies one finger pad flat, with little pressure. von Lanz and Wachsmuth (2003) describe its position as follows: "The pulse of the posterior artery can be felt in the medial malleolar groove, approximately halfway between medial malleolus and the Achilles tendon."

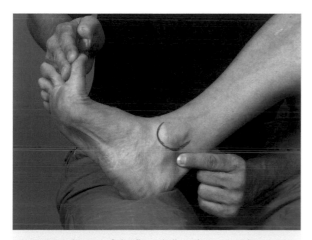

Fig. 7.20 Palpation of the flexor hallucis longus tendon.

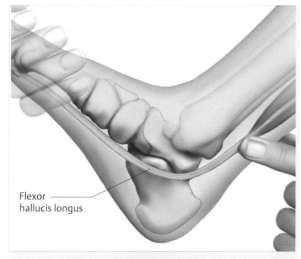

Flexor hallucis longus

Fig. 7.21 Palpation of the flexor hallucis longus tendon.

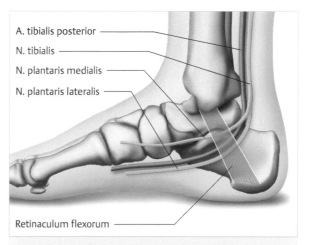

A. tibialis posterior
N. tibialis
N. plantaris medialis
N. plantaris lateralis

Retinaculum flexorum

Fig. 7.22 Illustration of the tibial artery and nerve.

After a short time of flat and patient palpation, the pulsation of the artery is felt. It can be followed for a short distance to proximal. In approximately 72% of the subjects studied by Yang et al. (2017), the bifurcation points of the artery were located within the tarsal tunnel.

Technique—Tibial Nerve

Directly next to the artery lies the tibial nerve, which passes through the tarsal tunnel and then divides into two branches (plantar nerves, Yang et al., 2017). The therapist attempts to identify the nerve by hooking around it (like with a guitar string), using a pointed palpation technique perpendicular to the structure. The nerve rolls away underneath the palpating finger when it has been exactly located. It is not possible to precisely identify the vein using palpation.

The relation of the position of the artery and the nerve is highly variable. The artery can be located proximal or distal to the nerve or even between the neural branches.

Technique—Tendon of the Tibialis Anterior

The palpation leaves the medial malleolus and concentrates on other structures on the medial side of the foot. The tendon of the anterior tibial muscle is a landmark for finding articular spaces on the medial edge of the foot.

The wide tendon of the tibialis anterior can be clearly demonstrated using dorsiflexion, adduction, and supination of the foot to contract the muscle (▶ Fig. 7.23). Its edges can be marked without any difficulty and followed distally down onto the medial edge of the foot. The tendon widens here, flattens, and eludes further palpation. This is the location of the joint space between the medial cuneiform and the base of the first metatarsal (MT).

Technique—Retinaculum Flexorum

The proximal edge of the retinaculum flexorum is palpable. The starting point is a location directly plantar and proximal to the medial tuberosity of the posterior process of the talus that can be palpated with a fingertip directed toward plantar and distal. When deep pressure is applied, the fingertip slides in a somewhat plantar and distal direction until a firm elastic edge can be distinctly felt. This edge becomes taut when the heel is everted (▶ Fig. 7.24).

Joint Spaces on the Medial Border of the Foot

The following joint spaces will be located (▶ Fig. 7.25 and ▶ Fig. 7.26):
- Talus—navicular, talonavicular joint, part of the TT joint line (Chopart joint).
- Navicular—medial cuneiform.
- Medial cuneiform—base of the first MT: part of the tarsometatarsal joint line (Lisfranc joint line).
- Head of the first MT—base of the first proximal phalanx, metatarsophalangeal joint; first metatarsophalangeal joint.

Technique

Talus—Navicular Joint Space

Using adduction and supination, the two prominent tendons on the medial side of the foot—tibialis anterior and tibialis posterior—become more pronounced and a fossa can usually be observed on the medial side of the foot. Its position and shape are slightly similar to the radial fossa of the hand.

The talonavicular joint space can be found in this fossa. The course of the articular space on the medial side of the foot is not perpendicular to the edge of the foot but inclines approximately 30° obliquely to plantar-proximal.

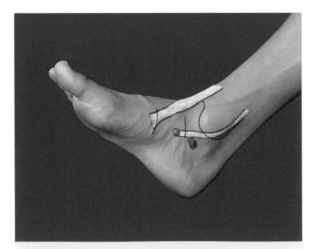

Fig. 7.23 Palpation of the retinaculum flexorum.

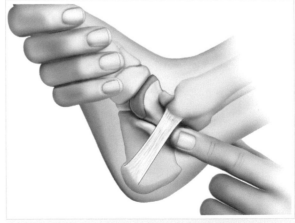

Fig. 7.24 Palpation of the retinaculum flexorum.

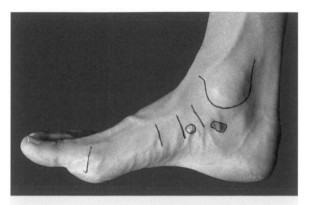

Fig. 7.25 Joint spaces on the medial border of the foot.

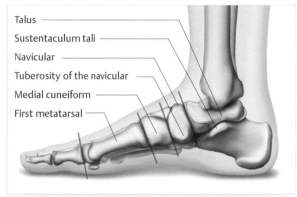

Talus
Sustentaculum tali
Navicular
Tuberosity of the navicular
Medial cuneiform
First metatarsal

Fig. 7.26 Topography of the medial joint spaces.

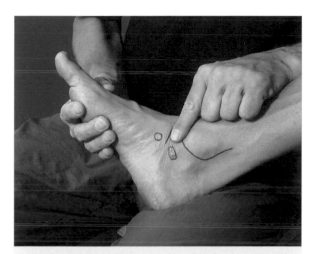

Fig. 7.27 Palpation of the talonavicular joint space.

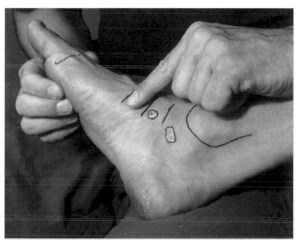

Fig. 7.28 Palpation of the joint space between the medial cuneiform and the first MT.

This joint space corresponds to the medial part of the TT (Chopart) joint line or of the transverse tarsal joints (▶ Fig. 7.27).

Tips

Another reliable method to locate the joint space involves finding the insertion of the tibialis posterior at the navicular tuberosity (see ▶ Fig. 7.15). The joint space is found immediately proximal to the tuberosity.

The navicular is not only accessible on the medial side. The therapist should keep in mind that it is equally as wide as the talus (see ▶ Fig. 7.59).

It is not possible to accurately differentiate the dorsal dimensions of the other tarsal bones from one another using either palpation or tests of joint play. It is, however, easy to differentiate between these bones and the sole of the foot: the palpating finger moves away from the firm resistance of the tarsal bones and encounters tissue of soft and elastic consistency.

Navicular—Medial Cuneiform Joint Space

The palpating finger slides into a shallow depression directly distal to the navicular tuberosity reminiscent of the anterior "V" of the AC joint. This indentation marks the joint space between the navicular and the adjacent medial cuneiform.

Medial Cuneiform—Base of the First Metatarsal Joint Space

It is very difficult to locate this joint space using palpation (▶ Fig. 7.28).

First, the joint space is small, and second, there is hardly any movement at this joint that could be used to locate it more accurately. This is typical of the joints along the tarsometatarsal joint line.

First Metatarsophalangeal Joint Space

The distal, prominent head of the first MT must first be located. It appears large and convex on the distal end of the first MT. The first metatarsophalangeal joint space lies

7

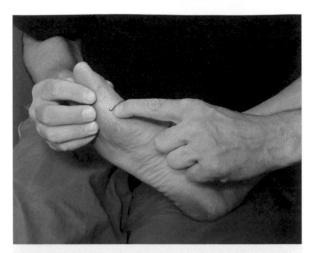

Fig. 7.29 Palpation of the first metatarsophalangeal joint space.

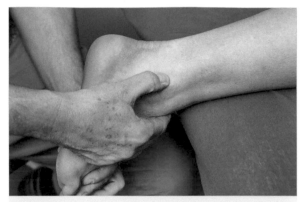

Fig. 7.30 Ottawa Ankle Rules—palpation of the posterior edge of the fibula.

distal to it (▶ Fig. 7.29). This must be emphasized because, without experience in palpation, there is a tendency to look for the articular space proximally.

Confirmation of Joint Space Location Using Movement

In the following section, the optimal technique will be described to confirm location of the joint space using movement.

With the exception of the talonavicular joint, only small movements can be made to confirm the position of the articular space. This technique must therefore accomplish three goals:
• To clearly fixate the proximal bones with a large area of contact so that the bones do not move (using the proximal hand).
• To palpate movement in the joint space (using the proximal hand).
• To facilitate small movements (using the distal hand).

The index or middle finger of the proximal hand is always used for palpation. The remaining fingers and the hypothenar eminence use a large area of surface contact to stabilize the bones proximal to the joint space, ensuring that the slight facilitated movement does not continue more proximally. The distal hand facilitates movement so that the edge of the distally positioned bone pushes against the palpating finger. Usually the direction of movement is adduction or extension.

7.2.4 Tips for Treatment

Using the Ottawa Ankle Rules

To lower the high costs of radiography for the assessment of ankle sprains, a group led by Ian G. Stiell at the University of Ottawa developed, in 1991, a set of prediction rules

(Stiell et al., 1992). These prediction rules were meant to be able to detect the presence or absence of fractures of the ankle and midfoot. Since then, the diagnostic reliability of these rules has been tested numerous times. In their systematic review, Bachmann et al. (2003) report a sensitivity of 96 to 99% and suggest that using the rules can reduce the number of unnecessary radiographs by 30 to 40%.

Using the Ottawa ankle rules (▶ Fig. 7.30) is very easy and the rules are mainly based on using palpation to provoke pain. If one of the following items is present, the likelihood of a fracture is very probable:
• Bone tenderness along the distal 6 cm of the posterior edge of the tibia.
• Bone tenderness along the distal 6 cm of the posterior edge of the fibula.
• Bone tenderness at the base of metatarsal V.
• Bone tenderness at the navicular.
• Directly following injury, the inability to bear weight for more than four steps.

Transverse Frictions in Inflammation of the Tibialis Posterior Synovial Sheath

Tendinopathy and irritation of the synovial sheath or of the insertion of the tibialis posterior are some of the most common soft-tissue lesions arising on the medial aspect of the foot and often occur in association with flatfoot deformities (Wilder and Sethi, 2004). In addition to the Achilles tendon and the tendons of the peroneal muscle, the tendon of the tibialis posterior is the most frequently affected (ibid.). In patients with clinically confirmed irritation, the prevalence, confirmed by MRI, of tendinosis was 52% and the prevalence of peritendinosis was 66% (Premkumar et al., 2002).
• The tendon is located using the previously described technique.
• The foot is placed under tension, without causing pain, and transverse frictions are applied. The foot is therefore positioned in abduction, pronation, and, if necessary,

some dorsiflexion. The preliminary tension stabilizes the structure while the technique is being administered and prevents it from rolling back and forth underneath the finger applying the frictions.

- The hand coming from dorsal palpates the entire accessible length of the tendon and synovial sheath. Transverse frictions are applied to the site that the patient indicates to be most painful (▸ Fig. 7.31).

Transverse Frictions in Cases of Tibialis Posterior Insertion Tendinopathy

- First the tendon is followed as far as its insertion and the full extent of the navicular tuberosity is found by circular palpation with the finger pad. The tuberosity is not the sole area of insertion for the tendon but is nevertheless the site of clinical interest.
- The finger applying the frictions must be able to push away the tendon to reach the insertion well (▸ Fig. 7.32). The necessary relaxation in the tendon is reached by positioning the foot in adduction with supination. This relaxes the abductor hallucis, which as a result permits contact with the tuberosity somewhat further to plantar.
- The technique involves applying pressure as the finger moves from plantar to dorsal. This should be performed with the distal hand, as the pad of the index finger is clearly able to come into contact with the tuberosity. The thumb of the hand applying friction hooks into the lateral edge of the foot and thus stabilizes its hold.

Joint-specific Techniques of the Talonavicular Joint

The transverse tarsal joints play a decisive role, in biomechanical collaboration with the talocrural joint and the talocalcaneal joint, in mobility and flexibility of the foot.

Malfunctions along the articular chain of the Chopart joint line can only be detected by tests of joint play in the articular connections involved. For this reason, knowing precisely the position and orientation of the articular space plays a decisive part.

The medial component of the transverse tarsal joints is the talonavicular joint, which should be examined and, if necessary, mobilized.

In this joint-specific technique, it is imperative that the therapist holds onto the tarsal bones as near to the joint as possible and mobilizes them exactly parallel to the joint space.

The navicular can slide back and forth to plantar (medial with supination) or dorsal (lateral and pronation) on the talus (▸ Fig. 7.33). In contrast to the other articular spaces that are accessible on the medial skeleton of the foot, the local excursions are quite large.

Posterior Tibial Artery

The quality of the tibial artery pulse provides information on the circulation and blood supply in the foot and toes and is important for the evaluation of peripheral occlusive arterial disease.

Tarsal Tunnel Syndrome

Pain provocation tests play the most important role in diagnosing tarsal tunnel syndrome, a compression neuropathy of the tibial nerve and its plantar branches (Abouelela and Zohiery, 2012). For the triple compression stress test, the ankle is placed in passive full plantar flexion and the foot in inversion, and pressure in the tarsal tunnel is increased. In addition, manual pressure is applied directly to the tarsal tunnel. Irritation of the posterior tibial nerve or its branches is present if the complaints (e.g., local pain) are triggered within 30 seconds. Abouelela und Zohiery (2012) report a test sensitivity of 86% and specificity of 100%.

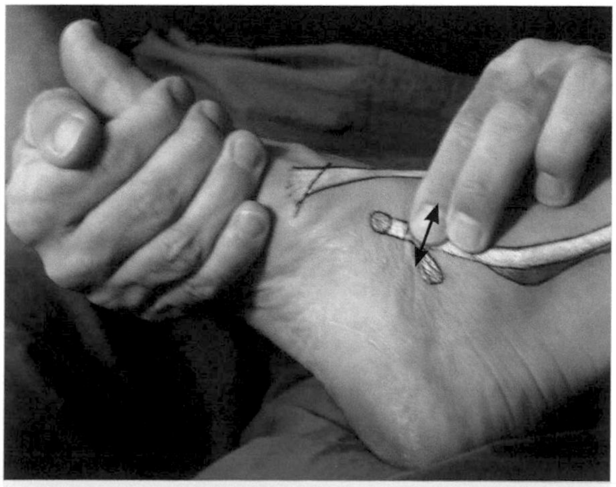

7

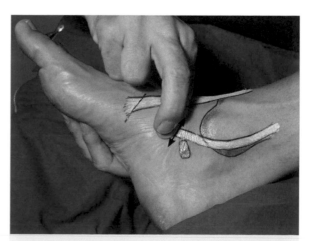

Fig. 7.31 Transverse frictions on the tibialis posterior—technique applied to the tendon.

Fig. 7.32 Transverse frictions on the tibialis posterior—technique applied to the insertion.

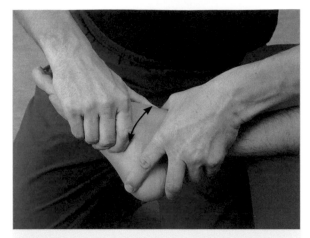

Fig. 7.33 The navicular gliding back and forth on the talus.

7.3 Palpation of the Lateral Border of the Foot

7.3.1 Summary of the Palpatory Process

All relevant osseous elevations will be located and demonstrated first, followed by the identification of the large tendons and their protective tendon sheaths. The important joint spaces will be located and an idea of the position of the ankle ligaments conveyed.

Starting Position

The therapist sits on the medial side of the foot. The patient's leg rests on the therapist's thigh to allow access to structures from a wide variety of directions while the foot remains mobile (▶ Fig. 7.34).

7.3.2 Overview of the Structures to be Palpated

- Lateral malleolus.
- Peroneal trochlea.
- Base of the fifth metatarsal.
- Peroneus longus and brevis.
- Calcaneocuboid joint.
- Fourth/fifth metatarsal—cuboid joint space.
- Dimensions of the cuboid.
- Position of the lateral ligaments.
- Anterior tibiofibular ligament.

Lateral Malleolus

The start of this palpation is comparable to the start of the palpation tracing around the malleolus on the medial side. As a reminder: Provocative palpation of the distal 6 cm of the posterior edge of the fibula is part of the

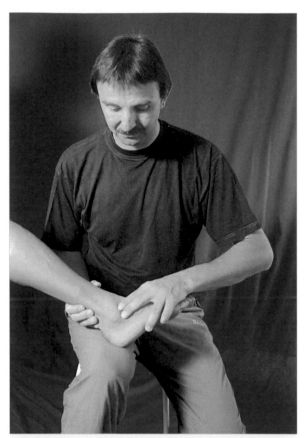

Fig. 7.34 Starting position for palpation of the lateral border.

Ottawa Ankle Rules (Chapter 7.2.4). All the important lateral ligaments of the ankle joints begin here. The superior peroneal retinaculum extends from the lateral malleolus toward the heel and prevents dislocation of the peroneal tendons.

Technique

The hand coming from distal performs transverse palpation with the finger pads to visualize the edges of the external malleolus, which is an easy task as the entire malleolus is very prominent (▶ Fig. 7.35). The transition onto the anterior border of the tibia can also be demonstrated by following the edge of the malleolus anteriorly. The distal end of the tibial ridge marks the joint space of the ankle. The neck and head of the talus are found immediately distal to this.

When speaking of the malleolus boundaries, the terms anterior and distal tip are used. Precise palpation of the edge shows that the lateral malleolus lies surprisingly far to medial.

Peroneal Trochlea

The peroneal trochlea is described as a small, tear-shaped elevation on the lateral aspect of the calcaneus. The

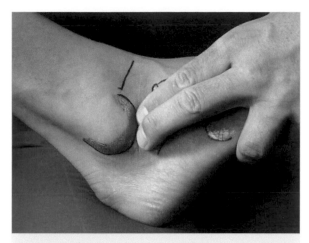

Fig. 7.35 Circling around the lateral malleolus.

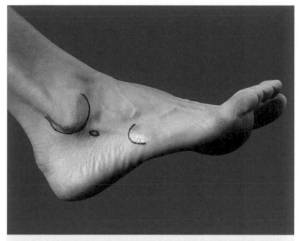

Fig. 7.36 Position of the most important osseous reference points on the lateral side of the foot.

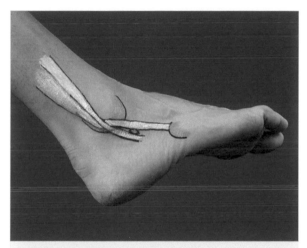

Fig. 7.37 Position of the peroneus tendons.

parallel tendons of the peroneal muscles separate at this point (▶ Fig. 7.36 and ▶ Fig. 7.37).

Technique

Plantar and somewhat toward the toes from the distal tip of the malleolus is a small, drop-shaped strip that varies in distinctness among individuals. For unambiguous identification, the peroneal tendons must be completely relaxed otherwise they are too prominent and make it impossible to spot the trochlea.

Base of the Fifth Metatarsal

The tuberosity of the fifth metatarsal, the thickening at the proximal end of the fifth metatarsal, is very easy to feel at the lateral edge of the foot. There are two possibilities for reliable identification:
- The therapist uses two to three fingertips and slides them from the heel to distal, in the direction of the fifth

toe. The first distinct, bony elevation encountered is the base of the fifth MT, also known as the tuberosity.
- The patient is asked to flex the foot with abduction and pronation, against a certain amount of resistance. This innervates the peroneal muscles and causes the tendons at the lateral edge of the foot to stand out. One of the tendons can be followed down onto the base of the fifth MT.

Another tendon has a flat insertion at this base, somewhat further dorsal and distal. This is the tendon of the peroneus tertius, which is not present in all individuals. Although misleadingly labeled as such, this muscle is not the third peroneus muscle, but rather a section of the extensor digitorum longus that has split off.

Tip

As a reminder: Applying direct pressure to the base of metatarsal V is part of the Ottawa Ankle Rules (Chapter 7.2.4).

Peroneus Longus and Brevis

Both of the peroneal muscles belong to the plantarflexor muscle group of the ankle. They run behind the flexion/extension axis of the ankle, traveling posterior to the lateral malleolus to reach the skeleton of the foot.

Technique

Palpating the Lower Leg

Both muscles originate laterally, on the fibula. The peroneus longus tendon travels from here superficial to the muscle belly of the peroneus brevis for a certain distance

7

and the tendons are on top of one another immediately proximal to the malleolus. The muscle bellies can be felt with direct, flat palpation with rhythmic flexion, abduction, and pronation. The tendon that can be palpated at this point is that of the peroneus longus. In comparison, the peroneus brevis tendon is significantly more difficult to reach, "hidden" beneath the longus tendon. Defining the boundaries between the muscle bellies and, further distal, the tendons on the one hand and the fibula or the tissue associated with the Achilles tendon on the other hand, can also be achieved with rhythmical muscle activity (▶ Fig. 7.38).

Palpating the Lateral Malleolus

Both tendons, lying one over the other, run in their own groove posterior and distal to the lateral malleolus. Here they are held in place by the retinaculum musculorumperoneorum superius, which varies considerably in width, thickness, and insertions and can be intensely stretched by inversion trauma (Ferran et al., 2006).

The retinaculum can be palpated with direct palpation and varying tension by extension, adduction, and supination. It is sometimes mistaken for the calcaneofibular ligament, which in its further course is in fact harder to palpate (not illustrated).

Injuries of the retinaculum have the clinical appearance of a tendon sheath pathology. The sheaths of the peroneal tendons extend 2 cm from proximal of the malleolus approximately to the peroneal trochlea. The synovial sheath of peroneus brevis may even be in contact with the capsule of the ankle. Capsule ruptures therefore often cause bleeding in the synovial sheath. Dislocations from this stabilized position within the guide channel occur primarily with trauma (Marti, 1977). However, the tendency to dislocation can also be congenital. The peroneus longus tendon can only be palpated here when the therapist approaches the malleolus from posterior. Deep in the

malleolar groove, palpation succeeds only with effort and vertical fingertips.

Palpation of the Superior Peroneal Retinaculum

From the distal posterior edge of the fibula, this structure continues toward the heel descending slightly plantarward to insert at the calcaneus directly after crossing the peroneal tendons. Directly posteriorly (further heelward), the lateral dorsal cutaneous nerve runs from the lower leg to the lateral foot (von Lanz and Wachsmuth, 2003). The therapist hooks the vertical fingertip around this structure deeper down. Trauma to the retinaculum is a possible complication affecting the ligament during a twisting trauma of the foot, and owing to a rupture and flat malleolar fossa (in 18% of all individuals; Ferran et al., 2006) can lead to peroneal tendon subluxation.

The superior edge of the retinaculum can be distinctly palpated. During palpation, the therapist's finger, directed plantarward, first slides on the distal lower leg over the peroneal tendons further plantarward. When the descending of the tendons into the peroneal tunnel can be felt, the therapist places the finger vertically. The therapist applies increasing pressure in the attempt to palpate the superior edge of the retinaculum, which becomes distinctly tightened when the heel is inverted (▶ Fig. 7.39).

If the injury to the retinaculum is not severe (not ruptured) transverse friction may offer pain relief.

Palpating the Lateral Border of the Foot

Both tendons run together to the trochlea peronealis. Proximally, the tendon of the brevis emerges from under the tendon of the longus. Their communal course ceases at the trochlea and the tendons separate. The peroneus longus tendon travels to the cuboid along the lateral border of the foot and then runs in a plantar and medial direction. This is the third change in direction for the tendon over its entire length. It is usually extremely difficult

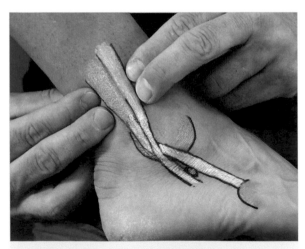

Fig. 7.38 Searching for the peroneus tendons on the distal lower leg.

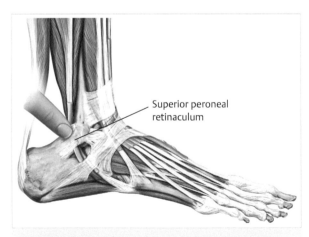

Superior peroneal retinaculum

Fig. 7.39 Palpation of the superior peroneal retinaculum.

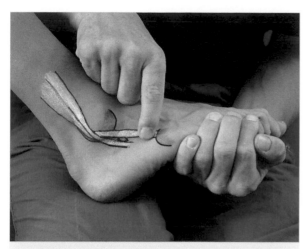
Fig. 7.40 Palpation of the peroneus brevis tendon.

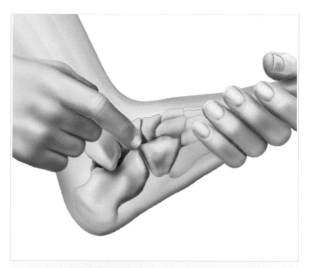
Fig. 7.41 Illustration of the palpation technique at the calcaneus.

to palpate the tendon on the lateral aspect of the foot and to differentiate it from the peroneus brevis tendon.

The peroneus brevis tendon can be easily traced with transverse palpation down onto its insertion (▶ Fig. 7.40). If it is not possible to observe or transversely palpate the tendon between the trochlea and the base of the fifth MT, the patient is asked to contract and relax their foot in abduction and pronation.

Calcaneocuboid Joint

Palpation now leaves the region surrounding the malleolus and concentrates on finding the other tarsal bones and their articulations. In particular, this involves identification of the cuboid and its articular contacts.

Before continuing, a few rules are listed below for this region:
- Approximately two-thirds of the length of the calcaneus lie posterior to the lateral malleolus and only one-third anterior.
- The cuboid is very small on the lateral edge of the foot (approximately 1 finger width).
- All dorsiflexor tendons lie on the talus.

The calcaneocuboid (CC) joint space is decidedly the most interesting joint space on the lateral border of the foot. This articular space is the outer portion of the Chopart joint line (transverse tarsal joint).

Technique

There are three methods for locating this joint space.
- Following the posterior edge of the calcaneus.
- Directly searching for the anterior calcaneal process.
- Estimating the dimensions of the cuboid.

The third is the most unreliable method and therefore not explained in detail here. The hypothesis is that the plantar cuboid is only 1 cm long (from the calcaneus to the base of metatarsal V). Therefore, if the finger follows the bone starting from the base, the CC joint space would have to be found here on the plantar side.

Method 1: Following the posterior edge of the calcaneus

The first method starts on the superior edge of the calcaneus. This edge can be found by first placing the foot in slight inversion (plantar flexion, adduction, and supination) and then palpating anterior to the lateral malleolus toward the sole of the foot. A sharp edge can be felt. The therapist should follow this edge distal and medial until the head of the talus prevents further palpation (▶ Fig. 7.41 and ▶ Fig. 7.42).

This is the point (tip of the calcaneus) of origin of the bifurcate ligament, which is usually injured here in an inversion trauma. Pressure to proximal (toward the heel) gives access to the tarsal sinus or canal. A line from this calcaneus tip, perpendicular to the outer edge of the foot (with the foot in neutral position), corresponds to the position of the CC articular space (▶ Fig. 7.43).

> **Tip**
>
> The location is confirmed using a minimal movement. The calcaneus is stabilized proximally by the palpating finger, and the distal hand facilitates slight abduction and pronation. The cuboid now slides back and forth to dorsal against the palpating finger and thus confirms the correct position of the articular space.

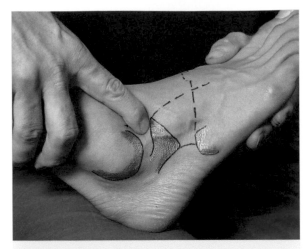

Fig. 7.42 Palpation of the tip of the calcaneus.

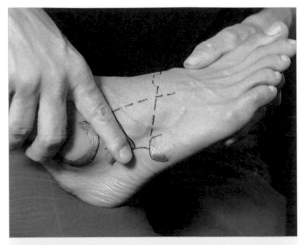

Fig. 7.43 Location of the CC joint space between the calcaneus and the cuboid.

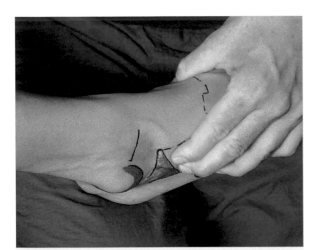

Fig. 7.44 Palpation of the distal calcaneus.

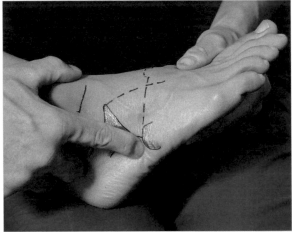

Fig. 7.45 Palpation of the base of the fifth MT.

Method 2: Locating the anterior calcaneal process.

The second method can be applied particularly well if the foot is very mobile. The distal end of the calcaneus bulges out significantly as the muscle bulk of the intrinsic toe extensors (digitorum brevis and hallucis brevis) attaches there. This end in particular clearly protrudes in mobile feet positioned in extensive inversion (Hall and Sheriff, 1993). It can now be palpated from distal quite simply as a projecting step and the therapist can find the articular space lying directly in front of it. The distal edge of the calcaneus appears here as a prominent, hard edge (▶ Fig. 7.44).

Correct identification is confirmed when the foot is passively returned to neutral or moved further into eversion (dorsiflexion, abduction, and pronation). The step is no longer palpable as the cuboid translates dorsally.

Fourth/Fifth Metatarsal—Cuboid Joint Space

The joints with the bases of the fourth and fifth MTs belong to the tarsometatarsal joint line. In general, all joints in this joint line have only very little mobility. The most stable articulations are found centrally, on the dorsum of the foot:
• Intermediate cuneiform—base of the second MT.
• Lateral cuneiform—base of the third MT.

The more mobile joints are found on the edges.

Technique

Location of these joints starts at the base of the fifth MT. The therapist comes from a proximal direction and hooks around the base (▶ Fig. 7.45). A line is then drawn medially from this point onto the base of the first MT.

Determination of its location has been described in the section "Local Palpation of the Medial Border of the Foot" above. This line is used for orientation, reflecting the position of the tarsometatarsal joint line fairly accurately.

The joint between the cuboid and the bases of the fourth and fifth MTs is roughly found along this line.

Dimensions of the Cuboid

- The cuboid articulates with the following bones:
  - *Calcaneus—proximally*: this joint has already been located.
  - *Fourth and fifth metatarsals—distally*: these joints are part of the tarsometatarsal joint line. Therapists are also already familiar with them.
  - *Navicular and lateral cuneiform—medially.*
- The navicular and lateral cuneiform have a true planar joint. It represents an important functional component of the transverse tarsal joints and plays an important role for the kinematic complex of this region. It should not be forgotten when searching for very local restrictions in mobility and should also be examined in joint play tests. A guiding line is needed to identify this joint space as it cannot be clearly palpated.
- Topographical anatomy is of help here, which states that this joint line lies along the elongation of the space between the third and fourth metatarsals. When the therapist slides the finger proximally along this space on the dorsum of the foot and follows the metatarsalia (and not the extensor tendons), the extended part of this line indicates the position of the joint space. On the plantar surface of the foot, the space between the second and third MTs is used to find the joint line.
- The joint space between the cuboid and the medially positioned bones articulating with it therefore extends from plantar-medial to dorsal-lateral. In other words, it extends at a right angle to the plane of the dorsum of the foot.

Several conclusions can be drawn about the cuboid following palpation and the use of guiding lines (▶ Fig. 7.46):
- It is definitely not shaped like a cube.
- The CC joint space is almost as wide as the joint space between the cuboid, the fourth MT, and the fifth MT.
- The cuboid is very narrow laterally, only around 1 finger width
- The muscle bellies of the intrinsic toe extensors lie superficial to the cuboid. On a slender foot, they look like a type of swelling. They originate on the calcaneus. The muscle bellies can be clearly demonstrated by strongly extending the toes.

Position of the Lateral Ligaments

The position and course of the ligaments on the lateral side of the ankle are similar in principle to those on the medial side (▶ Fig. 7.47). Of course, some differences exist:
- The ligaments are not as thick laterally.
- No ligament is present that originates from the lateral malleolus and crosses over the TT joint line.
- Certain sections of the ligaments can be reached very easily.

The **anterior and posterior talofibular ligaments** are part of the control and stability mechanisms of the talocrural joint.

The **posterior ligament** cannot be accessed as the peroneal tendons and their retinaculum lie on top of it. In addition, the talus insertion, the lateral tubercle of the posterior talar process, is located deep, where it cannot be palpated.

In comparison, the course and the insertion of the **anterior talofibular ligament** onto the fibula and talus can be easily accessed (▶ Fig. 7.48).

As this is one of the most commonly traumatized structures in the human musculoskeletal system, many

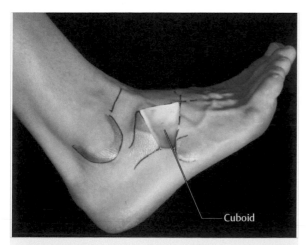

Fig. 7.46 Projection of the position of the cuboid.

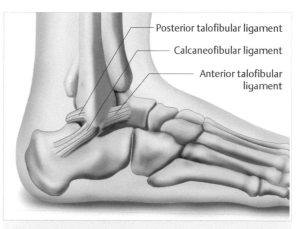

Fig. 7.47 Lateral ligaments.

Posterior talofibular ligament

Calcaneofibular ligament

Anterior talofibular ligament

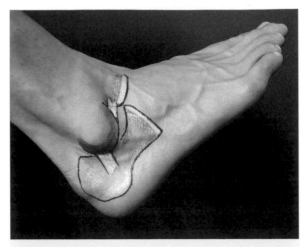

Fig. 7.48 Position of the anterior talofibular and calcaneofibular ligaments.

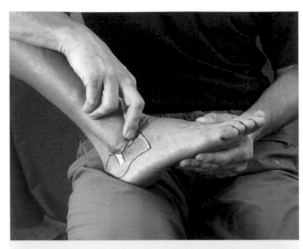

Fig. 7.49 SP for palpation of the anterior tibiofibular ligament.

physicians and therapists are interested in determining its exact location. It extends between the anterior tip of the lateral malleolus and the neck of the talus. According to anatomical literature, the length of the ligament is approximately 1 to 1.5 cm. When the outer edge of the foot is positioned at 90° to the leg, the ligament runs parallel to the lateral edge of the foot.

The third ligament, the **calcaneofibular,** extends between the distal tip of the fibula and the lateral aspect of the calcaneus, slanting downward by approximately 30° to posterior plantar. It forms a 120° angle with the anterior talofibular ligament and is about 6 to 8 mm wide. It is also difficult to access the entire length of this ligament. Only the fibular fixation is accessible when the foot is in passive flexion because in this foot position the peroneal tendons are clear of the insertion point. The ligament is reached in this position at the distal tip of the fibula, directly dorsal to the peroneal tendons.

Anterior Tibiofibular Ligament

This ligament can be accessed at three different locations:
• The insertion on the anterior tip of the malleolus.
• The insertion on the neck of the talus.
• Its course between these two fixed points.

The proximal hand is used for all three location procedures. The forearm rests on the leg of the patient. The distal hand is used to position the foot (▸ Fig. 7.49).

Technique

Insertion on the Malleolus

As the therapist is searching for the insertion onto bone, the ligament should be relaxed to allow free access to the malleolus. This is accomplished by placing the foot in a slightly everted position.

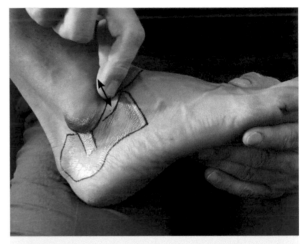

Fig. 7.50 Transverse frictions on the anterior tibiofibular ligament at the insertion on the malleolus.

The palpating finger is placed on the malleolus, with the middle finger exerting pressure on it from above. The forearm is extensively pronated during this movement (▸ Fig. 7.50).

Pressure is applied to the palpating movement from plantar to dorsal and reduced in the opposite direction.

Middle Section

The technique applied here corresponds to the previous description, with a few modifications:
• The forearm is not pronated as much.
• The finger pad is placed between the two bony fixed points.
• The distal hand moves the foot into an inverted position. This tightens the ligament and stabilizes it beneath the palpating finger. If a patient presents with injury to the structure following a varus-inversion trauma, the therapist should pay attention to pain-free positioning of the foot.

Insertion on the Talus

The procedure is characterized by:
- the foot being positioned in slight eversion to relax the ligament;
- the arm being positioned in slight supination;
- the pad of the index finger coming into contact with the neck of the talus (collumtali).

For reliable location of the insertion at the neck of the talus, an attempt is first made to palpate, with slightly flexed talocrural joint, a markedly projecting and pointed bony feature directly medial to the malleolus, which disappears in extension. This is the anterolateral boundary of the talar trochlea. Directly distal to it, the neck of the talus forms a concave surface, on which the ligament inserts.

7.3.3 Tips for Assessment and Treatment

Several examples demonstrate the application of accurate surface palpation of the lateral border of the foot. These include techniques treating ligamentous structures, synovial sheaths, and insertions, as well as manual therapy techniques that target the joints.

Transverse Frictions at the Anterior Tibiofibular Ligament

Transverse frictions for treatment are administered as described in the palpation above and will not be explained in further detail. The intensity and duration should merely be adjusted when treatment is the aim of the intervention.

Transverse Frictions at the Peroneus Brevis Tendon and Synovial Sheath

The technique is similar to the one used to locate the tendon between the peroneal trochlea and its insertion (see ▶ Fig. 7.40). To aid stabilization, the tendon should be stretched to a certain degree before frictions are applied. Therefore, the foot is positioned in adduction, supination, and, if necessary, some dorsiflexion (▶ Fig. 7.51).

The index finger transversely palpates and treats the structure with or without the help of the middle finger. The therapeutically effective pressure is applied during the movement from plantar to dorsal. The tendon sheath is reached with this technique, going between the peroneal trochlea and the lateral malleolus; the tendon is found between the trochlea and the insertion.

Transverse Frictions at the Insertion of the Peroneus Brevis

It is imperative that the peroneus brevis tendon is relaxed and does not impede free access to the base of the fifth MT. The proximal hand therefore moves the foot into an abducted and pronated position. The index finger of the distal hand is now used to palpate. The thumb hooks around medially and stabilizes this grip (▶ Fig. 7.52).

The insertion for the peroneus brevis is not on the side of the base, but rather on the proximal end. For this reason, the distal forearm is positioned in pronation so that the index finger is coming from a proximal direction and can push down on the insertion. The middle finger can be positioned on top of the index finger for support. The therapeutically effective movement is conducted by applying pressure from plantar to dorsal (▶ Fig. 7.53).

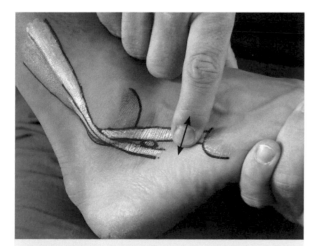

Fig. 7.51 Transverse frictions on the peroneus brevis—technique applied to the tendon.

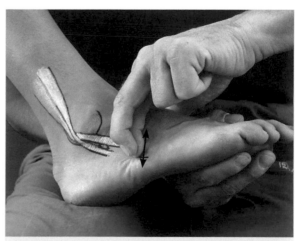

Fig. 7.52 Transverse frictions on the peroneus brevis—technique applied to the insertion.

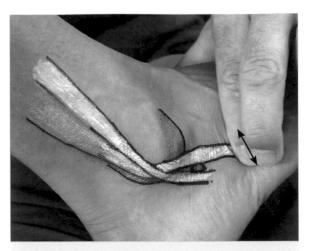

Fig. 7.53 Technique applied to the insertion—alternative view.

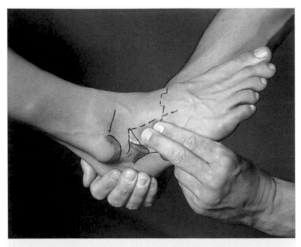

Fig. 7.54 Test of joint play at the calcaneocuboid joint.

Tip

If a thin structure should roll under the palpating finger during palpation along the tendon sheath, the tendon, or the insertion of the peroneal tendons, it is the cutaneus dorsalis lateralis, a branch of the superficial peroneal nerve. It can be reliably found directly on the dorsal side of the base of the fifth metatarsal. Uninterrupted transverse friction should take its position into account and avoid irritation.

Tests of Joint Play at the Transverse Tarsal Joints

This joint complex includes the talonavicular joint medially as well as the articulations between the cuboid and the calcaneus, navicular, and lateral cuneiform. It is crucial to know that both joints move simultaneously when the cuboid is being mobilized and that it is only the fixed component of the joint that decides which joint is being assessed and which joint may take part in the movement.

Therefore, the prerequisites for the successful application of techniques targeting the tarsal joints are:
- exact knowledge of the position of the respective tarsal bones;
- exact knowledge of the position and alignment of the joint spaces;
- experience and information regarding the applicable intensity and speed of the technique.

Calcaneocuboid Joint

The medial hand is used to stabilize the heel with a little valgus and the entire foot in a neutral position.

The lateral hand holds onto the plantar and dorsal aspects of the cuboid very pointedly (▶ Fig. 7.54).

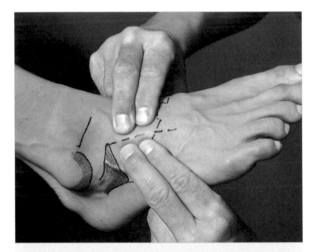

Fig. 7.55 Test of joint play at the "intermediate joint."

It should be remembered that the cuboid reaches to medial up to and including the fourth metatarsal, and plantar up to and including the third metatarsal. The lateral hand moves the cuboid to dorsolateral or plantarmedial parallel to the articular space.

From the Cuboid to the Navicular and the Lateral Cuneiform

The position of the fingers on the cuboid remains the same. The fixating hand now moves from the calcaneus to the navicular and the lateral cuneiform, both of which are found medially at the same level as the cuboid (▶ Fig. 7.55).

The cuboid is again mobilized in the same manner as above. The calcaneus is now permitted to follow this movement to some extent.

7.4 Local Palpation of the Dorsum of the Foot

7.4.1 Summary of the Palpatory Process

A main concern during palpation of the dorsum of the foot is finding the talus, the articulating surface for the ankle joint and the transverse tarsal joints.

Vascular and neural structures are also accessible on the dorsum of the foot and may be part of assessment and treatment.

Starting Position

An SP can be selected that corresponds to the descriptions seen in the palpation of either the medial or the lateral borders of the foot. It is important that the dorsum of the foot is freely accessible and the foot is able to move freely.

7.4.2 Overview of the Structures to be Palpated

- Joint space of the ankle.
- Neck and head of the talus.
- Blood vessels on the dorsum of the foot.
- Neural structures on the dorsum of the foot.

Joint Space of the Ankle

The joint space has already been successfully accessed when the outer borders of the medial and lateral malleoli are encircled. The thick tendons of the dorsiflexors make an accurate location procedure significantly more difficult. It is nevertheless very important that the articular space is exactly located when applying techniques that target the talocrural joint.

Technique

Similar to the procedure for the radiocarpal joint, the joint space is made accessible by relaxing the superficial soft tissues by passively positioning the ankle in slight dorsiflexion.

To demonstrate the entire width of the anterior edge of the tibia, the therapist can choose to access the joint from either the medial or lateral malleolus, using the index finger for palpation. The expected result of transverse palpation is a transverse bony edge that the finger hooks into. The talus is found immediately distal to this edge (▶ Fig. 7.56 and ▶ Fig. 7.57). To palpate between the tendons, it may be necessary to try out different spots and use a little more pressure.

Neck and Head of the Talus

Technique

Location from Lateral

In the section examining palpation of the lateral border of the foot, it has already been described how the fingers can push against the talus from a lateral position by first palpating the edge of the calcaneus (▶ Fig. 7.58). When this spot has been located the lateral extent of the talus becomes clearer. The tarsal sinus, entrance to the tarsal tunnel, is also located at this point.

Location from Medial

The talus can be accessed from medial at several points:
- Medial tubercle of the posterior process of the talus.
- Between the medial malleolus and sustentaculum tali.
- Between the medial malleolus and the navicular tuberosity.
- Between the sustentaculum tali and navicular tuberosity.

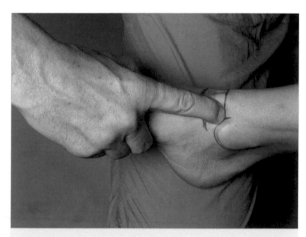

Fig. 7.56 Surface view of the site used to access the ankle joint.

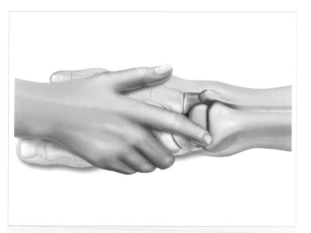

Fig. 7.57 Access to the talocrural articular space.

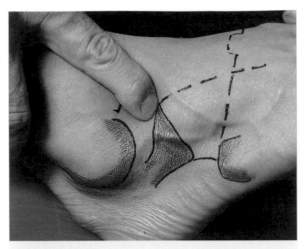

Fig. 7.58 Hooking around the talus from lateral.

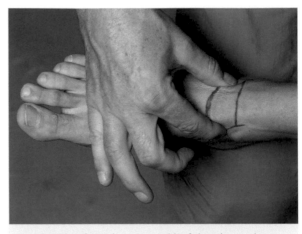

Fig. 7.59 Identifying the entire width of the talus on the surface.

The location of these bony reference points has already been extensively described in the section "Local Palpation of the Medial Border of the Foot," before.

Dorsal Talus

Two important points should be connected to illustrate the dimensions of the dorsal aspect of the talus: the lateral point, where the talus can be accessed, and the medial point, between the medial malleolus and the navicular tuberosity. The therapist can use thumb and index finger to hook around these two points (▶ Fig. 7.59 and ▶ Fig. 7.60). The distance between them illustrates the width of the talus (neck and head of the talus).

The therapist can now verify the two corresponding rules mentioned previously: all tendons belonging to the dorsiflexors of the ankle and the extensors of the toes are found on the dorsal surface of the talus as they pass over the ankle. There is no tendon dorsal to the calcaneus, thus the width of the talus can be easily recognized by the clearly visible tendons. The navicular is equally as wide as the talus and is found immediately distal to it.

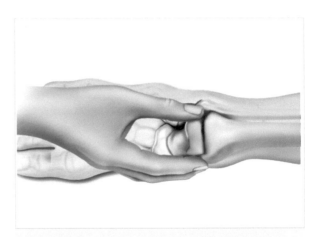

Fig. 7.60 Demonstration of the entire width of the talus.

Blood Vessels on the Dorsum of the Foot

Technique

Anterior Tibial Artery

The access in the ankle region that is used to locate the artery is fairly reliable. According to Netter (1992) and von Lanz and Wachsmuth (2004), the anterior tibial artery lies immediately lateral to the tendon of the extensor hallucis longus. Winkel (2004) states that its position is rather variable and recommends that therapists be patient and use only gentle pressure to locate the blood vessel.

The extensor hallucis longus tendon is therefore made visible using an isometric contraction. A finger pad is placed flat, applying only gentle pressure:

- laterally, between the tendons of the extensor halluces longus and extensor digitorum longus; and
- medially, between the tendons of the extensor hallucis longus and tibialis anterior, remaining there until the pulse can be clearly felt (▶ Fig. 7.61).

Once the artery has been found, its pulse can be followed proximally for some distance along the leg.

Dorsalis Pedis Artery

This artery is palpable in a distal direction (still parallel to the tendon of the extensor hallucis longus) until the midfoot region. As the dorsalis pedis artery it crosses under the tendon of the extensor hallucis and then passes to the surface distally between the first and second metatarsals. Here, it can be felt again with direct and very local flat palpation (▶ Fig. 7.62).

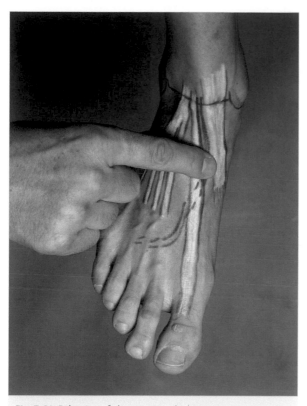

Fig. 7.61 Palpation of the anterior tibial artery.

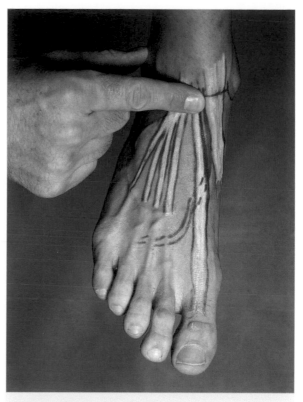

Fig. 7.62 Palpation of the dorsalis pedis artery.

Neural Structures on the Dorsum of the Foot

Both branches of the peroneal nerve cross dorsally over the ankle. They travel in different tissue layers and have only sensory qualities.

Technique

Deep Peroneal Nerve

The deep peroneal nerve accompanies the anterior tibial artery over its entire length. It becomes superficial in the distal leg as it exits the anterior compartment. Proximally, the nerve can be accessed with some effort, slightly superior to the joint space of the ankle. It is felt under fingertip palpation directly lateral to the anterior tibial artery (von Lanz and Wachsmuth, 2004) as a deep, rolling structure that does not pulse and exhibits no movement during muscle activity.

The nerve then disappears deeper into the dorsal fascia of the foot and can be neither accessed nor accurately located beneath the different tendons. It is significantly easier to palpate the nerve again on the distal metatarsus adjacent to the dorsalis pedis artery (▶ Fig. 7.63).

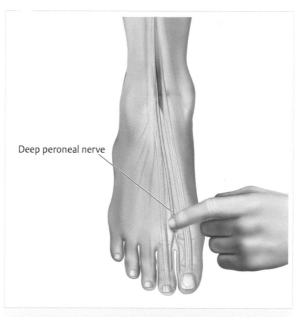

Deep peroneal nerve

Fig. 7.63 Location of the deep peroneal nerve.

Superficial Peroneal Nerve

Two peripheral nerves can be located on the dorsum of the foot that are not covered by the retinaculum. They are therefore easier to find and are sometimes visible as a fine, white line under the skin (▶ Fig. 7.61).

Both of them pass to the surface, approximately 1 hand width proximal to the talocrural joint through the fascia of the leg and are part of the superficial peroneal nerve:
- Medial dorsal cutaneous nerve.
- Intermediate dorsal cutaneous nerve.

In some cases, it is possible to find the branching of the superficial peroneal nerve into its two branches on the distal leg.

The entire length of these branches can be seen and palpated by passively positioning the foot in extensive inversion. It is often possible to follow the cutaneus dorsalis intermedius as far as the head of the fourth metatarsal.

A suitable palpation technique is a pointed, transverse palpation where the therapist once again attempts to hook around these structures as they would a guitar string (▶ Fig. 7.64).

Very often, the course of this cutaneous nerve runs via the anterior talofibular ligament. This means that in administering therapeutic transverse friction, the therapist must keep its course in mind. On the other hand, it is possible that as a result of surgery, the nerve is compromised by scarring or stretching. This can lead to pain and paresthesia at the lateral dorsum of the foot.

7.4.3 Tips for Assessment and Treatment

Techniques Targeting the Ankle Joint

A variety of manual therapy techniques fall back on the therapist's knowledge of local anatomy. This is not so much about the ability to grasp the tibia and fibula, but the ability to reach the talus near the joint. It is often observed that grip on the dorsum of the foot is too broad. This results in several joints moving and the technique does not exclusively act on the ankle joint.

Examples

Anterior-Posterior Glide of the Talus

This technique is suitable to improve dorsiflexion of the ankle. The accurate placement of the mobilizing hand on the talus guarantees successful treatment (▶ Fig. 7.65). The direction of push on the talus is directly vertical.

Anterior-Posterior Glide of the Tibia on the Talus

This technique, used for both assessment and to improve plantar flexion of the ankle, depends entirely on the complete stabilization of the talus during mobilization of the leg. A common mistake when conducting this procedure is to place the fixating hand too far from the talus (▶ Fig. 7.66).

Test of Range of Motion in the Talocalcaneonavicular Joint

Another example that can be used to clarify the application of local topographical knowledge is the testing of mobility in the TCN joint.

It is well known that the TCN joint is an extremely complex construction and is important for functional foot movements during weight-bearing. Range of motion is assessed in the following directions:
- Varus—medial and proximal tilting of the calcaneus.
- Valgus—lateral and distal tilting of the calcaneus.

This is quite difficult and depends on the therapist's sense of touch (▶ Fig. 7.67).The alignment of the tarsal canal,

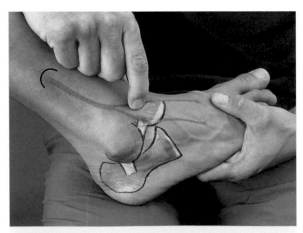

Fig. 7.64 Palpation of the branches of the superficial peroneal nerve.

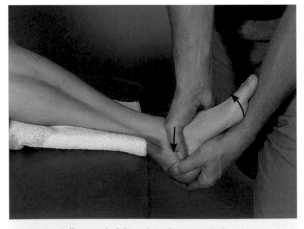

Fig. 7.65 Rolling and gliding the talus posteriorly.

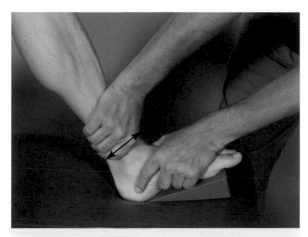

Fig. 7.66 Tibia and fibula gliding back to posterior.

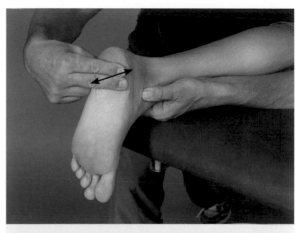

Fig. 7.67 Testing range of motion at the TCN joint.

which is aligned perpendicularly to the rotational axis of the TCN joint, provides orientation for the movement plane. To use this orientation for the range of motion test, the position of the tarsal tunnel is projected onto the sole of the foot. In so doing, the therapist looks for the following:

- The position of the tip of the calcaneus laterally, which is then marked on the lateral edge of the foot (▶ Fig. 7.41).
- The proximal aspect of the sustentaculum tali at the medial edge of the foot, which is then marked on the medial edge of the foot (▶ Fig. 7.12).

Test for Arterial Blood Flow

The arteries at the ankle and along the dorsum of the foot are palpated to assess the arterial supply in the foot. Therefore, finding the pulses of the foot is a useful skill for physicians and therapists.

Transverse Friction Without Endangering Neural Structures

There is a possibility of producing unintended irritation of a neural structure on the dorsum of the foot.

The superficial peroneal nerve and one of its branches (intermediate dorsal cutaneous nerve) can pass directly superficial to the anterior tibiofibular ligament (▶ Fig. 7.68).

This ligament is one of the most commonly injured ligaments in the musculoskeletal system and is therefore quite frequently subject to surgical intervention or treatment with local frictions.

The therapist may also irritate this neural structure during treatment with local transverse frictions. In both cases, sensory disturbances, pain, and, at times, paresthesia, indicate the presence of neural irritation.

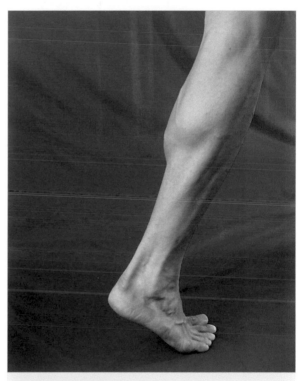

Fig. 7.68 Triceps surae and the Achilles tendon.

7.5 Local Palpation of the Distal Posterior Leg

7.5.1 Summary of the Palpatory Process

Palpation of the posterior aspect is only used to accurately identify the Achilles tendon and its insertion (▶ Fig. 7.68). The palpatory techniques and their therapeutic use merge here and are discussed together.

Starting Position

It is recommended that the patient be positioned in prone-lying with the foot hanging over the edge of the table. It is then easy to access the Achilles tendon, and the foot can move freely.

The therapist usually sits distal to the foot (▶ Fig. 7.69).

7.5.2 Overview of the Structures to be Palpated

- Borders of the Achilles tendon.
- Insertion of the triceps surae.
- Palpation of the tendon.

7.5.3 Borders of the Achilles Tendon

The collagenous parts of the triceps surae are bundled together in the Achilles tendon, the calcaneal tendon. The heads of the gastrocnemius form a tendinous plate. The soleus muscle radiates into this plate from anterior. Further to caudal, the fibers taper to a free-running tendon, approximately 15 cm long, that inserts on the tuberosity of the calcaneus.

The attachment onto the bone is by no means limited to one point. The tendon widens into a delta to half-moon shape on the entire width of the calcaneus (Doral et al., 2010). In an anatomical preparation it can also be distinguished on the lateral surfaces as far as the plantar side of the calcaneus .

The clinically most important section of the tendon lies between the aponeurosis and the proximal border of the calcaneus, approximately 2 to 6 cm proximal to its insertion. Eighty per cent of all Achilles tendon ruptures occur in this zone (Hess, 2010).

Technique

Side Borders

Starting at the calcaneal tuberosity, the therapist palpates proximally and attempts to mark the side borders of the tendon. This boundary is followed with perpendicular palpation to proximal until a distinct edge of the widening tendon can no longer be felt. The aponeurosis with the deeper-lying soleus begins at this point (▶ Fig. 7.70).

7.5.4 Insertion of the Triceps Surae

The Achilles tendon inserts on the proximal aspect of the calcaneal tuberosity, chiefly over the plantar two-thirds of this surface. The subcutaneous calcaneus bursa is located on the dorsal third.

Technique

The foot is positioned passively in extensive plantar flexion. Tension in the Achilles tendon is relieved by the approximation of the triceps surae.

This is now palpated from proximal to distal, with firm pressure applied. In several palpation steps from proximal to distal, the tendon is pushed away to anterior with a flat finger pad. The transition from tendon to tuberosity is identified by the sudden change from a firm-elastic feel to a significantly stronger form of resistance (▶ Fig. 7.71). The area of tendon insertion starts at this point. Bursae are found here both subcutaneous and underneath the tendon (subcutaneous calcaneal bursa and the bursa of the calcaneal tendon). If there is inflammation, pain can be provoked by this local pressure any fluctuation that can be felt under the palpating finger may indicate a swelling.

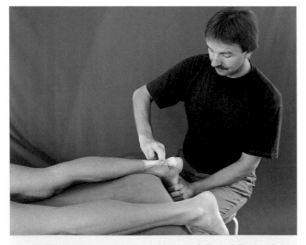

Fig. 7.69 Starting position for palpation of the Achilles tendon.

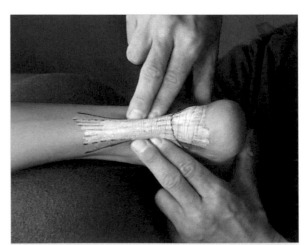

Fig. 7.70 Palpation of the borders of the Achilles tendon.

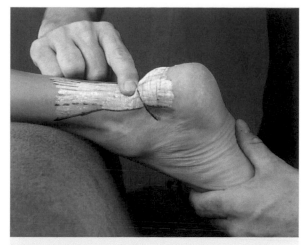

Fig. 7.71 Palpation of the insertion of the Achilles tendon.

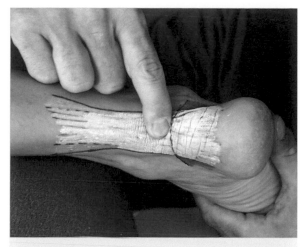

Fig. 7.72 Palpation of the insertion—detail of the technique.

> **Tip**
>
> The junction between the tendon and calcaneus can also be identified when the calf muscles are contracted. Significantly more pressure must be applied by the palpating fingers (▶ Fig. 7.72).

7.5.5 Palpation of the Tendon

Now that the clinically important areas have been identified in which tendinopathy, bursitis, and insertion tendinopathy may be found, the tendon itself will be palpated. The objective of the following palpation is finding painful spots within the tendon.

To find these spots, different variations of provocative transverse friction are used.

Technique

Method 1

This palpation technique uses the pincer grip by simultaneously using the pads of the thumb and the index finger (▶ Fig. 7.73). It is particularly suitable for the finding and treatment of conditions at the edge of the tendon.

The tendon is preloaded by passive extension of the foot. The fingers are moved anteriorly without applying pressure (toward the floor). The thumb and index finger pinch into the tissue. With sustained pressure, the fingers are then pulled posteriorly. This is the diagnostic (provocative) or therapeutically effective component of the technique.

▶ **Procedure**
- The tendon is prestretched by passive extension of the foot.

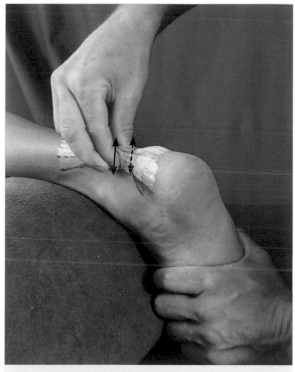

Fig. 7.73 Bilateral transverse frictions.

- The fingers are guided in an anterior direction (in spatial terms, downward) without applying pressure.
- The therapist pinches the thumb and index finger.
- The fingers are pulled in a posterior direction, maintaining this pressure. This is the diagnostically (provocative) and/or therapeutically effective component of the technique.

Tip

It is not permissible to rub the skin at any phase of the technique. Most likely, rubbing the skin will result in skin damage. The tendon is palpated in steps of 1 cm if this technique is being used diagnostically to identify the most affected part.

Method 2

Only the index finger is used in this method.

Once again, the therapist is sitting distal to the foot. The tendon is once more preloaded by maximal extension of the foot and fixed in this position. This tension is important so that the technique can be performed on a stabile tendon. The palpating finger would constantly slide off the tendon if the tendon were relaxed.

The palpating hand moves toward the side of the tendon. The middle finger is placed on top of the index finger, which is positioned on the tendon. The thumb rests on the malleolus on the side of the foot, stabilizing the hand.

In the illustrated example, the index finger maintains skin contact and moves medially without applying pressure. Pressure is applied to the tendon as the finger moves laterally (▶ Fig. 7.74).

As with the first method, this method is also used for both diagnosis and treatment.

This technique can be used to identify the most painful point by palpating the entire length of the tendon. From experience, this is approximately 2 cm proximal to the edge of the calcaneal tuberosity.

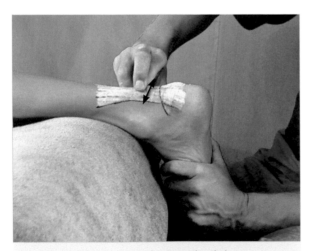

Fig. 7.74 Posterior transverse frictions—detailed view.

Bibliography

Abouelela AA, Zohiery AK. The triple compression stress test for diagnosis of tarsal tunnel syndrome. Foot. 2012; 22(3):146–149

Akiyama K, Takakura Y, Tomita Y, Sugimoto K, Tanaka Y, Tamai S. Neurohistology of the sinus tarsi and sinus tarsi syndrome. J Orthop Sci. 1999; 4(4):299–303

Athavale SA, Swathi, Vangara SV. Anatomy of the superior peroneal tunnel. J Bone Joint Surg Am. 2011; 93(6):564–571

Bachmann LM, Kolb E, Koller MT, Steurer J, ter Riet G. Accuracy of Ottawa ankle rules to exclude fractures of the ankle and mid-foot: systematic review. BMJ. 2003; 326(7386):417

Blair JM, Botte MJ. Surgical anatomy of the superficial peroneal nerve in the ankle and foot. Clin Orthop Relat Res. 1994(305):229–238

Dhillon MS. Fractures of the Calcaneus. Jaypee Brothers Medical Pub; first edition; 2013; p.10

Doral MN, Alam M, Bozkurt M, et al. Functional anatomy of the Achilles tendon. Knee Surg Sports Traumatol Arthrosc. 2010; 18(5):638–643

Ferran NA, Oliva F, Maffulli N. Recurrent subluxation of the peroneal tendons. Sports Med. 2006; 36(10):839–846

Hall RL, Shereff MJ. Anatomy of the calcaneus. Clin Orthop Relat Res. 1993 (290):27–35

Helgeson K. Examination and intervention for sinus tarsi syndrome. N Am J Sports Phys Ther. 2009; 4(1):29–37

Hess GW. Achilles tendon rupture: a review of etiology, population, anatomy, risk factors, and injury prevention. Foot Ankle Spec. 2010; 3(1):29–32

Hintermann B. Biomechanics of the unstable ankle joint and clinical implications. Med Sci Sports Exerc. 1999; 31(7) Suppl:S459–S469

Hudes K. Conservative management of a case of tarsal tunnel syndrome. J Can Chiropr Assoc. 2010; 54(2):100–106

Huson A. Joints and movements of the foot: terminology and concepts. Acta Morphol Neerl Scand. 1987; 25(3):117–130

Huson A. Biomechanics of the tarsal mechanism. A key to the function of the normal human foot. J Am Podiatr Med Assoc. 2000; 90(1):12–17

Johal KS, Milner SA. Plantar fasciitis and the calcaneal spur: fact or fiction? Foot Ankle Surg. 2012; 18(1):39–41

Landsmeer JM. Studies in the anatomy of articulation. The equilibrium of the "intercalated" bone. Acta Morphol Neerl Scand. 1961; 3:287–303

Lanz T von, Wachsmuth W. Praktische Anatomie, Bein und Statik. 2. Aufl. Berlin: Springer; 2003

Lundberg A. Kinematics of the ankle and foot. In vivo roentgen stereophotogrammetry. Acta Orthop Scand Suppl. 1989; 233:1–24

Marti R. Dislocation of the peroneal tendons. Am J Sports Med. 1977; 5(1):19–22

Matsui K, Takao M, Tochigi Y, Ozeki S, Glazebrook M. Anatomy of anterior talofibular ligament and calcaneofibular ligament for minimally invasive surgery: a systematic review. Knee Surg Sports Traumatol Arthrosc. 2017; 25(6):1892–1902

Netter FH. Farbatlanten der Medizin. Bd. 7: Bewegungsapparat I. Stuttgart: Thieme; 1992

Olexa TA, Ebraheim NA, Haman SP. The sustentaculum tali: anatomic, radiographic, and surgical considerations. Foot Ankle Int. 2000; 21(5):400–403

Padovani JP. [Anatomic and physiologic review of the lateral ligaments of the tibiotarsal joint and the lower peroneotibial ligaments]. Rev Chir Orthop Repar Appar Mot. 1975; 61(Suppl 2):1247–127

Premkumar A, Perry MB, Dwyer AJ, et al. Sonography and MR imaging of posterior tibial tendinopathy. AJR Am J Roentgenol. 2002; 178(1):223–232

Starck D. Vergleichende Anatomie der Wirbeltiere auf Evolutionsbiologischer Grundlage. Heidelberg: Springer; 1978

Stiell IG, Greenberg GH, McKnight RD, Nair RC, McDowell I, Worthington JR. A study to develop clinical decision rules for the use of radiography in acute ankle injuries. Ann Emerg Med. 1992; 21(4):384–390 van Langelaan EJ. A kinematical analysis of the tarsal joints. An X-ray photogrammetric study. Acta Orthop Scand Suppl. 1983; 204:1–269

Weigel B, Nerlich M. Praxisbuch Unfallchirurgie. Heidelberg: Springer; 2004

Wilder RP, Sethi S. Overuse injuries: tendinopathies, stress fractures, compartment syndrome, and shin splints. Clin Sports Med. 2004; 23(1):55–81

Winkel D. Nichtoperative Orthopädie und Manualtherapie. Anatomie in Vivo. 3. Aufl. München: Urban & Fischer bei Elsevier; 2004

Yang Y, Du ML, Fu YS, et al. Fine dissection of the tarsal tunnel in 60 cases. Sci Rep. 2017; 7:46351

Yao K, Yang TX, Yew WP. Posterior Tibialis Tendon Dysfunction: Overview of Evaluation and Management. Orthopedics. 2015; 38(6):385–391

7

Chapter 8

Soft Tissues

8 Soft Tissues

8.1 Significance and Function of Soft Tissues

Skin and muscles represent independent sensory input organs for treatment methods based on reflexes (connective-tissue massage) and energy flow (acupuncture) as well as locally applied treatment methods (e.g., Swedish massage).

Systematic palpation of these tissues has long been a topic of discussion. In connective-tissue massage, changes in skin consistency, for example, are attributed to specific disorders of the inner organs or the vertebral column. Classical massage treatment targets pathological muscle tension in particular. In these treatment methods, palpation is used for the purpose of assessment and also for monitoring progress. Massage is rarely used without previously palpating local or general hardening in the muscles.

Therapists must manually palpate through skin and muscles if they wish to reach deeper-lying structures. As an example, certain segmental tests and treatment procedures cannot be successfully conducted without moderate pressure being applied to deeper tissues. It would be easy to incorrectly interpret the patient's pain solely as a result of the applied pressure, if you were unable to assess the sensitivity of the different layers of tissue. Therapists should not only gain information about superficial tissue if, for example, they wish/intend to treat these tissue later (Swedish massage, connective-tissue massage), the sensitivity of superficial tissue should also be assessed in cases where the therapy involves applying sufficient pressure to penetrate deeper layers of tissue (manual therapy).

In particular, patients with chronic back symptoms are the least able to provide exact information about their symptoms. These patients are frequently affected by hyperalgesia (hypersensitivity to pain stimuli) or hyperesthesia (hypersensitivity to touch) as a result of central sensitization. They have difficulty describing the exact location of their symptoms, and the corresponding interpretation of tests that use direct pressure is unsuccessful.

When therapists are unable to recognize such changes, they tend to attribute the symptoms to the skin, the muscles, or bony parts, depending on which area their work mainly focuses on.

8.2 Common Applications for Treatment in this Region

Skin and muscle are frequently the tissue targeted in:
- Reflex-based treatment forms: connective-tissue massage, reflex zone therapy based on the work of Gläser and Dalicho, etc.

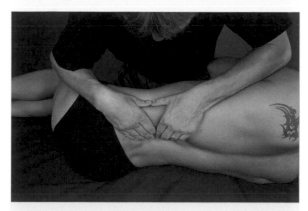

Fig. 8.1 Lumbar soft-tissue technique.

- Regional or locally applied techniques: Swedish massage, heat therapy, soft-tissue techniques in manual therapy (▶ Fig. 8.1), and more.

8.3 Required Basic Anatomical and Biomechanical Knowledge

Even beginners only need a short amount of time to gain the relevant prerequisite knowledge. Being able to initially orient yourself using general bony (▶ Fig. 8.2) and muscular structures (▶ Fig. 8.3) in the neck, back, and pelvis is sufficient. The techniques used to locate these structures will be described in the coming sections. Two prerequisites are the following:
- To be able to conduct an orienting and systematic palpation.
- To be able to describe the location of palpated structures well and to document these findings.

8.4 Summary of the Palpatory Process

8.4.1 Extent of the Palpation

The entire surface of the skin and the underlying muscles from the gluteal area to the occiput will be palpated. This includes the following muscles in particular: the glutei, erector spinae, latissimus dorsi, trapezius, rhomboids, infraspinatus, supraspinatus, and the deltoid.

8.4.2 Criteria for Palpation

What will be assessed:
- The surface of the skin.
- The consistency of tissue.
- Sensation.
- Pressure pain sensitivity.

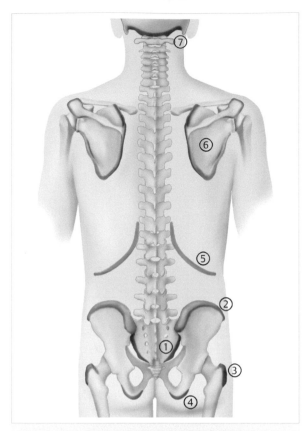

Fig. 8.2 Bony orientation. 1 = edge of the sacrum; 2 = iliac crest; 3 = greater trochanter; 4 = ischial tuberosity; 5 = all accessible spinous processes and ribs; 6 = borders, angles, and protruding processes of the scapula; 7 = from the occiput to the mastoid process.

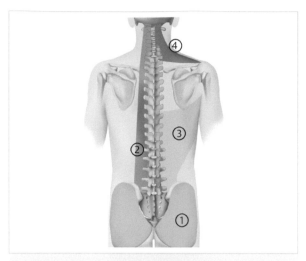

Fig. 8.3 Muscular orientation. 1 = gluteal muscles; 2 = erector spinae, especially multifidus lumborum, spinalis thoracis, semispinalis cervicis; 3 = latissimus dorsi; 4 = descending part of trapezius.

Memorize

Skin and muscles have their own terminology for consistency. The term turgor is used for the skin and tension for the muscles. Both of these terms are used in palpation to define the amount of tension that the displacing or pressurizing finger feels as resistance.

Surface of the Skin

The following characteristics are assessed: smooth/rough, dry/moist, warm/cold, hair growth, protrusions. Also check whether the changes are general or only found locally (compare with the other side of the body!).

Tip

As an exercise, try to write a list of adjectives describing the characteristics of the skin surface, for example, soft, coarse, elastic, tensed, thickened, parchmentlike, cracked.

Consistency of Tissue

The term consistency has many different meanings. It is used here as a standard to measure the compliancy of tissues when displaced or when pressure is placed on them. It is along these lines that the viscoelastic properties of tissue are assessed.

Sensation

Skin sensation is checked in passing when the surface of the skin and its consistency are being examined. It does not need to be assessed separately in clinical practice. The therapist will be made aware that the sensation needs to be assessed during the subjective assessment or when the patient informs them of sensory changes during palpation.

What Should the Therapist Pay Attention To?

Sensory deficits are rare in the trunk. They are more likely to occur in the joints of the limbs as a result of nerve-root compression or peripheral-nerve lesion. A hypoesthesia or an anesthesia in the region of the back is to be classified as dangerous! If one of these symptoms is encountered, it is necessary to clarify whether this is a familiar symptom or whether it should be investigated further.

Caution

Do not treat the back if the cause of sensory deficits has not been clarified!

Sensory deficits interfere with massages or other interventions (e.g., electrotherapy) as the patient cannot provide the therapist with important feedback regarding the appropriate dosage. Such treatment must be performed with appropriate caution.

When considering whether, and in what dosage, treatment should be administered, it is also important to identify possible hypersensitivity to touch (hyperesthesia) or pain stimuli (hyperalgesia). It is normal for tissue to be hypersensitive to pressure during wound healing in the acute, exudative stage. This is the result of peripheral sensitization. Pathological hyperesthesias or hyperalgesias develop secondary to chronic pain. This is the result of central sensitization in the dorsal horn of the spinal cord. Hypersensitive parts of the body transmit pain signals when touched roughly and can only be treated using techniques where minimal pressure is applied or large surface contact is made (e.g., stroking as part of classical massage). At times it may be appropriate not to treat manually at all (refer to van den Berg, 2003 to gain further knowledge of the physiology of chronic pain).

Sensitivity to Pressure that Causes Pain

The size of the area being treated and the selection, speed, and intensity of treatment techniques are chosen according to the pain sensitivity of the tissue, among other factors. It is also possible to estimate the expected results of muscle treatment by assessing whether the muscles are the source of pain. Ideally, the techniques described later in the book provoke pain in the patient's muscle tissue. If the techniques do not provoke pain in the muscles or if the skin or skeleton are the source of symptoms, the treatment of soft tissue will not result in any kind of pain relief.

8.5 Method and Techniques of the Palpatory Process

A specific methodology is available that enables palpation to be conducted comprehensively in a short period. This succession of techniques places increased stress on the tissue:

- **Skin**
  - Stroking the skin to assess its qualities.
  - Stroking the skin to assess its temperature.
  - Assessing the skin's consistency using displacement tests.
  - Assessing the skin's consistency using the lifting test.
  - Assessing the skin's consistency using skin rolling.
- **Muscles**
  - Assessing the muscles' consistency using transverse frictions with the fingers.

▶ Fig. 8.4 illustrates the procedure used to assess the consistency of the skin (left-hand side) and the muscles (right-hand side).

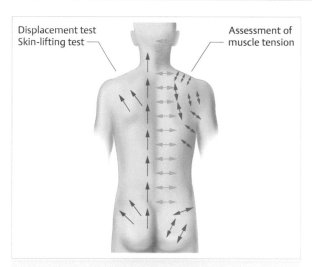

Fig. 8.4 Procedure used for skin and muscle palpation.

The techniques are conducted using different areas of the hand. These areas are suitable for the palpation of certain sensations due to their differing degrees of special receptor dispersion. For example, the most successful method for the palpation of skin temperature is to use the back of the hand or the posterior surface of the fingers. A large number of thermoreceptors are found here. The finger pads are used to detect fine differences in contour and consistency in tissue. The high density of mechanoreceptors makes the finger pads ideal for this purpose.

8.6 Starting Position

Neutral and relaxed pronation is appropriate when assessing the soft tissue of the posterior trunk. This should be standard for comparable assessment techniques. Of course, it is possible to alter this neutral starting position (SP) if necessary for certain treatment techniques or if it ensures that the patient is free of symptoms when lying. For example, padding is placed under the hip joint, pelvis, and abdomen in cases of arthritis. The following description depicts an ideal case scenario and applies to most of the SPs in Chapters 9–12.

During general inspection of the prone patient (▶ Fig. 8.5), the therapist determines whether the head, thoracic spine, thorax, lumbar spine, and pelvis are situated in a straight line without lateral shift or rotation:

- If possible, the head is positioned in neutral rotation. The nose is placed in the face hole of the treatment table.
- The arms are positioned next to the body; the fingers can be placed slightly under the pelvis. Alternatively, the arms may also be placed over the side of the table. The arms should never be positioned at head level. This tenses the thoracolumbar fascia, making palpation of structures more difficult at the transitional area

between the lumbar spine and the sacrum. In addition, it causes rotation of the scapula, which in turn alters the length of various muscles in the shoulder girdle.

- The distal lower leg rests on a foot roll, ensuring that the muscles of the lower leg and thigh are relaxed. The foot roll may be dispensed with if the rotation of the legs does not change the tension in the gluteal muscles.

Some frequently asked questions are: Should padding always be placed underneath the pelvis and abdomen and the head-end of the treatment table lowered? How much lordosis or kyphosis should be allowed or supported? What can therapists decisively orient themselves on in addition to what the patient feels? The answers can be found when you look at the patient's posture in standing. The general rule is: the curvature of the patient's spine in standing is also permitted in the prone position. This is achieved by altering the position of the treatment table or providing support with padding.

The therapist stands to the side of the treatment table opposite the side to be palpated. Naturally, the therapist pays attention to the height of the treatment table. The table should be sufficiently high to ensure an ergonomical standing position.

8.6.1 Difficult and Alternative Starting Positions

Observation and palpation findings in the prone position differ significantly from the vertical (e.g., sitting) and side-lying position. One reason for this is that gravity causes the skin to sag. The skin is therefore subject to some degree of preliminary tension. The back and neck muscles are more tense in unsupported sitting as they maintain the body's upright position. It is therefore difficult to feel changes in muscle consistency (e.g., increased muscle tension).

If you want to reduce the anti-gravity effect in the trunk and neck muscles, ensure that the weight of the head, arms, and, when necessary, the upper body rests on a supportive surface. This can be achieved by sitting on the side

of a treatment table and using appropriate padding. When the active muscle tension in the back and neck muscles is reduced, the body bends forward and hip flexion surpasses 90° (caution with recent total hip replacements [THRs]). This results in a flexed lumbar spine, with flexion continuing more or less up into the thoracic spine. This in turn increases the passive tension in all posterior fasciae and the trunk muscles and increases the resistance that the palpating finger has to work against.

Neutral Starting Position: Sitting

The neutral sitting position roughly imitates the curvature of the spine when the patient is standing upright. The best position to obtain this is unsupported sitting on the corner of a treatment table. This SP is generally not very stable. Description of a more stable SP in sitting follows below.

The patient sits on the treatment table with the thighs resting fully on the table. It is recommended that only patients with circulatory disorders and those with poor stability have the soles of the feet in contact with the floor. The knees are separated further than the width of the hips, facilitating pelvic tilt movements. This enables positioning of the lumbar lordosis. The thoracic and cervical curvatures are positioned to correspond with the curvatures in standing or are corrected when necessary. The patient's arms hang down loosely beside the body. The forearms or the hands rest on the thighs.

The therapist stands to the side of the patient and opposite the side to be palpated. The therapist should pay attention to the height of the treatment table, ensuring that the standing position is ergonomical.

Neutral Starting Position: Side-lying

This SP also attempts to reproduce the patient's natural spinal curvature (▶ Fig. 8.6). If the patient cannot adopt this position without pain, the position is naturally adapted to make it possible for the patient to remain in the side-lying position for a certain amount of time.

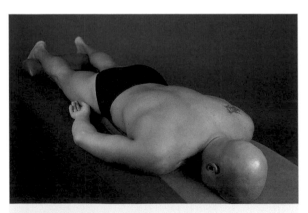

Fig. 8.5 Patient in prone position.

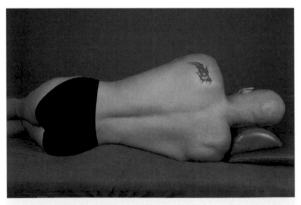

Fig. 8.6 Patient positioned in side-lying.

Otherwise the following short formula applies: no lateral flexion, rotation, forced kyphosis, or forced lordosis.

This is achieved by placing the patient in an easily accessible side-lying position and placing padding underneath the lumbar and cervical spines so that these sections of the vertebral column are no longer laterally flexed. This accommodation requires individual effort.

The upper body and the pelvis are then placed in neutral rotation: both sides of the pelvis and both shoulders lie on top of each other.

Both legs should rest on top of each other. The hip joints are not flexed more than 70° so that the lumbar spine is not forced out of its lordotic position. The knee joints are clearly flexed. Check the head position again.

The therapist stands facing the back of the patient. The therapist should check that the treatment table is high enough to ensure an ergonomic stance.

8.7 Palpation Techniques

8.7.1 Palpating the Surface of the Skin

The procedure for palpating the skin incorporates all posteriorly accessible parts of the skin. The palpation starts in the pelvic region, in particular over the sacrum and the iliac crests, and continues upward to the occiput. Attention is paid to the skin's quality and varying temperature (see also Chapter 1).

Technique Used for the Surface of the Skin

The qualities of the skin, its roughness, etc. are assessed by slowly stroking the skin systematically with flattened hands (▶ Fig. 8.7).

Technique Used to Assess the Temperature of the Skin

The back of the hand or the posterior side of the fingers are used to perceive the skin's temperature (▶ Fig. 8.8). The therapist pays attention to possible differences between the left- and right-hand sides and between neighboring superior and inferior regions. It is frequently observed that the pelvic or the lumbar region is colder without pathological cause.

8.7.2 Palpating the Quality of the Skin (Turgor)

The skin's consistency is dependent on the balance of fluid in the skin and can be ascertained using elasticity tests. The aim is to determine general elasticity of the skin and whether there are areas of differing elasticity that may provide the therapist with information about the skin's reflex response to pathological irritants such as internal organs.

When comparing sides during the assessment of skin consistency, it is important to pay attention to the location of assessment. It should be at the same distance from the vertebral column on both sides. Differences in distance result in different palpatory findings, which means the assessment is then unreliable.

8

Criteria

All tests consist of initially deforming the skin with minimal force and stretching the skin to the maximum. The degree of deformation reached is evaluated and the time it took to reach this stretch is observed. The skin is then mildly stretched in a rhythmic manner. The elasticity felt in the

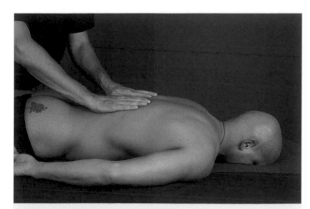
Fig. 8.7 Palpating the quality of the skin.

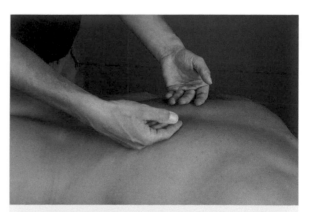
Fig. 8.8 Palpating the skin temperature.

skin's response is noted. There are principally no differences between this procedure, including the criteria applied, and the assessment of passive movement or joint play.

Full tissue deformation can only be successful with the appropriate intensity. This requires considerable concentration, especially when a beginner is palpating.

Displacement Test Technique

This is the simplest and least provocative test. The outstretched hand is placed on the surface of the skin. Minimal pressure is applied and the skin is pushed in a superior direction until the increasing tension in the skin restricts further movement (▶ Fig. 8.9). The therapist conducts this test in a rhythmic manner, paying special attention to the tissue's resistance to movement and the path that both hands follow over the body's surface.

The area to be assessed encompasses the sacral region, passes over the iliac crests in a lateral direction, runs paravertebral up to the cervicothoracic junction, and includes both scapulas (see also ▶ Fig. 8.4). This is the only test that can be used to gain information about the skin's consistency if the skin is extremely sensitive. Both of the following tests are more aggressive.

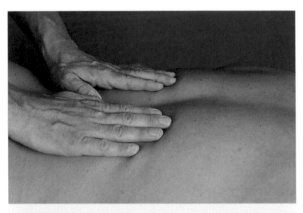

Fig. 8.9 Displacement test.

Skin-lifting Test Technique

The test on the next level of intensity deforms the skin perpendicular to the skin's surface. This test can also be performed bilaterally and simultaneously. The thumb and a few finger pads grasp a section of the skin and form a skin fold, which is then lifted away from the surface of the skin (▶ Fig. 8.10).

The same assessment criteria apply here: tissue resistance and the degree of motion. It is almost impossible to assess these criteria when patients are obese or have a high level of turgor. Also, it is frequently observed that it is impossible to lift up the skin in the lumbar region. This is purely a variation of the norm. The skin is usually lifted up several times paravertebrally from approximately S3 to T1.

Skin-rolling Technique

This technique combines skin lifting perpendicular to the body's surface and displacement parallel to it. It is very informative but is a fairly aggressive, more challenging technique, and can only be conducted on one side at a time.

Both hands are used to form a skin fold on one side of the body, similar to the skin-lifting test. Starting with the lumbosacral region, this skin fold is then quickly rolled paravertebrally in a superior direction (▶ Fig. 8.11). The therapist tries to keep the skin lifted as much as possible and not to lose the skin fold during the movement. The finger pads always pull new skin into the fold, and the thumbs push the fold upward in a superior direction.

8.7.3 Palpating the Consistency of Muscle (Assessment of Muscle Tension)

Most soft-tissue techniques on the trunk influence the pathologically altered muscle consistency (muscle tension). Only a positive result in the assessment of muscle tension justifies the use of soft-tissue treatment techniques (e.g., massage). Therefore, the state of the muscle must be systemically examined at the start of a treatment

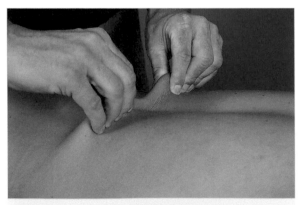

Fig. 8.10 Skin-lifting test.

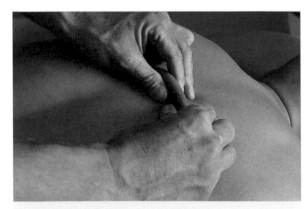

Fig. 8.11 Skin rolling.

series and also be included at the start of each treatment session. It is not enough to depend on information from the patient to accurately observe treatment progress.

The palpation of tissue resistance in muscles requires a certain intensity, appropriate technique, and a reliable procedure (see also ▶ Fig. 8.4). Muscle tension is palpated after the skin has been pushed against the body's fasciae. This prevents the skin from providing the therapist with further information. Furthermore, the amount of pressure applied depends on the size or the thickness of the muscle to be palpated.

The technique applied is, therefore, transverse friction using the fingers. This should be performed in the gluteal and the lumbar regions with the hand pushing down (with the aid of the other hand when necessary) so that deeper-lying muscles such as the piriformis can be reached. Palpation is performed in the thoracic, cervical, and scapula regions with both hands separate from one another to save time.

The palpating hands now "scan" the muscle tissue using large movements. An attempt is made to gain a general idea of the consistency. The tissue is only palpated at a local level if abnormalities have been identified during the general "scan." Local palpation of muscle is then conducted using small movements, assessing the muscle's precise condition and the extent of change. This way of proceeding saves time and is effective. If the palpation provokes pain, extra attention must be paid toward the hardened tissue (see the section "Interpreting the Muscle Consistency [Tension] Palpation Findings" below). Principally, global and local hardening of muscles can easily be found using intensive transverse palpation.

During the physical therapy training, palpation is introduced as a separate entity. Later on it is usually conducted in connection with the objective assessment. It is nevertheless recommended that beginners separate the results of observation and palpation to train the respective senses.

Techniques

- The therapist begins by pushing the fingers of one hand down onto the gluteal area at the edge of the sacrum and applies frictions.
- The hand moves transversely over the gluteus maximus and the underlying piriformis.
- The hand then moves laterally onto the small gluteal muscles (▶ Fig. 8.12a) in the space between the iliac crest and the greater trochanter.

8

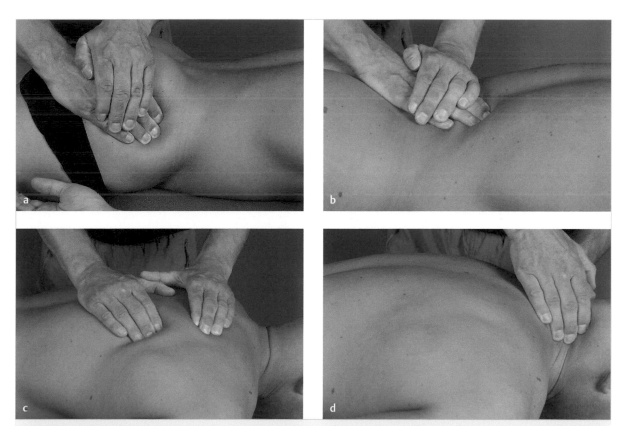

Fig. 8.12 a–d Assessing muscle tension.
a. In the gluteals.
b. In the lumbar region.
c. Along the scapula.
d. In the cervical region.

- The lumbar erector spinae are palpated paravertebrally (▶ Fig. 8.12b). If the back extensors are very well developed, the palpation will have to be separated into more medial and more lateral segments.
- The thoracic erector spinae are palpated paravertebrally until approximately the level of T1 is reached. The therapist will be able to use both hands simultaneously for the palpation from here onward most of the time. It is no longer necessary to place extra weight on the palpating hand to apply enough pressure to reach the deep tissues.
- The therapist moves along the medial border of the scapula in the area of the rhomboids and the transverse and ascending parts of the trapezius (▶ Fig. 8.12c).
- The infraspinatus and supraspinatus are assessed, moving laterally from a medial position over the scapula.
- The belly of the descending part of the trapezius is then palpated, returning in a medial direction.
- The paravertebral and suboccipital neck muscles are assessed next (▶ Fig. 8.12d).
- Tense adductors are expected to be found in patients with overloaded or painful shoulder joints. The palpation continues laterally along the scapula and the consistency of latissimus dorsi, teres major, and teres minor is felt. It is useful to also palpate the deltoids since a loss of muscle tone may be found here as a result of inactivity.

Tip

The lumbar extensors form a uniform muscle mass due to the osteofibrotic sheath consisting of the vertebral processes and the thoracolumbar fascia. A variety of techniques in classical massage or functional massages utilize this fact, pushing the complete muscle mass laterally away from the row of spinous processes. The back extensors are no longer a uniform muscle mass in the thoracic region:
- The amount of muscle decreases.
- The fascia ends approximately at the level of T7–T8.
- The spinalis is found directly adjacent to the spinous processes.

The palpating finger must not only overcome the skin to reach the muscles; it must also overcome the body's fasciae. These fasciae are not always of the same thickness in each section of the back (see Chapter 1). When the therapist is aware of how the fasciae are constructed, expectations regarding the consistency of the muscle tissue to be palpated will be correct.

8.8 Tips for Assessment and Treatment

The palpation of the posterior soft tissue is analyzed first. When the patient indicates pain, the therapist should consider how they can proceed systematically to clearly identify the tissue in which pain originates. Following this, the results of the individual palpatory findings are discussed. This section ends with examples of treatment, the main focus being on the treatment of muscles.

8.8.1 Differentiating between Tissues

How can you find out which tissue is affected?

The pressure applied during palpation is uncomfortable when the skin is hyperesthetic or hyperalgesic. It is also known that a certain amount of palpatory pressure, for example, onto the back extensors, is transferred as a slight movement onto the vertebral segment. How is it then possible to reliably find the affected tissue when pressure causes pain?

We will discuss this by using the example of paravertebral palpation along the middle thoracic spine. Visualize the situation with a patient. The therapist systematically palpates the back extensors from inferior to superior using transverse frictions. At the level of the scapula the patient reports the pressure to be very uncomfortable. The question is: does muscle hardening definitely cause the reported pain? The therapist must now differentiate between tissues to answer this question.

Is the skin sensitive to pressure? The therapist should have already gained information about this when assessing skin consistency. It can happen that something is overlooked, in which case the skin consistency test is repeated using the technique that stresses the skin the most: skin rolling. The therapist broadly rolls the skin over the affected area now and compares it to the other side. When the patient indicates the same symptoms as those that appeared during localized pressure, the skin is the source of pressure pain. More precise information about the condition of deeper-lying structures is not possible using palpation. If the muscles are treated (e.g., soft-tissue techniques or massage) despite the skin sensitivity, treatment must be conducted with caution and with a large area of surface contact.

Is the vertebral column causing the symptoms? The therapist places the flat hand directly over the vertebral column and pushes anteriorly, alternating between more pressure and less pressure while gradually increasing the overall pressure (▶ Fig. 8.13). If this is not precise enough, the therapist can use the ulnar side of the hand and the same technique on the spinous and transverse processes in the area of pain. The vertebral column is at least partially the source of symptoms if the patient indicates the same symptoms felt during the previous palpation.

Are the costovertebral joints sensitive to pressure? It can be difficult to differentiate a myogelosis (local muscle hardening) from a sensitive costovertebral joint in thin patients. Both are found very locally and are very firm. A myogelosis can mostly be pushed somewhat to the side. This cannot be expected with a rib. To make sure, the

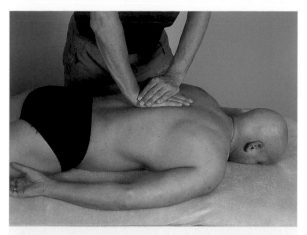

Fig. 8.13 Careful provocation of the thoracic spine.

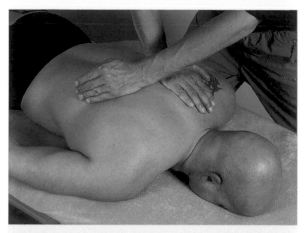

Fig. 8.14 Careful provocation of the costovertebral joints.

therapist places the ulnar side of their hand or thumb on the rib and pushes down onto the rib using a slow rocking motion and gradually increasing the pressure (▶ Fig. 8.14) (see also the section "Posterior Palpation Techniques," Chapter 11). If this is the most painful test, the source of symptoms can be found in an irritated or blocked costovertebral joint. Treating the muscle alone will most likely not result in permanent relief.

The therapist can be sure that the muscles are sensitive and are the cause of the patient's symptoms when the provocation of skin, vertebral column, and the costovertebral joints do not provide clear answers. Remember these differentiating tests, especially when soft-tissue treatment has not yet produced the desired result.

> **Tip**
>
> Determine whether there are any contraindications before applying pressure to the vertebral column or ribs.

8.8.2 Interpreting the Findings of Skin Surface Palpation

The most important questions following this are:
• Does the skin give you a reason not to test or treat deeper-lying structures? Possible reasons include diseases or injuries to the skin, but can also include rough, cracked, parched skin where strong deformations of the skin, as is the case during massages, are contraindicated. Acne, scarring, and lipomata also restrict the area that can be treated. The chronification of pain and disorders of the peripheral nervous system can cause hyperalgesia or hyperesthesia. The pressure from the therapist's hand may then be perceived as unpleasant. The treatment is questionable in this case.

• How much pressure can safely be applied when the use of a manual technique is possible?
• When classic massage treatment is used, how much of the massage product should be used?

8.8.3 Interpreting the Skin Consistency (Turgor) Palpation Findings

All three tests presented here should result in the same findings. Elasticity and sensitivity noted should be equal. The techniques should be reassessed or the patient questioned again if this is not the case. These tests stress the skin with different degrees of stretch (see also Chapter 1).

The sympathetic nervous system regulates the balance of fluids. Reflex changes to fluid accumulation are a sign of nociceptive afferents that are above or below threshold and arise from sections of a neurological segment (viscerotome, sclerotome, myotome). These changes may be seen during observation in the form of retracted skin or swelling. For further explanations, please read the relevant literature on reflexology. Certain changes in consistency, especially the retraction or adhesion of skin, can be positively affected by manual techniques (skin rolling, soft-tissue techniques to the thorax, etc.). Such findings are seen during the skin palpation of patients suffering from pulmonary and bronchial disorders (bronchial asthma, post-pneumonia).

8.8.4 Interpreting the Muscle Consistency (Tension) Palpation Findings

The assumption regarding "normally tensed" tissues and the corresponding palpable resistance is critical when interpreting the muscle consistency results. It can be assumed that muscle tissue yields quite a lot to pressure applied perpendicular to it and that the tissue has a soft and very elastic feel. Palpation on patients frequently results in completely different findings.

> **Memorize**
>
> Muscle-tissue consistency can change due to physiological and pathological reasons. It can be either softer or harder than expected.

Softer consistencies are seen in atrophies following immobilization or injury as well as in disorders of the nervous system that are accompanied by hypotonic paralysis.

Harder consistencies are interpreted as hardened muscles when the entire muscle or large parts of the muscle are affected. Smaller areas of hardening are identified as myogeloses or trigger points (see also Chapter 1).

Besides these harder consistencies, classified as pathological, there are also completely normal deviations from the expected consistency norm.

What Does it Mean When a Hardened Muscle Is Found?

Not every hardened muscle has to be treated. Painful, hardened areas that correspond to the patient's reported area of pain are of interest. Naturally, hardened muscles that hinder the access to deeper-lying structures (e.g., facet joints) are also of interest.

If the therapist finds an abnormally hardened area in a muscle during palpation, it is recommended that the therapist asks the patient the following questions to determine the pathological degree of the hardened area and its importance to the patient:

- **Question 1: Can you feel the hardened area?**
  - The therapist does not attach any meaning to the findings if the patient's answer is "no."
  - The therapist proceeds with the questioning if the patient's answer is "yes."
- **Question 2: Is the pressure that I apply to the hardened area uncomfortable?**
  - The therapist does not attach any meaning to the findings if the patient's answer is "no."
  - The therapist proceeds with the questioning if the patient's answer is "yes."
- **Question 3: Does the hardened area correspond to the area where your symptoms are?**
  - The therapist attaches little meaning to the findings if the patient's answer is "no."
  - The therapist makes a mental note of the findings if the patient's answer is "yes," classifying the findings as particularly important, and documents this on a body chart.

This list of questions enables the therapist to individually structure treatment using soft-tissue techniques or massage to target the symptoms. It also prevents the therapist spending too much time on less important areas of muscle. The therapist should pay particular attention to the following areas of hardening when planning treatment:

- Hardening that was conspicuous during the third question.
- Hardening that prevents access to deeper-lying structures.
- Hardening that is important for the familiarization with and the treatment before the application of manual therapy techniques.

8.9 Examples of Treatment

> **Memorize**
>
> Examples for massage therapy are presented below (Reichert, 2015).

8.9.1 Lumbar Functional Massage in Side-lying

Lateral flexion in the lumbar region must be pain-free for the patient and must be assessed before commencing the technique. In addition, any contraindications must be ruled out. However, the massage delivers especially great tension relief and effects mobilization, so that this extra preliminary effort is well worth it.

The contraindications are as follows:
- Any acute, painful symptoms in the lumbar spine.
- Pronounced instability in the lumbar spine.
- Arthritis and severe restrictions in mobility in a hip.
- Total hip replacement.
- All other contraindications for physical therapy.

Starting Position

The patient lies in a neutral side-lying position. The side to be treated is uppermost. The therapist places both hands paravertebrally, grasping the upper-lying back extensors. The superior end of the therapist's forearm rests lightly on the patient's thorax. The inferior end of the forearm rests on the pelvis between the greater trochanter and the iliac crest (▶ Fig. 8.15).

Technique

▶ **Phase 1.** The back extensors being treated are displaced laterally (in spatial terms toward the roof). The therapist achieves this by pulling the finger pads upward and slightly separating the thumbs.

▶ **Phase 2.** To intensify this technique, the therapist pushes the elbows against the areas of support. The more inferiorly positioned arm slides up to 80% during this movement. The role of the more superiorly positioned forearm is to prevent the thorax from moving with the rest of the body. Its job is not to force lateral flexion! The result should be lateral flexion of the lumbar spine (toward the right in this example). This combines the transverse stretch from phase 1 with a longitudinal stretching of the back extensors (▶ Fig. 8.16).

▶ **Phase 3.** The lower legs can be used as a lever to increase the range of lateral flexion in younger patients where lateral flexion is pain-free. The patient's lower legs hang over the edge of the treatment table (phase 3a, ▶ Fig. 8.17). The therapist pushes on the pelvis with the forearm and the patient lowers their lower legs (phase 3b, ▶ Fig. 8.18) → lateral flexion is increased immensely. Not every patient can be expected to undergo this enormous stress on the lumbar spine. There are, therefore, a few contraindications that should be observed with this technique.

Tip

The muscles in the area of the lumbosacral junction can be reached by changing the hand placement in each variation of this technique (▶ Fig. 8.19). Only the therapist's more superiorly positioned hand hooks medially around the back extensors. The more inferiorly positioned hand rests on the pelvis and facilitates lateral flexion only. It is no longer in contact with the back muscles.

The treatment effect can be intensified by using neurophysiological aids to increase the range of pelvic and leg motion (in phase 3), which increases the movement in the lumbar spine:
• Reciprocal inhibition for phase 2.
• Contract relax for phase 3.

Reciprocal Inhibition for Phase 2

The aim is to inhibit the upper-lying back extensors through activity in the lower-lying muscles. Therefore,

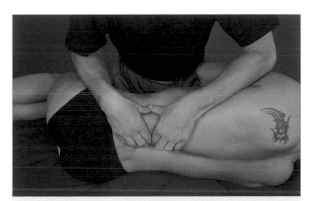

Fig. 8.15 Starting position for lumbar functional massage in side-lying.

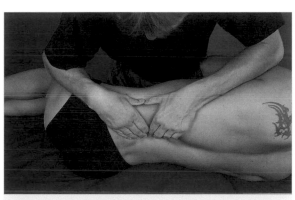

Fig. 8.16 Lumbar functional massage in side-lying, technique phase 2.

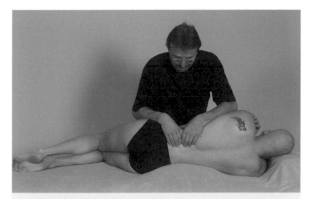

Fig. 8.17 Lumbar functional massage with side-bending, technique phase 3a.

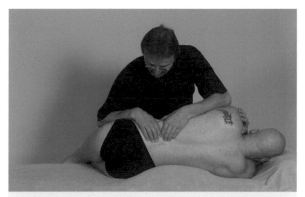

Fig. 8.18 Lumbar functional massage with side-bending, technique phase 3b.

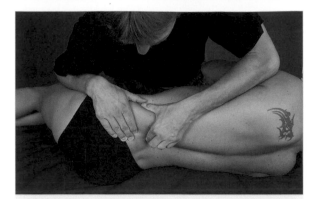

Fig. 8.19 Lumbosacral hand placement.

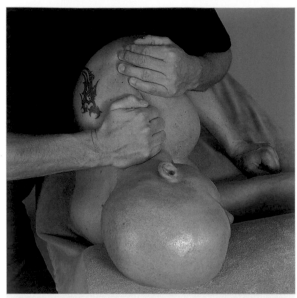

Fig. 8.20 SP for the functional massage of the trapezius in side-lying.

the therapist instructs the patient to move the upper-lying side of the pelvis inferiorly. The patient can only achieve this by activating the lower-lying lumbar muscles (and therefore inhibiting the upper-lying lumbar muscles). The patient begins to move at exactly the same moment when the therapist uses both arms to force lateral flexion.

Contract Relax for Phase 3

The relaxing effect following isometric muscular activity has been discussed in the literature. Neurophysiological evidence cannot be described at present. This principle functions though in clinical situations. It is therefore important that the patient becomes increasingly involved in the procedure by focusing on muscle tension and relaxation, and that the patient is given enough time to relax. During the phase 3 procedure, the patient lifts both lower legs to the level of the treatment table, then holds this for a few seconds, perceives the tension in the lumbar spine and the pelvis, lets the lower legs drop, and then feels the relaxation. It is only now that the therapist manually forces lateral flexion and changes the erector spinae's form.

8.9.2 Functional Massage of the Trapezius in Side-lying

The functional massage in side-lying is one of the most effective options to decrease tension in the frequently painful and tense descending fibers of the trapezius. The technique combines longitudinal stretching (movement of the shoulder girdle) with a manual transverse stretch. As patients are often unable to relax their shoulder girdle muscles, it is recommended to first passively protract, retract, elevate, and depress the scapula and move the scapula diagonally. At the same time the therapist can assess whether the necessary movements can be performed without causing pain in the shoulder girdle joints.

The technique itself starts with the trapezius in a slightly approximated position, followed by a diagonal movement of the shoulder. The hand molded over the trapezius applies an impulse or pressure onto the muscle belly in the opposite direction.

Starting Position

The patient lies in a neutral side-lying position and slides as close as possible to the edge of the treatment table next to the therapist, who stabilizes the patient with the body from a standing position.

One hand is resting on the shoulder joint and facilitates the shoulder girdle, while the other hand holds onto the descending fibers of the trapezius using the palmar grip (▶ Fig. 8.20).

Functional Massage

The muscle is approximated by slightly elevating and protracting the shoulder girdle (scapula moves forward and upward).

The thenar eminence pushes the muscle in an anterior direction without the hand slipping over the skin → transverse stretch.

The shoulder girdle is facilitated into an extremely depressed and retracted position (scapula moves backward and downward, ▶ Fig. 8.21) → longitudinal stretch.

The stretch is stopped if the muscle belly slips out from underneath the therapist's hand.

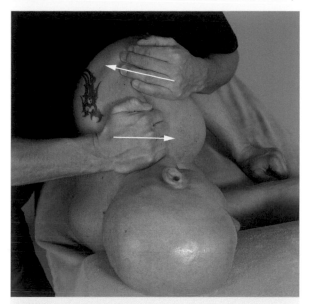

Fig. 8.21 Functional massage of the trapezius In side-lying, variation 1.

The effectiveness of this technique can be improved by prestretching the muscle farther using lateral flexion away from the side to be treated (the head-end of the treatment table is lowered, or the pillow is removed). The stretch is significantly more effective due to this.

Lateral flexion must be pain-free for the patient and must be assessed before commencing the technique. Another variation involves transverse deformation of the trapezius with depression and protraction and simultaneously pulling the muscle in a posterior direction.

Chapter 13.8 presents an additional cervical functional massage.

If the heel of the therapist's hand continuously rubs up against the superior angle of the scapula during the previously described technique, the scapula can be moved out of the way. This is achieved by passively elevating the arm to a sufficient extent (at least 90° of glenohumeral joint flexion) and maintaining this position. The scapula is placed in extensive external rotation, and the superior angle of the scapula moves inferiorly. There is now more space on the trapezius for the therapist's molding hand (variation according to Matthias Grötzinger).

Bibliography

Reichert B. Massage-Therapie. Stuttgart: Thieme; 2015
Gläser O, Dalicho WA. Segmentmassage. 4. Aufl. Leipzig: Thieme; 1972
Van den Berg F, Ed. Angewandte Physiologie, Band 4: Schmerzen verstehen und beeinflussen. Stuttgart: Thieme; 2003

8

Chapter 9

Posterior Pelvis

9 Posterior Pelvis

9.1 Significance and Function of the Pelvic Region

The pelvis is the kinetic and kinematic center of the musculoskeletal system. It is the center of the functional unit of the lumbopelvic-hip (LPH) region. The kinematic chains of the vertebral column and the lower limbs meet here. The pelvis must be able to withstand a variety of bio-mechanical demands, especially when the body is in upright position. Vleeming states (personal communication, 2002):

> ### Memorize
>
> "The body's core stability starts in the pelvis so that the three levers—legs and vertebral column—can be moved safely!"

The pelvis has adapted itself to these demands throughout the phylogenetic evolution (▶ Fig. 9.1):

The large, protruding ala of the ilium provides a large area for the attachment of soft tissues and therefore the muscular prerequisites for an upright posture in standing: gluteal, back, and abdominal muscles. This protruding area of the ilia envelops and protects several organs.

The sacroiliac (SI) joint has increased greatly in size; the ligamentous apparatus has become considerably stronger. The load-transferring area between the SI joint and the acetabulum or the ischial tuberosities has been reduced in length and strengthened.

The sacrum has remained in the same position in the sagittal plane, tilting inward toward the abdominal cavity. This allows lumbar lordosis and enhances shock absorption. Ligaments stabilize the sacrum's position.

Mobility in the SI joint is related to age and gender. The range of motion is governed by hormones, among other things, in females. Pelvic movement enables the birth canal to dynamically adapt during delivery.

The increase in hip-joint mobility, especially in extension, is also the result of phylogenetic development. The femoral head is integrated into the body's plumb line. During walking, the trochanter point is transported forward during the mid-stance phase.

The pelvic muscles have been strengthened and their endurance improved. This allows the body to economically maintain upright positions and ensures that standing on one foot is safe. The pelvis absorbs impulses arising from the legs and increases the range of hip-joint motion by rapidly transferring movement up into the lumbar spine.

In total, the phylogenetic adaptations are a good example of morphological and functional adaptation in the entire musculoskeletal system. These adaptations are shaped significantly by three aspects:
- Bipedal locomotion.
- Grasping function of the hands.
- Spatial adjustment of the head.

9.2 Common Applications for Treatment in this Region

The pelvis is frequently the focus of treatment for symptoms in the LPH region (lumbar spine, pelvis, hip) due to the intensive strain that the pelvis experiences during different tasks. Therapists have a special task when assessing patients: to find out why the patient is suffering from pain in the buttocks or the groin.

The following structures possibly generate pain (tissues that cause pain):
- Lumbar or inferior thoracic structures.
- The SI joints and their ligaments.
- Structures in the hip joint.
- Nerves in the gluteal region.
- Muscular components.

The last can be a primary or secondary source of pain and appear tensed and tender to touch.

Also, various internal organs are represented in the Head zones located in the skin of the gluteal region.

Certain assessment techniques and forms of treatment are thus applied to the gluteal region. Apparently, over 50 provocation and mobility tests have been described for the SI joint at an international level (Vleeming et al., 2006). Each study group for manual therapy uses their own individual test. International standardization is not yet foreseeable. When these tests are being conducted or the patient is being mobilized, it frequently makes sense that certain osseous reference points (iliac crests, anterior

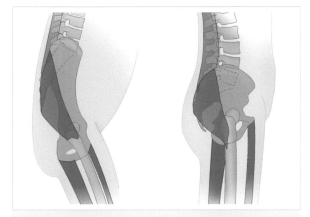
Fig. 9.1 The evolutionary development of the pelvis.

and posterior iliac spines) are palpated accurately and their position compared with the other side.

The sacrum and the ilium are often mobilized in opposite directions during assessment and treatment (▶ Fig. 9.2). It is very important that the hand position is well placed and secure.

Some peripheral nerves can be irritated locally as they pass through the gluteal region on their way to their target organ. In the case of the sciatic nerve, this can occur at two locations (▶ Fig. 9.3):

- Compression neuropathies caused by an extremely tense piriformis (piriformis syndrome).
- Friction at the ischial tuberosity and the hamstrings tendon of origin (hamstring syndrome; Puranen and Orava, 1988).

These problems can be confirmed using an accurate and detailed palpation with the application of pressure.

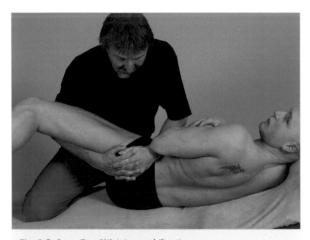

Fig. 9.2 Sacroiliac (SI) joint mobilization.

A piriformis compression syndrome occurs only when at least a portion of the sciatic nerve passes through the muscle belly of the piriformis. According to Vleeming (personally communication, 2003), the fibular part passes through the piriformis muscle belly in only 4 to 10% of all people (▶ Fig. 9.4). A sustained muscle contraction alone is not expected to compress the nerve as the muscle is smooth and fibrous on the side facing the nerve. Also, the 4-cm-long muscle belly cannot expand so much during contraction that it compromises or stretches the nerve.

The trigger-point treatment, based on the work of Travell and Simons (1998), is concerned with the location of locally hardened muscles that may act as independent pain generators. Dvořák et al. also dealt with the subject of tender points within manual diagnostics. These points provide the clinician with information regarding the spinal level of sacroiliac and lumbar aggravation (Dvořák et al., 2008).

Dvořák labeled tender points as tendinoses and zones of irritation. Local surface anatomy is used here to find the appropriate muscular structure or to link the point that is tender on palpation to its respective muscle.

Muscle pathologies are treated using classical massage techniques, such as kneading (▶ Fig. 9.5), local frictions (▶ Fig. 9.6), or a variety of specialized techniques. These techniques can be conducted more accurately when the therapist has a good knowledge of the available area and can correctly feel the muscular structure being sought.

Precise palpation is also used to confirm bursitis by applying local and direct pressure (▶ Fig. 9.7) (e.g., when presented with a type of snapping hip) or to perceive muscle activity in the pelvic floor directly medial to the ischial tuberosity (▶ Fig. 9.8).

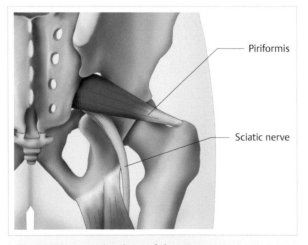

Fig. 9.3 Position and pathway of the sciatic nerve.

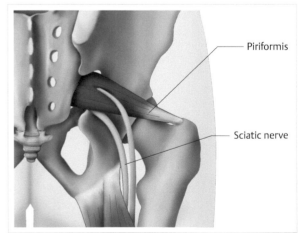

Fig. 9.4 Variations in the anatomy of the sciatic nerve.

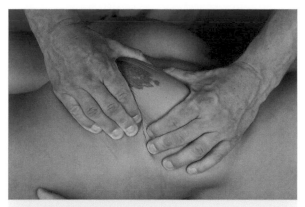

Fig. 9.5 Kneading the gluteal muscles.

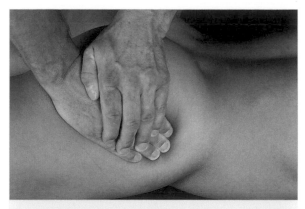

Fig. 9.6 Local frictions on the gluteal muscles.

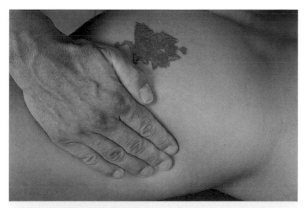

Fig. 9.7 Palpating for bursitis.

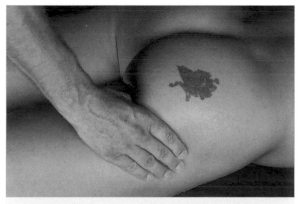

Fig. 9.8 Palpating for muscle activity in the pelvic floor.

9

9.3 Required Basic Anatomical and Biomechanical Knowledge

The pelvis is the anatomical and functional center of the "lumbopelvic region." Two movement complexes meet at the sacrum: the vertebral column and the pelvis. This means that vertebral movement is directly transmitted onto the pelvis, and vice versa.

Several points on the pelvis are of static and dynamic significance: the base of the sacrum, iliac crest, SI joint, pubic symphysis, and the ischial tuberosity. The different types of loading are dealt with here, for example, by transferring the load in sitting or standing. Important ligamental structures and muscles insert here.

Surprisingly, anatomical literature does not always agree on the bony compilation of the pelvis. Netter (2004) only includes the two pelvic bones. In total, the pelvis should be understood to be a bony ring consisting of three large parts: two pelvic bones (consisting of the ilium, ischium, and pubis) and the sacrum (▶ Fig. 9.9).

The different parts are joined together by mobile and immobile bony connections:

- Mobile: two SI joints and the pubic symphysis.
- Immobile: Y-formed synostosis in the acetabulum as well as a synostosis between the ischial ramus and the inferior

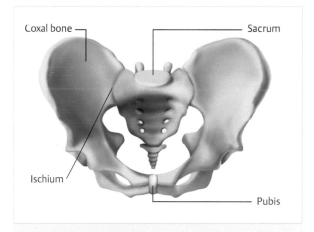

Fig. 9.9 Parts of the pelvis.

pubic ramus, the bony connection between the originally distinct sacral vertebrae at the transverse ridges.

The mobile connections allow a certain amount of flexibility in the pelvis, absorbing the dynamic impulses coming from a superior or inferior direction. Shock absorption is an important principle for the lower limbs and is continued in the pelvis. This flexibility also creates a gradual transition from the more rigid pelvic structures to the mobile lumbar segments.

9.3.1 Gender-based Differences

The gender-specific characteristics of the pelvis are presented in almost every anatomy book. In summary, these characteristics are based on the difference in form and are most distinctly seen in the ala of the ilium and the ischial tuberosities. In total, the male pelvis is described as being long and slender and the female pelvis as being wider and shorter. The dimensions of the female pelvis are therefore seen as a phylogenetic adaptation to the requirements of the birth canal during childbirth.

The differences in detail:
- The alae of the ilia are higher and more slender in the male pelvis.
- The inner pelvic ring, the level of the pelvic inlet, or the arcuate line tend to be rounder in the male pelvis and more transversely elliptical in the female pelvis.
- The two inferior pubic rami form an arch (pubic arch) in the female pelvis. It has been described as more of an angle (pubic angle) in the male pelvis.

Naturally, these different characteristics in the bony anatomy of the pelvis also have a meaning for local surface-anatomy. They determine what is to be expected topographically when searching for a specific structure (▶ Fig. 9.10):
- The iliac crests are readily used for quick orientation in the lumbar area. The most superior aspect of the iliac crest is found higher up in males than in females:
  - According to McGaugh et al. (2007), the line connecting the most superior aspect of the iliac crests (Jacoby's line)
    - is located at the level of the L4 spinous process in 59% of men. In 22% it is at the level of the L4/L5 interspinous space and in 14% at the level of the L5 spinous process.
    - in 46% of women, it is located at the level of the L4 spinous process, in 28% at the level of the L4/L5 interspinous space, and in 26% at the level of the L5 spinous process.
      However, identifying the L4 level requires very precise palpation of the bony edge. Chakraverty et al. (2007) and Pysyk et al. (2010) have cautioned that manual palpation tends to access a higher level (L3 or L3/L4)
  - As with the iliac crests, the anterior superior iliac spine (ASIS) is preferably located to determine levels within the pelvis. It can be assumed that the female ASISs are found significantly further apart than their male counterparts. Therefore, it is necessary to search for them more laterally.
- The inferior pubic rami meet at a significantly smaller angle in the male pelvis. It is therefore expected that

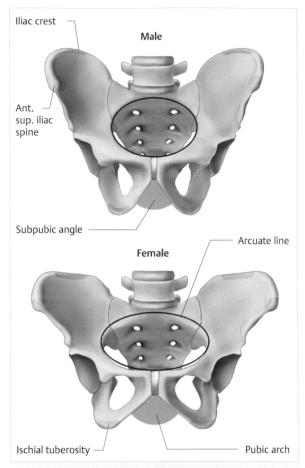

Fig. 9.10 Gender-based differences and bony reference points.

the ischial tuberosities can be palpated significantly more medially in the male pelvis than in the female pelvis.

9.3.2 Coxal Bone

The coxal bone is the largest fused bony entity in the musculoskeletal system once skeletal growth has been completed. Two surfaces extend superiorly and inferiorly from a central collection of bony mass in the acetabular area:
- Superior surface = ala of the ilium. This surface is entirely osseous. Its borders are strengthened by strong edges and projections (iliac crest and diverse spines). Although the middle of the ala of the ilium is osseous as well, it tends to be thinner and can be perforated in some cases.
- Inferior surface = the rami of the ischium and the pubis with a central collagen plate (obturator membrane).

When planes are drawn at a tangent over these superior and inferior surfaces, these planes are seen to be found at a 90° angle to each other (▶ Fig. 9.11).

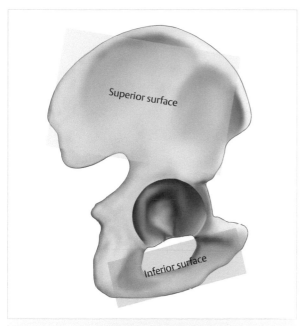

Fig. 9.11 Illustrating the planes on the coxal bone.

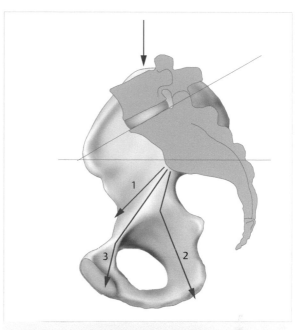

Fig. 9.12 Spongy thickening in the coxal bone.

The protruding edges, spines, and flattened areas of both surfaces of the coxal bone act as possible sites of origin or insertion for muscles and ligaments. Anatomical specimens show that the ilium is almost completely enclosed by the small gluteal muscles and the iliacus. The obturator membrane is likewise located between the obturator externus and the obturator internus. Thus, a series of active dynamic forces act on the coxal bone.

Other sections with significantly spongy thickening (▶ Fig. 9.12) can be identified in addition to the above-mentioned bony edges at the edge of both coxal bones and the central bony mass:

- The body's weight in standing is transferred from the SI joint to the acetabulum and vice versa along the arcuate line. The arcuate line divides the greater from the lesser pelvis (1).
- Weight is transferred in sitting between the SI joint and the ischial tuberosity (2).
- Pressure and tensile stresses are transmitted from the coxal bone onto the symphysis via the superior pubic ramus (3).

The weight of the body is transferred from the vertebral column onto the pelvis at the SI joint. This is approximately 60% of the entire body weight in an upright position.

9.3.3 Sacrum

The sacrum is the third and central part of the bony pelvis. It is well known that the sacrum is a fusion of at least five originally distinct vertebrae. The final ossification into a single bone occurs in the fifth decade of life. Remnants of cartilaginous disks are existent prior to this.

Location and Position

The location and position of the vertebral column's kyphotic section at the pelvis can be identified in the median cut of the pelvis. The recognizable tilt of the sacrum into the pelvic space can be calculated by using the angle between the transverse plane and a line extending from the end plate of S1 (Kapandji, 2006). This generally amounts to approximately 30° (▶ Fig. 9.13).

The sacrum's position has several consequences:

- It is the foundation for the lumbar lordosis and therefore the double "S" seen in the vertebral column.
- The tip of the sacrum points posteriorly and enlarges the inferior section of the birth canal.
- Vertical loading in the upright position is transformed less into translational movement and more into rotational movement (tendency to nutate). This is absorbed by the ligamentous apparatus.

The sacrum's distinctive form becomes evident in the posterior view (▶ Fig. 9.14). It is characterized by various structures:

- The S1 end plate (base of the sacrum).
- The sides of the sacrum:
  - S1 to S3 = auricular surface and the sacral tuberosities (neither are palpable).
  - S3 to S5 = edge of the sacrum (palpable).
- The connection between the inferolateral angles.

9

It is now apparent that the sacrum is not triangular in shape but rather trapezoid.

Detailed Anatomy

The posterior aspect demonstrates additional interesting details (▶ Fig. 9.15):

- S1 has not only received the vertebral body end plate, but also the superior articular processes. These form the most inferior vertebral joints with L5.
- Generally, it is possible to look through the bony model in four places on each side. The sacral foramina are found posteriorly and anteriorly at the same level and allow the anterior rami and the posterior rami of the spinal nerves to exit from the vertebral column and into the periphery.
- Long ridges are found over the entire remaining posterior surface. These ridges are formed by the rudiments

of the sacral vertebrae that have grown together. The median sacral crest is the most important of these ridges for palpation. The rudiments of the sacral spinous processes can be seen here as irregular protrusions and can be palpated well. All other crests and the posterior foraminae are hidden under thick fascia and the multifidus muscle.

Apex of the Sacrum and the Coccyx

The apex of the sacrum forms the sacrum's inferior border. It lies in the middle, slightly inferior to the line connecting the two inferolateral angles. The mobile connection to the coccyx is found here. This is interchangeably labeled a synovial joint or a synchondrosis (with the intervertebral disk) in literature (▶ Fig. 9.16; Rauber and Kopsch, 2003).

Great variations are seen in the construction of the inferior sacral area. The median sacral crest usually runs down to the level of S4. Normally no rudiments of the spinous processes can be observed at the S5 level. Instead, an osseous cleft can be seen: the sacral hiatus. According to von Lanz and Wachsmuth (2004a), this posterior cleft is only found in approximately 46% of the population at the level of S5 and extends to the level of S4 or S3 in

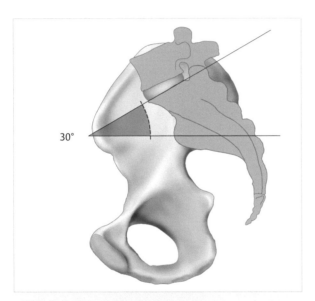

Fig. 9.13 Position of the sacrum.

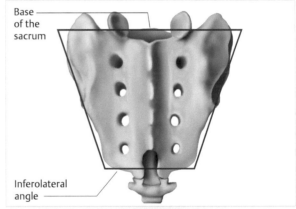

Fig. 9.14 General shape of the sacrum.

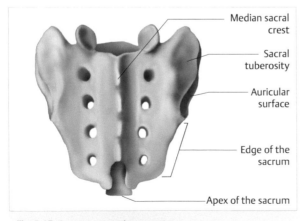

Fig. 9.15 Sacrum, posterior aspect.

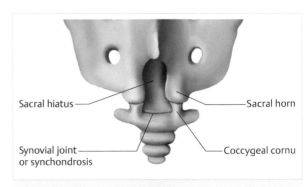

Fig. 9.16 Sacrococcygeal transition.

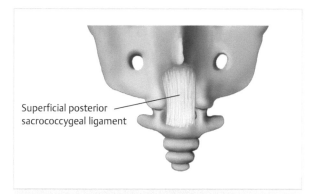

Fig. 9.17 Hiatus and membrane.

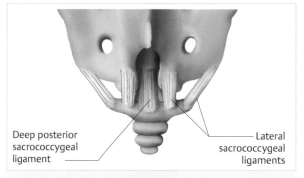

Fig. 9.18 Ligamentous connections between the sacrum and coccyx.

33.5%. This makes accurate palpatory orientation on the inferior sacrum significantly more difficult.

The S5 arch leading to the hiatus is incomplete and is covered by a membrane (▶ Fig. 9.17). Small osseous horns (sacral horns) form its borders on the side. These horns are easily palpable in most cases but vary greatly in size and are irregularly shaped. They face two small osseous protrusions in the coccygeal bone, the coccygeal cornua, which are also palpable.

The covering membrane at the level of S5 is a continuation of the supraspinous ligament and continues onto the coccyx as the superficial posterior sacrococcygeal ligament. The membrane covers the vertebral canal as it peters out inferiorly. It is palpated as a firm and elastic structure, which clearly distinguishes it from the osseous borders.

Additional ligamentous connections between the sacrum and coccyx are (▶ Fig. 9.18):
- The deep posterior sacrococcygeal ligament, the continuation of the posterior longitudinal ligament.
- The lateral sacrococcygeal ligament (intercornual and lateral sections), presumably continuations of the former ligamenta flava and the intertransverse ligament.

These ligamentous structures are traumatically overstretched when people fall onto their buttocks and especially onto the coccyx. Their tenderness on pressure can be treated successfully using transverse frictions to relieve pain when they are directly palpated.

9.3.4 The Pelvic Ligaments

The ligaments of the pelvis can be classified according to their position and function. We are therefore familiar with ligaments that:
- act to maintain contact between the surfaces of the SI joint:
  ○ interosseous sacroiliac ligaments, located directly posterior to the SI joints;
- restrict nutation and therefore stabilize the sacrum:
  ○ anterior sacroiliac ligaments (reinforce the capsule);
  ○ posterior sacroiliac ligaments;

  ○ sacrotuberous ligament;
  ○ sacrospinous ligament;
- can limit counternutation:
  ○ long posterior sacroiliac ligament.

The **anterior sections of the capsule** (anterior sacroiliac ligaments) are very thin (< 1 mm) and have little mechanical relevance (personal correspondence from the IAOM study group). They perforate easily when joint pressure is increased (arthritis). They are not stretched during the iliac posterior test (SI joint test) as the entire function of the ligament is found posterior to the joint.

The interosseus **ligaments** are very short, nociceptively supplied ligaments that act as pain generators in the presence of sacroiliac pathologies (e.g., instability or blockages). Their function is to maintain the traction in the respective SI joint.

It is easiest to understand the function of the **nutation restrictors** by looking at the stress on the sacrospinous and sacrotuberous ligaments when the body is in a vertical position (▶ Fig. 9.19). Approximately 60% of the body's weight bears down on the S1 end plate. This is positioned quite anterior to the nutation/counternutation axis so that the base of the sacrum tends to fall farther into the pelvic space. This tendency is counteracted by the posterior and anterior ligaments positioned very close to the joint. The tip of the sacrum tends to lever itself anteriorly and superiorly. This movement is counteracted by the sacrospinous and sacrotuberous ligaments.

The **long** posterior **sacroiliac ligament** (▶ Fig. 9.20) connects both posterior superior iliac spines (PSISs) with the respective edge of the sacrum. It is approximately 3 to 4 cm long, 1 to 2 cm wide, and extends inferiorly into the sacrotuberous ligament. It is the only ligament that counteracts counternutation. It has been described by Vleeming et al. (1996) and already published several times. It has also been mentioned by Dvořák et al. (2008).

The fibers of the multifidus muscle are noticeable as they extend medially into the ligament. A section of the ligament arises from the gluteus maximus on the lateral side.

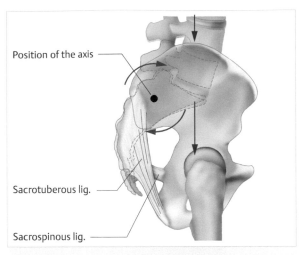

Position of the axis

Sacrotuberous lig.

Sacrospinous lig.

Fig. 9.19 Function of the nutation restrictors.

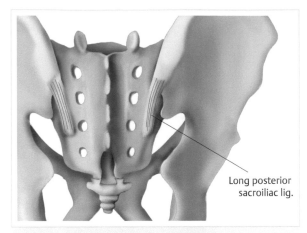

Long posterior sacroiliac lig.

Fig. 9.20 Long posterior sacroiliac ligament.

9.3.5 The Sacroiliac Joint

The significance of the pelvis as central element in the musculoskeletal system has already been described. To understand the exceptional significance of the SI joint, the functional relationship between the various kinematic chains should first be clarified.

First Kinematic Chain: The Sacrum as Part of the Vertebral Column

The L5, sacrum, and ilium form a kinematic chain. No bone moves without the others moving. It is nearly impossible to clearly attribute the effects of pathology and treatment to a specific level. The iliolumbar ligaments (especially the inferior short, stiff sections) are important for the linkages within this chain.

Second Kinematic Chain: The Sacrum as Part of the Lower Limbs

The largest SI joint movements occur when the hip joints are included in the movement symmetrically and without loading, such as is the case during hip flexion in supine position.

Third Kinematic Chain: The Sacrum as Part of the Pelvic Ring

The SI joint biomechanics are controlled by the symphysis. Extensive, opposing movements of the iliac bones primarily meet up at the symphysis. SI joint instability can also affect the symphysis. We therefore differentiate the SI joint instability types into those without loosening of the symphysis and those with loosening of the symphysis.

Few topics concerning the musculoskeletal system are discussed as controversially as the SI joint. Views and opinions about the SI joint vary between the individual manual therapy study groups as well as between manual therapists and osteopaths. The significance given to the SI joint therefore depends on each therapist's personal criteria and individual point of view.

Reasons for the Differences in Opinion about the SI Joint

Special Anatomical Factors

The construction of this joint cannot be compared with any "traditional" joint (▸ Fig. 9.21):
- It is a firm joint (amphiarthrosis) anteriorly and connects the bones posteriorly via a ligamentous structure (syndesmosis).
- The joint surfaces are curved at all levels and have ridges and grooves.
- The sacral joint surface is very thick, the iliac surface extremely rough.

SI Behavior during Movement

- The sacrum and the ilium always move against each other in a three-dimensional manner.
- Describing the position of the axes during these movements is extremely complicated.
- Movement primarily occurs around a frontotransversal (transversal) axis and is very slight (according to Goode et al. [2008], approximately a maximum of 2°). These movements are labeled nutation and counternutation (▸ Fig. 9.22). The extent of joint mobility is influenced by hormones, particularly in women (Brooke, 1924 and Sashin, 1930). Mobility also increases when SI joint disorders are present, for example, with arthritis.

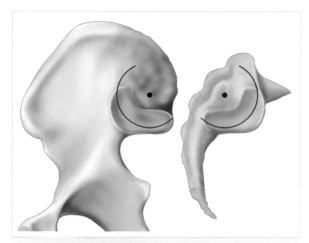

Fig. 9.21 Sacroiliac (SI) joint surfaces (according to Kapandji).

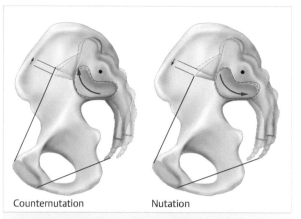

Counternutation   Nutation

Fig. 9.22 Sacroiliac (SI) joint movements (according to Kapandji).

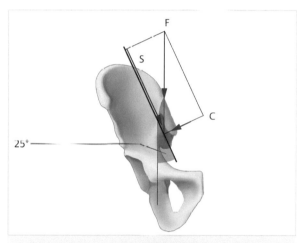

Fig. 9.23 Alignment of the SI joint surfaces (from Winkel, 1992). F = force, S = shear force, C = compression.

- The male SI joint starts to become immobile from around age 50 due to the formation of osseous bridges (Brooke, 1924; Stewart, 1984).

The complexity of this joint also makes it easy to understand why comparatively few good studies exist that examine standardized assessment methods and treatment techniques. More than 50 tests have been described for assessment alone.

Memorize

For these reasons, the SI joint remains obscure and difficult to comprehend—a mystical structure, a platform for experience and speculation.

9.3.6 Sacroiliac Joint Biomechanics

With an average surface area of 17.5 cm², the SI joint is the largest joint in the human body (Rana et al., 2015).

The SI joint is held together by its structure and the strength of tissues. This can be seen in the frontal plane by looking at the general alignment of the joint surfaces. According to Winkel (1992) the joint surfaces are tilted at approximately 25° from the vertical (▶ Fig. 9.23).

The sacrum's wedge shape permits the auricular surface to support itself on the similarly shaped iliac joint surface (force closure). Nevertheless, the joint's construction and the friction coefficient of the uneven and roughened surface are not sufficient to stabilize the sacrum's position.

It therefore becomes clear that additional strength is needed to keep the joint surfaces together (holding the joint together with the strength of tissues). In particular, this is the function of the interosseous sacroiliac ligaments. These ligaments lie immediately posterior to the joint surfaces and are made of short, very strong, and nociceptively innervated collagen fibers. The SI joint is held together more by the joint structure in males and the strength of tissues in females.

The interosseous ligaments are supported by muscular structures and other ligamentous structures that generally act as nutation restrictors. These structures therefore qualify as further SI joint stabilizers:
- The anterior abdominal muscles (especially the oblique and transverse sections) pull on the ilia anteriorly and place the interosseous ligaments under tension (▶ Fig. 9.24).
- The complex thoracolumbar fascia is considered an important stabilizer of the lumbosacral region (Vleeming and Dorman, 1995).
- The multifidus acts as a hydrodynamic strengthener. Its swelling during contraction tightens the thoracolumbar fascia.

9

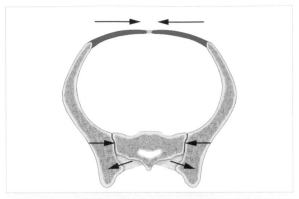

Fig. 9.24 Ventral tenseness of the ilia.

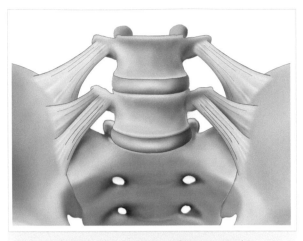

Fig. 9.25 Iliolumbar ligaments (according to Kapandji).

- The gluteus maximus originates on the posterior surface of the sacrum. The superficial fibers cross over the SI joint and likewise radiate into the thoracolumbar fascia.
- The piriformis originates on the anterior surface of the sacrum. It crosses over the SI joint.
- The pelvic floor muscles, for example, coccygeus and levator ani exert their force onto the posterior pelvis.
- The posterior and anterior sacroiliac ligaments, together with the sacrospinous and sacrotuberous ligaments, primarily restrict the nutation of the sacrum. Loading tightens these ligaments and likewise increases the compression of the SI joint.
- Several sections of the iliolumbar ligaments cross over the SI joint in the middle. Lumbar lordosis increases the SI joint surface compression (▶ Fig. 9.25).

Pool-Goudzwaard et al. (2001) described in a study the stabilizing role of the iliolumbar ligaments on the SI joint. Gradual transection of the ligaments resulted in a significant increase in SI joint mobility in the sagittal plane.

The ligaments also contribute to sacroiliac movements being transmitted onto the lower lumbar segments and vice versa. Movement within the pelvic ring and movement in L4-S1 must always be regarded as a kinematic chain.

Memorize

The dominating concept until several years ago was that the SI joint, as a classic amphiarthrosis, was not supplied with its own muscles. This presumption is correct as regards the mobility function. However, it can be put on record that force closure, in the form of a multitude of dynamized ligaments and muscles, holds the joint surfaces together and stabilizes the SI joint.

9.3.7 Ligament Dynamization in the Sacroiliac Joint

The interplay between muscles and ligaments near joints has been known for a long time now. The knee joint is a perfect example of this. The extension of muscles into capsular-ligamentous structures is called ligament dynamization. Two examples of pelvic ligaments are presented here to demonstrate how intensive the contact is between muscles and the functional collagen in this region.

Sacrotuberous Ligament

The sacrotuberous ligament is connected to the following:
- Gluteus maximus from a posterior direction.
- Biceps femoris from an inferior direction.
- Piriformis from an anterior direction.
- Coccygeus from a medial direction.

Vleeming and Dorman (1995) explain the functional significance of the sacrotuberous ligament, dynamized by the biceps femoris, on the SI joint as follows:

We know that the hamstring muscles are most active at the end of the swing phase during gait. The hamstrings slow down the anterior tibial swing a few milliseconds before heel contact, decelerating knee extension.

The long head of the tensed biceps femoris often merges with the sacrotuberous ligament via large bundles of collagen (also without contact with the ischial tuberosity) and dynamizes the ligament (▶ Fig. 9.26). The biceps femoris activity prevents the sacrum from fully nutating and stabilizes the SI joint directly before the landing phase.

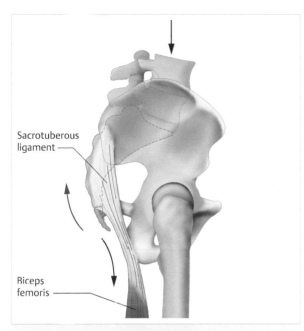

Fig. 9.26 Dynamization of the sacrotuberous ligament.

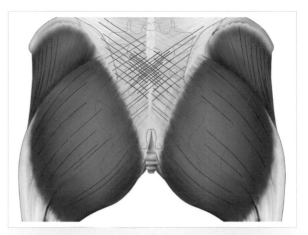

Fig. 9.27 Alignment of the collagenous fibers in the thoraco-lumbar fascia.

Thoracolumbar Fascia

The thoracolumbar fascia consists of three layers:
- Superficial layer—posterior layer.
- Middle layer—inserted on the lumbar transverse processes.
- Deep layer—anterior layer found anterior to quadratus lumborum and iliopsoas.

The posterior, superficial layer contains collagen fibers arising from several muscles that can tighten up this aponeurosis:
- Latissimus dorsi.
- Erector spinae.
- Gluteus maximus.

Each of the muscles is able to dynamize the fascia. The fascia forms a diagonal sling between the latissimus dorsi and the contralateral gluteus maximus (▶ Fig. 9.27). The force of the sling acts perpendicular to the joint surfaces, stabilizing the SI joint and the inferior lumbar spine during strong rotation. Consequently, the participating muscles and the fascia belong to the primary SI joint stabilizers. This sling can be especially trained using trunk rotation against resistance.

This fascial layer is also connected to the supraspinous ligament and the interspinous ligament up to the ligamenta flava. Vleeming (personal communication) comments on this: "The entire system is dynamically stabilized."

Muscles also dynamize the middle and deep layers. It is well known that the transversus abdominis tightens the middle layer (see also the section "Detailed Anatomy of the Ligaments," in Chapter 10).

The required background information on the pelvic muscles is given in the section "Palpatory Procedures for Quick Orientation on the Muscles" below.

9.4 Summary of the Palpatory Process

Two different approaches to the palpation of the posterior pelvic region will be explained below:
- Quick orientation.
- Local palpation.

The introductory quick orientation is used to obtain an initial rough impression of the location and shape of prominent bony landmarks that delineate the working area for diagnostic and treatment techniques in the region. Large muscles are defined and differentiated from one another in their position and course.

Local palpation aims to find important bony reference points (landmarks), to differentiate precisely between form and tissue, and to identify the path of peripheral nerves. To achieve this, palpatory techniques will be described and orienting lines will be drawn on the skin to point out structures that are difficult to reach or difficult to differentiate from other structures.

9.5 Palpatory Techniques for Quick Orientation on the Bones

First, the large structures in this region are searched to enable quick and effective orientation in the region of the bony pelvis (▶ Fig. 9.28):
- Iliac crest.
- Greater trochanter.
- Sacrum.
- Ischial tuberosity.

9

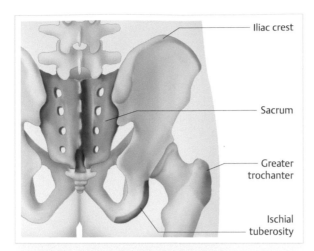

Fig. 9.28 Bony reference points.

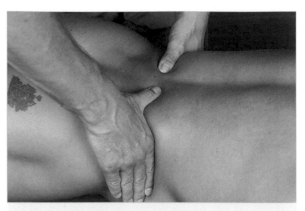

Fig. 9.29 Quick orientation: iliac crests.

Therapists should be aware of the location and dimensions of these structures for a variety of reasons. The bony landmarks constitute the border of the area of treatment for the gluteal muscles. When orientation is exact, the actual treatment area for this muscle, for example, using classical Swedish massage or functional massage techniques, becomes considerably smaller than perhaps originally expected. Those therapists that orient themselves less can apply massage techniques occasionally to the sacrum. Quick orientation restricts the area to be treated to the gluteal muscles and their insertions.

> **Memorize**
>
> These large osseous structures provide important clues for the precise local palpation that comes up later.

9.5.1 Starting Position

The patient lies on a treatment table in a neutral prone position. The sections of the body are positioned without lateral shift or rotation. The arms lie next to the body. The patient should avoid elevating the arms up to head level as this tightens the thoracolumbar fascia and makes the palpation of a variety of structures more difficult in the area of the lumbosacral junction. The head is positioned, when possible, in neutral rotation and the nose is placed in the face hole of the treatment table. The therapist stands on the side of the treatment table and opposite the side to be palpated. Please refer to the section "Starting Position," Chapter 8, for further details.

Iliac Crests

Locating the iliac crests is the quickest and most preferred approach for orientation in the LPH region. It is possible to roughly orient yourself in the lumbar region from here, find the lowermost rib, and locate the superior border of the pelvis.

Technique

The quick orientation can be conducted simultaneously on both sides of the patient's body. Both hands form a firm surface; the thumbs are abducted. The lateral sides of the hands are placed on the patient's waist and move in a medial direction while moderate pressure is being applied. This technique is continued until the tissue resistance significantly increases and eventually stops further movement (▶ Fig. 9.29).

Starting from this position, the hand is pushed in a variety of directions:

- Pressure in a medial direction → resistance is soft and elastic: pressure is being applied to the edges of the latissimus dorsi, quadratus lumborum, and erector spinae. This is approximately at the level of the L3/L4 spinous processes.
- Pressure in a superior direction → resistance becomes significantly firmer. The 12th or 11th rib is reached when coming from an inferior position.
- Pressure in an inferior direction → resistance becomes significantly firmer: pressure is applied onto the iliac crest when coming from a superior position = superior border of the pelvis.

When palpating the distance between the lowest rib and the iliac crest, we see that this distance is approximately two fingers wide and hence clearly smaller than on common skeletal models. This small distance clearly demonstrates the necessity of flexibility in the 11th and 12th ribs. The lowest ribs move closer to the iliac crests during extensive lateral flexion and must, at times, move out of the way in an elastic manner.

Tip

Start the palpation anteriorly if the soft tissue at the waist does not permit palpatory differentiation between the iliac crest and the lowest rib. Location of the anterior superior iliac spine is also possible and accurate in the prone position. The upper edge of the iliac crest can be followed from here until the posterior trunk is reached.

Greater Trochanter

The greater trochanter is the only part of the proximal femur that is directly accessible and is therefore an important point for orientation in the lateral hip region. It is the attachment site for many small muscles that come from the pelvis and elongates the lever arm for forces arising from the small gluteal muscles. The greater trochanter additionally provides therapists with the possibility of drawing conclusions about the geometry of the femur.

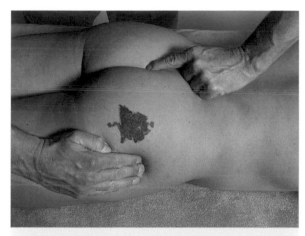

Fig. 9.30 Locating the greater trochanter.

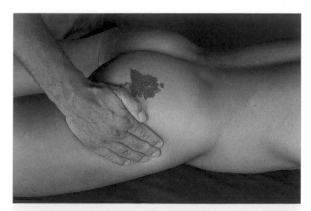

Fig. 9.31 Palpating the greater trochanter.

Technique

It is very helpful if the therapist can clearly visualize the topography of this region. Two additional aids can be used for orientation if it is difficult to picture the position of the greater trochanter accurately:

• The greater trochanter can be found at approximately the level of the tip of the sacrum. This is roughly found at the level of the start of the post-anal furrow at S5 (▶ Fig. 9.30).
• The trochanter is found approximately one hand-width inferior to the iliac crest.

The therapist places the flat hand on the lateral pelvis and expects to feel a large, rounded structure—bony and hard to the touch—when directly palpating it (▶ Fig. 9.31).

Tip

It is sometimes difficult to find the trochanter as this region may be obese in some patients. In these cases another aid is needed to confirm the location of the trochanter. The therapist can flex the knee on the ipsilateral side and use the lower leg as a lever, internally and externally rotating the hip joint. This results in the trochanter rolling back and forth underneath the palpating fingers and enables the lateral surface and the superior aspect to also be palpated well (▶ Fig. 9.32).

The superior tip of the greater trochanter is the point of insertion for the often tensed piriformis, among others (see also Chapter 9.8.3). The lateral surface is a good lead when manually determining the femoral neck anteversion (FNA) angle (see also Chapter 5).

Sacrum

The inferior tip of the sacrum is located at the start of the post-anal furrow and extends superiorly for approximately

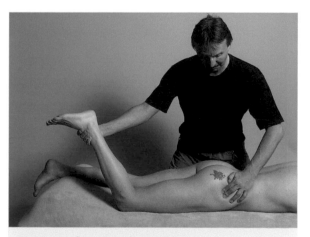

Fig. 9.32 Confirmation with movement.

225

one hand-width. As mentioned above, the sacrum is significantly wider than is commonly perceived or seen on skeletal models.

Technique

Several fingertips of one or both hands are placed perpendicular to the longitudinal axis on the area where the sacrum is suspected to be. This is several finger-widths superior to the post-anal furrow.

Transverse palpation is used. The sacrum feels like a flat, irregularly shaped structure. It always feels hard when direct pressure is applied to it during the assessment of consistency. A more precise differentiation of the structures on the sacrum will be described in the sections below. The transverse palpation proceeds in a lateral direction until the finger pads slide anteriorly (► Fig. 9.33).

The consistency assessment demonstrates a soft, elastic form of resistance. This is the edge of the sacrum, which is now followed along its entire length superiorly and inferiorly. The inferolateral angle of the sacrum is reached when palpating in an inferior direction.

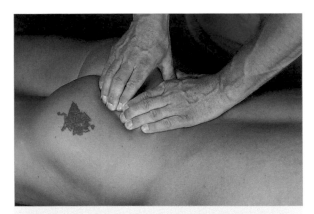

Fig. 9.33 Palpating the edge of the sacrum.

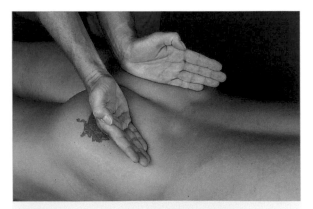

Fig. 9.34 Demonstrating the size of the sacrum.

Tip

Once the position of the two edges has been found, the medial edges of the hands can be used to show the entire length of the sacral edges. The entire width of this central structure in the bony pelvis is now recognizable (► Fig. 9.34). As will be explained later during precise palpation, the palpated edge does not correspond to the entire length of the sacrum (superior-inferior dimensions). The edge is only palpable from the inferior angle to the level of S3. The SI joint and the iliac crest are connected at the superior end.

Ischial Tuberosity

The ischial tuberosity is another large structure and a major important point for orientation. It is an important attachment site for thick ligaments (sacrotuberous ligament) and muscles (hamstrings).

Technique

The therapist uses a pinch grip (thumb medial), palpating along the gluteal fold in a medial direction until the thumb comes across the hard resistance of the tuberosity (► Fig. 9.35). The tuberosity is a surprisingly wide structure. Only the tip of the tuberosity is relevant for now.

9.6 Palpatory Procedures for Quick Orientation on the Muscles

The quick osseous orientation has determined the position of the muscular soft tissue in the gluteal region (► Fig. 9.36). The muscles extend between:

- Sacrum—medial.
- Iliac crest—superior.
- Ischial tuberosity—inferior.
- Greater trochanter—inferolateral.

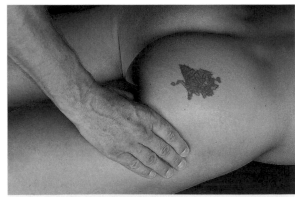

Fig. 9.35 Locating the ischial tuberosity.

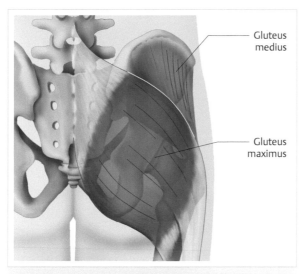

Fig. 9.36 Position of the gluteal muscles between the osseous boundaries.

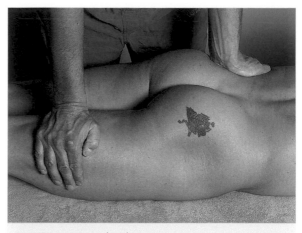

Fig. 9.37 Activity in the gluteus maximus.

In most cases it is impossible to recognize the borders or the protruding points of the buttock muscles or their insertions. Muscular activity is required to define the position and the borders of these muscles.

9.6.1 Starting Position

The neutral prone position described above is generally sufficient to gain access to the laterally lying muscles. Side-lying is another possible SP.

Gluteus Maximus

The most prominent muscular structure in the posterior pelvis is the large muscle of the buttocks. In most cases, the shape of the muscle belly can be clearly observed when the muscle is active. The medial and lateral borders of the muscle belly are well defined as this muscle largely contributes to the development of the post-anal furrow and the gluteal fold. The superior and inferior borders are significantly more difficult to define.

Technique—Middle of the Muscle Belly

The patient is asked to raise the leg off the treatment table to demonstrate the shape of the muscle. The second hand can be used to resist active hip extension if the muscle is not active enough to be located (▶ Fig. 9.37). If this is also not sufficient to define the muscle, the flattened hand is placed in the center of the buttock and the muscle is reactivated with hip extension.

Tip

If active extension, with or without resistance, is not sufficient in defining the shape of the muscle belly, the other functions of the gluteus maximus can be used. Repeated muscular contractions are used to emphasize the prominences and contours more clearly.

The gluteus maximus is a strong external rotator of the hip joint. Its action in the sagitto-transversal (sagittal) plane is the subject of controversy in the literature. As the superior parts of the muscle are found superior to the adduction-abduction axis, it remains questionable whether the muscle only adducts or whether it can also abduct the hip. Hip adduction is recommended to gain better differentiation to the small gluteal muscles.

The muscle activity is increased using the following method:
- The patient turns the tip of the foot outward and the heel inward before or during leg elevation.
- While maintaining the muscle activity in extension and external rotation, the therapist applies additional pressure from the inner side of the thigh and stimulates adduction (▶ Fig. 9.38).

The contours of the muscles protrude maximally using this method. The borders of the muscle can be specifically reached from the middle of the muscle belly.

Technique—Area of Origin

The origin (proximal area of attachment) is located using palpation moving in a superomedial direction. The muscle belly leads the palpation mainly onto the sacrum. The muscle's area of origin is often defined as the edge of the sacrum in the literature. However, it becomes noticeable that the therapist almost reaches the middle of the

9

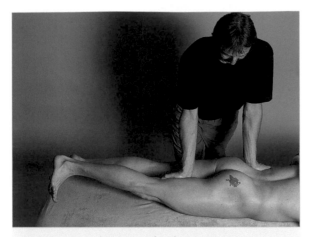

Fig. 9.38 Increased activity in the gluteus maximus.

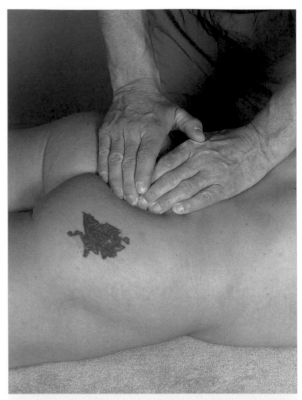

Fig. 9.39 Palpating the gluteus maximus—area of origin when relaxed.

sacrum and not the edge of the bone, as could be expected. This can be explained by looking at the anatomy of the superficial part of the muscle, which does not have a bony insertion. Rather, these parts of the muscle radiate into the thoracolumbar fascia.

Tip

The muscle's dimensions on the surface of the sacrum can be palpated more exactly by alternately relaxing (▶ Fig. 9.39) and tensing (▶ Fig. 9.40) the muscle.

Technique—Area of Insertion

The insertion of the gluteus maximus (distal area of attachment) is located by starting the palpation in the middle of the muscle belly and moving in an inferolateral direction. It is always found inferior to the greater trochanter.

It is also impossible to isolate the point of attachment here—the gluteal tuberosity—using palpation. If the muscle is followed along its length, using slow rhythmical activity if necessary, the palpation ends relatively laterally on the thigh (▶ Fig. 9.41). Again, the superficial sections of the muscles do not demonstrate bony attachments here. Rather, they radiate into the soft tissue. In this case, the soft tissue is the iliotibial tract. Dvořák et al. (2008) refer to these sections as the tibial portion. It is therefore not possible to clearly define the muscle in its inferolateral section.

Technique—Medial Edge

The medial boundary is easy to see and simple to palpate compared with the previously described techniques. Here the muscle forms the post-anal furrow. It covers the ischial tuberosity when the hip is extended.

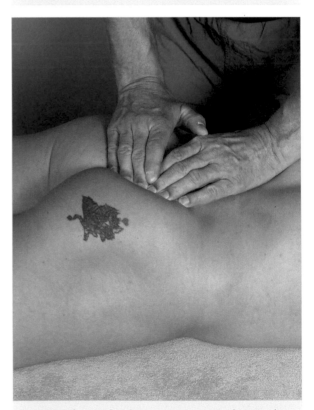

Fig. 9.40 Palpating the gluteus maximus—area of origin when active.

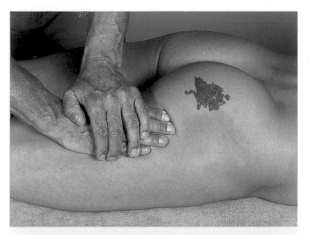

Fig. 9.41 Palpating the gluteus maximus—area of insertion when active.

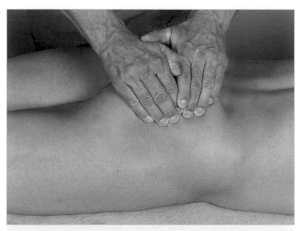

Fig. 9.42 Palpating the gluteus maximus—lateral edge.

Technique—Lateral Edge

It is admittedly very difficult to differentiate between the superolateral sections of the gluteus maximus and the small gluteal muscles. When relaxed, the gluteal region tends to present itself as a uniform, protruding form. Even when the gluteus maximus is tensed, the edge of the muscle is not clearly recognizable. It partially covers the posterior section of the gluteus medius.

It is not possible to differentiate the muscles through contraction with extension or external rotation only, as the posterior sections of the small gluteal muscles perform these actions as well. This leaves the therapist with the only option of working with adduction (the gluteus maximus) or abduction (gluteus medius and minimus).

The muscle is activated using extension and external rotation, and the muscle belly of the gluteus maximus is followed in a superolateral direction until the assumed region of the muscle border is reached (▶ Fig. 9.42). Adduction of the muscle is now additionally stimulated, causing the muscle belly of the gluteus maximus to protrude. Subsequently, abduction is conducted to emphasize the small gluteal muscles.

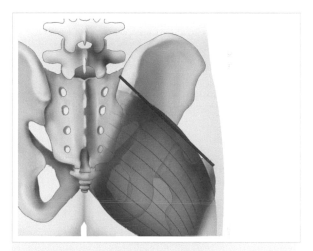

Fig. 9.43 Graphical illustration of the superolateral edge of the gluteus maximus.

muscle activity has already been described. The gluteus minimus is completely covered by the gluteus medius. It is therefore not possible to differentiate between these two muscles using palpation.

Technique

The palpating hand (when necessary with the second hand applying pressure to it) is placed on the side of the pelvis between the iliac crest and the tip of the trochanter. Pressure is applied deep into the tissue. The finger pads feel the expected soft consistency of the tissue (▶ Fig. 9.44). The position of the gluteus medius only becomes evident when it is activated with abduction. The patient does not have to expend a lot of effort for this. Normally only slight activity is sufficient.

This technique enables the therapist to easily palpate the entire length of the muscle between its origin (iliac crest) and its insertion (greater trochanter). Only the palpatory border anterolateral to the tensor fasciae latae

Tip
The recommendations of Winkel (2004) are to be followed should the attempt to locate the superolateral edge of the muscle fail. Based on his experience, this edge is located along the line connecting the PSIS with the tip of the trochanter (▶ Fig. 9.43).

Gluteus Medius

The muscle belly attaches itself directly onto the superolateral edge of the gluteus maximus muscle belly. An attempt to differentiate between these muscles using

9

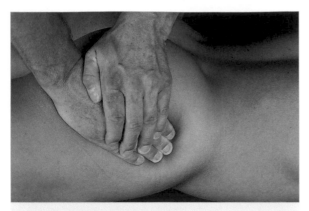

Fig. 9.44 Palpating the gluteus medius.

and medial to the gluteus maximus is more difficult in this SP.

> **Tip**
>
> When trying to differentiate between the gluteus maximus and the gluteus medius, the therapist can also attempt to reciprocally inhibit the gluteus maximus. The patient pushes the knee down into the treatment table (hip flexion) or lets the heel fall out to the side (internal rotation). The gluteus medius can be selectively observed by subsequently instructing the patient to abduct the hip.

Iliotibial Tract

This long and collagen-intensive reinforcement of the fascia in the thigh runs an interesting course (▶ Fig. 9.45):
- The proximal point of attachment is at the most superior part of the iliac crest.
- It passes lateral over the pelvis and the small gluteal muscles;
- over the greater trochanter, along the side of the thigh;
- lateral over the knee joint space, mainly inserting into the Gerdy tubercle (or the lateral condyle of the tibia).

The tract is placed under tension when:
- Muscle activity radiates from the superficial layer of the gluteus maximus;
- Muscle activity radiates from the tensor fasciae latae;
- The muscle belly of the gluteus medius protrudes during activity;
- The muscle belly of the vastus lateralis protrudes during activity (the most effective form of tension, according to personal correspondence from Vleeming).

Technique

During the palpation of the muscle belly of the gluteus medius (▶ Fig. 9.44) from medial to lateral using transverse

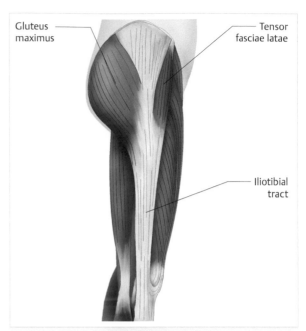

Fig. 9.45 Position of the iliotibial tract.

frictions, the palpating hand encounters an area of firm consistency. The difference is especially apparent in athletes. When the entire area of firm consistency is palpated, the therapist palpates a structure that is two to three fingers wide between the trochanter and the iliac crest.

> **Tip**
>
> It is impossible to successfully differentiate using muscle activity because it is the difference between soft and firm consistencies that makes the position of the tract distinct. Muscle activity removes the soft consistency during palpation.

9.7 Local Palpation Techniques

9.7.1 Summary of the Palpatory Procedure

The iliac crest is a common point used for orientation when the pelvis is being palpated. Starting from here, therapists orient themselves when ascertaining the level of structures in the lumbar area, start searching for the PSIS, and compare sides to ascertain whether the left- and right-hand sides are found at differing heights and whether a pelvic obliquity is present. Additional precise palpation of the sacrum also starts at the PSISs. The diagnostic benefits of palpating the PSISs to assess mobility or determine sacroiliac asymmetry or dysfunction are limited. Various authors have questioned the diagnostic reliability of these tests (Laslett, 2008). Considering the range of motion of the SI joint of 2 to 4° around the X-axis, the PSISs constitute only a few millimeters of movement in this range of motion. Due to the high tension placed on the soft tissues, palpating the PSISs with the patient standing is very challenging. Reliable interpretation of the PSIS movements, for example, in lumbar flexion (standing flexion test), is thus even more difficult. In contrast, the validity and reliability of the pain provocation test tend to be more satisfactory (Laslett, 2008).

Locating the two PSISs is the first step to reliably differentiate between the sacral and lumbar spinous processes.

All other accessible sections of the sacrum will be palpated during later sections of the palpatory procedure. Muscular activity in the multifidus and the location of important pelvic ligaments follow. Finally, several lines will be drawn on the pelvis to clarify the position of other muscular and neural structures.

Starting Position

The patient lies in a neutral prone position on the treatment table, with a face hole. The sections of the body are positioned without lateral shift or rotation. The arms are lying next to the body. Elevation of the arms to the level of the head should be avoided as it tenses the thoracolumbar fascia and impedes palpation of different structures in the area of the lumbosacral junction. If possible, the head is not positioned in rotation. The therapist stands to the side of the treatment table opposite the side to be palpated. Please see the section "Starting Position," in Chapter 8 for further details.

9.7.2 Ilium—Iliac Crest

The iliac crest has already been located during the quick orientation. It is now necessary to accurately palpate its superior border.

Technique

The palpation changes to a perpendicular palpation once the iliac crest has been found. The hand is positioned here superior to the iliac crest and the finger pads push down against the iliac crest at a right angle (▶ Fig. 9.46).

9.7.3 Ilium—Posterior Superior Iliac Spine (PSIS)

The significance of the PSIS has already been emphasized in the summary of the palpatory procedure. The PSIS's exact layout can be determined using two different techniques. One common misconception should be discussed first. Therapists often connect the PSIS to the location of the "dimples," the indentations in the skin over the posterior pelvis. This is definitely not correct. The PSISs are not found at the level of these dimples; they are found on average approximately 2 cm inferior and lateral to these indentations. The much-cited "dimples" are found where the gluteal and lumbar fasciae connect with deeper layers.

Technique—Variation 1

The perpendicular technique is used again when locating the iliac crest (as described above). The iliac crest is palpated centimeter by centimeter in a medial direction (▶ Fig. 9.47). The palpation increasingly turns in an inferior direction to reach and, when necessary, mark that most inferiorly located section of the PSIS (▶ Fig. 9.48).

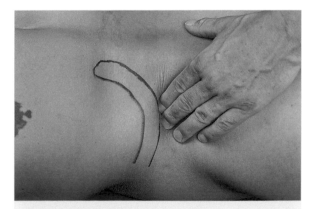

Fig. 9.46 Local palpation of the iliac crest.

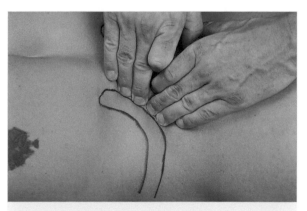

Fig. 9.47 Locating the PSIS—variation 1: SP.

Technique—Variation 2

A transverse palpation of the iliac crest is conducted. The thumb moves with a sweeping, low-pressure, transverse movement from inferior to superior across the crest (▸ Fig. 9.49 and ▸ Fig. 9.50), where the therapist expects to feel a round structure.

This palpation gradually moves in a medial and inferior direction (▸ Fig. 9.51 and ▸ Fig. 9.52).

Finally, the therapist should focus on the point where the structures no longer feel rounded, but instead feel flat and slanted (▸ Fig. 9.53 and ▸ Fig. 9.54). At this point the fingers are no longer on the iliac crest but are already located over the lateral edge of the sacrum. The

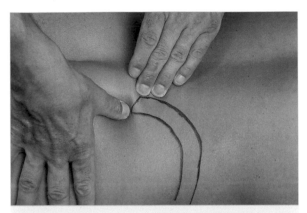

Fig. 9.48 Locating the PSIS—variation 1: final position.

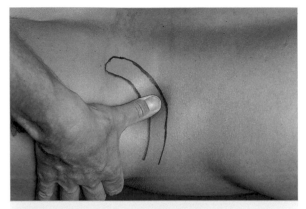

Fig. 9.49 Locating the PSIS—variation 2: SP.

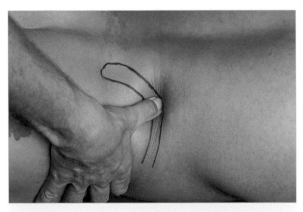

Fig. 9.50 Locating the PSIS—variation 2: final position.

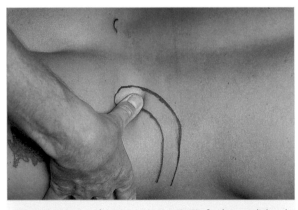

Fig. 9.51 Locating the PSIS—variation 2: SP; further medial and inferior.

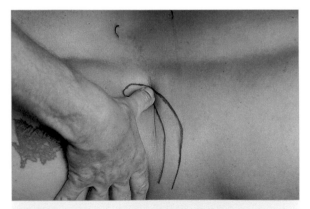

Fig. 9.52 Locating the PSIS—variation 2: final position; further medial and inferior.

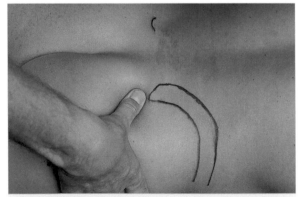

Fig. 9.53 Locating the PSIS—variation 2: SP; edge of the sacrum.

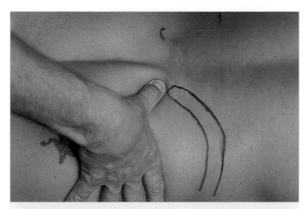

Fig. 9.54 Locating the PSIS—variation 2: final position; edge of the sacrum.

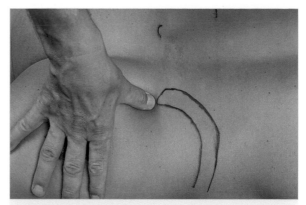

Fig. 9.55 Locating the PSIS—variation 2: inferior edge of the PSIS.

transitional area between the iliac crest and sacrum should be visualized again:

- Slightly further superior: rounded palpation of the iliac crest.
- Slightly further inferior: flattened slant of the edge of the sacrum.

The thumb is now positioned over the edge of the sacrum, points in a superior direction, and hooks around the iliac crest. This technique is used to mark the inferior edge of the PSIS (▶ Fig. 9.55).

Tip

In this technique it is especially important to carry out a rather large movement with the thumb. The iliac crest is a very wide structure that requires a wide movement to feel its rounded contour.

Memorize

Accurate location of the PSIS is the crucial palpatory technique on the posterior pelvis. If you are unable to clearly identify it, all further attempts to clearly define structures are bound to fail.

Information on Pathology

The exact location of the PSIS can cause patients pain under certain circumstances, especially when locating the inferior aspect of the PSIS. This is most likely due to the long posterior sacroiliac ligament being sensitive to pressure, which can indicate the presence of a pathological SI joint.

Technique—Palpation in Standing

Locating the PSIS in the standing position is much more difficult than in the prone position. The increased tension

in the gluteal and multifidus muscles makes distinct palpation cumbersome. The thumb must palpate with more pressure to feel the bony shapes and determine the differences in consistency between tense soft tissues and bones (▶ Fig. 9.56).

Tip

Palpation can first be conducted on one side in difficult cases using technique variation 2 and a lot of pressure. To do this, the therapist stands more to the side of the patient and stabilizes the pelvis anteriorly.

In other cases, flexion of the vertebral column and the associated iliac bone movement (as in the standing flexion test) can be helpful. The spines can become more obvious during this movement.

9.7.4 Sacrum—S2 Spinous Process

The line connecting the two PSISs allows the therapist to accurately locate the S2 spinous process (▶ Fig. 9.57). Starting from this position, the lumbosacral junction and the other sacral spinous processes can be correctly located.

Technique

To correctly depict these structures, both PSISs are first located using the thumbs. The spinous process of S2 is located at the middle of the line connecting the PSISs. It is quite large and can usually be clearly palpated as a roughened area over the sacrum (▶ Fig. 9.58).

9.7.5 Sacrum—Median Sacral Crest

Three different ridges are located on the posterior side of the sacrum and represent the rudiments of the sacral spinous and articular processes. Most of the posterior aspect of the sacrum is so densely covered with ligamentous structures that only the median sacral crest can be palpated with certainty. The spinous process has been

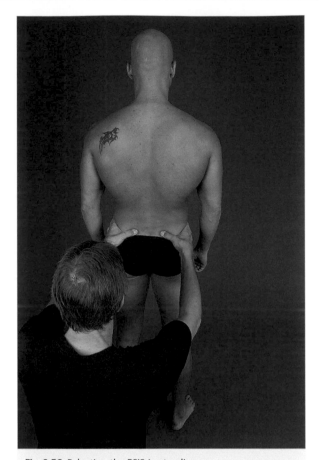

Fig. 9.56 Palpating the PSIS in standing.

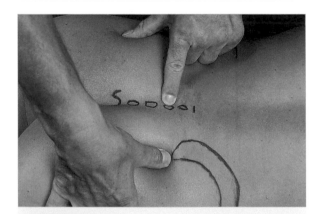

Fig. 9.58 Locating S2.

reduced to the level of a tubercle. Considerable variation is found in its shape:
- The shape of the S1 spinous process varies greatly between individuals. It can be felt as an obvious or slight elevation superior to S2, or may be completely absent. The S1 spinous process is still going to play an important role for palpation later on. First, the SI joint extends superiorly to a limited extent; second, palpation of the lumbar spine starts here.

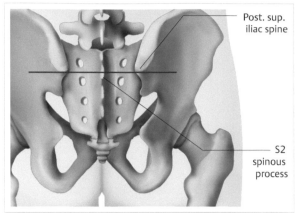

Fig. 9.57 Level allocation: both PSISs—S2 spinous process.

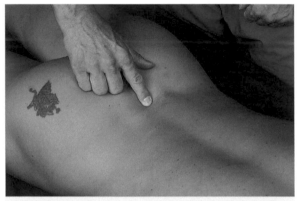

Fig. 9.59 Locating S1.

- The S5 spinous process is always absent. The laminae of the original S5 vertebra are not closed and therefore do not unite posteriorly to form a structure resembling the spinous process.

Technique

The location of the S2 spinous process can be accurately found by connecting both PSISs (see above). Subsequent palpation is performed using small circular movements, preferably with the pad of the index or middle finger, moving directly superior and inferior away from the S2:
- *S1:* the palpating finger points in a superior direction (▶ Fig. 9.59). If the S1 spinous process is palpable, the neighboring superior structure will be the L5 spinous process (see the section "Local Bony Palpation," Chapter 10).
- *S3, S4:* the palpating finger points in an inferior direction (▶ Fig. 9.60). The shape of the elevations along the median sacral crest also varies among individuals. One variation is that they simply form one large structure. The level of S5 can then be accurately located.

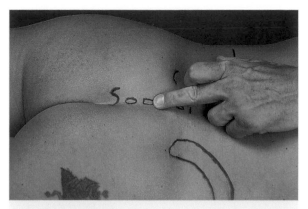

Fig. 9.60 Locating S3.

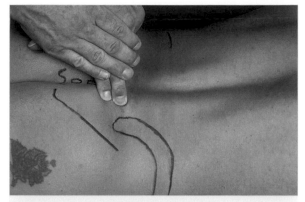

Fig. 9.61 Palpating the multifidus when active.

9.7.6 Sacrum—Insertion of the Multifidus

The fibers of the lumbar multifidus are evident on the posterior surface of the sacrum directly next to the midline. Its collagen fibers merge with the rear ligaments, for example, with the long posterior sacroiliac ligament.

The action of the multifidus is similar to a hydrodynamic reinforcement of the thoracolumbar fascia. The multifidus swells up during contraction and tightens the fascia from the inside outward, like a bicycle tire becoming more taut when the inner tube is pumped up. Several palpating finger pads are placed directly next to the mid-line over the sacral surface. The patients slightly increases their lordosis (▶ Fig. 9.61). The consistency of the tissue to be palpated becomes distinctly firmer when it is activated.

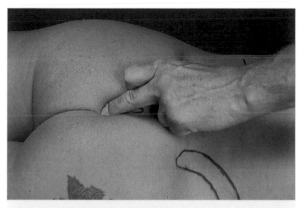

Fig. 9.62 Palpating the sacral hiatus.

9

Technique

Several palpating finger pads are placed directly next to the mid-line over the sacral surface. The patients slightly increases their lordosis (▶ Fig. 9.61). The consistency of the tissue to be palpated becomes distinctly firmer when it is activated.

9.7.7 Sacrum—Sacral Hiatus

The palpating finger searches for the different prominences found along the median sacral crest. The therapist should expect to feel irregular prominences during the palpation. This changes when the level of S5 is reached. A small flattened area is felt.

Technique

The middle finger pad is preferably used. It points in an inferior direction, slides down from S4, and moves onto a small, flattened plateau (▶ Fig. 9.62). The sacral hiatus and its covering membrane, representing the level of S5, are felt here.

Tip

There are two different methods available to confirm the correct location:

- Pressure is applied in an anterior direction. The covering membrane is being palpated when the tissue yields elastically and no hard bony resistance is felt (▶ Fig. 9.63).
- The finger pads collide with protruding bone when they are moved to the left and right. More circular palpation demonstrates that these elevated structures are osseous processes (▶ Fig. 9.64). These are the sacral horns, the rudiments of the S5 vertebral arch laminae. Their shape and size vary between individuals. A difference between left and right may even be seen in the same patient. It is not possible to detect the inferior sacral borders precisely as the sacral horns also face the protrusions in the coccyx bone. The horns will be searched for again during the further course of precise palpation of the pelvis.

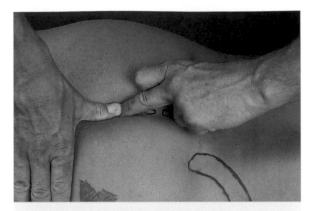

Fig. 9.63 Applying pressure to the membrane.

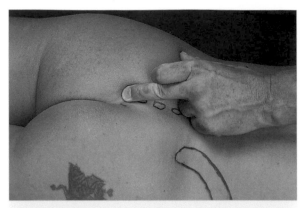

Fig. 9.64 Locating a sacral horn.

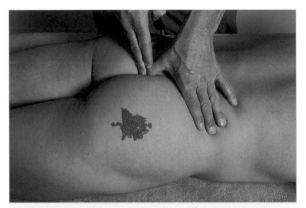

Fig. 9.65 Assessing the consistency at S4.

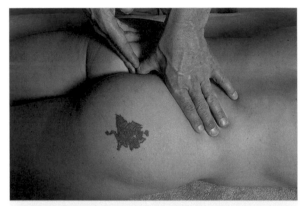

Fig. 9.66 Assessing the consistency of the coccyx.

9.7.8 Sacrum—Sacrococcygeal Transition

The apex of the sacrum and its mobile articulation with the coccyx is found directly inferior to the hiatus.

Technique

The fingers are placed at a steep angle to the sacral hiatus and the finger pads palpate. The fingers slide inferiorly into a transverse groove directly inferior to the hiatus. This is where the sacrum connects to the coccyx.

The sacrum and the coccyx are further differentiated from one another by assessing consistency. The resistance is quite firm when direct pressure is applied to the sacrum (safest at the S4 level) (▶ Fig. 9.65). Inferior to the joint, the coccyx reacts to pressure with more elasticity (▶ Fig. 9.66).

Information on Pathology

People who have fallen and compressed their coccyx may still experience pain when they are palpated here. This is due to an overstretching of the ligamentous connections that stabilize the joint. These ligaments (lateral sacrococcygeal ligaments) originate from the posterior aspect of the sacral horns. Local transverse frictions at the origin are used as treatment to relieve pain.

9.7.9 Sacrum—Inferolateral Angles of the Sacrum

The inferolateral angles of the sacrum are found at the level of the sacral horns. The distance between these two angles demonstrates how wide the inferior part of the sacrum is. It is apparent that the sacrum is not triangular but is shaped more like a trapezoid. The inferolateral angles of the sacrum can be reached using three different techniques.

Technique—Variation 1

The pad of the middle finger is used to palpate the membrane covering the sacral hiatus again. Index and ring fingers are slightly spread out to the side and rest on the surface of the buttocks. The inferolateral angles of the sacrum are found underneath these finger pads (▶ Fig. 9.67). This variation is especially used for quick orientation.

Technique—Variation 2

The inferior edge of the sacrum is palpated by moving laterally from the sacral apex. The inferolateral angle is

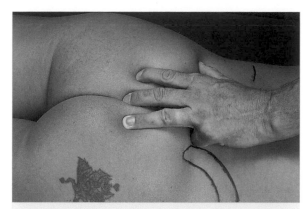

Fig. 9.67 Locating the inferolateral angle of the sacrum—variation 1.

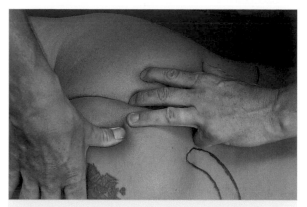

Fig. 9.68 Locating the inferolateral angle of the sacrum—variation 2.

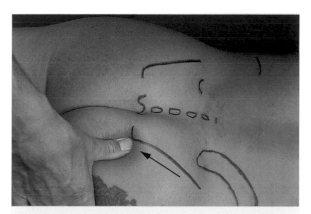

Fig. 9.69 Locating the inferolateral angle of the sacrum—variation 3.

situated at the point where the palpating finger changes direction and palpates more superolaterally (▶ Fig. 9.68).

Technique—Variation 3

This technique is used for quick orientation at the sacrum to detect the edges of the sacrum. The finger pads or the medial edge of the hand are used for this technique, palpating along the edge of the sacrum in an inferior direction until the edge of the sacrum clearly turns in a medial direction (▶ Fig. 9.69).

Tip

The presence of strong collagenous structures makes the precise palpatory location of the inferolateral angle, as conducted in the second and third technique variations, significantly more difficult. Therefore, firm pressure must be applied to the respective edges of the sacrum during palpation. The consistency assessment of palpated structures is likewise very important. The neighboring ligaments are very firm, yet somewhat elastic, when directly pressed down upon.

9.7.10 Sacrotuberous Ligament

One of the most strongly collagenous structures in the musculoskeletal system connects each edge of the sacrum—especially at the level of the inferolateral angle—with the corresponding ischial tuberosity: the sacrotuberous ligament.

Technique

The two important bony structures, the inferolateral angle of the sacrum and the ischial tuberosity, have already been found (▶ Fig. 9.70). The ligament is almost as wide as a thumb and is located between these two bony reference points. Transverse palpation with the thumb or pressure from the index finger is used to palpate. The ligament is very firm, but nevertheless elastic when directly palpated (▶ Fig. 9.71).

As this ligament belongs to one of the most important nutation restrictors, it is not fully tightened in the supine position and yields somewhat elastically when direct pressure is applied to it.

9.7.11 Long Posterior Sacroiliac Ligament

Another ligament in the sacroiliac ligamentous apparatus can be directly accessed and used for diagnostic purposes. The long posterior sacroiliac ligament connects the PSIS with the corresponding edge of the sacrum. It is approximately 3 cm long, almost one finger-width wide, and merges with the sacrotuberous ligament. It is the only ligament that restricts counternutation. As already stated, it is one area of insertion of the multifidus.

The ligament can be reached using transverse palpation directly inferior to the PSIS and is felt as a rounded structure (▶ Fig. 9.72 and ▶ Fig. 9.73). The further course of the ligament (after approximately 2 cm) as it heads toward the edge of the sacrum can only be palpated vaguely.

9

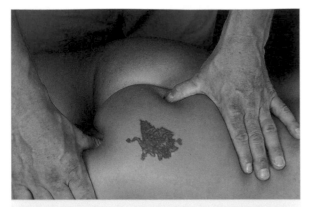

Fig. 9.70 Sacrotuberous ligament—locating the fixed points.

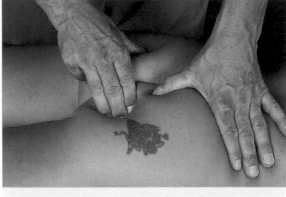

Fig. 9.71 Sacrotuberous ligament—direct palpation.

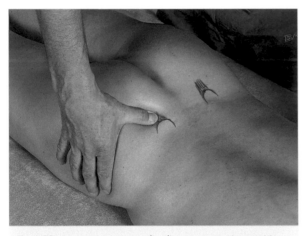

Fig. 9.72 Long posterior sacroiliac ligament, starting position.

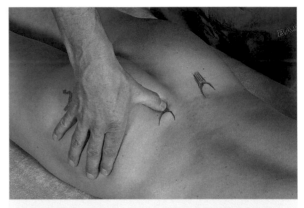

Fig. 9.73 Long posterior sacroiliac ligament, final position.

According to Vleeming (2002), pain on transverse palpation of the ligament immediately inferior to the PSIS is considered a pathological finding and indicates the presence of a pathological SI joint.

9.8 Orienting Projections

Several structures in the posterior pelvis cannot be palpated at all or can only be palpated using aids. Therefore, therapists need to project structures onto the surface of the skin and mark guiding lines to orient themselves. First a guiding line is marked between a PSIS and a sacral horn. This is the foundation for all further projections and palpations.

9.8.1 Posterior Inferior Iliac Spine (PIIS)

The connecting line is halved by a 2-cm-long line that is marked at a right angle. The end of this second line is the starting point for the local palpation of the PIIS.

Technique

A thumb is placed on this point and pushes anteriorly with ample pressure. The other thumb can be used for support when necessary. The thumb tries to move in a superior direction. Hard bony resistance is felt. The therapist now hooks around the PIIS, coming from an inferior direction (▶ Fig. 9.74).

The PIIS is always found at the level of the S3 spinous process and represents the inferior border of the SI joint. The joint surface is only approximately 1 cm away from the palpation at this point, which can be better understood when viewing an anatomical specimen.

Tip

This technique can be somewhat unpleasant for patients as the palpation must be conducted using firm pressure. This is mostly tolerated as it is impossible to endanger truly sensitive structures, for example, vessels or nerves.

9.8.2 Sacroiliac Joint Projection

It is now possible to transfer the exact position of the joint onto the surface of the skin to better visualize the joint's spatial dimensions and size.

The posterior projection of the joint space is found approximately 2 cm lateral and parallel to the line connecting the PSIS and the sacral horn (▶ Fig. 9.75).

Technique—Projection

- A connecting line is marked again if necessary.
- The PIIS is found and the S3 spinous process located in the sacral mid-line.
- The S1 spinous process is identified using palpation. The level of the S2 spinous process can also be confirmed, if necessary, by connecting the two PSISs.
- A line is marked parallel and approximately 2 cm lateral to the connecting line.
- The positions of S3 and S1 are transferred onto this parallel line.

This results in the SI joint's position, alignment, and superior/inferior level being projected onto the posterior surface of the body (▶ Fig. 9.76). It is now evident that the edge of the sacrum can only be palpated between the inferolateral angles at the level of S5 and the PIIS (at the level of S3). The SI joint is found superior to this and makes direct palpation impossible.

9.8.3 Piriformis

This muscle is said to be of significant importance in various pathological conditions. The assessment of its consistency has a type of monitoring function. Its location can therefore be important in the assessment or, in some cases, the treatment of symptoms in the LPH region.

The muscle is located in two steps. Its position is first projected onto the surface of the skin, followed by the palpatory assessment of consistency (▶ Fig. 9.77).

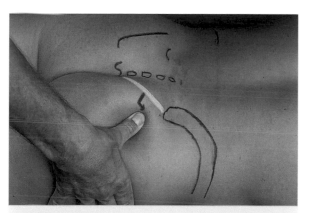

Fig. 9.74 Palpating the posterior inferior iliac spine (PIIS).

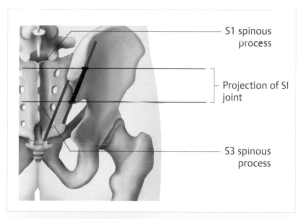

S1 spinous process

Projection of SI joint

S3 spinous process

Fig. 9.75 Position of the sacroiliac (SI) joint, posterior aspect.

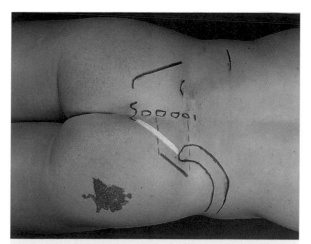

Fig. 9.76 Projecting the sacroiliac (SI) joint onto the skin.

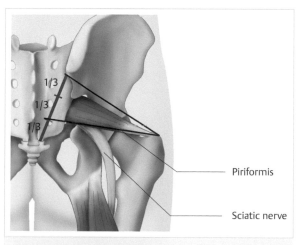

1/3
1/3
1/3

Piriformis

Sciatic nerve

Fig. 9.77 Position of the piriformis.

9

Technique—Projection

- The muscle's position is clarified by first drawing a line between the PSIS and the sacral horn. This line is now cut into thirds.
- The superior tip of the greater trochanter is needed as a further bony reference point. Its location has already been described (see the section "Greater Trochanter" above).
- A line is drawn from the inferior aspect of the PSIS to the tip of the trochanter. This line represents the superior border of the piriformis.
- A line is drawn between the tip of the trochanter and the point between the middle third and the superior third of the divided connecting line. This line illustrates the inferior border of the piriformis.
- The result is a slender triangle with its base positioned medially and the tip laterally (▶ Fig. 9.78).

Technique—Palpation

After the location of the piriformis has been projected onto the skin, the muscle belly can be directly palpated. Two to three fingers push down onto the center of the triangle. The finger pads are used for palpation and firm pressure is applied. The therapist is looking for a rounded structure. This structure's consistency is somewhat firmer than its direct surroundings.

> **Tip**
>
> The edge of the sacrum is located approximately 2 to 3 cm lateral to the line connecting the PSIS and the sacral horn. The approximately 4-cm-long muscle belly is searched for directly lateral to this. This mostly corresponds to the center of the triangle. The muscle turns into an inserting tendon further laterally, which cannot be palpated.

Information on Pathology

This muscle is frequently pathologically dense and tender to pressure when lumbar, SI joint, or hip and thigh symptoms are present.

A piriformis syndrome is referred to when a permanent increase in muscle tension irritates the sciatic nerve. This diagnosis is apparently supported when trigger points are discovered in this muscle.

Mercer et al. (2004), in their literature review, investigated a multitude of differing recommendations dealing with the palpation of these sensitive points in the muscle. They furthermore examined the position and shape of the piriformis on 10 bodies in a study, applying the palpatory procedures recommended in literature to locate the piriformis. Only two methods were found to be reliable. They looked at the inferior edge of the muscle belly in relation to the tip of the coccyx and found that this distance varied by up to 2 cm.

9.8.4 Sciatic Nerve and the Gluteals

The position and the further pathway of the thickest of all peripheral nerves (sciatic nerve) (▶ Fig. 9.79) can likewise be accurately projected onto the surface of the skin. Direct palpation leads the palpating finger onto the nerve, which cannot be felt as such. It is too relaxed in the supine position and lies slightly corrugated in the tissue. This results in the nerve yielding somewhat to direct palpation, and it cannot be identified as an independent structure. The nerve can normally cope well with direct and firm pressure. Palpation is painful only when a true neuritis is present.

Projection—Exit Point Out of the Pelvis

The sciatic nerve passes underneath the piriformis for several centimeters and emerges at a point that can be very well described using the lines already present. The connecting line demonstrating the inferior boundary of

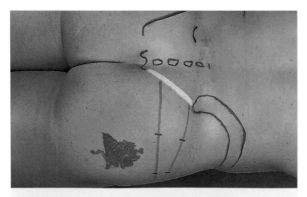

Fig. 9.78 Projection of the piriformis—muscle belly.

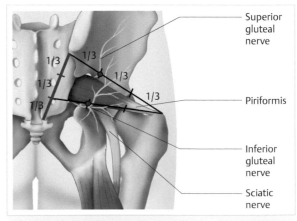

Fig. 9.79 Position of important nerves in the gluteal region.

the piriformis is divided into three. The nerve emerges from underneath the muscle at the intersection between the medial and medial third, exiting the pelvis posteriorly (▶ Fig. 9.80).

Technique—Palpation

The exact location can be reliably confirmed using palpation. The thumb or another finger applies moderate pressure to the tissue in an anterior direction.

The correct position has been found when the therapist additionally pushes in a superior direction and the movement is restricted by a firm, elastic structure. This is the muscle belly of the piriformis. While pressure is still being applied in an anterior direction, additional movement in a medial direction results in the palpating finger pushing against the hard edge of the sacrum (▶ Fig. 9.81).

This confirmed palpation marks the infrapiriform foramen. This is where the inferior gluteal nerve—the motor supply for the gluteus maximus—also travels to the surface. The posterior femoral cutaneous nerve is another neural structure that passes through this foramen. Some of its rami are found posterior to the ischial tuberosity, and some are found inferior to the ischial tuberosity as they travel in a medial direction.

Projection—Further Pathway in the Pelvis

The sciatic nerve's further pathway along the posterior pelvis can be determined using two more bony reference points (▶ Fig. 9.82). Local palpation confirms the nerve's pathway projected onto the skin for orientation.

The required reference points have already been found:
• Ischial tuberosity.
• Greater trochanter.

Another line is marked between the tip of the ischial tuberosity and the tip of the greater trochanter and cut in half.

The middle of this line is connected to the previously found exit point for the sciatic nerve under the piriformis. This enables the therapist to project the pathway of this approximately thumb-wide neural structure onto the skin (▶ Fig. 9.83).

Projection—Further Pathway in the Thigh

The further pathway of the nerve can be visualized as traveling from the middle of the line between the tuberosity and the trochanter, extending down the posterior thigh, and ending in the middle of the popliteal fossa.

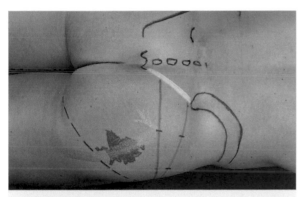

Fig. 9.80 Projection of the sciatic nerve as it exits the pelvis.

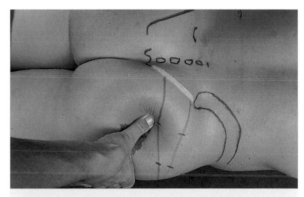

Fig. 9.81 Palpating the sciatic nerve at its exit point.

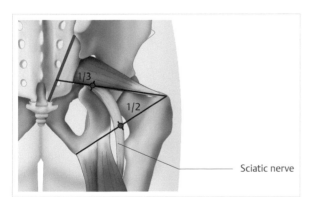

Fig. 9.82 Pathway of the sciatic nerve in the pelvis.

Sciatic nerve

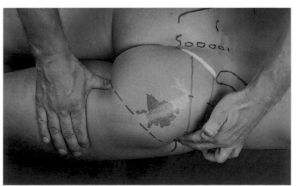

Fig. 9.83 Projection of the sciatic nerve pathway.

9

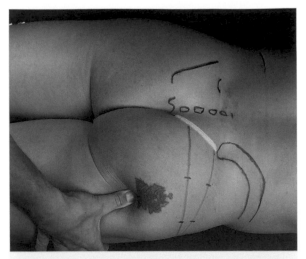

Fig. 9.84 Palpating the sciatic nerve at the ischial tuberosity.

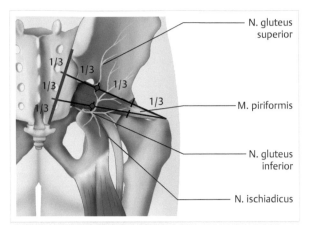

Fig. 9.85 Exit site for the superior gluteal nerve out of the pelvis.

Significant pressure can be applied halfway along the above-mentioned line. The deeper tissues are simultaneously penetrated and pressure is applied directly onto the nerve. The finger is then pushed in a medial direction and immediately feels the bone of the ischial tuberosity (▶ Fig. 9.84). The pathway of the sciatic nerve can be seen on anatomical specimens as running directly lateral to the tuberosity.

The nerve even forms a groove along the side surface of the tuberosity as we age. It is well known that the nerve divides into its two branches approximately one hand-width proximal to the popliteal fossa. The tibial nerve and the common peroneal nerve can be palpated well in the popliteal fossa (see also Chapter 6.9).

The nerve's narrow passage between the tuberosity and the trochanter is described earlier in the Chapter 5.3.3.

Projection—Superior Gluteal Nerve

The small gluteal muscles are innervated by the superior gluteal nerve. This nerve exits the pelvis posteriorly at the same point as the previous neural structures. The correct location of this nerve can also be confirmed using the same method for palpation (▶ Fig. 9.85).

The upper line indicating the superior border of the piriformis is divided into three. Again, the exit point for the nerve is found at the intersection between the medial and middle thirds. This point can be verified by applying pressure in an anterior direction and moving in a superior direction against the muscle belly of the piriformis and moving medially against the hard edge of the sacrum. This marks the suprapiriform foramen.

9.9 Tips for Treatment

SI joint mobilization requires great manual strength, best applied by the largest bony leverage that can work on the pelvis. The necessary reference points can be found using the quick bony orientation, for example, the iliac crests, the ischial tuberosity, and the edge of the sacrum.

Several ligamentous structures can also cause **sacral pain** when irritated. The long posterior sacroiliac ligament indicates functional disorders in the SI joint. Over-stretched ligamentous connections to the coccyx are frequently the source of pain following a fall onto the buttocks.

Local soft-tissue pain is difficult to diagnose. Pelvic pain must first be identified as pain that is not being referred or projected. Now, the attempt is made to locate and identify the affected tissue. Bursitis, peritrochanteric insertion symptoms, a tense piriformis, or even piriformis syndrome are examples of local sources of pain. An exact palpatory technique identifies the affected structure quite well and supplements the results of the functional assessment wisely.

Exercises for the pelvic floor muscles are widely based on perception. Tactile feedback from the pelvic floor muscles directly medial to the ischial tuberosity helps patients to develop a feel for voluntary activity more quickly.

Bibliography

Brooke R. The sacro-iliac joint. J Anat. 1924; 58(Pt 4):299–305

Chakraverty R, Pynsent P, Isaacs K. Which spinal levels are identified by palpation of the iliac crests and the posterior superior iliac spines? J Anat. 2007; 210(2): 232–236

Dvořák J. Manuelle Medizin. Bd. 1, Diagnostik. Berlin: Springer; 1998

Dvořák J, Dvořák V, Gilliar W, Schneider W, Spring H, Tritschler T. Musculoskeletal Manual Medicine. Diagnosis and Treatment. 5th ed., Stuttgart-New York: Thieme; 2008

Kapandji IA. Funktionelle Anatomie der Gelenke. 4. Aufl. Stuttgart: Thieme; 2006

Lanz T von, Wachsmuth W. Praktische Anatomie, Rücken. Berlin: Springer; 2004

Laslett M. Evidence-based diagnosis and treatment of the painful sacroiliac joint. J Manual ManipTher. 2008; 16(3):142–152

McGaugh JM, Brismée JM, Dedrick GS, Jones EA, Sizer PS. Comparing the anatomical consistency of the posterior superior iliac spine to the iliac crest as reference landmarks for the lumbopelvic spine: a retrospective radiological study. Clin Anat. 2007; 20(7):819–825

Mercer SR, Cullen B, Lau P, et al. Anatomy in Practice: Palpation of Piriformis. Abstract Booklet. Australian Association of Anatomy and Clinical Anatomy. Department of Anatomy and Cell Biology. University of Melbourne; 2004

Netter FH. Atlas of Human Anatomy; 3rd ed. Teterboro, New Jersey: Icon Learning Systems; 2004

Pool-Goudzwaard AL, Kleinrensink GJ, Snijders CJ, Entius C, Stoeckart R. The sacroiliac part of the iliolumbar ligament. J Anat. 2001; 199(Pt 4):457–463

Puranen J, Orava S. The hamstring syndrome. A new diagnosis of gluteal sciatic pain. Am J Sports Med. 1988; 16(5):517–521

Pysyk CL, Persaud D, Bryson GL, Lui A. Ultrasound assessment of the vertebral level of the palpated intercristal (Tuffier's) line. Can J Anaesth. 2010; 57:46–49

Rana SH, Farjoodi P, Haloman S, et al. Anatomic Evaluation of the Sacroiliac Joint: A Radiographic Study with Implications for Procedures. Pain Physician. 2015; 18(6):583–592

Rauber A, Kopsch F. Anatomie des Menschen. Bd. I: Bewegungsapparat. 3. Aufl. Stuttgart: Thieme; 2003

Reichert B. Massage-Therapie. Stuttgart: Thieme; 2015

Sashin D. A critical analysis of the anatomy and the pathological changes of the sacroiliac joints. J Bone Joint Surg Am. 1930; 12:891–910

Stewart TD. Pathologic changes in aging sacroiliac joints: a study of dissecting-room skeletons. Clin Orthop Relat Res. 1984(183):188–196

Travell JG, Simons DG. Handbuch der Muskel-Triggerpunkte. Obere Extremität, Kopf und Thorax. Stuttgart: Fischer; 1998

Vleeming A, Dorman TA. Self-locking of the sacroiliac articulation. Spine. 1995; 9::407–18

Vleeming A, Pool-Goudzwaard AL, Hammudoghlu D, Stoeckart R, Snijders CJ, Mens JM. The function of the long dorsal sacroiliac ligament: its implication for understanding low back pain. Spine. 1996; 21(5):556–562

Vleeming A, de Vries HJ, Mens JM, van Wingerden JP. Possible role of the long dorsal sacroiliac ligament in women with peripartum pelvic pain. Acta ObstetGynecolScand. 2002; 81(5):430–436

Vleeming A, Albert HB, Östgaard HC, Stuge B, Sturesson B. Evidenzfür die Diagnose und Therapie von Beckengürtelschmerz – EuropäischeLeitlinien. Physioscience. 2006; 2:48–58

Vleeming A, Schuenke MD, Masi AT, Carreiro JE, Danneels L, Willard FH. The sacroiliac joint: an overview of its anatomy, function and potential clinical implications. J Anat. 2012; 221(6):537–567

Winkel D, et al. Das Sakroiliacalgelenk. Stuttgart: Fischer; 1992

Winkel D. Nichtoperative Orthopädie und Manualtherapie. Anatomie in Vivo. 3. Aufl. München: Urban & Fischer bei Elsevier; 2004

9

Chapter 10

Lumbar Spine

10 Lumbar Spine

10.1 Significance and Function of the Lumbar Spine

The embryonic curves change during early childhood development in two sections of the vertebral column. The lumbar spine represents one of these sections. The mobile sections of the vertebral column (cervical and lumbar spines) become lordotic. The thoracic spine and the sacrum remain in their original kyphosis. The cervical and lumbar spines also possess deep prevertebral muscles (e.g., psoas major, adductor longus).

10.1.1 Supporting the Weight of the Body

From a kinetic point of view, the lumbar spine supports the weight of the upper body, the head, and the arms. As already described, approximately 60% of the body's weight in an upright posture is transmitted from the lumbar spine onto the S1 end plate. The lumbar spine adapts to this loading with wider and more solid material in the bones, collagen, and fibrous cartilage (structural stability/force closure).

10.1.2 Spatial Alignment of the Upper Body

The lordotic sections of the spine provide spatial orientation for the parts of the body they support. The lumbar spine supports, props up, and turns the upper body. The cervical spine supports and aligns the head in relation to its surroundings.

10.1.3 The Importance of Stability for Standing and Lifting

The intervertebral disks, ligaments, and muscles are in particular responsible for stability in the vertebral column and achieve this using compression and tension banding. The erector spinae are not very active in the upright posture. Their activity increases when the body's center of gravity moves anteriorly, for example when:
• The upper body bends forward.
• The cervical spine is flexed.
• An arm is elevated.

It is important that the tissues provide the mobile parts of the chain with force closure to enable controlled movement. For this reason, science of human movement states that: "stiffness is a precondition for movement." In a multisegmental system such as the vertebral column, stability is maintained by reducing the range of available mobility in individual segments so that the entire system can move harmoniously. The trunk extensors become inactive after approximately 60° of trunk flexion due to the ligamentous structures taking over the job of decelerating movement. The thoracolumbar fascia is the most important ligamentous structure (see ▶ Fig. 10.32).

10.1.4 Movement in the Trunk

The lumbar spine is an organ designed for flexion, with movement mainly occurring in the sagittal plane. It is just as natural to move out of the lordosis to bend the trunk backward and forward as it is to develop the lordotic form when standing. The lumbar spine is anatomically constructed and equipped for flexion. It is irrelevant whether the movements are proper flexion or just a straightening out of the lordosis for palpation.

Certain anatomical structures assist the lumbar spine in its movement in the sagittal plane:
• The alignment of the lumbar vertebral joints superior to L5 makes extensive movement in the sagittal plane possible (▶ Fig. 10.1).
• Thick intervertebral disks make extensive tilting movements possible in the lumbar segments.
• Structures that decelerate movement and absorb forces: ligamenta flava, interspinous ligaments, thoracolumbar fascia.

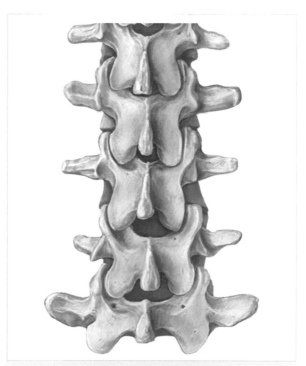

Fig. 10.1 Schematic illustration of the alignment of the lumbar zygapophysial joints (ZAJs). Compare this to ▶ Fig. 10.9.

- The exceptionally strong intrinsic muscles of the lateral tract (iliocostalis, longissimus).

10.1.5 Development of Energy Needed for Locomotion

According to Serge Gracovetsky (1989), the impulse for walking arises in the lumbar spine and is based on the mobility and activity in the muscles that cause rotation (the multifidi and external oblique). The legs only follow and reinforce this movement. Examples from evolution (fish, amphibians) demonstrate how important lateral flexion is for locomotion. In human beings, the lumbar spine uses lateral flexion and coupled rotation to transfer the trigger for locomotion onto the pelvis and the legs, whereby a lumbar lordosis and a certain walking speed are important. The impulse and energy arise solely in the legs when gait is slow; this requires a great deal of strength.

10.1.6 Junction between the Rigid and Mobile Vertebral Column

The junction between the lumbar spine and the sacrum is a region of anatomical and pathological turbulence. Anatomical variations in the number of vertebrae (e.g., hemisacralization) as well as a multitude of pathological conditions are frequently found here. This distinctive feature is probably due to typical biomechanical loading in addition to the lumbar spine acting as the junction between the freely mobile vertebral column and the rather rigid pelvis, in particular the sacrum.

This region is supported by different anatomical structures:

- The alignment of the L5-S1 zygapophysial joints.
- Strongly reinforced ligaments or ligaments that have been additionally developed (anterior longitudinal ligament, iliolumbar ligaments).
- Thoracolumbar fascia with its various collagenous layers and muscular dynamization.

10.2 Common Applications for Treatment in this Region

Most symptoms in the lumbar region are directly or indirectly related to the intervertebral disks. It is a known fact that the primary and most secondary intervertebral disk pathologies tend to be found in the lower lumbar segments of L4/L5 and L5/S1. The primary intervertebral disk symptoms range from internal rupturing to the different forms of protrusions and prolapses of intervertebral disk substance (▶ Fig. 10.2). These symptoms possess a large potential for self-healing. The initial physical therapy management of acute back pain aims to assess the primary pain and relieve affected neural structures, thereby

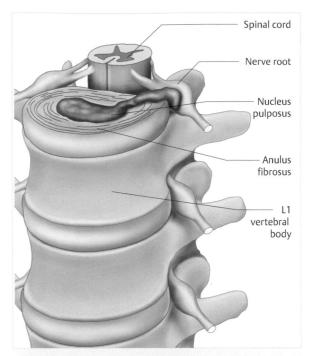

Fig. 10.2 Intervertebral disk prolapse.

supporting self-healing. The first inflammatory stage ends after a few days. Physical therapy then addresses the increased muscle tension, adaptive postures, immobilization, decreased proprioception, and, when necessary, the repositioning of the intervertebral disk substance.

The therapeutic approaches to treatment always address the entire lumbar spine. Precise palpation techniques only have limited use here. For instance, it is generally not necessary to ascertain which segment is affected by provoking pain with palpation or assessing the local mobility. It is important to assess whether there is excessive muscle tension in the paravertebral muscles for the treatment of subacute disk-related symptoms. This provides therapists with a sensible basis when they are deciding which treatment to use. When patients present with these sets of symptoms, therapists are therefore required to systematically palpate the muscles and have knowledge of surface anatomy (see the section "Palpating the Consistency of Muscle [Assessment of Muscle Tension]" in Chapter 8).

The *secondary pathological intervertebral disk conditions* behave completely differently. Surface anatomy is often required in this case. Degenerative changes to the lumbar disks cause a surprisingly large range of symptoms. The intervertebral disks can be the source of pain and can be responsible for the involvement of sensitive ligamentous and neural structures (▶ Fig. 10.3).

These types of pathological disorders are mainly in the form of local segmental instability, chronic intervertebral disk irritation, disorders and diseases in the

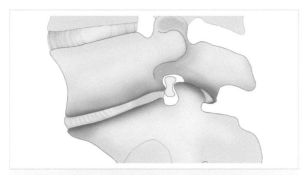

Fig. 10.3 Types of pathological changes possible as a result of intervertebral disk degeneration.

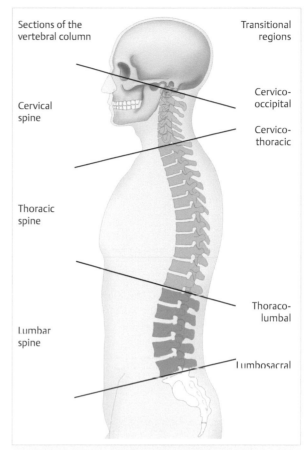

Fig. 10.4 Anatomical sections of the vertebral column.

zygapophysial joints, and varying degrees of stenoses. Of course, combinations of these pathological conditions are possible. Just think of the neighboring hypermobile and hypomobile segments that are frequently present.

There are several different approaches to therapeutic management. The main aim of these approaches is pain relief and stabilization. Detailed anatomical orientation is an important foundation for segmental assessment and for the reliable use of local segmental techniques.

The roles of surface anatomy here are the following:
- To locate the affected segments using pain provocation.
- To identify the affected segments by differentiating them from the neighboring segments (locating their level).
- To assess the segmental stability and mobility using angled or translation tests.

Competence in palpation is obtained from the consequential use of surface anatomy. It enables the therapist to provide exact information on the functional characteristics of the lumbar spine and therefore substantiates the treatment plan and the targeted use of pain-relieving and/or mobilizing techniques.

10.3 Required Basic Anatomical and Biomechanical Knowledge

The following information represents only a selection of information available on local anatomy and biomechanics. Several areas, such as the construction and function of the intervertebral disks or neuroanatomy, are not discussed in order to stay on the topic of surface anatomy. These sections primarily discuss the anatomical details required for palpation. A basic knowledge of movement segments according to Junghanns is of advantage.

10.3.1 Anatomical Definitions

The inferior section of the freely moveable vertebral column, the lumbar spine, usually consists anatomically of five freely moveable vertebrae. However, this is not the case in every individual. As already mentioned above, the lumbosacral junction is quite variable and anatomically turbulent. Töndury (1968, in von Lanz and Wachsmuth, 2004a) wrote about the entire spectrum of variation in the anatomy with respect to the anatomical boundaries of all sections of the vertebral column (▶ Fig. 10.4): "Only approximately 40% of all people have their boundaries in the normal location." The boundaries between the thoracic spine and the lumbar spine as well as the lumbosacral junction are of interest here.

When S1 is separated from the sacrum, it takes on the role of a lumbar vertebra and is labeled anatomically as lumbarization. This results in the lumbar spine possessing six vertebrae. The anatomist defines the superior variation or sacralization as the fusion of L5 with the sacrum. This can be present partially or on both sides (▶ Fig. 10.5). In this case, only four freely mobile vertebrae exist. It becomes quite confusing when the therapist considers that there is even more variety in the number of sacral vertebrae. The terms refer therefore to the possible variations (lumbarization or sacralization) in the freely moveable lumbar vertebrae (von Lanz and Wachsmuth, 2004a):

10

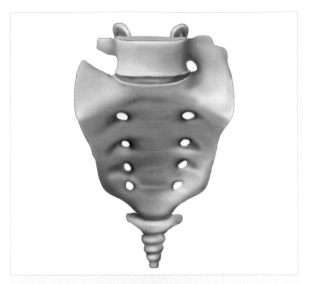

Fig. 10.5 Hemisacralization.

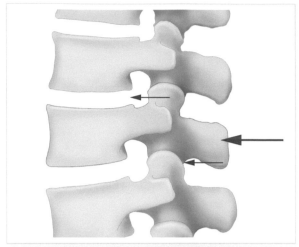

Fig. 10.6 Posteroanterior pressure displaces the vertebra.

- Five lumbar vertebrae → common number in the lumbar spine.
- Four lumbar vertebrae →hemi-/sacralization in 3 to 12%.
- Six lumbar vertebrae → hemi-/lumbarization in 2 to 8%.

How Does this Affect Palpation?

A focus of surface anatomy along the vertebral column is defining the exact location, the level of a structure. Topographical knowledge provides the therapist with expected norms. These norms are transferred onto the living body during palpation. What does it mean when our confidence in topographical orientation—our knowledge of anatomy that we learn during training—becomes lost in the variation?

Variations in the anatomy of the lumbar spine make it difficult to locate the L5 spinous process. When three protruding and pointed spinous processes are found at the lumbosacral junction, it is difficult to differentiate between L5 and S1 by simply looking at their shape. What options exist to confirm the location of a structure when no movement in L5 on S1 can be felt, as is seen when mobility is restricted or when hemisacralization is present? How can therapists remain confident that palpation is correct when the suspected S1 spinous process moves on S2? Is the location incorrect or is a lumbarization present?

Fortunately, constants also exist in anatomy. Certain structures have a constantly recurring shape, always react to pressure in the same way, and behave typically when they move (changes due to pathological conditions are not included here):
- The L5 spinous process is always smaller than the L4 spinous process.

- The T12 spinous process is always smaller than the L1 spinous process.
- Posteroanterior pressure applied to a spinous process moves the vertebra slightly anteriorly (▶ Fig. 10.6).
- Rotation (in a coupled movement pattern) in one segment leads to the development of a palpable step between two neighboring spinous processes.

10.3.2 Shape of the Inferior Lumbar Vertebrae and Intervertebral Disks

From an anatomical point of view, the lumbar lordosis is supported by the wedge-shaped construction of the vertebral bodies, especially at L5 and most notably at the L5/S1 intervertebral disk (Bogduk, 2000) (▶ Fig. 10.7).

The lumbar spine is usually positioned in its physiological lordosis when it is being palpated. This is independent of the patient's starting position (SP) (prone, side-lying). It may be the most natural position, but it does make the palpatory process more difficult. A lordotic lumbar spine offers certain conditions for palpation:
- The palpation demonstrates that the superior section of the sacrum is definitely tilted anteriorly and its angled surface can be distinguished.
- When the erector spinae are prominent, all spinous processes can only be reached at their tips and somewhat to the side.
- The L5 spinous process is mostly found deep in the tissues and in close proximity to L4 and S1.
- The thoracolumbar fascia and the back extensors are relatively relaxed.

Further sections will explain which lumbar spine positions are favorable or less favorable for precise palpation.

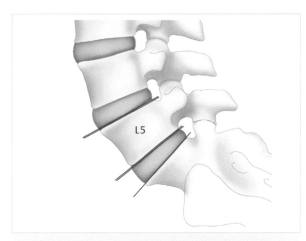

Fig. 10.7 Wedge shape of the vertebrae and intervertebral disks.

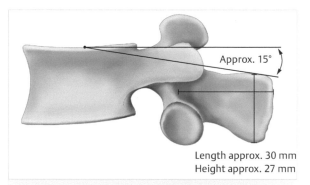

Fig. 10.8 Length and shape of a lumbar spinous process.

10.3.3 Detailed Anatomy of Bony Structures

The thick vertebral bodies (VBs) are generally shaped like a bean or a kidney. Each VB is a tube made of the bone's cortical substance filled with the bone's spongy substance. The VB is enclosed superiorly and inferiorly by hyaline end plates. These end plates are nowadays included functionally as a part of the intervertebral disk (Bogduk, 2000). The vertebral arch connects immediately posterior onto the vertebral body. All vertebral processes are attached to the arch:

• Spinous process.
• Superior and inferior articular processes.
• Costal processes.

Spinous Processes

These processes point directly posterior and are strongly developed (► Fig. 10.8). They are the only osseous structure in the lumbar spine that the palpating finger can reach with certainty. The shape of the lumbar spinous processes is typical and can be well differentiated from the neighboring sections of the vertebral column during palpation.

Aylott et al. (2012) demonstrate that the length and width of the spinous processes increase with age (approx. 0.5 mm/10 years for both length and width). Aylott measured an average height (superior-inferior dimension) of 27 mm for the L1 to L4 spinous processes in men. The height of the L5 spinous process was only 17 mm. All of the measurements were around 3 mm less in women. The study conducted by Shaw et al. (2015) on approx. 3000 cadaveric lumbar vertebrae provides additional information about the length of the L1 to L4 spinous processes (from the edge of the vertebral foramen to its tip), stating an approximate length of 30 mm, while the L5

spinous process is 25 mm. Slope at L1 to L4 was approximately 15° and at L5 approximately 24° (► Fig. 10.8).

Thus, the following observations can be made about the L5 spinous process: It is shorter, and has a shorter and steeper slope than the other lumbar spinous processes (Shaw et al., 2015). When palpating the L5 spinous process it almost seems to point posteriorly. It can generally be well located. The therapist may get confused between neighboring spinous processes when the S1 spinous process is pronounced. This can make it more difficult to allocate a segment to a specific level.

The Shape and Alignment of the Lumbar Spinous Processes

The novice therapists may initially be surprised by the size and morphology of the lumbar spinous processes. The L1-L4 spinous processes are rather broad (superior-inferior dimensions) and have an exceptionally irregular shape with indentations along their posterior aspect, giving them an undulating appearance (► Fig. 10.9). The spinous processes are often expected to be smaller than they actually are.

Bursae are regularly found between the neighboring lumbar and thoracic spinous processes. As with the other sections of the vertebral column, the therapist should not expect the lumbar spinous processes to always form a straight line. The lumbar spinous processes can protrude laterally away from the mid-line by up to a few millimeters and up to 1 cm in the thoracic spine and still be seen as a normal variation in anatomy.

The palpatory differentiation of spinous processes by locating the interspinous space is made considerably more difficult by their undulating form. Aids must be used once again to ensure that structures have been allocated to the correct level. Provided the condition of tissues does not make palpation difficult in study partners and patients, the long spinous processes can be correctly differentiated from the pointed L5 and the T12 spinous processes after gaining some experience. The T12 spinous process is likewise very thin.

10

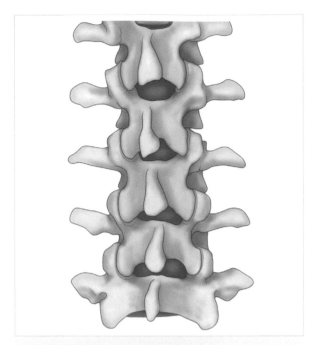

Fig. 10.9 Irregular row of spinous processes.

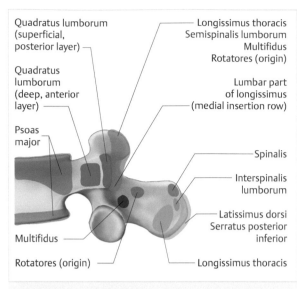

Fig. 10.10 Muscular attachments (from Dvořák, 1998).

Therapists and physicians often directly connect the position of the spinous processes with a local pathological condition. A spinous process that deviates from the midline is mostly interpreted as a rotational malpositioning of the respective vertebra. However, this cannot always be the case due to the large variation in anatomy. A palpatory finding must always be supported by local mobility tests and provocation tests to conclude the presence of a segmental pathological condition.

Lumbar Transverse Processes

The lumbar transverse processes are remnants of ribs from the times of somitic composition. This arrangement can still be observed in the thoracic spine and is the reason why the transverse process is labeled the costal process. All transverse processes are strongly developed and extend directly sideways from the vertebral arch. According to von Lanz and Wachsmuth (2004a), the L3 costal process is the widest. In rare cases (4–8%), L1 can possess an oversized process that is described in literature as a lumbar rib (von Lanz and Wachsmuth, 2004a). This makes it more difficult to differentiate the thorax from the lumbar spine when using palpation.

A multitude of muscles attach onto the transverse processes (Dvořák et al., 1998). As with the spinous processes, the transverse processes are therefore perfect levers for acting forces moving the lumbar vertebrae into lateral flexion and rotation (▶ Fig. 10.10). The transverse processes separate the posterior intrinsic back muscles topographically from the anterior deep abdominal muscles (e.g., psoas major).

Muscular or dynamized connective-tissue structures are currently regarded as functionally very important in the stabilizing treatment of the lumbar spine. These structures insert on the costal processes:
- Transversus abdominis over the middle layer of the thoracolumbar fascia.
- Quadratus lumborum.
- Multifidus.
- Longissimus.

The attempt to reach the transverse processes using palpation is only conclusive on slender people. The transverse processes are located several centimeters anterior to the superficial surface of the back and are completely covered by the thick, prominent back extensors. Only the tips of the L3 and possibly the L4 transverse processes can be reached. This is achieved by applying significant posteroanterior pressure lateral to the back extensors and superior to the iliac crests, then palpating in a medial direction in the hope of coming across a hard structure.

The purpose of this maneuver is questionable, alongside the technical difficulties associated with this procedure. This technique is not suitable for diagnosing the alignment of the structure or for the selective provocation of pain and will therefore not be discussed later.

Zygapophysial Joints

These are some of the most important functional parts of the vertebra. The largest variety of terms is also used to describe these joints (e.g., facet joints, vertebral joints). The thickness and construction of intervertebral disks enable segments to move. In principle, the zygapophysial joints (ZAJs) determine how this potential for movement is used. The alignment of these joints dictates the direction and partially the range of segmental movement. It is well known that the superior articular process of the inferiorly positioned vertebra (more concave) forms a ZAJ with the inferior articular process of the superiorly positioned vertebra (more convex) (▶ Fig. 10.11).

The **position of the lumbar joint facets** between T12/L1 and L4/L5 is uniformly described in manual therapy literature (Dvořák et al., 1998): In relation to the vertebral bodies, the superior joint surfaces are arranged upright and converge at an average angle of 45° from posterolateral to anteromedial (▶ Fig. 10.12). This angle gradually decreases in the more superior vertebrae (Bogduk, 2000).

This results in the lumbar spine's affinity to movement in the sagittal plane, enables the lumbar spine to laterally flex, and prevents axial rotation. The latter movement can best be visualized by looking at the axes for lumbar movement found in the disk (see the section "Basic Biomechanical Principles" below).

The L5/S1 joint facets orient themselves more in the frontal plane, somewhat increasing this segment's ability to axially rotate.

The **principle of anatomical variation** continues in the lumbar ZAJs.

Joint surfaces of the same level can be shaped differently with different spatial alignment without being pathological. Individual differences in the shape of the ZAJs between sides is labeled "facet tropism" (Jerosch and Steinleitner, 2005) (▶ Fig. 10.13). This means that the previously described spatial alignment of the joint surfaces is to be understood as only representing the average and that there are differences between the left and right side in each segment.

The ability to palpate the vertebral column is mainly used to assess segmental mobility and to ascertain the level of individual structures. To be able to do this, the therapist must be aware of the possible range of motion in the sections of the vertebral column.

The influence of differently formed joint facets on the palpation during movement will be clarified later. It can be presumed that facet tropism does not affect the degree of symmetrical movement in the lumbar spine (flexion and extension). When the anterior tilt of the vertebra is different on the left and right side during flexion, this cannot be felt because sagittal movement is simply perceived as an opening or closing of the spinous processes (▶ Fig. 10.14). A difference in movement between the sides where the vertebra moves asymmetrically does not change the palpable range of motion.

This is different for asymmetrical lateral flexion or rotation movements, where the effect of differently formed joint positions and shapes is important. The range of motion in segmental lateral flexion and rotation to the left and to the right can therefore differ, even in healthy

10

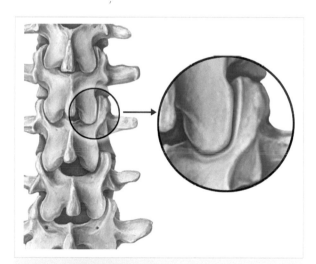

Fig. 10.11 Zygapophysial joint (ZAJ).

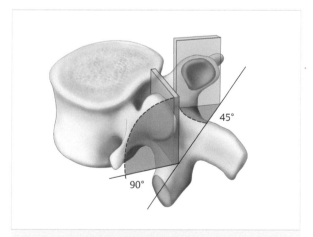

Fig. 10.12 Alignment of the lumbar zygapophysial joints (ZAJs).

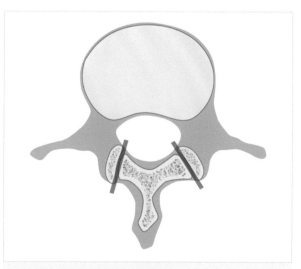

Fig. 10.13 Facet tropism.

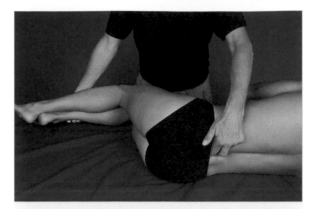

Fig. 10.14 Palpating flexion and extension.

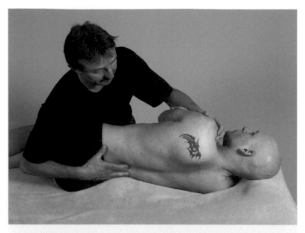

Fig. 10.15 Palpating lateral flexion and rotation.

segments. For this reason, the therapist compares sides when assessing the range of local motion while still being aware of what is happening in the neighboring segments (▶ Fig. 10.15).

The ZAJs and their capsules stand out in anatomical specimens with their astoundingly large ball-like form. Their position is approximately at the level of the inferior edge of a spinous process. To palpate the ZAJs, the therapist must overcome a layer several centimeters thick (25–35 mm) consisting of the thoracolumbar fascia and the multifidus (Bjordal et al., 2003) (▶ Fig. 10.16). In my opinion, it is not possible to locate the joint by palpating the contours, feeling the different consistencies of the tissues, or through the use of palpation under movement. Pain can be provoked by applying pressure to the soft tissue. However, it is not possible to definitely attribute the pain on pressure to the involvement of the ZAJs.

10.3.4 Detailed Anatomy of the Ligaments

Four ligamentous systems can be differentiated from one another in the lumbar spine:
- Vertebral body ligaments.
- Columns of segmental ligaments.
- Additional lumbar ligaments.
- Thoracolumbar fascia.

Vertebral Body Ligaments

Both longitudinal ligamentous columns accompany the entire vertebral column: the *anterior and the posterior longitudinal ligaments.* These ligaments are also part of the basic ligamentous structures found in a segment (▶ Fig. 10.17).

The **anterior longitudinal ligament** (ALL) is found anterior to the foramen magnum and extends down to the sacrum where it attaches inseparably onto the periosteum. It becomes increasingly wider more inferiorly. Superficial layers skip over four to five vertebrae. Deeper

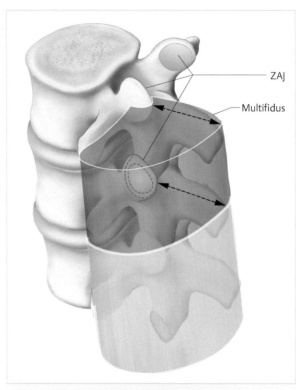

Fig. 10.16 The position of the lumbar zygapophysial joints (ZAJs) under the muscles.

layers connect two neighboring vertebrae (Bogduk, 2000). All sections of the ligament are attached to the middle of the vertebral body and are not firmly connected to the intervertebral disk's anulus fibrosus. This ligament helps to restrict lumbar extension and prevent an increase in lordosis.

The **posterior longitudinal ligament** (PLL) is also made up of two layers. The superficial layer runs in a longitudinal direction and is thin. The deep layer runs in a transverse direction and is wider. It connects to the anulus

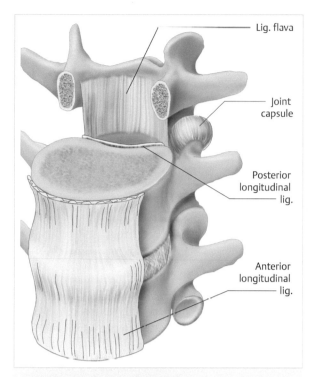

Fig. 10.17 Vertebral body ligaments.

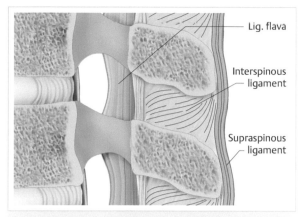

Fig. 10.18 Ligamenta flava and the supraspinous and interspinous ligaments.

fibrosus, reinforcing the disk. This ligament passes from the occiput to the coccyx, just like the anterior longitudinal ligament. The ligament has special nomenclature in its upper cervical section and at the lumbosacral junction. In comparison to the ALL, the PLL possesses a high number of nociceptors and acts as an alarm bell for certain pathological conditions in the intervertebral disk.

Columns of Segmental Ligaments

A row of short ligaments is found between the vertebral arches and the protruding processes, each connecting two vertebrae.

In young people, the **ligamenta flava** (▶ Fig. 10.18) are mainly made of elastic fibers. They extend between the laminae of the vertebral arch and line the posterior side of the vertebral canal. These ligaments are under tension even in an upright posture. When the trunk is flexed, these ligaments are placed under increasing tension, save energy, and help the vertebral column to return to an upright posture, therefore reducing the required muscle power. The anterior section of the zygapophysial joint capsules is formed by the ligamenta flava.

The **intertransverse ligaments** are quite thin and membranelike in the lumbar spine. They connect the transverse processes—called the costal processes here—and are placed under tension when contralateral lateral flexion and rotation are performed.

The **interspinous ligaments** (▶ Fig. 10.18) stretch between the spinous processes of two neighboring vertebrae. The literature describes the alignment of the fibers quite differently. The details vary from a vertical alignment, via the anterosuperior course of fibers (Netter, 2004), to the posterosuperior course of fibers (Bogduk, 2000), demonstrating the need for clarification in descriptive anatomy. All authors agree that these ligaments limit flexion and rotation.

The **supraspinous ligament** (▶ Fig. 10.18) is found superficial to the spinous processes and is basically the only ligament that can be palpated in the lumbar spine. This structure should not be seen as a ligament. Rather, it should be viewed as a doubling of the thoracolumbar fascia. Vleeming commented on this (personal communication, 2003): "The supraspinous ligament is really an anatomical specimen artifact."

The following relationships are currently being discussed:

- The superficial layers of this fascia meet at the midline.
- The connecting line is reinforced with ligament-like structures.
- A section is attached to the periosteum of the spinous processes.
- The other section is found in the interspinous space, forms the interspinous ligaments, and even extends into the ligamenta flava deep inside the movement segment.

As already described, it is very difficult to palpate the posterior aspect of the spinous processes due to their irregular contours and undulating shape. The presence of the supraspinous ligament makes it even more difficult to feel the interspinous space when searching for the boundaries to the neighboring vertebra using palpation. The supraspinous ligament is absent between L5 and S1 (Heylings, 1978, in Bogduk, 2000). This may contribute to

10

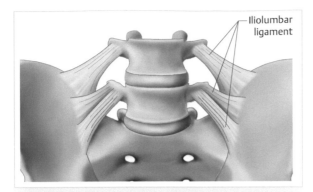

Fig. 10.19 Iliolumbar ligaments (simplified illustration).

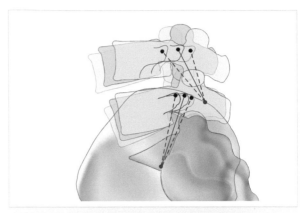

Fig. 10.20 Iliolumbar ligaments (simplified illustration).

the fact that the lower edge of L5 can be palpated well (see the section "Local Bony Palpation" below).

Additional Lumbar Ligaments

The **iliolumbar ligaments** (▶ Fig. 10.19) are the most important complex of ligaments that have contact with the lumbar spine but arise elsewhere. They run from different points on the L4 and L5 costal processes to the anterior aspect of the iliac crest and the ala of the ilium. The individual sections vary in their construction and are connected to the lumbar segmental ligaments and the sacroiliac ligaments (Pool-Goudzwaard et al., 2001).

The iliolumbar ligaments are also described in the anatomical literature (von Lanz and Wachsmuth, 2004a) as a continuation of the intertransverse ligaments, partially as a reinforcement of the thoracolumbar fascia (middle layer), as well as fibrotic parts of the quadratus lumborum. The position of these structures becomes apparent when the ligament is seen on an anatomical specimen. They are hidden beneath the several-centimeters-thick layer of intrinsic back muscles and lie in a tight corner between the transverse processes and the pelvis.

Individual fibers run along the frontal plane and restrict lateral flexion and rotation at L4-S1. The fibers are also arranged in a variety of ways in the sagittal plane (▶ Fig. 10.19 and ▶ Fig. 10.20), limiting flexion and extension (Yamamoto et al., 1990) and helping to prevent the lowermost free vertebra from gliding anteriorly (Bogduk, 2000).

Muscle activity can most likely assist the deep lumbar stability to a large extent by placing these ligaments under tension.

The iliolumbar ligaments help to control lateral flexion and rotation, especially at L5-S1. This action must be considered when palpating during movement.

Some textbooks (Chaitow, 2001) recommend palpating these ligaments for diagnostic purposes.

Readers should form their own opinion as to whether diagnostically conclusive palpation through the thoracolumbar fascia and the erector spinae, 5 to 7 cm deep, is possible.

Thoracolumbar Fascia

The collagenous fibers of the thoracolumbar fascia define the appearance during the inspection of an anatomical specimen of this region. The significance of the sacroiliac (SI) joint has already been described in Chapter 9 on "Posterior Pelvis." It is mentioned there that the superficial parts of the gluteus maximus radiate into the fascia. The collagenous fibers of the latissimus dorsi and gluteus maximus cross over the mid-line when they do this and are connected diagonally with each other (see the section "Ilium—Posterior Superior Iliac Spine" in Chapter 9).

More dynamizing structures are added to this in the lumbar region:

- Superficial layer: serratus posterior inferior.
- Middle layer:
  - Transversus abdominis.
  - Internal oblique.
  - Quadratus lumborum.
  - Erector spinae.

The **superficial layer of the fascia,** the aponeurotic area of origin for the latissimus dorsi, extends from the thoracolumbar junction to the iliac crests, covering the entire lumbar spine and sacral areas. The latissimus aponeurosis turns into a solid ligamentous plate (▶ Fig. 10.21). According to Vleeming (personal communication), the tensile loading capacity amounts to 500 kg and the plate is up to 1 cm thick.

The fibers within the fascia have a meshlike construction and do not only correspond to the continuation of the latissimus fibers that come from a superolateral position and point inferomedially. The fascia is at its widest at the level of L3, where it measures approximately 12 cm in width. It is narrowest at the level of T12.

Below T12, the fibers radiate into the fascial fibers on the contralateral side. They continue over the sacrum as the posterior sacroiliac ligament.

The **middle fascial layer** is also a solid aponeurosis. It stretches between the most inferior ribs, the L1-L4 costal processes, and the iliac crests (▶ Fig. 10.22). It separates the back extensors from the quadratus lumborum. In contrast to the superficial layer, the middle layer appears to be a site of origin for the lateral tract muscles and the quadratus lumborum. The foundation for this strong tendinous plate is the aponeurosis, which is the site of origin for the transversus abdominis (von Lanz and Wachsmuth, 2004a). The fibers from the internal oblique, in particular, radiate into this.

Barker et al. (2006) found in a study that the tension in the middle fascial layer significantly increases segmental stiffness and the resistance to flexion. According to their conclusions, tension in the fascia plays a significant role in segmental stability.

Richardson et al. (1999) also state that the multifidus and transversus abdominis provide basic stability for the lumbar spine (▶ Fig. 10.23). They described the relationship between delayed activation of the transversus abdominis and lumbar symptoms.

The muscle is normally activated approximately 4 ms before the trunk or the limbs start moving. Core stability is first built up before proceeding with further action. The muscle is activated too late in patients suffering from back pain. Based on these results, Richardson et al. (1999) developed an exercise program that is currently a source of discussion and used for therapeutic approaches.

Both layers of the thoracolumbar fascia are connected immediately lateral to the back extensors at the lateral raphe (▶ Fig. 10.24). Both of the fascial layers and the serratus posterior inferior form an osteofibrous channel with the vertebral arch and the processes. This channel is the guiding sheath for the erector spinae. The anatomy of this can be recognized by looking at the loose connective tissue superior to the sacrum positioned between the back extensors and the fascia. The osteofibrotic guiding sheath bundles up the back extensors and holds these muscles on the vertebral column when the muscles contract.

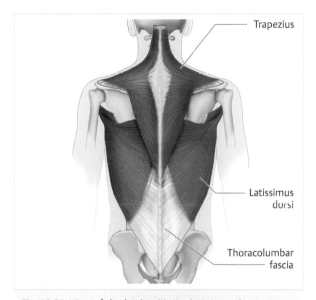

Fig. 10.21 View of the fascia with the latissimus dorsi.

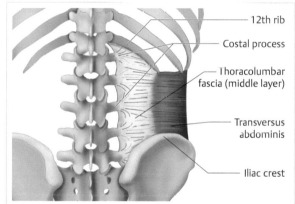

Fig. 10.22 Middle layer of the thoracolumbar fascia with transversus abdominis.

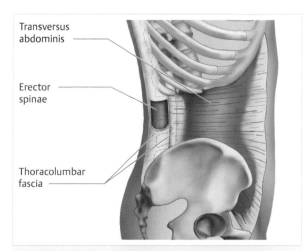

Fig. 10.23 Transversus abdominis.

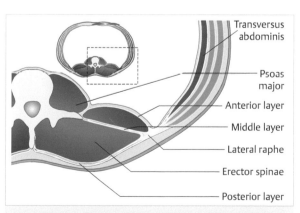

Fig. 10.24 The three layers of the thoracolumbar fascia.

10

The back extensors protrude more than the spinous processes. Together with the firm sheath of fascia on both sides, they form a type of depression over the row of spinous processes. The depth of this can differ depending on the lumbar lordosis form and the bulk of the back extensors. This means that the spinous processes can be reached here quite easily.

The osteofibrotic sheath turns the back extensors into a uniform muscle packet. Its medial side can be completely pushed away from the row of spinous processes and displaced laterally. This characteristic is taken advantage of in the different classical massage and functional massage techniques (▶ Fig. 10.25).

The compact fibrotic layer is up to 1 cm thick and raises a question about the accessibility of the muscular structures. The compact fascia prevents the muscle from being directly palpated when the therapist wishes to assess the muscles' consistency with palpation.

The positioning of patients during diagnosis and treatment is affected by the compact superficial fascia and a number of muscle fibers merging directly and indirectly into it. The patients should be placed in an SP that maximally relaxes or tenses the structure, depending on the aim. The minimal requirements for relaxation in the lumbar region are the physiological lordosis and not allowing the arms to be fully raised in the prone or side-lying positions.

10.3.5 Detailed Anatomy of the Muscles

Only the muscles that are important for the palpation of the lumbar region will be described in the following text:
- Latissimus dorsi.
- Intrinsic back muscles—medial tract.
- Intrinsic back muscles—lateral tract.
- Action of the lumbar muscles.

The innervation through the lateral branch of the dorsal ramus of the spinal nerve belonging to the segment is typical for this intrinsic muscle group. In terms of function, all superficial back muscles belong to the upper extremity and are generally innervated by a ventral ramus (to the brachial plexus) of a spinal nerve.

Latissimus Dorsi

This muscle was ontogenetically a gill muscle. The site of origin of the latissimus dorsi has been relocated quite inferiorly. As a consequence, its innervation from the thoracodorsal nerve (C6-C8) was relocated with the muscle.

The nomenclature for its sites of origin is divided into thoracic, lumbar, iliac, costal, and scapular areas. Its aponeurosis of origin is identical to the superficial layer of the thoracolumbar fascia (▶ Fig. 10.26). The thoracic site of origin is generally stated to be at the T7-T8 level but can vary greatly. The iliac origin is likewise very variable. The side edge of the site of origin is generally sought at the level of the most superiorly protruding part of the iliac crest (von Lanz and Wachsmuth, 2004a), though it may also be found further medial or lateral.

The 3- to 4-cm-wide and approximately 8- to 10-cm-long tendon of insertion travels together with the teres major's tendon of insertion toward the crest of the lesser tubercle at the humerus.

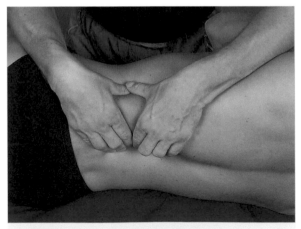

Fig. 10.25 Lumbar functional massage.

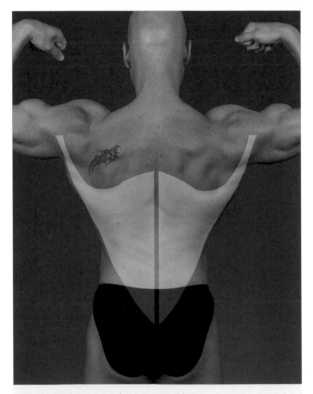

Fig. 10.26 Latissimus dorsi on an athlete.

Its function is not limited to the open kinematic chain, it also acts as a strong adductor to move the body around a fixed point in a closed chain (e.g., when a person supports themselves on parallel bars). Together with the teres muscles, it decelerates the forward swing of the arms during gait. Activity in the latissimus dorsi dynamizes the superficial layer of the thoracolumbar fascia and can therefore affect lumbar stability.

Aside from toned and very slender people (▶ Fig. 10.26), most people have a thin latissimus dorsi. This means that the muscle belly rarely presents itself with a clearly definable contour. Only the lateral edge can be palpated in the thoracic area during contraction (see the Tip box in Chapter 11).

Intrinsic Back Muscles—Medial Tract

The medial tract consists of sections that run over one segment and sections that are multisegmental. It lies close to the vertebral column in the triangular depression between the spinous and transverse processes (▶ Fig. 10.27). The muscles originate and insert into the processes of the lumbar vertebrae. The posterior aspect of the sacrum is the only exception here. The medial tract muscles are mostly covered by voluminous muscle bellies and the aponeuroses of origin for the muscles in the lateral tract (longissimus). The muscle groups belonging to the medial tract are typically innervated by the medial branch of the dorsal rami arising from the spinal nerve that belongs to the segment.

The small muscles mostly run over **one segment**. They can finely position the lumbar vertebrae and assist in the development of the necessary axial compression for the approximation of vertebrae with the use of tissue strength. The transversospinales appear to be functionally more important than the straight system. Von Lanz and Wachsmuth (2004a) have commented on this: "The transversospinales muscle strand represents the most important tensile system in the vertebral column."

The muscular sections of this system extend over three to six segments and are most clearly developed in the lumbar region. They are labeled the multifidus lumborum

(▶ Fig. 10.28). The origin can be followed to the third sacral vertebra in the space between the median sacral crest and the intermedial sacral crest. As described in the section "Sacrum—Insertion of the Multifidus" in Chapter 9, contractions in this muscle can also be palpated there. In von Lanz and Wachsmuth (2004a), it is further said: "Its mass of flesh represents a slab oriented in the sagittal plane. Its side surfaces are rounded and appear as a swelling bulge as soon as the aponeurosis of origin for longissimus is separated from the spinous processes."

The sections of the longissimus are quite thin and tendonlike in the lower lumbar and sacral regions. The multifidus can therefore be palpated very well and is sometimes visible directly paravertebrally (approximately 1.5 cm adjacent to the spinous process) from the sacrum up to the level of L3 (▶ Fig. 10.29). It becomes more difficult superior to this as the covering muscle becomes thicker.

The advantage of the muscle being palpable becomes obvious when the stabilizing function of the multifidus is being trained. The patient can attempt to selectively contract the multifidus using palpation for feedback. Hochschild (2001) labels the multifidus as the "key muscle for the segmental stabilization of the lumbar spine."

Intrinsic Back Muscles—Lateral Tract

The lateral tract of the back extensors is made up of two strong individual muscles in the lumbar region. These muscles represent the largest section of the palpable paravertebral muscles (▶ Fig. 10.30):

• Longissimus (lumbar part, thoracis, cervicis, capitis).
• Iliocostalis (lumbar part, thoracic part, cervicis).

The layout of both of these lateral tract muscles in the individual sections of the vertebral column results in the muscles being divided into many sections. The longissimus is the only muscle that extends with one section to the skull. This muscle group is typically innervated by the

10

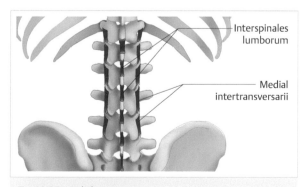

Fig. 10.27 Medial tract.

Interspinales lumborum

Medial intertransversarii

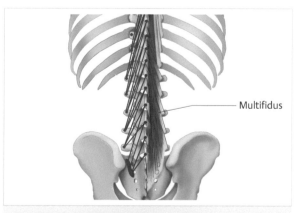

Fig. 10.28 Multifidus lumborum.

Multifidus

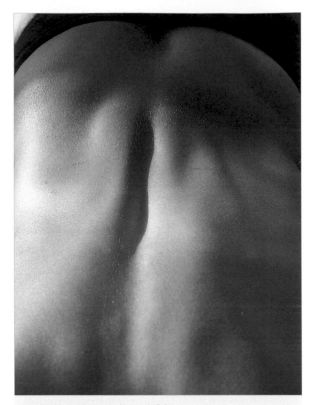

Fig. 10.29 Activity in the multifidus.

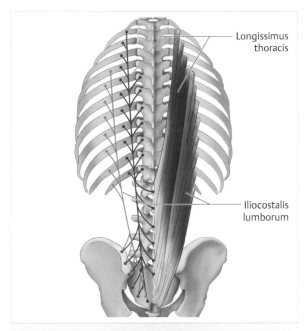

Fig. 10.30 Lateral tract of the intrinsic back muscles.

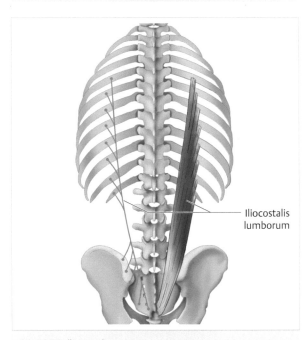

Fig. 10.31 Iliocostalis.

lateral branch of the dorsal rami arising from the spinal nerve that belongs to the segment.

The **longissimus** is found more medial and inserts with spikes only. These spikes are noticeable on the ribs. It lies on top of the medial section of the multifidus. It forms a thin tendinous plate in the lower lumbar region, which allows activity in the multifidus to be felt directly adjacent to the vertebral column. Its origin extends over the posterior surface of the sacrum between the intermedial sacral crest and the lateral sacral crest.

The **iliocostalis** (▶ Fig. 10.31), on the other hand, is located lateral and more superficial. Its origin extends from the lateral aspect of the sacrum to the iliac crest, covering the medial section of the quadratus lumborum. The muscle originates and inserts further onto the ribs and the rudiments of the ribs only. Both layers of the thoracolumbar fascia meet lateral to the muscle belly.

The Actions of the Lumbar Muscles

Bilateral activity in the back extensors controls and moves the trunk in the sagittal plane. The back extensors tense quickly on both sides when the trunk is displaced anteriorly and work eccentrically until approximately 60° flexion (▶ Fig. 10.32). The gluteus maximus helps to control **trunk flexion**. The back extensors do not have any active function beyond 60° flexion. The back extensors' passive resistance to stretch, the thoracolumbar fascia, and the ligaments found posterior to the movement axis now take over the action of stabilizing the trunk.

Activity, especially activity arising from the medial tract and the tension in passive structures, results in a build up of axial compression. This should be seen as the approximation of the vertebrae using tissue strength. This

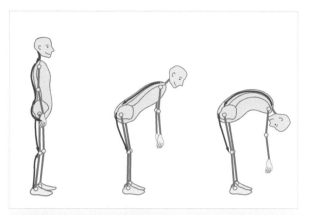

Fig. 10.32 Bending the trunk forward / slings of muscles shown during trunk flexion. The thoracolumbar fascia and the posterior ligaments carry the weight of the upper body in the right figure.

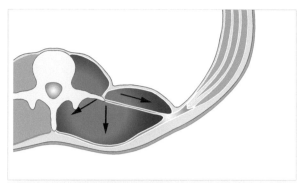

Fig. 10.33 Pumping up the thoracolumbar fascia.

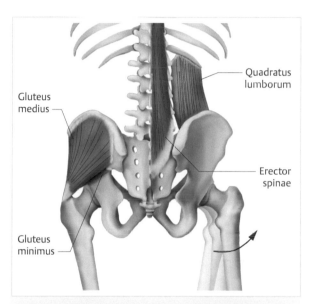

Fig. 10.34 The synergy of the back extensors—small gluteal muscles. The trunk is displaced to the left, the right trunk muscles and the left gluteals work together.

activity increases the stability in the vertebral column, which is intrinsically a mobile chain. The psoas stabilizes anteriorly when the trunk is extended, especially in the upper lumbar section.

One of the most important functions of the intrinsic back muscles is to tighten up the **thoracolumbar fascia** from inside outward (personal communication, Vleeming, 2006). This can be compared with pumping up a bicycle tube (▶ Fig. 10.33) and is achieved when the muscle belly becomes thicker during contraction. This illustrates the therapeutic use of hypertrophic back extensors.

The intrinsic back muscles are only slightly active in the **upright standing** position when the body weight is distributed evenly between the two legs. It is only in the thoracic region that constant activity is necessary to prevent falling. This is due to the weight of the thorax always pulling the vertebral column into flexion (Klein-Vogelbach, 2000).

Shifting the body's weight from both legs onto one leg, for example, onto the left leg, results in unilateral activity in an entire synergy on the right side (▶ Fig. 10.34):
- Erector spinae.
- Quadratus lumborum from the deep abdominal muscle group.
- Internal and external obliques from the side trunk wall muscles.

This activity in the muscles aims to prevent the pelvis from lowering on the right side. This occurs in cooperation with the small gluteals on the weight-bearing side (on the left here).

The back and the lateral trunk wall muscles have several functions during walking:
- They provide the impulse for walking (according to Gracovetsky, 1989) using rotation and lateral flexion.

Alternating concentric (start of the swing phase) and eccentric (end of the swing phase) activity causes lateral flexion in particular.
- They act as antagonists to the abdominal muscles. The arms swing during walking and give the upper body a rotational impulse. This movement has to be decelerated by the abdominal muscles. The tendency to flex during abdominal muscle contraction is counteracted by the extending strength of the back muscles.

In total, the muscle activity in standing and during walking is shaped by the constant change from concentric to eccentric activity. This should be integrated into the therapeutic concept for stabilizing treatment: vertical position and alternating activity with impulses for rotation and lateral flexion.

10

10.3.6 Basic Biomechanical Principles

The **lumbar segment** is a kinematic chain consisting of three links—one intervertebral disk and two zygapophysial joints. The three components all affect each other. In a healthy segment, the axes for movement are found in the disk (▶ Fig. 10.35). This results in little translational movement and a lot of tilting. A loss of height in the intervertebral disk shifts the axes and more shear forces develop (White and Panjabi, 1990).

Symmetrical Movement

The joint surfaces glide together (convergent movement) during extension (extension, lordosis) and away from each other (divergent movement, ▶ Fig. 10.36) during flexion (flexion, flattening out of the lordosis).

Asymmetrical Movements

Lateral flexion is inevitably combined with rotation in all sections of the vertebral column. Rotation likewise always occurs with simultaneous lateral flexion. This is known as a coupled movement. The direction of the associated movement in the lumbar spine changes according to whether the vertebral column is positioned in flexion or extension.

Coupled and Combined Movements

When the functional section from T10/T11 to L5/S1 is flexed, lateral flexion is automatically accompanied by an ipsilateral axial rotation:
- Flexion and lateral flexion to the right with rotation to the right (▶ Fig. 10.37).
- Flexion and lateral flexion to the left with rotation to the left.

In the extended position (e.g., physiological lordosis), lateral flexion is automatically accompanied by contralateral axial rotation. This applies to all segments:
- Extension and lateral flexion to the right with rotation to the left (▶ Fig. 10.38).
- Extension and lateral flexion to the left with rotation to the right.

Movements are always coupled in the same direction in older patients.

This coupling of movements occurs automatically during active and passive movements unless the therapist decides to consciously position the lumbar spine differently. Every other combination of rotation and lateral flexion is labeled as combined, or not coupled. Manual therapy uses combined positioning in the vertebral column to lock a joint as firmly as possible.

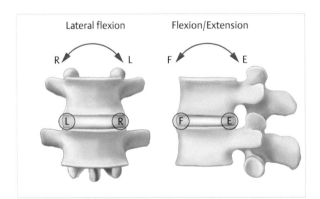

Fig. 10.35 Position of the movement axes.

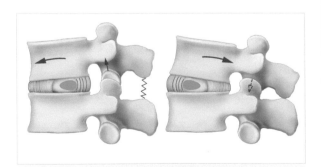

Fig. 10.36 Divergence and convergence.

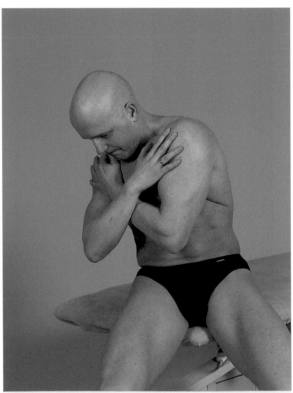

Fig. 10.37 Coupled position in flexion.

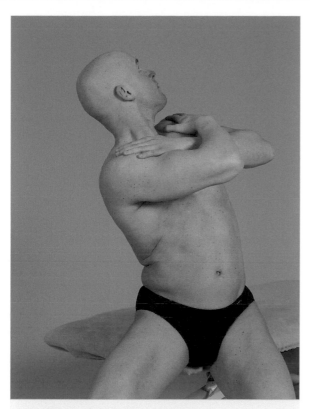

Fig. 10.38 Coupled position in extension.

Symmetrical and coupled movements can be used to assess segmental movement and to diagnose a restriction in mobility (see the section "Local Segmental Mobility Using Coupled Movements" below).

10.4 Overview of the Structures to be Palpated

Projections are used for orientation by defining the level of a structure and using connecting lines in the prone SP:
• Connection between the iliac crest (Jacoby's line) and PSIS.
• Lumbosacral cross.

Local bony palpation is used for the location of the lumbar spinous processes:
• Palpating from an inferior position via the S2 onto L5 spinous processes.
• Locating additional lumbar spinous processes.
• Palpating from a superior position via the T11 spinous process.

10.5 Summary of the Palpatory Process

Determining the exact level of an affected segment is vital for some tests and treatment techniques. Therapists can only orient themselves in the lumbar region when the spinous processes have been palpated correctly. This is, and will always be, no simple task, even after the therapist has gained some experience. The therapist should therefore know how to approach the palpation of the lumbar spinous processes. It helps to be able to visualize the expected form and consistency of structures and to use a couple of aids to confirm the correct location.

To correctly and specifically locate lumbar structures, several techniques are needed that have already been described in Chapter 9:
• Locating the iliac crest, described in "Palpatory Techniques for Quick Orientation on the Bones" (Chapter 9) and "Local Palpation Techniques" (Chapter 9).
• Locating the posterior sacroiliac spine (PSIS), described in the section "Local Bony Palpation" below).

There are vague but also rather precise methods available to therapists for orientation in the lumbar spine using palpation. The appropriate technique is used depending on the purpose and on the amount of time available. The following palpatory procedure involves the methods available for quick orientation when attempting to locate the level of L4 and S2.

The spinous process is the only directly accessible part of the lumbar vertebra. All other parts remain palpatory speculation. The ZAJ and the transverse process are found beneath centimeter-thick muscles. They can only be indirectly reached and, at times, pain may be provoked when the therapist applies pressure here. The spinous process is therefore the only reliable starting point available for the location of levels, pain provocation, and the assessment of segmental mobility. It is therefore necessary to exactly identify and label the spinous process.

10.6 Starting Position

The prone position is preferable. The patient is positioned in individual physiological lordosis. "Individual physiological" refers to the curvature seen when the patient is standing. This position is mainly achieved with the patient lying flat on the stomach. This results in a mid-position between extension and flexion that is suitable for the assessment of segmental mobility. Padding underneath the abdomen and pelvis flex the lumbar spine, and the spinous processes are moved further away from one another. This opens up the interspinous space, and the posterior soft tissues (supraspinous ligament and multifidus) are placed under more tension. The palpation tends to become more difficult depending on the amount of padding used.

Positioning the lumbar spine in an extreme lordosis, for example, with the patient using the elbows for support, approximates the spinous processes to an extent that makes it almost impossible to differentiate individual spinous processes to determine the level of a structure.

10

When in the prone position, it is generally not recommended to place padding underneath the abdomen before starting to palpate. It will not always facilitate location of the spinous processes. The interspinous spaces are very narrow and extremely difficult to differentiate from one another. A narrowing of the interspinous spaces by additionally increasing the lordosis before starting palpation is therefore to be avoided. All other types of patient positioning alter the typical movement pattern during segmental tests.

10.6.1 Positioning in the Frontal Plane

The therapist should ensure that the patient's pelvis is not shifted to one side when they are lying on their stomach. The pelvic shift corresponds to a lateral flexion that is initiated from inferior and particularly involves the lower lumbar segments.

The neutral prone position in this plane is not essential when the spinous processes are only being located and differentiated from one another. A non-neutral position changes the movement pattern when palpation is combined with the assessment of segmental mobility.

10.6.2 Positioning in the Transverse Plane

The therapist should also ensure that the vertebral column is not rotated before starting to palpate. Once the patient has adapted the prone position, the therapist checks whether both of the anterior superior iliac spines (ASISs) are in contact with the treatment table or are found with at least the same distance to the table. Rotation in the pelvis can be corrected if necessary.

Further comments and figures related to the prone position can be found in Chapter 8.

10.6.3 Difficult and Alternative Starting Positions

Neutral Side-lying

The more painful side is usually positioned uppermost for assessment and treatment. The therapist must ensure that the entire vertebral column is positioned with its natural or individually determined curvature. The presence of lateral flexion should be corrected using padding.

Vertical Body Positions

The sitting or standing SP always compounds the palpation of the spinous processes or the deep-lying structures due to activity in the muscles. The advantage of these SPs is the greater variety of coupled movements possible compared with the prone position. When the spinous processes can be palpated well in sitting, accurate information regarding segmental mobility can be gained.

10.7 Palpation Techniques

10.7.1 Orienting Projections

Only a few reference points are needed to locate a level relatively precisely when the therapist wishes to quickly orient themselves at the lumbosacral junction.

Connection between the Iliac Crest and the Posterior Sacroiliac Spine (PSIS)

The iliac crest is located on one side using one of the two previously described techniques (Chapter 9.7.2). The technique variation using the perpendicular palpation from superior is recommended. The most superior point on the iliac crest is marked on the skin to secure the palpation results. This step is repeated on the other side.

Both marks are then connected. An interspinous space is sought at the point where the connecting line meets the body's mid-line (see ► Fig. 10.39).

The specifications regarding the spinous process that will be found here are documented very differently in the literature. Chakraverty et al. 2007 found that there is considerable variability in localization by palpation and with imaging. When women and men are palpated, the result varies between processus spinosus from L3 to L4, most often at L3. With imaging in both men and women, the Jacoby line is obtained between processus spinosus L4 to L4-L5, most often processus spinosus L4. The Kappa agreement between the results of palpation and imaging

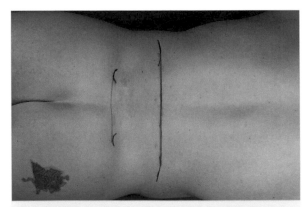

Fig. 10.39 Connecting the iliac crests and the posterior sacroiliac spines (PSISs).

(x-ray) = 0.05. The palpated level was on average 1–2 levels higher than x-rayed. These results were confirmed by a review by Cooperstein and Troung 2017.

The next step involves locating the PSIS and marking its most inferior boundary (lower edge) on the skin. The techniques for this have been described in Chapter 9.7.3. The lower edges of both PSISs are connected with a line. This line always (in 81%, McGaugh, 2007) passes over the S2 spinous process (▶ Fig. 10.39).

Lumbosacral Cross

A line is drawn between the right iliac crest and the left PSIS and another line between the left iliac crest and the right PSIS (▶ Fig. 10.40). In most cases, the point where these two lines meet indicates the position of the L5 spinous process. This quick method for orientation delivers more reliable results than locating the level by connecting the two iliac crests.

10.7.2 Local Bony Palpation

The aim is to correctly locate the lumbar spinous processes. This is achieved by following the steps below:
- Coming from an inferior position via the S2 spinous process.
- Locating additional lumbar spinous processes.
- Coming from a superior position via the T11 spinous process.

All spinous processes of the functional section of the lumbar spine will be located. This extends from T10/T11 to L5/S1.

Palpating from an Inferior Position via the S2 Spinous Process

Locating the lumbar spinous process from an inferior position is the most common and reliable method. The reliability of the palpatory findings, especially for L5 and L4, depends on the exact location of the PSIS and the S2 spinous process. This has been described in detail in Chapter 9.7.3. The palpation is now continued in a more superior direction.

Step 1: The inferior edges of both PSISs are located. The line connecting these two points marks the position of S2 (▶ Fig. 10.41). This rudimental spinous process is usually perceived as a significant elevation when palpated. The technique used here is where the finger pads palpate using slightly circulating movements.

Step 2: The finger pads slide approximately 1 cm superiorly and search for a small, rounded elevation that represents the remainder of the S1 process (▶ Fig. 10.42). In doing so, the fingers move anteriorly down a slanting slope. A large amount of variation is seen in S1; everything is possible. S1 can be as large as S2, it can be only a minimally palpable elevation, or be completely absent.

Step 3: The L5 spinous process is found approximately 1 finger width (patient's index finger) superior to S1. Its lower edge is reached by sliding the finger pads superiorly over the slanting sacrum until the tips of the fingers come across an explicitly hard object (▶ Fig. 10.43). The inferior edge of L5 is mostly felt to be a step superior to the L5-S1 interspinous space.

10

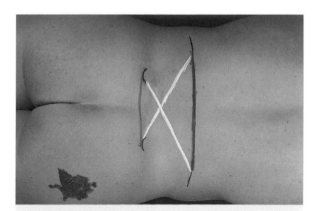

Fig. 10.40 Lumbosacral cross.

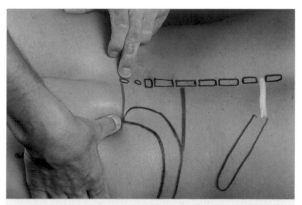

Fig. 10.41 Location of the S2 spinous process.

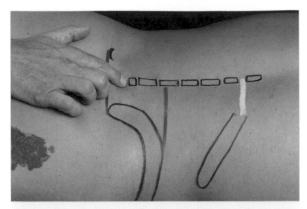

Fig. 10.42 Location of the S1 spinous process.

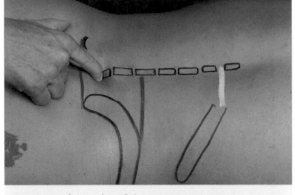

Fig. 10.43 Inferior edge of the L5 spinous process.

Comments on Pathology

In cases of severe spondylolisthesis in L5-S1, a local increase in the lordosis with the formation of a step can be palpated between L5 and S1 on slim patients (ski jump on phenomenon; Wittenberg et al., 1998). This palpatory result can be reached in the prone or standing SP.

> **Caution**
>
> These conclusions may not be reversed! Not every palpated step has to indicate the presence of a spondylolisthesis.

Confirming the Palpation Using the Shape and Size of Structures

Based on the anatomy described, it is normally expected that the L5 spinous process has a smaller and rounded shape that juts out posteriorly. The L1-L4 spinous processes are very long (superior-inferior dimensions). Despite this anatomical knowledge, it may be confusing and difficult to locate L5, especially when the S1 spinous process has a distinct form. In this case, its shape and size are similar to L5.

Confirmation Using the Assessment of End Feel

Using anteriorly directed pressure to differentiate between L5 and S1 is diagnostically conclusive. The medial side of the hand is placed on the point where the therapist assumes S1 to be. The other hand is placed on top of it (▶ Fig. 10.44). The therapist then pushes the hand in an anterior direction using slow oscillations. If pain is not provoked by this, the therapist pushes down firmly one more time to clearly assess the posteroanterior end feel.

The same maneuver is performed over the point where the therapist assumes L5 to be. The thumb is first placed over the point to emphasize the pointed spinous process

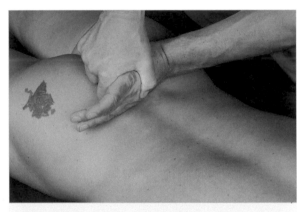

Fig. 10.44 Posteroanterior pressure on S1.

(▶ Fig. 10.45). The thumb is then reinforced using the medial side of the other hand or the thenar eminence (▶ Fig. 10.46). Rhythmical posteroanterior pressure is then reapplied and the sequence finishes with the end feel being assessed by firm pressure.

The results of both of the posteroanterior pushes are now compared. It is expected that S1 will only minimally yield to pressure and that its end feel will be almost hard. L5 usually yields significantly more to pressure and has a firm-elastic end feel.

> **Tip**
>
> Naturally, this differentiation technique should not be performed if the therapist suspects it will provoke pain.

Confirmation Using Movement

Another option is to feel the way L5 moves when posteroanterior pressure is applied. The therapist starts by searching for the assumed position of the L5/S1 interspinous space with a fingertip. Both of the neighboring spinous processes should be felt. The thumb or the

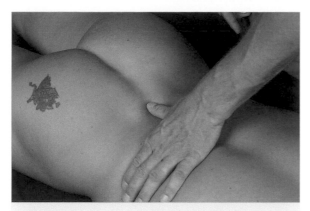

Fig. 10.45 Assessment of end feel at L5—phase 1.

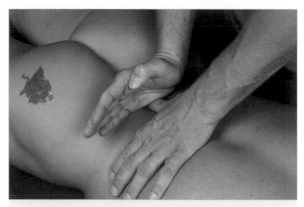

Fig. 10.46 Assessment of end feel at L5—phase 2.

hypothenar eminence is then used to apply pressure to the superiorly located spinous process. It is expected that the superiorly lying spinous process moves anteriorly and the inferior spinous process stays still. This attempt at differentiation between the assumed location of S1 and S2 results in no movement. This technique is also used to differentiate between the other lumbar spinous processes (see section "Locating Additional Lumbar Spinous Processes").

Tip

Both of the last tests for confirmation are based on the presumption that L5 moves anteriorly when a postero-anterior pressure is applied and that S1 remains immobile. Regardless of how helpful and informative both of these tests may be, some inaccuracy remains. These tests are not useful when variations in the anatomy are present in terms of hemisacralization or restriction in segmental movement at L5/S1. In this case, the position of L5 can only be confirmed by comparing its size to L4 and L3. These spinous processes are usually significantly longer than L5.

Summary

- Locate the PSIS and the S2 spinous process.
- Palpate in a superior direction from S2 onto S1.
- Palpate the inferior edge of the L5 spinous process.
- Confirm its position using a posteroanterior pressure with the assessment of end feel.
- Confirm its position using posteroanterior pressure with movement.
- When necessary, confirm its position by locating the first long spinous process (L4).

Locating Additional Lumbar Spinous Processes

The other lumbar spinous processes can be sought after the L5 spinous process has been located as correctly as possible. The therapist can be sure that the respective spinous process has been located correctly by:
- Examining its shape and size;
- Using movement to confirm the position.

As has already been mentioned, the L1-L4 spinous processes are rather broad and have an extremely irregular shape with indentations along their posterior aspect, giving them an undulating appearance. The waves formed by the spinous processes are found on the sides and posteriorly and imitate the presence of an interspinous space. To precisely locate the interspinous space, the therapist palpates along the side of the spinous process until a gap becomes apparent. It is less reliable to palpate posteriorly as the supraspinous ligament is solid, fibrotic, and may be tensed, preventing the therapist from gaining access to the expected gap.

Step 1: The inferior edge of L5 is marked using a short line. The therapist palpates to the side of this in a superior direction. The space between the L4 and L5 spinous processes is felt after a few millimeters (▶ Fig. 10.47). For good measure, the finger should be kept on the inferior edge of L5 for the moment. If the therapist is unable to find the inferior edge of L4, it is possible to start the procedure again from L5. The suspected location of the inferior edge of L4 is marked.

Step 2: The same technique is used to locate the L3 spinous process: the finger remains over L4/L5 and the next superiorly lying interspinous space is sought (▶ Fig. 10.48). All further spinous processes can be found using this method.

10

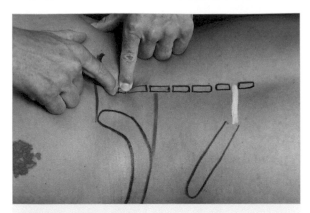

Fig. 10.47 Palpating L4/L5.

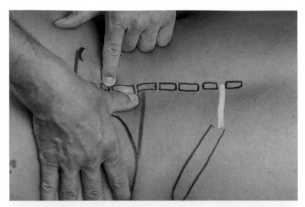

Fig. 10.48 Palpating L3/L4.

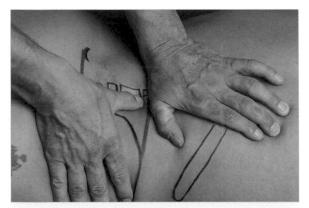

Fig. 10.49 Confirmation with movement.

Tip

The posteroanterior push does not have to be particularly strong. It is the returning movement, not the downward movement, that can be felt best. The posteroanterior push should therefore be released very quickly to ensure that the tip of the palpating finger can gain clearer information. When the anatomy of a patient makes location difficult, this technique may have to be repeated several times to confirm the correct palpation of the interspinous space. It is helpful to mark the superior and inferior edges of the spinous process so that the therapist can always proceed from a confirmed point. All spinous processes in the functional section of the lumbar spine can principally be found and marked on the skin using this method. The thoracolumbar junction is reached when the size of the spinous processes changes abruptly. The spinous processes are more pointed again superior to T12.

Palpating from a Superior Position via the T11 Spinous Process

Locating the T11 spinous process via the 12th rib is ideal for quick orientation in the thoracolumbar region. The tips of the 12th rib hang freely in the posterolateral trunk wall. **Step 1:** To find the 12th rib, the therapist first orients themselves on the lumbar back extensors and then moves laterally in the space between the iliac crest and the inferior costal arch. This space usually measures only 2 finger widths (▶ Fig. 10.50).
Step 2: A perpendicular technique is used next to confirm the position of the iliac crest (▶ Fig. 10.51). The therapist then turns the palpating fingers in a superior direction, attempts to locate the inferior edge of the 12th rib (▶ Fig. 10.52), and encounters a very firm structure relatively quickly.

Tip

Therapists should not let the length of the L4-L1 spinous processes unsettle them. They should trust their instincts.

Step 3—Confirmation with movement: To confirm the correct location of an interspinous space, the therapist moves the segment. The movement can be felt by the palpating finger. An interspinous space has been correctly located when the superiorly lying spinous process moves and the inferior spinous process remains immobile. This is achieved by placing a finger pad posteriorly over the interspinous space. The confirmation of the L3/L4 interspinous space is demonstrated in ▶ Fig. 10.49. The thumb pad applies oscillating posteroanterior pressure to the L4 spinous process superior to the position where the therapist assumes the interspinous space to be. The palpating finger pad can feel the superior spinous process moving up and down in the interspinous space.

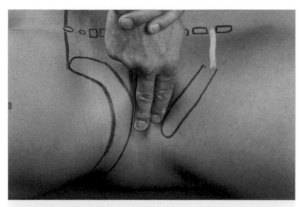

Fig. 10.50 Iliac crest and the 12th rib.

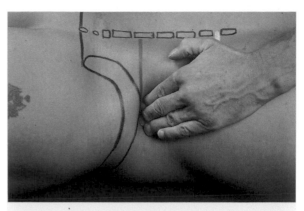

Fig. 10.51 Confirming the position of the iliac crest.

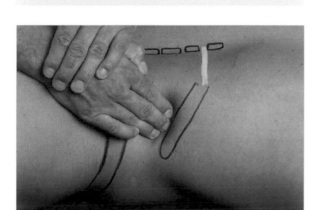

Fig. 10.52 Locating the 12th rib.

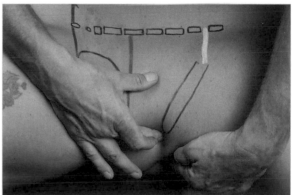

Fig. 10.53 Tip of the 12th rib.

10

Tip

It is important that the therapist palpates rather medially, near the back extensors. The therapist will palpate the 11th rib if they palpate too laterally. On pressure, the 12th rib does not have the typical hard osseous consistency. As already mentioned, this rib is relatively mobile and hangs freely in the trunk wall, making it more mobile than the ribs with direct or indirect contact to the sternum (1st—10th ribs). The 12th rib must be able to move out of the way of the iliac crest when extensive lateral flexion is being performed.

Step 3: This step involves confirming the location of the 12th rib. The inferior edge of the palpated rib is followed laterally along its length until the end of the rib is felt (▶ Fig. 10.53). The palpable end of the next superiorly lying rib should be located more laterally in the trunk wall.

Step 4: The palpating finger slides medially over the rib until the muscle mass of the erector spinae prevents the finger from maintaining direct contact with the rib (▶ Fig. 10.54). This point corresponds to the level of the T12 transverse process. The T11 spinous process is seen to be correctly located when the next superiorly lying spinous process above the level of the 12th rib and the T12 transverse process is found (▶ Fig. 10.55).

Step 5: Moving from here, the therapist can orient himself more inferiorly into the lumbar region or further superiorly into the thoracic spine (▶ Fig. 10.56).

Tip

Reliably locating the level depends very much on whether the 12th rib has been followed far enough medially. If this is not done accurately, the therapist will arrive at one level lower than expected. When the T11 spinous process has been correctly found, the next inferiorly located spinous process (T12) is pointed and short and the L1 spinous process is, in turn, very long.

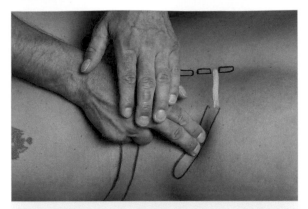

Fig. 10.54 Palpating in a medial direction.

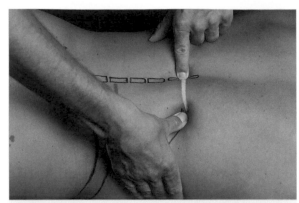

Fig. 10.55 Locating the level of the T11 spinous process.

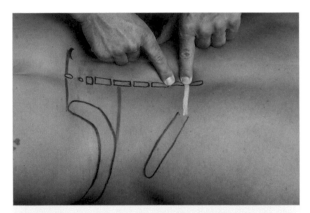

Fig. 10.56 Continuing palpation in the thoracolumbar region.

10.8 Tips for Treatment

10.8.1 Research Findings on Reliable Lumbar Palpation

The palpation of lumbar spinous processes is a standard procedure for both physicians and therapists (Nyberg and Russel Smith, 2013). It appears to be an indispensable skill for diagnosis and treatment (Kilby et al., 2012, Merz et al., 2013). Of the manipulative physical therapists surveyed by Carlesso et al. (2013) in Canada, 99% use this palpation.

The reliability and validity of the palpation of lumbar spinous processes is the subject of debate in the literature.

Downey et al. (1999) assess it very positively. Their study shows that physical therapists have 92% agreement for locating the randomly nominated spinal level of patients. For the study, the patients were in a relaxed prone position and were palpated by trained manipulative physical therapists.

Kilby et al. (2012) compare the agreement of manual palpation by experienced manual therapists of different lumbo-pelvic bony points with ultrasound images of the bony landmarks.

An Intra-class Correlation Coefficient (ICC) of 0.81 for all structures and 0.83 for the location of the L4 spinous process suggested that manual palpation may have acceptable validity.

Merz et al. (2013) carried out a validity study for palpation of the L5 vertebra with the patient in the sitting SP by an experienced physical therapist using three different techniques by comparing with location radiograph. The following techniques were used to locate the L5 vertebra:
• via the iliac crests.
• via the posterior superior iliac spine.
• through motion palpation.

The authors concluded that the accuracy of each single technique ranged from 45 to 61% and the combination of all three techniques ranged in accuracy from 69 to 83%.

The results of a study conducted by Mieritz and Kawcuk (2016) show that compared to diagnostic ultrasound for locating lumbar spinous processes, palpation is inferior, although the authors concede that the effort and time required for ultrasonic imaging is significantly higher than for manual palpation.

Schneider et al. (2008) conducted a study to determine the reliability of palpation of restricted lumbar segmental motion. The interrater reliability of two experienced doctors of chiropractic was 0.17. The kappa values for palpation for segmental pain provocation showed fair to good reliability (kappa values up to 0.73).

A study conducted by Brismée et al. (2005) evaluates interrater reliability of three experienced manual physical therapists performing motion testing of the L4 to L5 spinal segment of young subjects in side-lying position (▶ Fig. 10.60). Segmental rotation was determined in a coupled movement pattern. The testers were asked to indicate whether the greatest amount of segmental rotation was produced by lumbar lateral flexion either ipsilateral or contralateral to the direction of rotation. For this particular task, which involved determining which of the two segmental movements would produce the greatest segmental rotation, a maximum of 4% agreement was reached. Therefore, manual movement palpation is not recommended for this task.

Therapists and physicians use pain provocation and the assessment of stability and mobility as part of their diagnostic repertoire in the clinical assessment of the lumbar spine. Several reliable local segmental tests have emerged from this. The techniques, criteria, and interpretation of these tests will be described in the next section.

10.8.2 Test for Rotation (Transverse Vertebral Pressure)

The lumbar test for rotation (also called transverse vertebral pressure) is used in the local assessment of segments to assess the mobility and, in particular, the presence of hypermobility in axial rotation.

Technique

One thumb pad stabilizes the inferior spinous process from the side. The superior spinous process is pushed in the opposite direction (▶ Fig. 10.57), resulting in rotation. The test is concluded with the assessment of end feel. All spinous processes are tested on one side first, followed by the other side. This test is the most important for segmental hypermobility as axial instability is also the primary form of segmental instabilities.

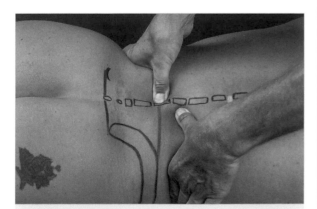

Fig. 10.57 Segmental test for rotation (transverse vertebral pressure).

Criteria

Is it possible to move the superior spinous process, and what type of end feel does it have? Does pain appear during this test and can this then be used to locate the painful segment?

Interpretation

T10 to T12: Slight rotation is expected here. The end feel is firm-elastic. A lack of rotational mobility is to be classified as restricted range of motion.

T12 to L5: No rotation should be possible here. A hard-elastic end feel is to be evaluated as normal. Rotational movement is to be interpreted as hypermobility.

L5 to S1: Due to the different position of the joint facets, some rotation is possible in this segment. The end feel is firm-elastic. Loss of mobility represents hypomobility in the segment.

10.8.3 Posteroanterior Segmental Joint Play

The posteroanterior push applied to a vertebra is one of the most common manual therapy techniques. It can be applied either to the spinous process or to the transverse process. Two segments always move when the therapist pushes the vertebra anteriorly (▶ Fig. 10.58). The pressure on the spinous process results in the ZAJ superior to the spinous process opening up and the capsule is placed under tension. The inferior ZAJ surfaces are compressed.

Aim

The assessment of segmental mobility, especially the presence of hypermobility, and pain provocation.

10

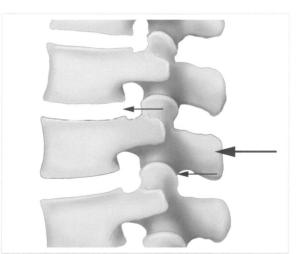

Fig. 10.58 The effect of posteroanterior pressure applied to the spinous process.

Criteria

The therapist pays attention to the range of motion, the quality of the end feel, and the aggravation of pain.

Procedure

The medial edge of the hand is usually placed perpendicular to the lordosis when pressure is applied to the spinous process (▶ Fig. 10.59). The L5 spinous process can be reached locally using a thumb (see ▶ Fig. 10.45).

Interpretation

The vertebra is expected to move a certain distance when posteroanterior pressure is applied to it. Healthy segments do not react to pressure, and the assessment of end feel is not sensitive. Some experience is required to allocate the yielding of a vertebra to pressure to a pathological condition in the neutral prone position. When the patient supports themselves on their elbows and adopts end-range lumbar extension, a hard-elastic end feel is classified as normal.

10.8.4 Palpation during Flexion and Extension Movements

This test addresses a variety of ways to palpate in side-lying. The patient is placed in neutral side-lying in preparation for these tests. Generally, the lumbar spine requires some padding; it is advantageous when the pelvis and legs are lying on a slippery surface.

Aim

To palpate how the segment moves when the hips are bilaterally moved into flexion and extension.

Criteria

The therapist pays attention to the opening and closing of the interspinous spaces.

Procedure

The therapist locates the L5 spinous process from an inferior position, as previously described. A finger pad is placed in the L5/S1 interspinous space and another in the L4/L5 interspinous space. It is possible to place the finger pads directly on top of or adjacent to the interspinous space. Starting with moderate hip flexion, the patient is moved gradually into more or less hip flexion. Both finger pads palpate the movement in the spinous processes at the same time (▶ Fig. 10.60).

Interpretation

The therapist pays attention to the interspinous spaces, for example, by palpating the interspinous spaces from inferior to superior (i.e., L5/S1 first, followed by L4/L5) as they open up during hip flexion and close during hip extension. When two neighboring vertebrae move simultaneously and no opening of the interspinous space can be detected, this is classified as hypomobility. This technique is suitable for finding the resting position of a segment. In this case the spinous process is positioned so that the interspinous space is neither fully opened nor fully closed. The resting position is most often found at approximately 70° flexion for L5/S1 and approximately 90° for L3/L4.

10.8.5 Anteroposterior Segmental Joint Play

Aim

This test attempts to slide two vertebrae on each other using translation.

Criteria

- The range of translation movement, especially the sudden increase in mobility in one segment.
- This test primarily assesses segmental hypermobility.

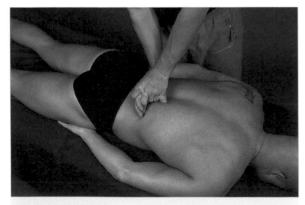

Fig. 10.59 Posteroanterior segmental joint play.

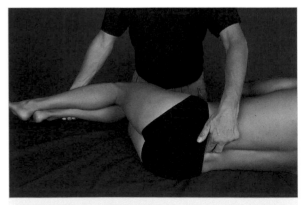

Fig. 10.60 Opening and closing of the interspinous spaces.

Procedure

The segment to be tested is located and placed in its resting position using the previously described technique.

Both of the neighboring spinous processes are located posteriorly using the finger pads and are stabilized by applying slight posteroanterior pressure. The fingertips on the inferior spinous process extend into the interspinous space (▶ Fig. 10.61).

The therapist's forearms stabilize the trunk and pelvis. Their hip comes into contact with the patient's knee joint. A straight movement is then made several times by alternately pushing the legs posteriorly and pulling the inferiorly placed spinous process and the pelvis anteriorly.

The position of the neighboring spinous process at the interspinous space is then palpated during the pull and the push. Can a distinct step be found here?

The segments L5/S1, L4/L5, and L3/L4 are assessed. It is possible to limit the translation movement to one segment by positioning the vertebral column. This is achieved by pushing the uppermost shoulder posteriorly until this movement reaches the segment directly superior to the segment to be tested. The segment is now locked in a coupled position.

Interpretation

Approximately 1 mm of translation movement from maximal posterior to maximal anterior is classified as normal. The L5/S1 segment is expected to be somewhat firmer due to the stabilizing function of the iliolumbar ligaments.

10.8.6 Local Segmental Mobility Using Coupled Movements

The best option to assess the presence of hypomobility in one segment is to evaluate how a segment moves using coupled movements. This can be used to test all segments of the functional lumbar spine (T10/T11 to L5/S1).

Aim

To use a coupled movement in lordotic side-lying by sliding the uppermost shoulder backward. A fingertip is used to palpate the interspinous spaces during this, starting with T10/T11.

Criteria

The coupled movement results in rotation with a palpable displacement of the spinous processes in relation to each other. The therapist observes whether the rotation causes the development or the increase of an interspinous step at the segment being assessed.

Procedure

- The patient lies in neutral side-lying with a slight lordosis. Sufficient padding is placed under the lumbar spine so that slight lateral flexion is present. The index or middle finger of one hand is placed over an interspinous space. The fingertip extends past the interspinous space, and the finger pad stabilizes the inferior spinous process (▶ Fig. 10.62 and ▶ Fig. 10.63).
- The other hand is used to push the uppermost shoulder posteriorly and introduces the coupled movement. The example shown in the figures demonstrates rotation to the left with lateral flexion to the right in an extended lumbar spine (▶ Fig. 10.64).
- As soon as the inferior process starts moving beneath the finger pad, the therapist stops moving the shoulder and assesses whether a step has developed between the spinous processes.
- The shoulder is then rotated back to neutral, a more inferior segment is sought, and the test is repeated.

Interpretation

The development of a step between two neighboring spinous processes at the end of the rotation is a sign of nor-

10

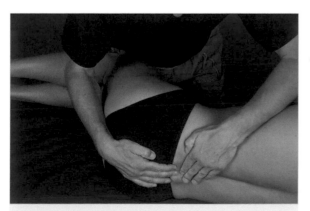

Fig. 10.61 Anteroposterior segmental joint play.

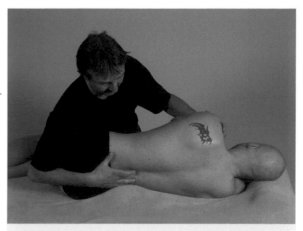

Fig. 10.62 Palpation with coupled movement—starting position.

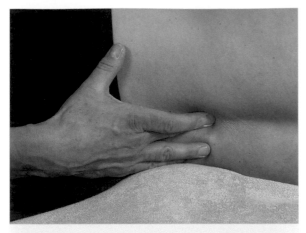

Fig. 10.63 Palpation with coupled movement—detailed view.

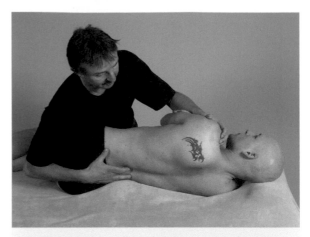

Fig. 10.64 Palpation with coupled movement—end position.

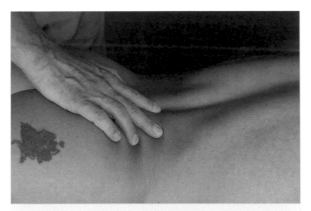

Fig. 10.65 Palpating the contraction of the lumbar multifidus.

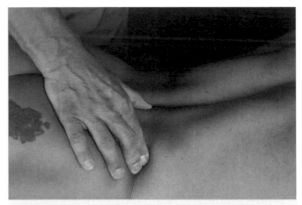

Fig. 10.66 Palpating the width of the entire erector spinae.

mal mobility. The superior spinous process usually rotates before the inferior spinous process. Experienced therapists can attempt to conduct the segmental mobility assessment in the sitting SP. Coupling is stronger in the weight-bearing position than in an SP without loading. This position, however, makes it considerably more difficult to feel how the structures move. Tension in the paravertebral muscles impedes the clear palpation of the interspinous spaces. It is also possible to assess how the vertebrae move in a coupled movement with flexion.

10.8.7 Training the Multifidus

According to current physical therapy concepts, the multifidus, in combination with the transversus abdominis and the thoracolumbar fascia, plays a decisive role in the stabilization of lumbar segments and the SI joint.

Treatment may therefore aim to recruit and train the multifidus. It makes sense to initially stimulate only the lumbar multifidus without stimulating the lateral-lying large sections of the erector spinae. Muscles can only be consciously contracted when the person is able to perceive the contraction. Tactile feedback regarding the degree of contraction is helpful.

Procedure

The muscle belly can be palpated paravertebrally from its origin on the posterior aspect of the sacrum (Chapter 9.7.6) to approximately the level of L3 when it is slightly tensed and the lumbar lordosis is increased (▶ Fig. 10.65). It measures 1 to 2 finger widths, depending on how well trained it is. Its contours can be visually differentiated from the neighboring longissimus and iliocostalis in slender people.

To comprehend the real dimensions of the multifidus, the significantly larger lateral tract of the erector spinae (iliocostalis and longissimus) can be made palpable for comparison. The head, and, when necessary, a small section of the upper body, is raised so that the compact consistency of the tense back extensors can be palpated from medial to lateral until the soft tissue next to the back extensors is palpated. The therapist can see the actual width of the back extensors by placing the thumb and index finger on either side of the muscles at the approximate level of L3 (▶ Fig. 10.66).

Bibliography

Aylott CE, Puna R, Robertson PA, Walker C. Spinous process morphology: the effect of ageing through adulthood on spinous process size and relationship to sagittal alignment. Eur Spine J. 2012; 21(5):1007–1012

Barker PJ, Guggenheimer KT, Grkovic I, et al. Effects of tensioning the lumbar fasciae on segmental stiffness during flexion and extension: Young Investigator Award winner. Spine. 2006; 31(4):397–405

Bjordal JM, Couppé C, Chow RT, Tunér J, Ljunggren EA. A systematic review of low level laser therapy with location-specific doses for pain from chronic joint disorders. Aust J Physiother. 2003; 49(2):107–116

Bogduk N. Klinische Anatomie von Lendenwirbelsäule und Sakrum. Berlin: Springer; 2000

Brismée JM, Atwood K, Fain M, et al. Interrater reliability of palpation of three-dimensional segmental motion of the lumbar spine. J Manual ManipTher. 2005; 13:215–220

Carlesso LC, Macdermid JC, Santaguida PL, et al. Beliefs and practice patterns in spinal manipulation and spinal motion palpation reported by canadian manipulative physiotherapists. Physiother Can. 2013; 65(2):167–175

Chaitow L. Palpationstechniken und Diagnostik. München: Urban & Fischer; 2001

Chakraverty R, Pynsent P, Isaacs K. Which spinal levels are identified by palpation of the iliac crests and the posterior superior iliac spines?. J Anat. 2007;210(2):232–236

Cooperstein R, Truong F. Systematic review and meta analyses of the difference between the spinal level of the palpated and imaged iliac crests. J Can Chiropr Assoc. 2017;61(2):106–120

Downey BJ, Taylor NF, Niere KR. Manipulative physiotherapists can reliably palpate nominated lumbar spinal levels. Man Ther. 1999; 4(3):151–156

Dvořák J. Manuelle Medizin. Bd. 1, Diagnostik. Berlin: Springer; 1998

Gracovetsky S. The Spinal Engine. Springer-Verlag, Wien, New York, Clin Biomech (Bristol, Avon). 1989; 4(2):127

Heylings DJ. Supraspinous and interspinous ligaments of the human lumbar spine. J Anat. 1978; 125(Pt 1):127–131

Hochschild J. Funktionelle Anatomie – Therapierelevante Details. Bd. 2. Stuttgart: Thieme; 2001

Jerosch J, Steinleitner W, Eds. Minimalinvasive Wirbelsäulen-Intervention. Aktuelle und innovative Verfahren für Praxis und Klinik. Köln: Dt. Ärzteverlag; 2005

Kapandji IA. Funktionelle Anatomie der Gelenke. 4. Aufl. Stuttgart: Thieme; 2006

Kilby J, Heneghan NR, Maybury M. Manual palpation of lumbo-pelvic landmarks: a validity study. Man Ther. 2012; 17(3):259–262

Klein-Vogelbach S. Funktionelle Bewegungslehre. Rehabilitation und Prävention. Bd. 1. Berlin: Springer; 2000

Lanz T von, Wachsmuth W. Praktische Anatomie, Rücken. Berlin: Springer; 2004

Leonhardt H, Tillmann B, Töndury G, Zilles K, Eds. Rauber/Kopsch: Anatomie des Menschen. Bd. I, Bewegungsapparat. 2. Aufl. Stuttgart: Thieme; 1998

McGaugh JM, Brismée JM, Dedrick GS, Jones EA, Sizer PS. Comparing the anatomical consistency of the posterior superior iliac spine to the iliac crest as reference landmarks for the lumbopelvic spine: a retrospective radiological study. Clin Anat. 2007; 20(7):819–825

Merz O, Wolf U, Robert M, Gesing V, Rominger M. Validity of palpation techniques for the identification of the spinous process L5. Man Ther. 2013; 18(4):333–338

Mieritz RM, Kawchuk GN. The accuracy of locating lumbar vertebrae when using palpation versus ultrasonography. J Manipulative PhysiolTher. 2016; 39(6):387–392

Netter FH. Atlas of Human Anatomy; 3rd Ed. Teterboro, New Jersey: Icon Learning Systems; 2004

Nyberg RE, Russell Smith A, Jr. The science of spinal motion palpation: a review and update with implications for assessment and intervention. J Manual ManipTher. 2013; 21(3):160–167

Pool-Goudzwaard AL, Kleinrensink GJ, Snijders CJ, Entius C, Stoeckart R. The sacroiliac part of the iliolumbar ligament. J Anat. 2001; 199(Pt 4):457–463

Render CA. The reproducibility of the iliac crest as a marker of lumbar spine level. Anaesthesia. 1996; 51(11):1070–1071

Richardson C, Jull G, Hodges PW, et al. Therapeutic exercise for spinal segmental stabilisation in low back pain. Edinburgh: Churchill Livingstone; 1999

Schneider M, Erhard R, Brach J, Tellin W, Imbarlina F, Delitto A. Spinal palpation for lumbar segmental mobility and pain provocation: an interexaminer reliability study. J Manipulative PhysiolTher. 2008; 31(6):465–473

Shaw JD, Shaw DL, Cooperman DR, Eubanks JD, Li L, Kim DH. Characterization of lumbar spinous process morphology: a cadaveric study of 2,955 human lumbar vertebrae. Spine J. 2015; 15(7):1645–1652

Vleeming A, Albert HB, Östgaard HC, et al. Evidenz für die Diagnose und Therapie von Beckengürtelschmerz – Europäische Leitlinien. physioscience. 2006; 2:48–58

White AA, Panjabi MM. Clinical Biomechanics of the spine, 2nd ed, Philadelphia: Lippincott; 1990

Willard FH, Vleeming A, Schuenke MD, Danneels L, Schleip R. The thoracolumbar fascia: anatomy, function and clinical considerations. J Anat. 2012; 221(6):507–536

Wittenberg RH, Willburger RE, Krämer J. Spondylolyse und Spondylolisthese. Orthopade. 1998; 27:51–63

Yamamoto I, Panjabi MM, Oxland TR, Crisco JJ. The role of the iliolumbar ligament in the lumbosacral junction. Spine. 1990; 15(11):1138–1141

10

Chapter 11

Abdominal Region

11

11 Abdominal Region

11.1 Significance of the Region

The abdominal wall provides the anterior and lateral cover of the visceral organs. The muscle tone of the abdominal muscles is functionally opposed to the diaphragm. During inhalation and contraction, muscle tone relaxes slightly. It increases during exhalation. The abdominal muscles support and effect an abdominal press. Owing to the great distance of the rotational axes of the lumbar and thoracic segments and the very good lever, the oblique abdominal muscles, compared to parts of the back extensors, are very good trunk rotators.

The activity of the abdominal wall muscles clamps the hip bones ventrally and thus contributes to the stability of the sacroiliac joints. In an electromyography (EMG)-supported study, Cowan et al. (2004) demonstrate the relationship between groin pain and delayed onset of transversus abdominus, confirming a positive effect of the abdominal muscles on the stability of the symphysis. The activity of the abdominal muscles therefore plays a role in the treatment of symphyseal instabilities, such as those occurring during and after pregnancy. The significance of timely activity of the transverse abdominal muscle for lumbar stability has already been discussed in the Chapter 10.3.5 on functions of the lumbar muscles.

11.2 Common Applications for Treatment in this Region

Abdominal massage is used in adults and young children to promote overall relaxation. The ability of abdominal massage to promote bowel activity is also known. Colon massage is a very effective method for supporting bowel activity in an atonic colon (Reichert, 2015), although its use has largely been supplanted by drug therapy.

Individuals with spinal cord injury have impaired vegetative functions such as bowel movement and micturition. Patients with paraplegia may have to learn to manually trigger the bladder.

Respiratory therapy commonly focuses on respiratory depth and rhythm. The initial goal is to instruct the patient to perform relaxed abdominal breathing, which is the normal form of breathing during low physical activity. Abdominal breathing also has a calming effect, serves as a suction/force pump for venous transport in the abdominal region, and slightly shifts the abdominal organs as an additional stimulus for intestinal peristalsis.

Manual lymph drainage is the most suitable therapy for treating impaired lymph drainage from the leg and groin. For a better preparation of the lymphatic drainage, a deep abdominal drainage should be carried out in advance. The section below aims to provide precise and in-depth guidance for therapeutic understanding of the abdominal region, such as those required for colon massage and manual lymph drainage.

Muscle recruitment and strengthening play an important role both in treating patients with deep back, pelvic, and groin complaints as well as in postpartum pelvic floor exercises. Prior to the actual strengthening, the patients' perception of their body must be sensitized and the proper timing of the activity must be fine-tuned.

In Western Europe, the abdomen is seldom the object of massage or physical therapy. Therapeutic diagnostics of functional impairment of the internal organs tends to be performed by observing tissue changes as defined by dermatomes. Palpation and auscultation of the abdominal and pelvic region tend to be performed by internists or surgeons. In Traditional Chinese Medicine (TCM), however, this is quite different. Abdominal wall diagnosis plays a key role in TCM (Greten, 2017). Inspection and palpation focus on pain and guarding or tension of the abdominal wall, among other things, the muscle tone at the intercostal arch, the upper abdomen, the periumbilical region, and the lower abdomen.

When it comes to palpating the groin region, Winkel (2004) states that the therapist is not directly responsible for performing specific palpation to confirm an inguinal hernia. However, when examining the groin region, the therapist must not overlook an inguinal hernia.

11.3 Required Knowledge (Topographic and Morphologic)

In the section below, anatomical aspects of the abdominal wall and the internal organs are presented if they are of therapeutic interest and are palpable. For this reason, various organs are not described below. For more detailed information, the anatomical literature in this book's reference list may be consulted. To enhance description and understanding of the positions of muscles and organs, the trunk wall is subdivided into regions using lines and levels.

11.3.1 Boundaries of the Abdominal Wall

- Superior boundary: Inferior margin of the thorax with the intercostal arch and xiphoid process
- Inferior boundary: Iliac crest, inguinal ligaments, and pubic symphysis
- Lateral boundary: Medial axillary line (▶ Fig. 11.1)

11.3.2 Regions of the Abdominal Wall

- It is easiest to subdivide the regions of the abdominal wall by designating structures to the left and to the

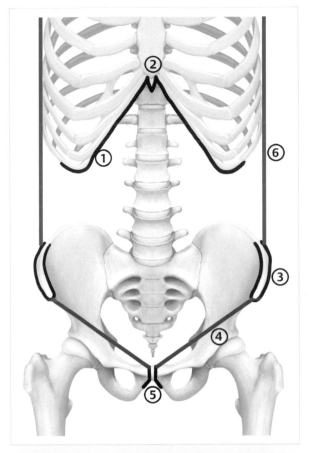

Fig. 11.1 Boundaries of the abdominal wall: 1 = costal arch, 2 = xiphoid process, 3 = iliac crest, 4 = inguinal ligament, 5 = pubic symphysis, 6 = medial axillary line.

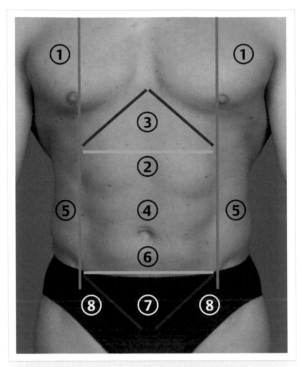

Fig. 11.2 Regional divisions of the abdominal wall: 1 = medioclavicular line, 2 = subcostal plane, 3 = epigastric space, 4 = umbilical region, 5 = lateral abdominal region, 6 = interspinous plane, 7 = pubic region, 8 = inguinal region.

right of the linea alba—the tendinous, abdominal section of the anterior median line where the rectus sheaths meet. In some women, this line becomes pigmented in the second trimester of pregnancy. The darker color becomes significantly lighter or disappears completely after the pregnancy (Schmailzl and Hackelöer, 2002).

- Two lines connecting bony structures are used to subdivide the abdominal region transversely.
- The connecting line of the inferior margins of the 10th rib shows the position of the subcostal plane.
- The epigastric space, which contains the hepatic field and the gastric field, is located above this plane. Superior to the subcostal plane, the medial abdominal region is located with the umbilical region and the lateral abdominal regions. This subdivision is undertaken by the medioclavicular line, where the lateral margins of the abdominal rectus muscles are approximately located.
- The anatomical literature does not agree on the second transverse subdivision of the abdominal region. Some authors, such as Rauber and Leonhardt (1987), connect the highest points of the iliac crests. Here, the

interspinous plane, the line connecting the two anterior superior iliac spine (ASIS), is demonstrated. Superior to this plane, the inguinal regions are located laterally and at the center, the pubic region.

▶ Fig. 11.2 shows the subdivision of the abdominal regions.

11.3.3 Deep and Superficial Abdominal Muscles

The deep abdominal muscles are the muscles that delimit the abdominal region posteriorly (▶ Fig. 11.3):
- Psoas major and minor muscles.
- Quadratus lumborum muscle.

Psoas Major and Minor Muscles

The psoas muscles are primarily known as the agonists of hip flexion. In the closed chain, the psoas major muscle, in conjunction with the abdominal muscles, serves to elevate the trunk from the supine position. During this activity, it exerts enormous lordotic tension on its origin sites, the L1–L4 vertebral bodies, transverse processes, and vertebral disks. With the compressive force component that arises additionally, it is known in the realm of physical therapy as an "evil muscle" with a generally negative impact on the lumbar spine, although this reputation is unjustified. With its unilateral innervation, it contributes to active lateral bending of the lumbar spine.

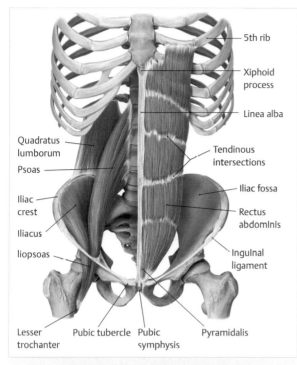

Fig. 11.3 Deep abdominal muscles and rectus muscles.

Quadratus Lumborum Muscle

This multilayer muscle stretches between the 12th rib, the lumbar transverse processes, and the iliac crest. It combines several functions. It supports forced exhalation and provides synergy for lateral bending (in both cases, by lowering the 12th rib). During walking, it controls the position of the pelvis in the frontal plane and in so doing works together with the contralateral gluteus minimus muscles. Its stabilizing influence on the lumbar spine and the layers of the thoracolumbar fascia was debated for a certain time but never consistently or conceptually implemented. Ploumis et al. (2011) describe the relationship between muscle atrophy of the back extensor muscles and the deep abdominal muscles in patients with chronic low back pain.

The superficial abdominal muscles delimit the abdominal space laterally and anteriorly. On each side there are three flat and one subdivided muscle. From superficial to deeper-lying these are:

- Rectus abdominis (▶ Fig. 11.3)
- External oblique (▶ Fig. 11.4)
- Internal oblique (▶ Fig. 11.5)
- Transverse abdominal (▶ Fig. 11.6)

Together, these muscles, in interaction with the pelvic floor and the diaphragm, are responsible for exerting adequate pressure on the internal organs and ensuring

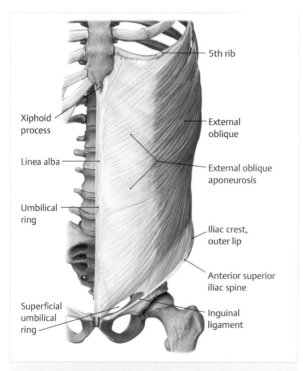

Fig. 11.4 External oblique.

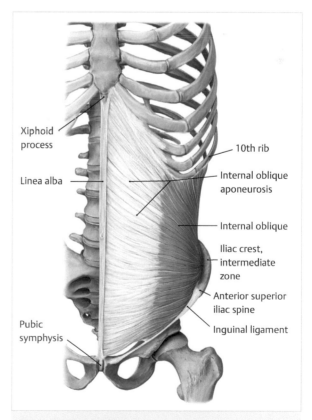

Fig. 11.5 Internal oblique.

11

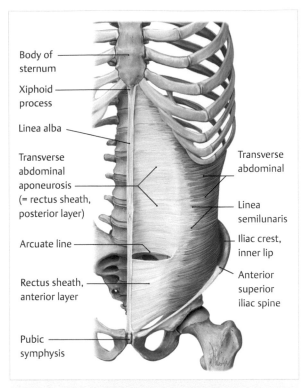

Body of sternum

Xiphoid process

Linea alba

Transverse abdominal aponeurosis (= rectus sheath, posterior layer)

Arcuate line

Rectus sheath, anterior layer

Pubic symphysis

Transverse abdominal

Linea semilunaris

Iliac crest, inner lip

Anterior superior iliac spine

Fig. 11.6 Transverse abdominal.

separate innervation of the individual muscle bellies. This enables the rectus abdominis muscles to alternatively pull the rib cage inferiorly and/or set the pelvis upright.

External Oblique

This flat muscle developed from the external intercostal muscles (▶ Fig. 11.4) after the ribs withdrew from the abdominal region in the course of evolution. Rauber and Leonhardt (1987) describe that its fibers generally extend from superior-lateral to inferior-medial, like the trajectory of a hand being slid into a pants pocket. It arises from the 5th to 12th ribs with muscular attachments (Schünke et al., 2005). As it does so, the attachments interdigitate with those of the serratus anterior at what is referred to as Gerdy's line (Schünke et al., 2005). They become particularly prominent when the muscle is forced to exert flexion and rotate the trunk heterolaterally against resistance.

Internal Oblique

This muscle's fibers embody the continuation of the internal intercostal muscles and also have their basic superolateral to inferomedial course (▶ Fig. 11.5).

The muscle belly of the internal oblique is generally covered by the external oblique and is thus not actually directly palpable. With the external oblique of the contralateral side, it completes an anterior diagonal muscle loop.

Transverse Abdominal

The section on the thoracolumbar fascia has already discussed (Chapter 10.3.4) this structure's position and lumbar impact in detail. The muscle's stabilizing effect is based on the connection between the linea alba and the lumbar transverse processes via the thoracolumbar fascia (▶ Fig. 11.6). If the anterior side of the muscle has a stable base, it can reverse the fixed point and mobile points and impact the lumbar spine rather than the abdomen.

Directly medial to the anterior superior iliac spine (ASIS), its aponeurosis can be accessed unimpeded with palpating fingers. When working with patients, this access is used when practicing deliberate recruitment of the muscle. To perceive its activity, the therapist only has to ask the patients to pull in their belly button.

The muscle bellies of all flat abdominal muscles are located on the lateral wall of the trunk. Anteriorly and medially, they each transition into an aponeurosis that inserts into either the linea alba and/or the iliac crest. Between the medial border of their muscle bellies and the outer edge of the rectus abdominalis muscle on one side the linea semilunaris is located around the level of the medioclavicular line (▶ Fig. 11.2). Lower-lying organs, especially the portions of the colon, can be accessed at this point without the resistance of the muscle bellies.

they are held together. When lifting heavy objects, the abdominal region forms a firmly encased stable soft tissue bladder through exhalation.

The abdominal press actively exerts pressure on the intestines (Schünke et al., 2005). This supports, for example, the emptying of the rectum (defecation), the bladder (micturition), and the stomach (vomiting). During the expulsive phase of labor, the abdominal press supports the contractions of the uterus (bearing down pains).

These muscles control the posture of the upright upper body. During forced walking, they, along with the oblique back muscles, limit the rotation movements of the upper body. The transverse and oblique abdominal muscles are stretched over the iliac bones and thus help stabilize the sacroiliac joints (Chapter 9.3.6). The influence of the transverse abdominal muscles on the deep lamina of the thoracolumbar fascia and consequently on lumbar stability has already been mentioned a number of times (see the section on thoracolumbar fascia in Chapter 10.3.4).

Rectus Abdominis Muscles

Both of the rectus abdominis muscles run at the level of the 3rd to 7th ribs to the pubic tubercle next to the symphysis (▶ Fig. 11.3). They lie in a connective tissue sheath formed by the aponeuroses of the flat abdominal muscles. These aponeuroses meet at thelinea alba, which separates the two rectus muscles. The transverse intersections evoke the earlier development of ribs and permit

The oblique muscles contract during lateral bending on the same side against resistance (Rauber and Leonhardt, 1987). With the direction of the trunk rotation, the two oblique muscles can be distinguished:
- Trunk rotation toward the contralateral side = external oblique.
- Trunk rotation toward the ipsilateral side = internal oblique.

11.3.4 Organs of the Abdominopelvic Cavity

Abdominal Cavity

The abdominal cavity is bordered by the rib cage, diaphragm, abdominal muscles, vertebral column, and the iliac bones (Frick et al., 1992). In an inferior direction, it continues as the pelvic cavity, which is finally closed by the pelvic floor. The abdominal cavity contains the intestinal organs, as well as the liver and pancreas, which are both glands. Like the mediastinum in the thoracic cavity, the abdominal cavity also has a connective tissue compartment for large conductive pathways (e.g., aorta) behind the abdominal cavity.

The peritoneum completely encloses the organs located in the abdominal cavity and separates the organs and the abdominal wall by a gap. The inside of the peritoneum produces a serous fluid that lubricates the shifting of the organs against each other and the wall. A few milliliters of fluid are sufficient for this. Since only low volumes of gases occur in the organs of the abdominal cavity, they are not compressible, but are highly deformable. Every change in the shape of an organ causes the shape and position of the adjacent organ to change.

Shifts occur through abdominal breathing and changes in body position or posture, for example. The muscle tone of the abdominal and pelvic floor muscles is regulated such that the peritoneum can ideally surround the organs without compressing them. When there are changes in the volume of the abdominal cavity through the filling of the stomach and bowels and/or through breathing, the muscle tone of the abdominal muscles adapts accordingly.

Anatomy textbooks on the internal organs set the separation of the upper and lower abdomen at around the level of L2 (Rauber and Leonhardt, 1987; Frick et al., 1992). This corresponds approximately to the position of the inferior edge of the transverse part of the colon.

The *upper abdomen* extends through the curvature of the diaphragm from the level of T9 to the level of L2 and is mostly enclosed by the thorax. Located here are the liver, gallbladder, spleen, the largest part of the pancreas, stomach, and upper part of the duodenum. The *lower abdomen* extends from the level of L2 to the pelvic inlet plane (S1 – symphysis): lower part of the duodenum, head of the pancreas, and small and large intestines.

Upper Abdomen

The position of the organs in the upper abdomen (▶ Fig. 11.7) is dependent on breathing and posture. Age-related loss of elasticity of the lungs causes the organs to drop. Precise determination of the position of the lungs is only possible with imaging techniques (Rauber and Leonhardt, 1987).

Stomach

The stomach is where the enzymatic degradation of food through gastric acid takes place. Resorption plays only a minor role in this process. Gastric acid destroys bacteria in food and thus has an important protective function.

The shape and position of the stomach are highly variable. Rauber and Leonhardt (1987) describe its position as running asymmetrically in the upper abdomen from the upper left to the lower right. Most of the stomach is located on the left of the median plane. The stomach opening (cardia) is located at around the level of T11. Anatomical descriptions report three different most common shapes. In the lower half of the epigastric region, the stomach can be palpated on the left of the median plane.

Spleen

The spleen is a lymphatic organ that can influence blood composition in multiple ways:
- As an important immune organ, it is filled with specific defense cells.
- It removes old red blood cells ("lymph node of the bloodstream") and stores platelets.

The approximately fist-sized organ is shaped like a coffee bean. It is 10 to 12 cm long, 6 to 8 cm wide, and weighs 150 to 200 g. A fibrous capsule delimits the otherwise soft tissue from its surroundings. The spleen is located in a fossa behind the stomach and is located directly in front of the 9th to 11th ribs and directly below the diaphragm. The longitudinal axis falls laterally following the course of the 10th rib. The spleen has two surfaces facing the diaphragm and the bowels. The anterior pole does not usually protrude beneath the ribs. If the spleen is enlarged, this pole is difficult to access and the patient must breathe in deeply (Rauber and Leonhardt, 1987) while in the left semi-side-lying position (▶ Fig. 11.36).

Liver

As a multifunctional organ, the liver, weighing around 2,000 g, is the body's largest gland and an important storage and excretory organ. The most important functions of the liver are as follows:
- Producing bile as an exocrine product for emulsion of fats in the duodenum.

11

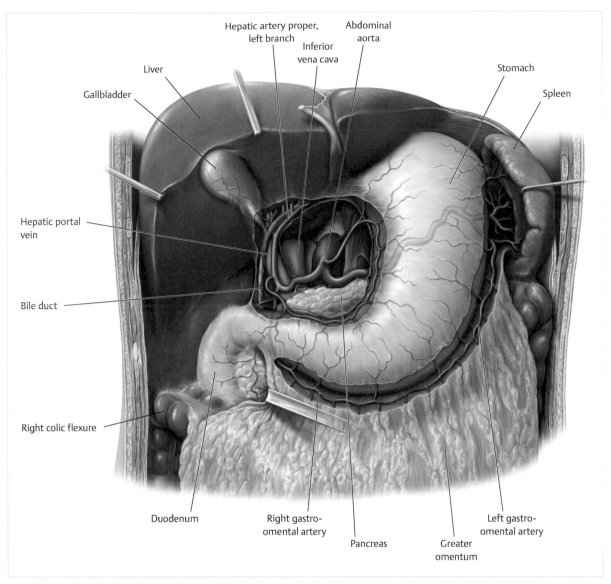

Fig. 11.7 Organs of the upper abdomen.

- Synthesizing the body's own substances from low-molecule components.
- Storing up to 1 L of blood and 400 g of glycogen. This corresponds to a caloric value of around 1,600 kcal.
- "Detoxifying" the blood, for example, converting ammonia into urea.

The liver occupies the largest space in the upper abdomen. It is mainly located on the right of the median plane behind the ribs. Enclosed in a firm connective tissue capsule, it has a smooth exterior. The shape of the liver is primarily determined by the adjacent organs. Rauber and Leonhardt (1987) report that the typical triangular shape is present in only 65% of all people. The superior surfaces adjoin the interior thorax and diaphragm. The third side (visceral fascia) faces the intestines. The inferior margin starts at the lateral right in the plumb-line of the medial axillary line and rises parallel to the costal arch in a left medial direction. Directly inferior to the xiphoid process in the upper epigastric region (hepatic field) it lies directly on the abdominal wall and can be accessed by applying pressure.

The movements of the liver are primarily dependent on breathing. As the lungs are connected with the diaphragm and the chest wall, the liver is firmly attached to the diaphragm through adhesive strength. The diaphragm thus "carries" the entire weight of the liver and in doing so relieves the rest of the intestines and the pelvic floor. Due to the attachment to the diaphragm, the liver follows its movements during breathing. In Rauber and Leonhardt (1987), the movement mechanism is described as follows: During exhalation, the diaphragm and liver are pressed into the rib cage through the contraction of the abdominal wall muscles and, at the same time, are sucked into the rib cage by the "pull of the lungs." The extent of this movement is dependent on the depth of the breath and can be between 1.5 and 7 cm. The superior border is at the level of the fourth intercostal space during exhalation.

Gallbladder

The gallbladder measures 8 to 12 cm by 4 to 5 cm. It is a sac that collects bile and discharges it as needed. The portion closest to the abdominal wall is the fundus of the gallbladder at the inferior margin of the liver. It is located in the corner between the exterior margin of the rectus abdominis and the right costal arch and thus lies on the colon at the right colic flexure.

Lower Abdomen

Large Intestine

The primary activities taking place in the large intestine are the resorption of water and salts, as well as thickening and fermentation of the intestinal contents. Slow peristalsis moves the intestinal contents, with only few movements effectively directed analwards. Frick et al. report that only two to three of these movements a day are especially pronounced (1992). In addition to local stretches and contractions, peristaltic waves occurring at a rhythmic interval of three to six per minute play an important role in the transportation of the intestinal contents.

The **large intestine** is divided into three **parts** (▶ Fig. 11.8): caecum, colon, and rectum. The large intestine is approximately 110 to 165 cm long and extends from the ileocecal valve (Bauhin's valve) to the anal canal and rectum. Bauhin's valve was named after Caspar

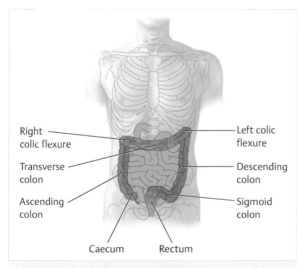

Fig. 11.8 Large intestine.

Bauhin (1560–1624), professor of medicine and anatomy in Basel (Rauber/Kopsch).

The nomenclatures "large intestine" and "small intestine" do not always accurately describe the actual structure. Rauber and Leonhardt (1987) point out that when the large intestine is contracted, it can be thinner ("smaller") than the small intestine. The special structural features of the large intestine are three thin longitudinal ribbons of muscle (taeniae coli), transverse constrictions, and bulges in the wall (haustra of colon).

The **caecum** is approximately 6 to 8 cm long and its position varies widely. Its position is generally described as medial and superior to the ASIS. It is located directly below the abdominal wall, to which it is fused, and the iliacus. The ileocecal valve forms the junction of the terminal ileum and the ascending colon. The appendix (vermiform appendix) is around 1 finger length long and the diameter of a pencil and is positioned medial at the inferior end. Its position also varies widely. It is frequently found on the posterior caecum. The appendix is known as the site of acute or chronic inflammation. Its common position was described by Charles McBurney (1845–1914), a surgeon in New York. The so-called McBurney's point is located on a line between the ASIS and the navel and at this point, on the border of the lateral third (McBurney, 1889).

The **colon** is commonly **subdivided** as follows: ascending colon, transverse colon, descending colon, and sigmoid colon (S-shaped part).

The **ascending colon** is directly connected to the caecum and extends to below the liver. It lies on the right posterior abdominal wall and is attached to it. With the right-angled right colic flexure, it passes directly into the transverse colon. The colic flexure is covered by the liver and, according to Rauber and Leonhardt (1987), its location varies between T3 and L4.

The course of the **transverse colon** avoids the overlying liver and stomach and is thus located below the hepatic and gastric fields of the epigastric area. It therefore runs in a convex arch inferiorly, ascending slightly toward the left up to below the spleen, where the left colic flexure is located. The flexure has a sharp bend and presents natural resistance to the movement of the intestinal contents. It is attached to the diaphragm with ligaments. The overall length can be seen between the angle of the right rectus margin and costal arch up to the angle of the left rectus margin and costal arch. This means that the transverse colon can only be directly accessed through the rectus abdominis muscles. The position of the transverse colon is highly dependent on body position (it is higher while lying than standing), how full the abdominal cavity is (pregnancy), and the extent to which the transverse colon itself is filled. The position of the left colic flexure varies between T10 and L3. The Cannon-Böhm area is located medial to the left colic flexure and on the transverse colon and constitutes the termination of the innervation area of the vagus nerve.

11

The **descending colon** descends retroperitoneally from the left colic flexure to the iliac crest, where it becomes the sigmoid colon between the iliac crest and the level of S1. Several small intestinal loops are situated between this part of the colon and the anterior abdominal wall.

The **sigmoid colon** is 45 cm long on average (Rauber and Leonhardt, 1987). Its location is also dependent on how full it is. It curves on itself toward the right and then bends downward into the pelvic space.

At the level of S2 to S3, the sigmoid becomes the **rectum**. It is 12 to 15 cm long and initially lies on the anterior side of the sacrum. While the term "rectum" may suggest that the structure is straight, this is not the case; it has three bends and terminates in the anal canal, which is 3 to 4 cm long.

Pelvic Cavity

The pelvic cavity contains the urinary bladder, the rectum, and the internal sex organs. Its inferior side is closed by the muscle and connective tissue plates of the pelvic floor.

Urinary Bladder

As the only accessible organ of the pelvic cavity, only the urinary bladder will be discussed here. It is located below the peritoneum, behind the symphysis, and on the pelvic floor (▶ Fig. 11.9). In the female pelvic cavity, the uterus is located directly behind the urinary bladder, while in the male pelvic cavity, the rectum is in this position. Superiorly, the sigmoid colon lies on the urinary bladder.

The size of the urinary bladder obviously depends on the extent to which it is filled. While up to 700 mL of urine can be deliberately retained, the urge to urinate sets in starting with 350 mL. As the bladder fills, the vertex of the bladder rises to over the symphysis. If muscle tone is weak, bladder emptying may be impaired, which can lead to urinary retention.

Abdominal Aorta

The abdominal aorta is located in the retroperitoneal space. It enters the abdominal cavity through the aortic hiatus at the level of T12. Further below, it runs in front of the lumbar vertebral bodies somewhat left of the median plane. In the abdominal cavity, it gives off a number of paired and unpaired branches. At the level of L4, it is divided into two pelvic arteries (common iliac arteries) that course along the medial borders of the psoas major muscles. These finally become the femoral arteries, which course below the center of the inguinal ligament into the anterior thigh area.

The proximity to the lumbar vertebral bodies allows the pulsation of the aorta to be felt posterior to the spinous processes with the patient in prone position. If very distinct pulsation of the aorta can be felt while palpating the abdominal wall (left next to the median line) of the patient in supine position, the aorta should be examined for a possible aneurysm (Ferguson, 1990).

11.3.5 Anatomy of the Groin

The area of the groin comprises the transition from the abdominal cavity to the proximal thigh. Deep in the groin, large muscles and important vessels leave the abdominal cavity and enter the thigh (▶ Fig. 11.10). To this end, the space below the inguinal ligament is divided into separate sections for the iliopsoas muscle and femoral nerve and the femoral artery and vein (Chapter 5).

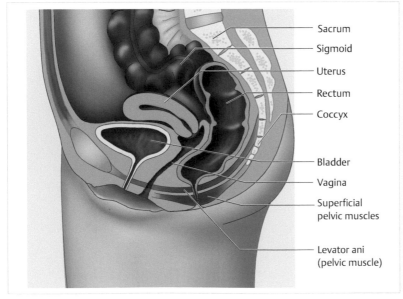

Sacrum

Sigmoid

Uterus

Rectum

Coccyx

Bladder

Vagina

Superficial pelvic muscles

Levator ani (pelvic muscle)

Fig. 11.9 Position of the bladder in the median section.

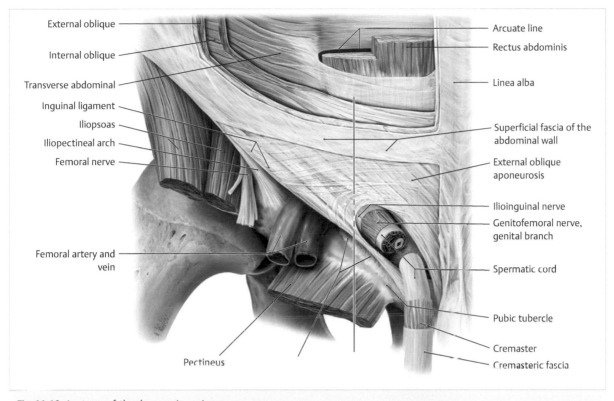

External oblique

Internal oblique

Transverse abdominal

Inguinal ligament

Iliopsoas

Iliopectineal arch

Femoral nerve

Femoral artery and vein

Pectineus

Arcuate line

Rectus abdominis

Linea alba

Superficial fascia of the abdominal wall

External oblique aponeurosis

Ilioinguinal nerve

Genitofemoral nerve, genital branch

Spermatic cord

Pubic tubercle

Cremaster

Cremasteric fascia

Fig. 11.10 Anatomy of the deep groin region.

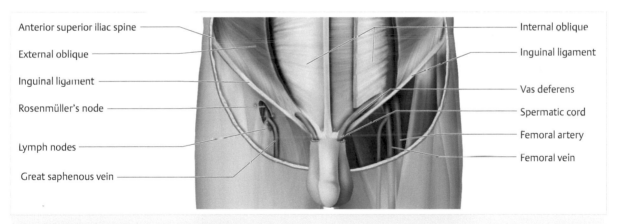

Anterior superior iliac spine

External oblique

Inguinal ligament

Rosenmüller's node

Lymph nodes

Great saphenous vein

Internal oblique

Inguinal ligament

Vas deferens

Spermatic cord

Femoral artery

Femoral vein

Fig. 11.11 Anatomy of the superficial groin region.

11

On the surface, the transition at the inguinal ligament is distinct (▶ Fig. 11.10). Here, the fascia of the abdominal wall muscles is interwoven with the fascia of the thigh (fascia lata) (▶ Fig. 11.11). At the center of the groin are several inguinal lymph nodes and the superficial greater saphenous vein enters the deep-lying femoral vein. Medially, the structures of the inguinal canal appear at the surface.

The inguinal canal runs above the medial half of the inguinal ligament (▶ Fig. 11.12). It starts deep and laterally with its deep inguinal ring entering through the fascia of the transverse abdominal muscle. This is around 1 cm above the mid-inguinal point (halfway between the ASIS and the pubic tubercle). Here, the conductive pathways running to the testes combine to form a cable having the diameter of a little finger.

In the course toward medial, the canal penetrates the fascia of the internal and external obliques. With the external oblique, it forms the superficial inguinal ring around 1 cm superior to the pubic tubercle. Inferiorly, the inguinal ligament delimits the canal. The posterior wall is formed by the transverse abdominal and the anterior wall by the obliques (Winkel, 2004).

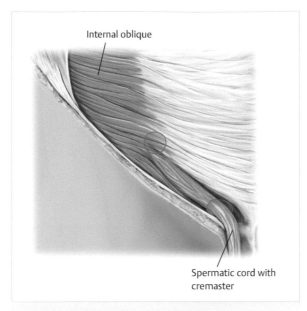

Fig. 11.12 Inguinal canal.

The content of the inguinal canal is described in the literature by Mann (Frick et al., 1992; Schünke et al., 2005) as follows:

- Ilio-inguinal nerve and genitofemoral nerve (branch)
- Spermatic cord: The firm spermatic cord, which is reinforced with different fascia, contains the following:
  ○ Cremaster
  ○ Vas deferens (spermatic duct)
  ○ Various blood vessels (testicular veins)
  ○ Various fascia

The structures of the female inguinal canal primarily comprise the following: ilio-inguinal nerve, round ligament of uterus, and the above-listed vessels and fascia. They run to the labia majora.

11.4 Summary of the Palpatory Process

The section below starts with a general orientation of the abdominal wall and then discusses deeper palpation of the abdomen and groin.

The bony landmarks framing the abdominal cavity are easy to find, and offer a foundation for dividing the abdominal wall into different regions through orienting projections. The most effective sites for palpating the activity of the abdominal wall muscles will then be discussed. The deep palpation of the abdomen is primarily intended to make the therapist secure when performing deep abdominal massage and detect potential pathological conditions. Secure palpation of the inguinal canal complements the descriptions of palpation of the groin in the section on the anterior thigh.

11.5 Overview of the Structures to be Palpated

11.5.1 Bony Structures

- Xiphoid process.
- Costal arch and tips of the 11th and 12th ribs.
- ASIS and inguinal ligament.
- Pubic symphysis.

11.5.2 Orienting Projections

- Anterior axillary line.
- Medioclavicular line.
- Inferior thoracic aperture.
- Epigastric space.
- Inguinal ligament.
- Spinous plane and promontory.
- Linea alba.

11.5.3 Muscles

- Rectus abdominis.
- Linea semilunaris.
- Regional subdivision of the central abdomen.
- Transverse abdominal.
- External oblique.
- Internal oblique.
- Abdominal aorta.
- L3 vertebral body and psoas major.

11.5.4 Palpation of the Colon

- Colon points according to Vogler with differentiation of pathological conditions.
- Inferior margin of the liver.
- Inferior margin of the spleen.

11.5.5 Palpation of the Groin Region

- Superficial inguinal ring.
- Palpation of inguinal hernias.

11.6 Starting Position

To complement the description of the starting positions (SPs) for palpation of the trunk, the neutral SP in supine position is described (▶ Fig. 11.13). It is particularly well suited for palpation of the thorax (Chapter 12.8.2) and the abdominal cavity. All of the structures are easy to access. Muscle activity required to confirm the position of muscle bellies can be performed effortlessly by the patient. The abdominal wall is relaxed enough to access bony structures and organs.

In the neutral supine position, the patient's upper body is generally rather flat. Thin padding is placed under the

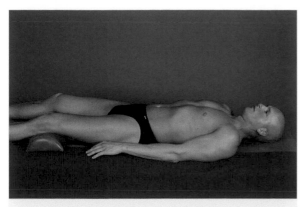

Fig. 11.13 Starting position in supine position.

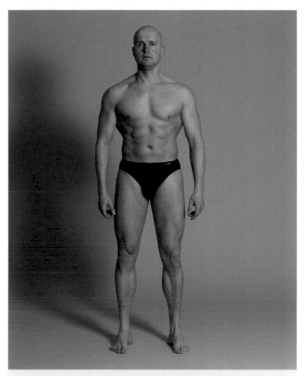

Fig. 11.14 Starting position while standing.

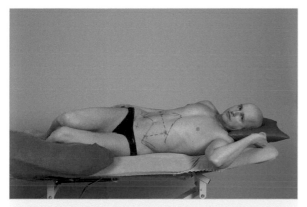

Fig. 11.15 Starting position in semi-side-lying position.

head. The patient's arms are relaxed and lie next to the body. A thin roll is placed under the knees to ensure slight lumbar lordosis. If the patient requests the head be raised higher and the knees be padded more thickly, there is nothing wrong with that. However, raising the head part of the table causing significant flexion of the cervical spine should be avoided, because the proportions of the upper abdominal cavity, in particular, and the borders of the thorax will considerably shift, and it may no longer be possible to access all of the deeper-lying structures. Similarly, especially thick padding under the legs that causes considerable pelvic tilt should be avoided.

11.6.1 Difficult and Supplementary SPs

Other possible SPs for palpation of the abdomen and groin include the bipedal stand, with equal weight-bearing on both sides, as well as the semi-side-lying position (▶ Fig. 11.14 and ▶ Fig. 11.15). The bipedal stand permits palpation of the bony reference points of the pelvis (ASIS and iliac crest) during weight bearing. Many physicians and therapists consider the determination of the position of these bony points to be key diagnostic factors.

The semi side lying position with the patient turned toward the left side is required in palpations described below only for the purpose of provoking a painfully enlarged spleen (see the following section 11.10.4 "Locating the Descending Point"). The position is characterized by sufficient padding of the upper body, pelvis, and legs. The most important goals are stability with simultaneous relaxation of the trunk muscles.

11.7 Palpation of the Bony Structures

11.7.1 Preparation

In order to access the area deep inside the abdomen, the patient must be asked to report any possible contraindications. Palpation must be soft using the entire flat hand on the upper and lower abdomen.

> **Caution**
>
> Ensure that the palpating hands are warm. Cold hands often cause guarding.

The therapist uses a flat hand to apply moderate pressure to different places in order to feel the tension of the abdominal wall. If the patient has not reported anything

11

abnormal, there should not be any perceivable differences in tension.

The back of the hand is used to feel the temperature of the abdominal wall. It is normal for both regions of the abdomen to have the same temperature.

If palpation using a flat hand has already triggered pain and guarding or differences in tension or temperature can be felt, the patient should be referred to a physician for further diagnosis. The presence of large volumes of subcutaneous fat compromises the reliability of these assessments. An additional possibility for recognizing a contraindication for deep palpation will be described later when looking for the points of colon massage. Every deep palpation should begin with the patient simultaneously expelling air.

11.7.2 Xiphoid Process

The palpation starts from the median with further orientation in an inferolateral direction (▶ Fig. 11.16).

The reliable starting point for complete palpation of the costal arch is found by continuously following the ster-

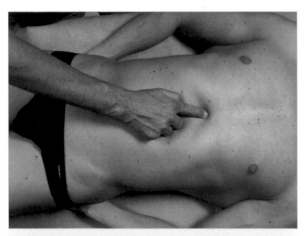

Fig. 11.16 Xiphoid process.

num while applying direct pressure posteriorly from superior to inferior until the palpating finger slides off bony structures and the carefully applied pressure is met with soft counter pressure. If the finger is hooked around superiorly, it is now located inferior to the tip of the sternum. Now the palpating finger is located in the epigastric space, which contains the hepatic field on the left and gastric field on the right. Indirect access to these organs is therefore good. Reliable palpation can also be conducted starting from the opposite end.

11.7.3 Costal Arch

Further palpation in an inferolateral direction, in a transverse direction against solid structures, now follows the costal arch, which consists of the costal cartilage of the 10th to 8th ribs. High-performance athletes occasionally report pain at the insertion of the abdominal muscles or fractures of the interchondral connections of the individual costal cartilage. The lateral condition causes hypermobility of the affected costal cartilage and is referred to as slipping rib syndrome in the literature (Udermann et al., 2005; Kumar et al., 2013).

The palpating finger consistently follows the costal arch in a lateral direction and meets the cartilaginous tip of the 11th rib. If the finger hooks around the inferior edge and continues further in an inferolateral direction, the tip of the 12th rib will be reached (▶ Fig. 11.17 and ▶ Fig. 11.18). If the finger were to continue following the structure, the palpation would end between the iliac crest and the inferior margin of the 12th rib (Chapter 10).

11.7.4 Anterior Superior Iliac Spine (ASIS) and Inguinal Ligament

The dominant bony orientation of the inferior abdominal wall is the ASIS. The pubic region extends between the spines of the two sides and the inguinal region, in each case from an ASIS to the symphysis (▶ Fig. 11.19).

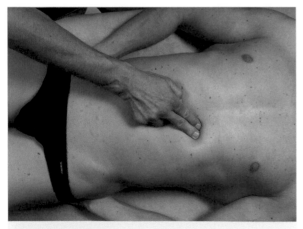

Fig. 11.17 Costal arch.

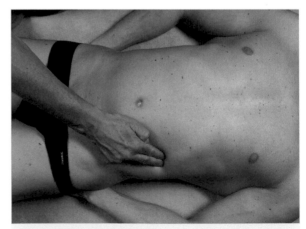

Fig. 11.18 Tip of the 11th rib.

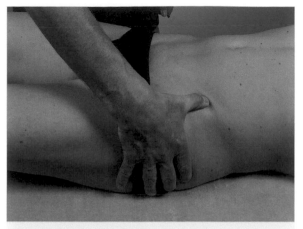

Fig. 11.19 Anterior superior iliac spine (ASIS).

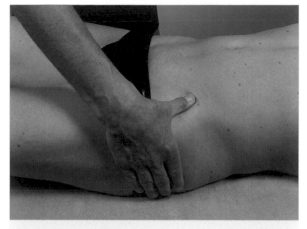

Fig. 11.20 Inguinal ligament.

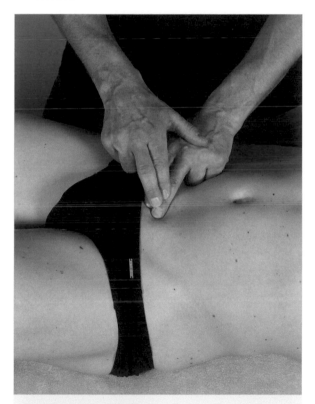

Fig. 11.21 Pubic symphysis.

Similar to the palpation of the posterior superior spine (Chapter 10), the therapist first follows the round contours of the iliac crest with transverse and generous palpation across the iliac crest. The end of the iliac crest, and in turn the ASIS, and the beginning of the inguinal ligament, is reached when the round movement of the palpating finger drastically changes to flat palpation (▶ Fig. 11.20). The chapter on the hip and groin region (Chapter 5) describes the location of further structures of the groin and thigh region.

11.7.5 Pubic Symphysis

The anterior pelvic girdle connection is around 40 mm long and has an oval articular surface that is 30 to 35 mm long. There is a 10- to 12-mm gap between the bony parts of the pubic bone (Becker et al., 2010). The symphysis is tilted by around 30 to 40° from a superoanterior to an inferoposterior direction compared to the longitudinal axis of the body. Its superoanterior end delimits the abdominal cavity (▶ Fig. 11.21).

It can be accessed when the connection between the two ASIS (interspinous plane) is searched in the center (linea alba). If moderate pressure is applied inferiorly and deeply, it can be identified based on the bony resistance. Small back-and-forth movements of the palpating finger allow the narrow space between the branches of the pubic bone to be felt as a small gap, even through the reinforcing ligaments.

11.8 Orienting Projections

The orienting projections that are possible due to bony palpation are presented next. Before commencing with palpation of the muscles, the abdomen is divided into regions using lines and planes.

11.8.1 Epigastric Region

- **Anterior axillary line:** At the level of the anterior axillary fold. It is delimited by the pectoralis major muscle (not illustrated).
- **Medioclavicular line:** In men, this line often runs through the nipples and is then referred to as the mamillary line.
- **Inferior thoracic aperture:** This aperture is demonstrated by the subcostal plane, a connecting line of the margins of the inferior costal arch, which can be found on the inferior margin of the cartilage of the 10th rib.

11

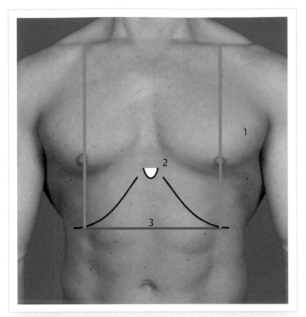

Fig. 11.22 Inferior thoracic aperture. 1 = medioclavicular line, 2 = xiphoid process, 3 = subcostal plane.

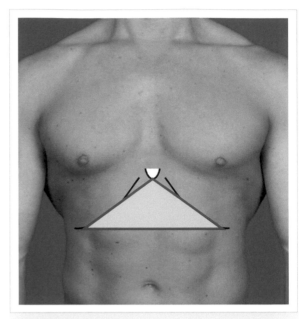

Fig. 11.23 Epigastric triangle.

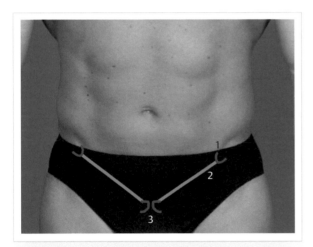

Fig. 11.24 Inguinal ligament. 1 = anterior inferior iliac spine, 2 = inguinal ligament, 3 = pubic symphysis.

These inferior margins can be reached when the medioclavicular lines meet the costal arches (Schünke et al., 2005; ▶ Fig. 11.22).

- **Epigastric region (epigastric triangle):** Lines are drawn from the endpoints of the subcostal plane to the xiphoid process. The area bordered by these three lines is the epigastric triangle (▶ Fig. 11.23).

11.8.2 Lower Abdomen

- **Inguinal ligament:** When locating the boundary between the lower abdomen and the thigh, the inguinal

ligament offers good orientation. Since it is not an actual ligament in the usual sense, but rather the connecting line of the fascia of the flat abdominal muscles, it cannot be clearly determined as an independent structure. For this reason, the bony fixed points (ASIS and pubic tubercle) must be connected with a line (▶ Fig. 11.24).

- Anatomists have described the connection of the two ASIS as the interspinous plane (Schünke et al., 2005). It identifies the position of the promontory of the sacrum, the anterior edge of the sacral base. The connections from the ASIS to the navel are important orientation aids for finding the first and fourth colon points. Both lines should be of the same length. If they are not, it must be assumed that the patient's pelvis is laterally shifted in supine position. This may also be a sign of pelvic obliquity or scoliosis (▶ Fig. 11.25).

11.8.3 Anterior Median Line

The linea alba runs in the center, between both muscle bellies of the rectus and the navel, and divides the abdomen into a left and a right half. In terms of pathology, diastasis recti and hernias are seen at this line (▶ Fig. 11.26).

11.9 Muscles

11.9.1 Rectus Abdominis

The rectus sheath gives both individual muscles a connective tissue capsule, so that the medial and lateral contours of the muscle bellies are either visible or can be felt during muscle activity. The tendinous intersections that pass

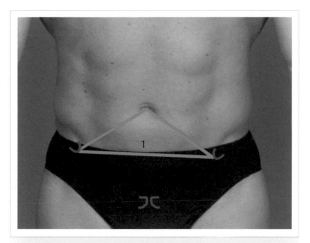

Fig. 11.25 Connection of the two anterior superior iliac spine (ASIS). 1 = interspinous plane.

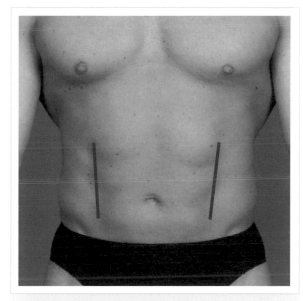

Fig. 11.27 Lines of the linea semilunaris.

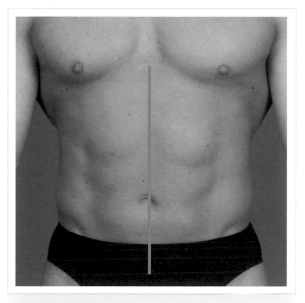

Fig. 11.26 Linea alba.

and continue only as fascia in the direction of the linea alba and also form the rectus sheath. This line, referred to as the linea semilunaris (Williams, 2009), is located somewhat medial to the medioclavicular line. At this line, which is also called the "semilunar line," the abdomen is covered only by fascia and access to deeper-lying structures is easier (▶ Fig. 11.27).

11.9.3 Regional Subdivision of the Central Abdomen

The last orienting projection of the abdominal wall describes the region of the umbilicus (navel). The semilunar lines between the flat abdominal muscles and the muscle bellies of the rectus muscles, as well as the subcostal and interspinous plane, surround a central abdominal region around the navel: the umbilical region. The area lateral to each semilunar line is referred to as the lateral abdominal region (▶ Fig. 11.28).

Transverse Abdominal

Therapists use secure palpation as a feedback method for muscle activity in abdominal drawing (in maneuvers). Approximately 2 cm medial to the ASIS on the interspinous plane, the coverage of the transverse abdominal by other muscles is lowest. Moderate deep pressure allows muscle contraction to be distinctly felt when the patient is asked to pull in their navel.

External Oblique

Midway between the iliac crest and the 12th rib and directly lateral to the muscle space (14 cm lateral to the

transversely across the muscle are best palpated during slight muscle activity. They are generally located at the level of the navel, at the level of the xiphoid process, and at the center of this distance (Williams, 2009). In rare cases, they show left–right symmetry and are located at the same level. The site 1 cm lateral and 2 cm inferior to the navel allows for reliable recording of muscle activity with EMG and is therefore also the most reliable location for palpation (Yang et al., 2017).

11.9.2 Linea Semilunaris

Between the rectus and the muscle bellies of the obliques, a line marks the point at which the muscle bellies of the flat abdominal muscles (transverse and obliques) terminate

11

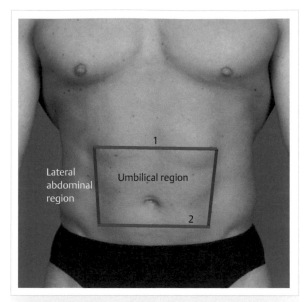

Fig. 11.28 Regional subdivision of the central abdomen. 1 = subcostal plane, 2 = interspinous plane.

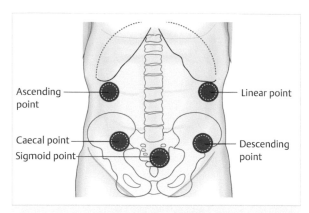

Fig. 11.29 Colon points according to Vogler.

linea alba) is the best place to palpate the activity of this powerful trunk rotator when the patient rotates the trunk to the opposite side.

Internal Oblique

Boccia and Rainoldi (2014) describe the most reliable option for palpating isolated activity. Palpation should be carried out exactly 2 cm below the most prominent point of the ASIS, just medial and superior to the inguinal ligament.

Abdominal Aorta

Dictated by the position of the abdominal aorta, palpation begins at the left of the vertebral column after all possible contraindications have been ruled out. In adults, the navel corresponds approximately to the position of the L3–L4 vertebral disk and is thus further superior thanks to the aortic bifurcation in the common iliac arteries at the level of L4. The aortic bifurcation is nearly precisely 2 cm inferior and left of the navel (Williams, 2009). By applying moderate pressure posteriorly and distinctly medially, the direct pulsation should be easy to feel in thin patients. If this pulsation is easy to feel in a corpulent individual, this is a sign of possible aortic dilation or even aortic aneurysm (Williams, 2009). In emergency medicine, palpation of the pulsation on the abdominal wall is also used to diagnose an aortic aneurysm rupture.

Psoas Major

Palpation begins again at the semilunar line, this time starting from the right side, again at the level of the navel

or somewhat superior to it. Using slowly increasing and yet firm pressure in a posterior and medial direction, the bony resistance of the L3 vertebral body should first be palpated. It can be assumed that the inferior vena cava will evade the gradual increase in pressure. Lateral to the L3 vertebral body, the muscle belly of the psoas major is then palpable. It responds to the direct pressure very firmly but still elastically. The iliacus can be accessed from the first and fourth colon points, as will be described later.

11.10 Palpation of the Colon

Manual treatments are very helpful for regulating intestinal motility. In addition to abdominal massage, colon massage according to Vogler is mainly used to treat defecation disorders resulting from atonia or spastic bowel muscles (Reichert, 2015). Vogler describes the treatment at five set points (▶ Fig. 11.29), where the colon can be reliably accessed and with the exception of the fifth point, no other organs need to be compressed to do so (Krauß, 1986):

1. Cecal point.
2. Ascending point.
3. Linear point (left colon flexure).
4. Descending point.
5. Sigmoid point.

The palpation of the colon at the first four points may also be used for diagnostic purposes. Normally, as the flat hand palpates along the colon, it meets consistent elastic resistance. Locally increased resistance is a sign of increased filling or spasms of the large intestine. Differentiation of inflammation in the area of the pressure point is described below.

11.10.1 Locating the Cecal Point

It marks the transition between the caecum and the ascending colon. On a line between the right ASIS and the

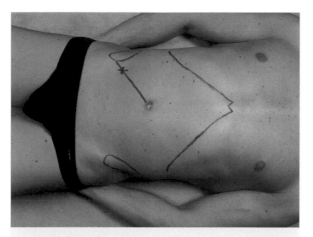

Fig. 11.30 First colon point.

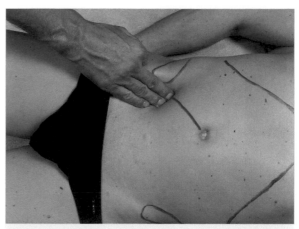

Fig. 11.31 Palpation at the cecal point.

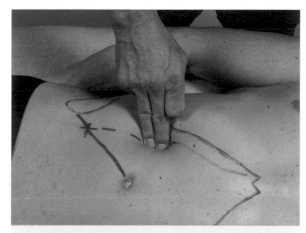

Fig. 11.32 Hand position of the second colon point.

navel, a point 2 finger widths superomedial to the ASIS is sought. It is located on the semilunar line lateral to the margin of the rectus (▶ Fig. 11.30).

The colon can be reached by pressing two or three finger pads posteriorly until somewhat firm resistance is encountered. If the patient's abdomen is relaxed, the pressure may be unaccustomed, but should not be unpleasant or painful. If the palpating finger is oriented deeply in an inferolateral direction, part of the iliacus will be reached.

▶ Differentiation from a Pathological Condition. If the palpation should cause sensitivity to pressure, it must be clarified whether the patient has a spastic colon or appendicitis, which is a contraindication for manual therapy of the colon (▶ Fig. 11.31).

If inflammation were present, the patient would already report pain and show guarding. If the therapist suddenly rebounded the fingers, the pain would substantially increase. Further medical examinations are then

required. The site described by Charles Heber McBurney in 1891 is still used today to diagnose appendicitis and as an access point for laparoscopy (Grover et al., 2012).

11.10.2 Locating the Ascending Point

The second point is located on the semilunar line around 2 finger widths below the costal arch and reflects the position of the right colic flexure (▶ Fig. 11.32).

Using two or three flat finger pads, if pressure is applied posteriorly the same consistency is expected as that at the first point, that is, with little resistance and high elasticity.

▶ Differentiation in the Case of Sensitivity to Pressure and Increased Firmness. If the patient presents with these clinical signs, the question is whether it is merely a case of a highly filled, possibly spastic, colon, or whether the patient has a pathological liver or gallbladder condition. To differentiate between these conditions, the therapist attempts to locate the inferior margin of the liver.

To do this, the therapist uses three or four flat finger pads and presses hard on the second colon point, first posteriorly and then superiorly, until the fingertips encounter increased resistance (very firm and somewhat elastic). This margin is generally easy to recognize, because the liver has the firmest tissue encountered during palpation of the abdomen.

The margin is normally smooth and round but not sharply circumscribed. The length of the inferior margin of the liver varies widely. Gilbert (1994) describes that the inferior margin protrudes up to 1 cm below the costal margin. He considers the presence of the liver 2 cm or more below the costal margin to be abnormal (▶ Fig. 11.33).

Since the liver "hangs" below the diaphragm, it follows its length during breathing. This mechanism is used to confirm the position of the inferior liver margin. The

11

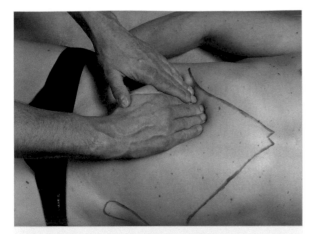

Fig. 11.33 Palpation of the hepatic margin 01.

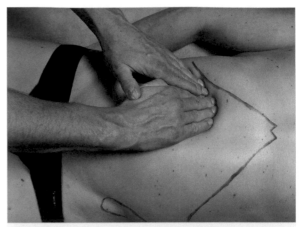

Fig. 11.34 Palpation of the hepatic margin 02.

therapist palpates the assumed margin, first with the patient breathing calmly and then requesting the patient to exhale deeply, while following the liver with the fingertips in a superior direction. When the patient inhales, the margin of the liver presses against the fingertips and thus confirms the correct location (▶ Fig. 11.34).

If this maneuver does not provoke any pain, spasticity or fullness of the colon at the right colic flexure is responsible for the unpleasant feeling of pressure during palpation of this point. If the pressure of the liver against the palpating fingers produces pain during deep inhalation, this may indicate a pathological condition (e.g., inflammation of the liver or gallstones). For this reason, this point is then omitted during a colon massage and a medical examination is advised.

▶ **Tips on Pathology.** In this way, experienced physicians can draw conclusions about the size and consistency of the liver. If the liver is severely enlarged, palpation must start in a position that is sufficiently inferior. During deep inhalation, pain on pressure provoked medial to the medioclavicular line may also be caused by a pathologically changed gallbladder (Murphy's sign). This clinical sign, with a specificity of 93.6%, has a high diagnostic value as well as a highly reliable predictive value for a pathological condition if it is determined (Trowbridge et al., 2009).

If the liver is pathologically enlarged, it can protrude very far down into the right abdominal cavity. An enlarged liver may be caused by venous congestion or cirrhosis of the liver, among other reasons.

If palpation causes pain on pressure, the cause is more likely to be a pathological condition of the gallbladder. A medical examination is urgently advised if pain on pressure occurs. When delivering manual colon therapy, the position of the margin of the liver must always be examined in order to reliably locate the colic flexure.

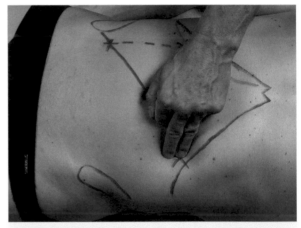

Fig. 11.35 Third colon point.

11.10.3 Locating the Linear Point

This point represents the position of the left colic flexure and is located in nearly a mirror image to the ascending point on the left side. Using palpation, it can be located in the superior continuation of the semilunar line to the costal arch. In contrast to the ascending point, palpation can begin directly at the costal arch (▶ Fig. 11.35).

▶ **Differentiation of Enlarged Spleen in the Presence of Sensitivity to Pressure and Increased Firmness.** The question is whether it is merely a case of a highly filled, possibly spastic, colon, or whether the patient has a pathological condition of the spleen. To differentiate between these conditions, the therapist attempts to locate the inferior margin of the spleen. The bean-shaped lymphatic organ has a posterolateral position in the peritoneum and measures approximately 11 × 7 × 3 cm. The longitudinal axis drops parallel to the alignment of the 9th and 11th ribs (Rauber and Leonhardt, 1987).

Since the spleen is connected to the diaphragm, it also follows the raising and lowering during exhalation and inhalation. When the patient is in the semi-side-lying position, the abdominal wall relaxes even more.

The therapist uses the fingertips of one hand to place moderate pressure below the left costal arch. During deep inhalation, the spleen moves from a posterolateral to an anterolateral direction, so that the inferior margin of the spleen moves against the fingertips. The therapist performing palpation recognizes this through a significant increase in pressure at the fingertips (▶ Fig. 11.36 and ▶ Fig. 11.37). The spleen is not palpable in healthy individuals. If the spleen is pathologically enlarged, it can be accessed below the left costal arch.

If this maneuver does not provoke any pain, spasticity or fullness of the colon at the left colic flexure is responsible for the unpleasant feeling of pressure during palpation of this third point.

11.10.4 Locating the Descending Point

Similar to the location of the cecal point, the descending point is also located around 2 finger widths on a line between the left ASIS and the navel. This palpation point is also located lateral to the rectus margin, so that little soft tissue covering the area between the skin and colon will impede palpation (▶ Fig. 11.38).

11.10.5 Locating the Sigmoid Point

The sigmoid point is located directly superior to the symphysis (▶ Fig. 11.39). The differences between palpation of this point and the previously described points are quickly apparent:

- Deep pressure is applied on the linea alba, directly superior to the symphysis.
- Deep pressure reaches the bladder, depending on how full it is, and in women, possibly also the uterus.

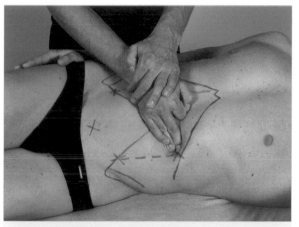

Fig. 11.36 Palpation of the spleen 01.

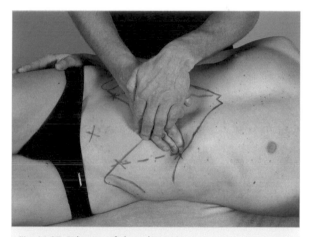

Fig. 11.37 Palpation of the spleen 02.

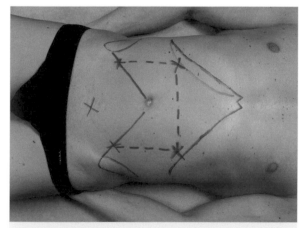

Fig. 11.38 Fourth colon point.

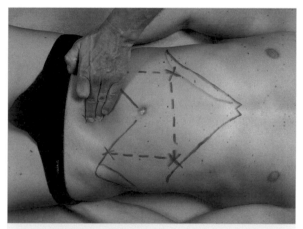

Fig. 11.39 Fifth colon point.

11

For this reason, it is advisable to use soft, increasing pressure.

11.11 Palpation of the Groin Region

In terms of structure, the inguinal canal is a hiatus, a virtual space between different layers of fascia and aponeuroses (Williams, 2009). It is the connection between two inguinal rings:

- The deep inguinal ring is an opening in the fascia of the transverse abdominal. It is located 1 to 1.5 cm superior to the center of the inguinal ligament.
- The superficial inguinal ring is created by an opening of the aponeurosis of the external oblique (Winkel, 2004). It is located superior to the transition of the medial to center third of the inguinal ligament. The superficial ring is the weaker of the two inguinal rings. Its lateral margin is stronger than the medial margin.

Starting from the deep inguinal ring, the inguinal canal runs medially. Fibers of the fascia of the transverse and internal oblique muscles accompany the sensitive structures through the canal. Size and shape vary in accordance with age: In newborns, the rings are located nearly on top of each other and the canal is very short. In adults, it is 3 to 5 cm long. In men, the canal is longer and the opening of the superficial ring is larger (Williams, 2009).

11.11.1 Technique and Expectations

With the patient in the supine position, the lower abdomen is undraped to allow improved access to the symphysis. The bony reference points, ASIS and pubic tubercle, are located. This demonstrates the course of the inguinal ligament. Palpation begins at the pubic tubercle and is oriented at the inguinal ligament up to the transition of the medial to the center third (▶ Fig. 11.40 and ▶ Fig. 11.41).

Applying direct pressure posteriorly and superiorly, the palpating fingertip makes its way through the subcutis to the abdominal wall, which becomes distinct through slight muscle activity (by asking the patient to pull in the navel). The superficial inguinal ring is reached when a round, pliable place on the abdominal wall is palpated. In a patient with an enlarged superficial inguinal ring, it feels as though the finger would be able to penetrate the abdominal cavity. In a patient with a hernia, a bulge is encountered. In men, Schiebler et al. (1999) recommend locating the spermatic cord and following it superiorly until the abdominal wall is reached. The ring should then be palpable directly lateral to the spermatic cord with the little finger.

The correct location of the palpation can be confirmed by the palpating finger meeting the firmer boundary of the ring in a lateral direction, while the medial boundary is much softer.

11.11.2 Palpation of Inguinal Hernias

The palpation of the groin region to confirm or exclude an inguinal hernia is one of the therapist's primary tasks. When examining the groin region, the therapist must not overlook an inguinal hernia.

- A lateral, indirect inguinal hernia is the protrusion of abdominal cavity contents through the deep inguinal ring. The hernial sac runs from the deep inguinal ring and through the inguinal canal and to the superficial inguinal ring. The incidence of inguinal hernia is higher in younger people.
- A medial, direct inguinal hernia is the protrusion of abdominal cavity contents through the superficial inguinal ring. The hernial sac pushes through the abdominal wall on a direct path to the superficial inguinal ring. It occurs more commonly in older individuals and in men is not related to the spermatic cord.
- In 15% of individuals, combined inguinal hernias occur that have both a lateral and a medial hernial sac.

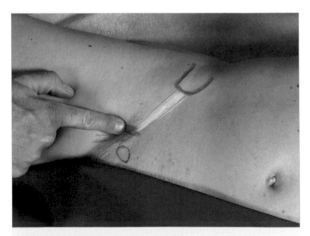

Fig. 11.40 Locating the inguinal canal.

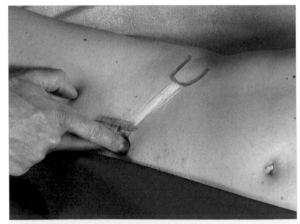

Fig. 11.41 Palpation of the inguinal canal.

Symptoms during coughing, lifting, and pressing, as well as constipation and stool retention, and also problems during urination are reported by the patient. These symptoms may be accompanied by vegetative symptoms and fever. A bulge may be detected during inspection. The palpation of the hernias is limited to the superficial inguinal ring. If a hernia is discovered during palpation, the palpation should be extended to the scrotum or labia majora (Winkel, 2004). The extent to which the hernia can be repositioned is often the critical factor for surgery. Imaging (e.g., ultrasound) can be used to differentiate a hernia from inguinal lymph nodes and can determine the type of tissue.

Bibliography

Becker I, Woodley SJ, Stringer MD. The adult human pubic symphysis: a systematic review. J Anat. 2010; 217(5):475–487

Boccia G, Rainoldi A. Innervation zones location and optimal electrodes position of obliquus internus and obliquus externus abdominis muscles. J Electromyogr Kinesiol. 2014; 24(1):25–30

Cowan SM, Schache AG, Brukner P, et al. Delayed onset of transversus abdominus in long-standing groin pain. Med Sci Sports Exerc. 2004; 36(12):2040–2045

Ferguson CM. Inspection, auscultation, palpation, and percussion of the abdomen. In: Walker HK, Hall WD, Hurst JW, eds. Clinical Methods: The History, Physical, and Laboratory Examinations. 3rd ed. Chapter 93. Oxford: Butterworth-Heinemann; 1990

Frick H, Leonhardt H, Starck D. Taschenbuch der gesamten Anatomie. Spezielle Anatomie II. 4. Aufl. Stuttgart: Thieme; 1992

Füeßel H, Middeke M, Duale Reihe Anamnese und klinische Untersuchung. 6. Aufl. Stuttgart: Thieme; 2018

Gilbert VE. Detection of the liver below the costal margin: comparative value of palpation, light percussion, and auscultatory percussion. South Med J. 1994; 87(2):182–186

Greten J. Kursbuch traditionelle chinesische Medizin: TCM verstehen und richtig anwenden. 3. Aufl. Stuttgart: Thieme; 2017

Grover CA, Sternbach G. Charles McBurney: McBurney's point. J Emerg Med. 2012; 42(5):578–581

Krauß H. Periostbehandlung, Kolonbehandlung: zwei reflextherapeutische Methoden (nach Vogler), 6. Aufl. Stuttgart: Enke; 1986

Kumar R, Ganghi R, Rana V, Bose M. The painful rib syndrome. Indian J Anaesth. 2013; 57(3):311–313

Leonhardt H, Tillmann B, Töndury G, Zilles K, Eds. Rauber/Kopsch: Anatomie des Menschen. Bd. I, Bewegungsapparat. 2. Aufl. Stuttgart: Thieme; 1998

McBurney C. Experience with early operative interference in cases of disease of the vermiform appendix. NY Med J. 1889; 50:676–684

Ploumis A, Michailidis N, Christodoulou P, Kalaitzoglou I, Gouvas G, Beris A. Ipsilateral atrophy of paraspinal and psoas muscle in unilateral back pain patients with monosegmental degenerative disc disease. Br J Radiol. 2011; 84(1004):709–713

Rauber A, Leonhardt H, Eds. Anatomie des Menschen: Lehrbuch und Atlas. Band 1 – Bewegungsapparat. Stuttgart: Thieme; 1987

Reichert B. Massage-Therapie. Stuttgart: Thieme; 2015

Schiebler TH, Schmidt W, Zilles K. Anatomie: Histologie, Entwicklungsgeschichte, makroskopische und mikroskopische Anatomie, Topographie. 8. Aufl. Heidelberg: Springer; 1999

Schmailzl KJG, Hackelöer BJ. Schwangerschaft und Krankheit: Wechselwirkung, Therapie, Prognose. Stuttgart: Thieme; 2002

Schünke M, Schulte E, Schumacher U, et al. Prometheus, Lern Atlas der Anatomie, Allgemeine Anatomie. Stuttgart: Thieme; 2005

Trowbridge RL, Rutkowski NK, Shojania KG. Does this patient have acute cholecystitis? JAMA. 2003; 289(1):80–86 Review. Erratum in: JAMA 2009; 302: 739

Udermann BE, Cavanaugh DG, Gibson MH, Doberstein ST, Mayer JM, Murray SR. Slipping rib syndrome in a collegiate swimmer: acase report. J Athl Train. 2005; 40(2):120–122

Vogler P, Krauß H. Periostbehandlung, Kolonbehandlung. Stuttgart: Thieme; 1986

Williams PL. Gray's Anatomy. 40th ed. Edinburgh: Churchill Livingstone; 2009

Winkel D. Nichtoperative Orthopädie und Manualtherapie. Anatomie in Vivo, 3. Aufl. München: Urban & Fischer bei Elsevier; 2004

Yang Y, Du ML, Fu YS, et al. Fine dissection of the tarsal tunnel in 60 cases. Sci Rep. 2017; 7:46351

11

Chapter 12

Thoracic Spine and Thoracic Cage

12 Thoracic Spine and Thoracic Cage

12.1 Significance and Function of the Thoracic Region

The thoracic region is one of the stable and comparatively rigid sections of the vertebral column. Initially, this may appear to be more of a disadvantage. However, on taking a closer look at the functions of the thoracic region it becomes clear that stiffness is actually an advantage.

The thoracic spine and the thorax have the following functions:
- Protective function.
- Supportive function.
- Junction between the cervical and lumbar spines.
- Respiration.

12.1.1 Protective Function

The thoracic spine, combined with the thoracic cage and the sternum, provides a stabile bony cage that protects the heart, lungs, and other important organs. Small and large mechanical stresses can be absorbed by this stabile, yet elastic, construction. The vertebral canal is very narrow, almost completely enclosed by bones, and home to a large section of the spinal cord.

12.1.2 Supportive Function

In addition to maintaining our upright posture, this section of the body must be stable enough to absorb all impulses arising in the arms. Large muscles, such as the latissimus dorsi and pectoralis major, and the scapulothoracic joint surfaces transmit large compressive and tensile loads. Without this central stability we would be unable to carry the weight of our arms, let alone that of larger loads. At the same time, the lateral tract of the erector spinae muscles is very strong in the lumbar region, but gradually loses its effectiveness more superiorly. Other strong muscles such as the spinalis provide the strength for thoracic extension.

12.1.3 Junction between the Cervical and Lumbar Spines

The thoracic mobility supports extensive arm movements —though not to the same extent as in the lumbar spine where mobility optimizes leg movement. Nevertheless, full arm elevation is only possible up to approximately 150° when the thoracic region is unable to move into extension. The expected range is generally 180°. Arm elevation causes movement from the cervicothoracic junction down to approximately T6/T7:
- in the form of extension (with bilateral arm elevation); or
- in the form of extension with rotation (when one arm is elevated).

This knowledge is useful when locating the level of thoracic symptoms. Can thoracic symptoms also be provoked using extensive arm elevation?

Extensive external and internal rotation at one shoulder joint is transmitted onto the thoracic spine as rotation. Bilateral rotation causes the thoracic spine to flex (with internal rotation) or extend (with external rotation).

From a biomechanical point of view, the thoracic spine has to act as a connection, passing on movement between the cervical spine and the lumbar spine:
- The predominant functional movement in the cervical spine is rotation.
- Flexion and extension are the dominating movements in the lumbar spine.

The cervical spine and the lumbar spine couple lateral flexion and rotation in their own specific way.

Anatomically, the mobile sections of the vertebral column can be well differentiated from one another. The thoracic spine stands out as the section that supports the ribs. Functionally, there is a fluent transition between its sections. Both lordotic sections extend functionally into the thoracic section of the vertebral column. It is therefore expected that extensive cervical movements can be palpated down to approximately T4–T5. Lumbar movements are carried over to approximately the level of T10–T11. The real thoracic spine is found between these points.

12.1.4 Respiration

In healthy people, quiet respiration is completely controlled by activity in the diaphragm. Forced respiration is supported by movement in the thorax. Respiratory movements are the result of the following:
- Elasticity in the thoracic cage.
- Mobility in the costovertebral joints.
- Supportive movements in the thoracic spine.
- Activity in different intrinsic muscles and the accessory muscles of inhalation.

The extensive costal joint movements associated with forced respiration are very important for the diagnostic process. Does deep inhalation or exhalation provoke back pain?

12.1.5 How Does this Affect Palpation?

The upper thoracic segmental movement associated with extensive arm elevation can be palpated well. An example of this is seen when the therapist places several finger pads over the cervicothoracic junction on the left side of the spinous process. The therapist can then feel the

12

spinous process's rotation to the left when the right arm moves into full elevation.

Respiratory movements can also be palpated. The opening and closing of the intercostal spaces provides information on the mobility of the ribs at their articular connections to the vertebral column and the flexibility of the intercostal muscles.

Different techniques can be used to palpate the thoracic segments during movement to assess the presence of restricted mobility. While clear rules exist explaining the relationship between lateral flexion and rotation in the lumbar spine and the cervical spine, it is not possible to set fixed rules for the mid-thoracic region. There is so much variation between individuals that functional relationships have to be newly assessed every time.

12.2 Common Applications for Treatment in this Region

The thoracic spine and the thorax are the home for the sympathetic nervous system. It is well known that the central region of the sympathetic nervous system is found in the lateral horn of the thoracic spinal cord. Important thoracic organs are represented in the large Head zones. This close relationship between viscerotomes and dermatomes can be used for diagnosis. Treatment not only affects these organs via the reflexes, it can also affect the neurovegetative control of the head and arms. Preganglionic fibers extend from the upper thoracic segments into the cervical sympathetic chain ganglions. The thoracic spine and the thorax are therefore an ideal location to apply mechanical (Swedish massage, connective-tissue massage, manual therapy), thermal, or electrical stimuli to affect sympathetic nervous system activity. These forms of intervention are the recurring topic of discussion in the treatment of chronic musculoskeletal pain.

The thoracic spine and the thorax are also often directly affected by the almost violent interventions used in open thoracic surgery. In older patients, these joints become rigid as part of the adaptive aging process. During this type of surgery, thoracic segments and costal joints are placed in extreme positions and are then forced into inactivity for weeks on end. In such a case, it takes a lot of effort to train a thorax to breathe properly again. A variety of respiratory parameters are used here for diagnosis: the frequency, rhythm, and direction of respiration, as well as the range of thoracic motion between maximal inhalation and expiration. The compression of the thorax and the mobilization of soft tissues are important manual techniques used in respiratory therapy that require certain basic palpatory dexterity.

Pain and restricted mobility in the costal and vertebral joints not only lead to restrictions in respiration, they also strongly interfere with daily tasks. Hypomobility in connection with pain plays an important role here. In no other section of the vertebral column is the assessment of

segmental mobility and extremely localized mobilization as important as in the thoracic spine (▶ Fig. 12.1).

Three large groups of pain origin are observed:
- Acute and chronic internal ruptures of the intervertebral disk.
- Painful hypomobility in the zygapophysial joints (ZAJs).
- Painful hypomobility in the costovertebral joints (costal joints).

Hypermobility is rarely seen to be a cause of symptoms. For a long time intervertebral disks were not considered a possible source of thoracic symptoms until it became clear that not only protrusions and prolapses, but also internal rupturing of the anulus fibrosus may be a possible source of symptoms. It is recommended that the sudden development of thoracic pain first be treated as an intervertebral disk problem. Axial unloading techniques have been successfully used here (▶ Fig. 12.2).

Specific regions display a higher frequency of certain pathological conditions (personal correspondence from the International Academy of Orthopedic Medicine [IAOM] study group):
- T1–T4: costovertebral joints > acute problem with the intervertebral disk > pathological ZAJ.
- T5–T8: acute problem with the intervertebral disk > pathological ZAJ > costovertebral joints.
- T9–T12: acute problem with the intervertebral disk > costovertebral joints > pathological ZAJ.

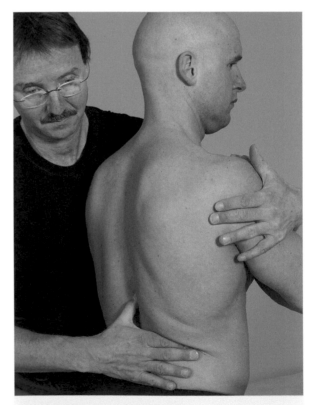

Fig. 12.1 Assessment of local mobility.

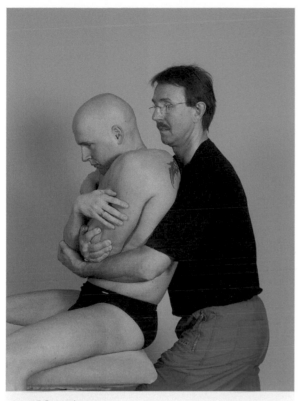

Fig. 12.2 Axial traction.

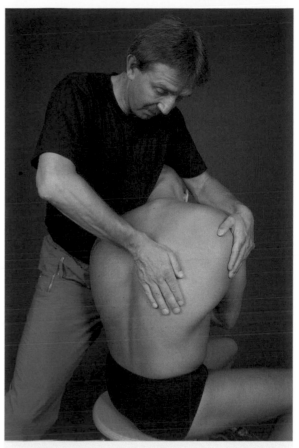

Fig. 12.3 Diagnosing the position of the ribs.

The first four costovertebral joints are very rigid and tend to be more hypomobile. A link to strenuous arm activity, or a one-off exertion of force, for example, carrying a very heavy weight, or sudden shortness of breath, is often seen as a cause of symptoms. The role of palpation is to accurately locate a level to provoke the costovertebral joints and to ascertain the position of structures during inhalation and expiration (▶ Fig. 12.3).

Symptoms arising from the costovertebral joints are often felt between the shoulder blades. They are also often felt on top of the shoulder. A large portion of the pain in the trapezius probably arises from the first rib being blocked in a position of inhalation.

12.3 Required Basic Anatomical and Biomechanical Knowledge

12.3.1 Functional Divisions in the Thoracic Spine

The thoracic spine differs anatomically from the other sections of the vertebral column due to its connection to the 1st–12th ribs on each side. The functional thoracic spine is not a single unit:
- The upper thoracic spine belongs to the cervical spine. Extensive cervical movements are carried on down to T4/T5.

- The lower thoracic spine belongs to the lumbar spine. Lumbar movements are carried on up to T10/T11. Flexion and extension are especially possible in this section.
- Based on this, the "real" thoracic spine is only found between T5 and T10.

On further inspection, these sections can also be differentiated from one another morphologically (▶ Fig. 12.4). The shape of the two upper thoracic vertebrae is more similar to a cervical vertebra while the lower thoracic vertebrae gradually take on the shape of a lumbar vertebra. Only the spinous processes in the middle section of the thoracic spine slant down typically at a steep angle.

12.3.2 Anatomical Characteristics of the Thoracic Spine

In the next section, only the typical morphological characteristics of the thoracic vertebra will be discussed. All further important information regarding the parts of a movement segment can be read in Chapter 10 in "Required Basic Anatomical and Biomechanical Knowledge."

12

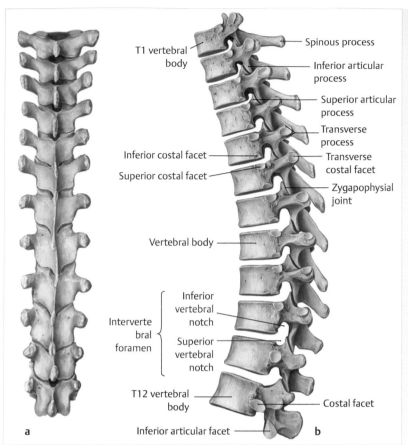

T1 vertebral body

Spinous process

Inferior articular process

Superior articular process

Transverse process

Inferior costal facet

Superior costal facet

Transverse costal facet

Zygapophysial joint

Vertebral body

Interverte bral foramen

Inferior vertebral notch

Superior vertebral notch

T12 vertebral body

Costal facet

Inferior articular facet

a   b

Fig. 12.4 View of the thoracic spine.

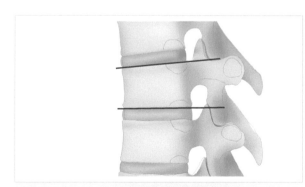

Fig. 12.5 Wedge shape of the vertebral body.

The Thoracic Vertebral Body

The thoracic kyphosis is not only a result of posture, it is also caused by anatomy. The lumbar lordosis is directly related to the wedge-shaped construction of the intervertebral disks at L4/L5 and L5/S1 and the L5 vertebral body. It is the wedge shape of the vertebral body that causes the kyphotic form (▶ Fig. 12.5). The superior and inferior end plates of the vertebrae are always parallel to one another in one segment. When examined, it can be seen that the vertebral body is more heart shaped. This is

probably an adaption to the very anteriorly located center of gravity for this section of the body.

Most thoracic vertebrae have two articular surfaces on each side that form a joint with the head of the ribs via the disk in the socket (joint of head of rib or costovertebral joint).

The Thoracic Intervertebral Disk

The thoracic intervertebral disks are quite thin and therefore adjust to the comparatively small movements in a segment. The heads of the ribs stabilize the disk on the sides. The posterolateral direction for a thoracic prolapse (not likely) is therefore occupied by bone. It is very unlikely that intervertebral disk substance will cause nerve-root compression. The intervertebral foramina, with their exiting spinal nerves, are found significantly superior to the intervertebral disk. This is another reason why spinal nerves are rarely affected by a thoracic prolapse.

The Vertebral Foramen

The vertebral foramen is round and, in comparison to the other sections of the vertebral column, very narrow (▶ Fig. 12.6). As the laminae of the thoracic vertebral arch

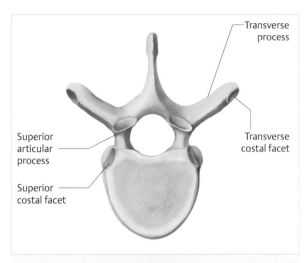

Fig. 12.6 View of a thoracic vertebra.

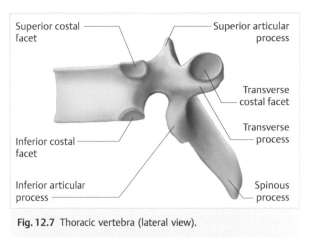

Fig. 12.7 Thoracic vertebra (lateral view).

are very high, the foramen is almost completely enclosed by bone from all sides. The spinal cord takes up almost the entire diameter of the foramen and cannot make way for other masses that may intrude on this space (e.g., fracture, bleeding, or intervertebral disk prolapse). The dura mater and the spinal cord have a particularly high chance of being compressed when these pathological conditions are present in the thoracic spine.

Spinous Process

The thoracic spinous process is known to be very long and points in an inferior direction (▶ Fig. 12.7). Its shape is the typical characteristic of a thoracic vertebra.

The length and the angle of the spinous process vary between the upper, middle, and lower thoracic sections. The slant results in a significant difference in the level between the tip of the spinous process and the corresponding transverse process. This difference is summarized in the "finger rule." This rule is used to locate the structures belonging to the same vertebra that can be reached using palpation.

The spinous processes overlap, especially in the mid-thoracic spine. This means that when the thoracic spine is brought into extension, the spinous processes come into contact with each other quickly here and compression increases. Small bursae absorb the friction while the spinous processes slide a little over one another and restrict extension. The thoracic spine is locked in this position.

How Does this Affect Palpation?

In a neutral starting position (SP), the very long **spinous processes** can be easily palpated and differentiated from one another. It is very simple to draw the outline of the tips on the skin. The sitting position is the only position where the active, tensed muscles may make it harder to access the spinous processes. Furthermore, the therapist must be aware that no spaces exist between the spinous processes. The tip of the superior spinous process lies on the posterior side of the inferior spinous process.

The **locked position of the thoracic spine** resulting from the overlapping thoracic spinous processes in extension is not a suitable SP to palpate segmental mobility. The segments are able to move better when the thoracic spine is slightly flexed—the resting position for the thoracic spine. The therapist should therefore ensure that the thoracic spine is always positioned in a slight kyphosis for all SPs.

The **"springing test,"** the posteroanterior pressure on the spinous processes, is not suited to assessing mobility in the thoracic spine. Pressure on these long processes does not result in translation movement. The vertebra tilts backward instead.

Transverse Process

The anatomical study conducted by Cui et al. (2015) clearly shows that the length of the traverse processes (measured from the base to the tip), at approx. 17 mm, remains nearly constant in all thoracic vertebrae (T1–T10). The transverse processes of T1 and T10 are the shortest. However, the transverse processes appear to become increasingly shorter from cranial to caudal, because they increasingly point more posteriorly. In T1, this posterior tilt angle is approx. 24° and the angle more or less continuously increases down to T10 to up to approx. 64°. The length of the T1 transverse process is of particular interest when searching for the costovertebral joint between the first rib and T1.

Each transverse process has a small joint facet on its anterior aspect that forms the costotransverse joint with a rib. The spatial orientation of the transverse process determines the position of the common axis for both costovertebral joints (see also "Mechanics of the Costovertebral Joints," see ▶ Fig. 12.14 below).

12

How Does this Affect Palpation?

The direct paravertebral area is covered by less muscle mass in the thoracic spine than in the lumbar spine. This enables the therapist to confidently access the transverse process and provides an extra lever to affect segmental mobility. The question is, how does the therapist find the transverse process belonging to a specific vertebra? This is achieved using two different methods:
- Each transverse process is found at the level of the accessible medial end of a rib. When counting the ribs from the 12th rib up to the 8th rib, for example, and consistently following this rib in a medial and cranial direction, the level of the T8 transverse process is reached.
- Locating a spinous process and overcoming a difference in height. The difference in position between the spinous process and the transverse process conforms to the finger rule. The therapist can reliably locate the level of a transverse process by first palpating the localized tip of the corresponding spinous process.

Tip

Finger rule

The typical thoracic vertebra is constructed with a difference in height between the spinous process and the transverse process. The extent of this difference varies almost from segment to segment. The therapist attempts to determine this difference by using the patient's index finger during palpation (▶ Fig. 12.8).

When the therapist wishes to access the corresponding transverse process, they move a specific number of finger widths in a superior direction from the lower edge of the spinous process:
- T1, T2 spinous processes: plus 1 finger width.
- T3, T4 spinous processes: plus 2 finger widths.
- T5-T8 spinous processes: plus 3 finger widths.
- T9, T10 spinous processes: plus 2 finger widths.
- T11, T12 spinous processes: plus 1 finger width.

Facet Joints

The alignment of the thoracic ZAJs is quite different from that seen in the lumbar region. In relation to the end plates, the superior joint processes are tilted upright at an average angle of 70° and are tilted 20° anteriorly on the sides (▶ Fig. 12.9). This means that the processes lie in a perfect circular arc around the rotation axis found in the disk. Rotation is therefore not significantly restricted by either the ZAJ or the ribs and is evenly distributed between all segments (excluding the thoracolumbar junction) (White and Panjabi, 1990).

How Does this Affect Palpation?

Segmental rotation is suitable for the assessment of segmental mobility and also for restoring this mobility with the use of appropriate techniques.

12.3.3 Thorax

The bony thorax is formed by 12 pairs of ribs and the sternum. Two kinematic chains meet at the point where the ribs connect to the vertebrae (▶ Fig. 12.10):
- Vertical kinematic chain = thoracic spine.
- Horizontal kinematic chain = costovertebral joints.

The two kinematic complexes affect one another with their mobility and stability. The thorax affects the thoracic spine by increasing its stiffness and reducing its range of motion, for example, during lateral flexion (White and Panjabi, 1990). This is advantageous when concentrating on the protective and supporting functions of the thoracic spine.

Construction of a Rib

A rib is a curved long bone that seeks contact with the sternum as it turns downward from posterior to anterior. It is made up of different sections (▶ Fig. 12.11).

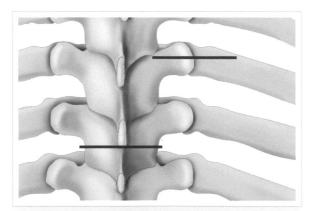

Fig. 12.8 Difference in height between the spinous process and the transverse process.

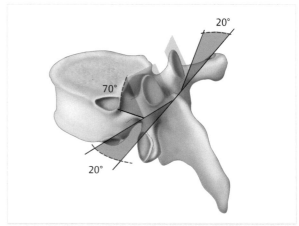

Fig. 12.9 Alignment of the thoracic zygapophysial joint (ZAJ).

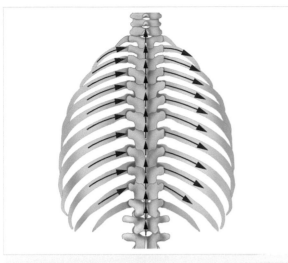

Fig. 12.10 Kinematic chains: thoracic spine and thorax.

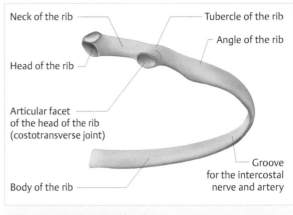

Fig. 12.11 Construction of a rib.

How Does this Affect Palpation?

- The tubercle of the rib can sometimes be palpated. It is found directly adjacent to the tip of the transverse process.
- The angle of the rib is the largest curve in the rib and extends the most posteriorly. The easiest point to feel the rib is at its angle near the vertebral column.
- The superior edge of the body of the rib is rounded; the inferior edge is more sharp-edged. With this knowledge, the therapist can assess whether malpositioning is present in fixed inhalation or expiration during the palpation of the thorax.

Articulations between the Ribs and Sternum

The ribs are divided into three groups based on the different types of contact with the sternum (► Fig. 12.12):
- Direct contact with the sternum: the true ribs—1st–7th ribs.
- Indirect contact with the sternum: the false ribs—8th–10th ribs.
- No contact with the sternum: the floating ribs (mobile ribs)—11th and 12th ribs.

The 11th and 12th ribs end without bony contact in the wall of the trunk and demonstrate a firm-elastic consistency on direct pressure. Their length varies considerably.

The connecting cartilage of the 8th to 10th ribs forms the costal arch. Both costal arches meet at the epigastric angle on the xiphoid process of the sternum. The distance between the costal cartilages of the 10th ribs demonstrates the size of the inferior thoracic aperture. The connection between the costal cartilage and its superior

neighbor is not particularly stabile. Subluxations can occur due to trauma ("slipping ribs," Migliore et al. 2014).

Most of the costosternal junctions to the true ribs are small true joints, very firm and resilient. The second rib is usually attached to the sternal angle (junction between the manubrium and the body of the sternum). Hardly any variations in anatomy are evident here.

Articulations between the Ribs and the Vertebrae

Differences are made depending on which parts of the rib or the vertebra articulate (► Fig. 12.13):
- *Costovertebral joints (joint of the head of the rib):* the head of the rib articulates with two vertebral bodies and the disk. Exceptions are the 1st, 11th, and 12th ribs. Only a vertebral body is seen here.
- *Costotransverse joints:* the tubercle of the rib forms a joint with the transverse process of the corresponding vertebra. Exceptions are the 11th and 12th ribs. No joints exist here.

The superior four ribs share very firm articulations with the vertebrae and tend to be more hypomobile. The first rib in particular stands out in clinical practice.

Mechanics of the Costovertebral Joints

The axis of movement couples both joints functionally and passes through the neck of the rib. The transverse process differs in length and spatial alignment in the upper, middle, and lower thoracic spine. It determines how far posterior and lateral the costotransverse joint is located. Ultimately, it determines the position of the rotational axis for movements of the ribs during inhalation and expiration (► Fig. 12.14).

The length and alignment of the transverse processes in the upper thoracic spine (T1–T7) causes the rotational axis to be aligned more in the frontal plane. This results

12

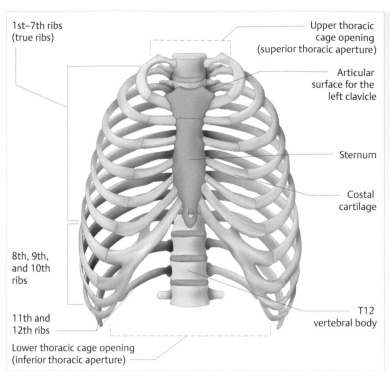

1st–7th ribs
(true ribs)

Upper thoracic
cage opening
(superior thoracic aperture)

Fig. 12.12 Divisions of the ribs.

Articular
surface for the
left clavicle

Sternum

Costal
cartilage

8th, 9th,
and 10th
ribs

11th and
12th ribs

T12
vertebral body

Lower thoracic cage opening
(inferior thoracic aperture)

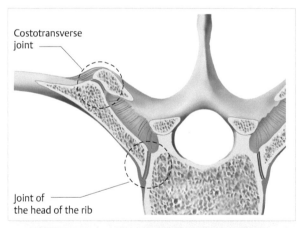

Costotransverse
joint

Joint of
the head of the rib

Fig. 12.13 The joints between the ribs and the vertebrae.

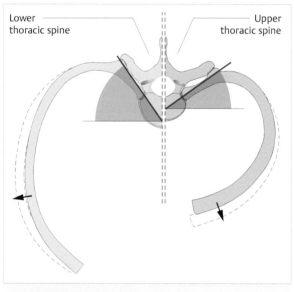

Lower
thoracic spine

Upper
thoracic spine

Fig. 12.14 Costovertebral joint mechanics.

in elevation and expansion of the thorax in the sagittal plane due to the mechanics of the ribs. The more sagittally oriented axes in the middle and lower thoracic spine enable the thorax to expand in a lateral direction.

Forced inhalation (▶ Fig. 12.15) always results in intercostal spaces widening in every section of the thorax. The intercostal spaces become narrower during expiration (▶ Fig. 12.16). This movement pattern allows diagnosing through palpation with movement. Movements of the arm have similar effects on the intercostal spaces:

• Arm elevation with flexion raises the upper thorax in a more anterior direction and opens up the upper intercostal spaces.

• Arm elevation with abduction raises the lower thorax in a more lateral direction and opens up the lower intercostal spaces.

The rotation of the ribs around the longitudinal axis in the neck of the rib during deep inhalation and expiration results in the inferior or superior edges of the ribs facing slightly outward.

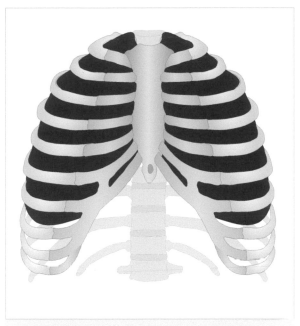

Fig. 12.15 Thorax in the position of inhalation (source: Kapandji, 2006).

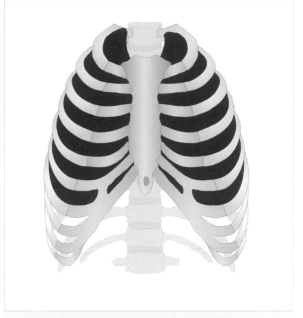

Fig. 12.16 Thorax in the position of expiration (source: Kapandji, 2006).

How Does this Affect Palpation?

The inferior or superior edges can be felt at the end of forced inhalation and expiration. The edges are not palpable during quiet respiration. The relationship of structures to one another is interesting when the ribs are pathologically fixed in a position of inhalation or expiration. When the therapist assesses the position of structures, it is noticeable that the blocked rib has another form in comparison to its neighboring mobile ribs (see the section "Assessment of the Costovertebral Joints" below).

Interaction of Movement between Costovertebral Joints and the Thoracic Segments

As described above, two kinematic chains meet: The vertical chain of thoracic movement segments and the horizontal chain of the ring-like rib segments. Vertical and horizontal chains, meaning the thoracic movements and costovertebral movements, have reciprocal influence.

When the cervical spine moves from the neutral position (slight kyphosis) in a certain direction, the thoracic cage remains in its resting position momentarily before it moves along.

During thoracic extension, a relative expiration position of the costovertebral joints initially occurs.

Practical assessment: Compare the thoracic movements with the patient sitting and breathing in and out deeply (a) in neutral position and (b) in extended thoracic spine position. In extension, expiration decreases (since

the thorax is already in relative expiration) and the extent of inhalation increases (since the thorax starts from relative expiration). Many patients with shortness of breath support themselves in thoracic extension in order to exploit this mechanism for deepened inhalation.

During thoracic flexion, a relative inhalation position of the costovertebral joints thus initially occurs.

Practical assessment: Compare the thoracic movements with the patient sitting and breathing in and out deeply (a) in neutral position and (b) in flexed thoracic spine position. In flexion, inhalation decreases (since the thorax is already in relative inhalation) and the patient would have to increase the extent of expiration (since the thorax starts from relative inhalation), if the abdominal contents did not naturally resist the movement of the thorax.

In the case of lateral flexion of the thorax, for example, to the right, the costovertebral joints on the concave side (in this case, on the right) achieve a relative inhalation position, and on the convex side (in this case, on the left), achieve a relative expiration position.

Practical Benefits

When examining a patient with thoracic spinal pain, the therapist can use these interactions to distinguish between the thoracic pain generators and pain from the costovertebral joints. According to IAOM doctrine, local segmental mobilizations should not be carried out without the mobilization of the associated rib ring segment in expiration and vice versa.

12

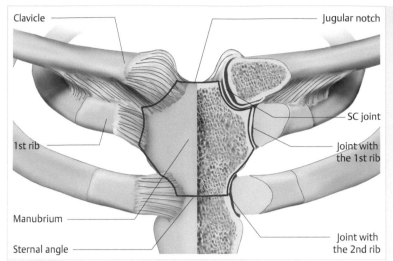

Clavicle

Jugular notch

Fig. 12.17 Manubrium of the sternum.

SC joint

1st rib

Joint with the 1st rib

Manubrium

Sternal angle

Joint with the 2nd rib

In respiratory therapy, the patient can be placed in the appropriate position, such as the tripod position or "C positioning," to enable the kinematic prerequisites for certain respiratory volumes or controlled breathing.

Detailed Anatomy of the Anteriorly Positioned Bones

▶ Fig. 12.17 is used in many anatomy books and shows the anatomy of the manubrium as the superior section of the sternum with its articular connections. The edge of the manubrium is equipped with many notches. The jugular notch is the most superiorly lying notch. The medial ends of the clavicles form the sternoclavicular (SC) joints lateral to this. The cartilage of the first rib has an articular connection to the manubrium immediately inferior to the SC joint. The sternal angle is found at the level of the connection to the second rib. This connection is described at times in anatomical literature as an articulation or as a synchondrosis. The manubrium moves on the body of the sternum as the thorax moves during respiration.

How Does this Affect Palpation?

The jugular notch is a reliable orientation point to access the manubrium from a superior position. The level of the notch also corresponds to the level of T2 (see the section "Anterior Palpation Techniques" in Chapter 13). It is easy to reach the SC joint from here (see the section "Sternoclavicular Joint Space" in Chapter 2).

The medial end of the first rib is found immediately inferior to the clavicle and extends posteriorly from here with a tight curve. It is very difficult to palpate. In comparison, the sternal angle is easy to reach and can be marked with confidence. The second rib is found at the same level without fail. The first five intercostal spaces can be reliably reached from here.

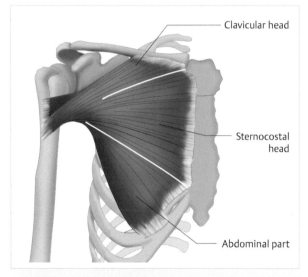

Clavicular head

Sternocostal head

Abdominal part

Fig. 12.18 Pectoralis major.

Detailed Anatomy of the Anterior Muscles

The anterior thorax is dominated by the pectoralis major (▶ Fig. 12.18). It is divided into three functional sections that are difficult to differentiate from one another anatomically. Their denominations refer to the surface of origin:
- Medial half of the clavicle: clavicular head.
- Manubrium and the body of the sternum, first to sixth costal cartilages: sternocostal head.
- Anterior rectus sheath: abdominal part.

How Does this Affect Palpation?

All edges of the muscle are palpable and also visible at times when active. The boundaries between the

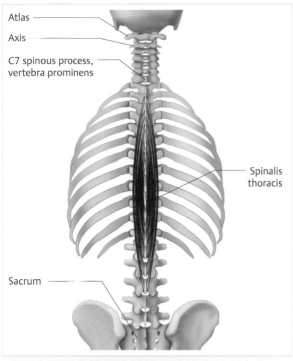

Atlas

Axis

C7 spinous process,
vertebra prominens

Spinalis
thoracis

Sacrum

Fig. 12.19 Spinalis thoracis.

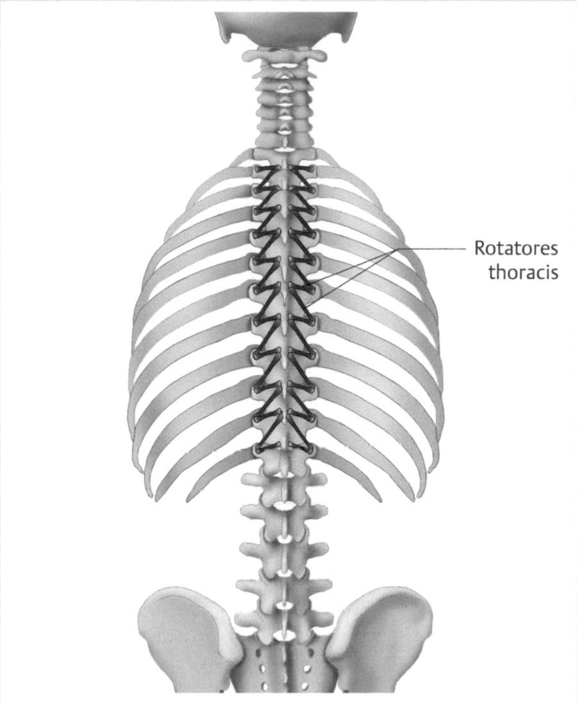

Rotatores
thoracis

Fig. 12.20 Rotatores thoracis.

individual sections are not distinctly recognizable. The rough muscle bundles that can be palpated do not usually correspond to the functional divisions.

12.3.4 Thoracic Back Muscles

Intrinsic Back Muscles

Within this group arising from the medial tract of the intrinsic back muscles, two muscle systems are unique to this region:
- Spinalis thoracis: represents the straight, spinal system.
- Rotatores thoracis: from the oblique, transversospinal system.

The interspinales muscles from several segments unite to form the spinalis thoracis (▸ Fig. 12.19). This muscle can only be found in the thoracic part of the vertebral column. It extends from L1–L3 to C7–T1 and is found directly adjacent to the row of spinous processes. The transition to the semispinalis cervicis is almost completely smooth. It forms the bulge of paravertebral muscles in the neck region and is consciously disregarded here.

The cross-section of the lateral tract gradually decreases here. The spinalis thoracis takes over its function of supporting the weight of the trunk against gravity. It also appears to be the muscle that has enough strength to extend the thoracic spine into extension.

The spinalis plays the most important role in the interplay between the extensors when correcting the posture of a strongly kyphotic thoracic spine.

How Does this Affect Palpation?

In the lumbar region, a depression is palpated directly next to the row of spinous processes before the palpating fingers rest against the medial side of the erector spinae muscle mass. This is not possible in the thoracic region. When palpating laterally from the tip of the spinous processes, the therapist immediately encounters a spinalis muscle approximately of 1finger width. Enormous muscle tension is frequently found here, which often feels unpleasant when direct pressure is applied to it.

The **rotatores thoracis muscles** (▸ Fig. 12.20) are short muscles found very deep in the tissue. They are in close contact with the ZAJs (from von Lanz and Wachsmuth, 2004a). The decisive factor for the exact terminology used for the muscles is their length:
- Extending over one segment: rotatores brevis.
- Extending over two segments: rotatores longus.

Their prominence corresponds well to the ability to rotate to almost the same extent in all thoracic segments. The actions of the rotatores thoracis include the extremely differentiated fine adjustment of position and the local stability of the thoracic movement segments.

12

Some authors call the rotatores muscles "monitoring muscles." This means that these muscles tense when disturbances in segmental mobility are present and can provide the therapist with information regarding pathology when they palpate (Dvořák et al., 1998). However, the author doubts whether clinicians are actually able to selectively palpate the rotatores and to clearly perceive increased tension in this muscle group. When examined on an anatomical specimen, their deep position hidden beneath several other muscles is revealed.

Extrinsic Back Muscles

The thoracic section of the back is dominated superficially by the latissimus dorsi and the most important representatives of the thoracoscapular muscle group. The latter muscle group extends from the trunk (from the row of spinous processes) to the scapula and belongs functionally to the upper limb. This consists of in particular:
- The descending and transverse parts of the trapezius.
- The rhomboids.

The originating fibers of the **latissimus dorsi** extend to the level of T7–T8 (see ▶ Fig. 12.21), and therefore also to the thoracolumbar fascia. The thoracolumbar fascia additionally receives fibers from the serratus posterior at this point. In comparison to the lumbar region, the latissimus

dorsi fibers do not cross the mid-line in the thoracic region. All further information about this muscle can be found in the section "Detailed Anatomy of the Muscles" in Chapter 10.

How Does this Affect Palpation?

The superior sections of the muscles can be recognized only in very muscular and very slim people. It is highly unlikely that this muscle can be reliably differentiated from other structures. Generally, the lateral edge can be demonstrated and palpated on toned people when their arm is active in extension.

According to von Lanz and Wachsmuth (2004), the most important parts of the **trapezius** for this section (▶ Fig. 12.21) have the following anatomical course:
- Ascending part: the fibers converge from their origin on the T4–T11/T12 spinous processes onto the medial end of the spine of the scapula, where they are evident posteriorly. Here they meet with the posterior fibers of the spinal part of the deltoid muscle.
- Transverse part: this part generally passes from the C7–T3 spinous processes to the upper edge of the spine of the scapula (lateral half). This is the thickest part of the trapezius. It becomes a prominent bulge when the scapula is adducted toward the vertebral column.

The therapist can generally note that the origins of this very superficially located muscle do not always have to involve attachment to both sides of the spinous processes. The fibers from both sides can merge into one another without bony contact; they sometimes form an aponeurosis that glides freely over the spinous processes, especially at the cervicothoracic junction. Bursae are frequently found on anatomical specimens. These bursae reduce friction. The question is: could bursitis also be a possible cause for gradually developing local symptoms in this area?

The junction between both parts of the muscle can only rarely be identified as a gap on anatomical specimens and is therefore not of interest for palpation. The inferior edge of the ascending part can be palpated when the muscle is active. The superiorly running fibers angled from medial to lateral become distinct when this part of the trapezius pulls the scapula posteriorly and inferiorly against resistance. Therefore, the hand palpates from an inferior position, perpendicular to the edge of the muscle, and hooks into the muscle.

12.4 Overview of the Structures to be Palpated

The goal of the palpation is to localize and identify all relevant bony structures and a number of important muscles. This includes:
- all spinous processes
- all transverse processes

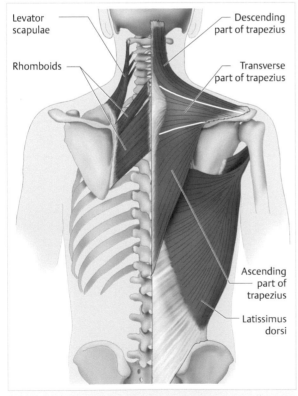

Levator scapulae

Rhomboids

Descending part of trapezius

Transverse part of trapezius

Ascending part of trapezius

Latissimus dorsi

Fig. 12.21 Extrinsic back muscles.

- all posterior ribs, insofar as palpable
- parts of the sternum
- ribs 1 and 2, anteriorly
- intercostal spaces

A variety of SPs are used here for palpation. The treatment examples should demonstrate how useful it is to apply surface anatomy precisely and to link this in with the daily clinical practice.

12.5 Summary of the Palpatory Process

The cervicothoracic junction is located in the sitting SP first and later with the patient pronated. All further sections of the thoracic segments and the ribs will be described after this. The sections of the sternum and the ribs are the subject of local palpation techniques anteriorly. The spatial alignment of some of the ribs will now become clear. The ability to conduct these techniques, especially the intercostal palpation, is the basis for the assessment of movement in the thorax during respiration.

The palpation of the scapula with its individual sections will not be discussed here (see section "Palpation of Individual Structures" in Chapter 2).

Correct palpation in the cervicothoracic region is used as a starting point to access the middle area of the thoracic spine and the posterior thorax. These regions could also be reached by starting inferiorly with the location of the 12th rib or the lumbar spinous processes. This has already been described in Chapter 10.

12.6 Starting Position

All SPs used here have been described in detail in Chapter 8.6. The therapist is a new element in the description of the SP in sitting. The therapist stands to the side of the patient, mostly opposite the side to be palpated. If it is necessary to move the head to confirm the correct location of a structure, the therapist facilitates the head movement with one hand and the other hand is used to palpate.

12.6.1 Difficult and Alternative Starting Positions

The SPs are always classified as difficult when access to the sought structure is obstructed, strong muscle activity prevents the therapist from being able to recognize a bony point precisely, or when the supportive surface is not large enough to provide a stable position for the patient. These positions can be encountered during clinical work with patients.

▶ **Examples**
- Palpating the cervicothoracic junction in the supine or side-lying position.
- Palpating the segmental thoracic mobility in sitting during movement.

12.7 Posterior Palpation Techniques

The exact palpation of the cervicothoracic junction is equally as important as the correct location of the posterior sacroiliac spine (PSIS) on the pelvis or the C2 spinous process in the upper cervical spine. It enables thoracic structures to be reliably accessed from a superior position and the lower cervical spine from an inferior position. The aim is to precisely visualize the C6–T1 spinous processes as well as the position of the first rib from posterior. This is followed by the location of all thoracic spinous processes and their relationship to their transverse processes and the corresponding ribs. This section concludes with several examples of assessment and treatment of the thoracic spine and the ribs that demonstrate how useful hands-on palpation is.

12.7.1 Cervicothoracic Junction in the Sitting Starting Position

The following technique aims to differentiate the thoracic and the cervical spines from one another. This cannot be done by locating the longest spinous process. The presumption that the longest spinous process corresponds to the vertebra prominens (C7) is misleading. The T1 spinous process is often the longer of the two.

Several of the following techniques require extensive cervical spine movement, which is not possible with every patient. They are only helpful when a certain amount of movement is available in the cervicothoracic region. When there are enormous restrictions in mobility in this region, differentiation is almost impossible. The only option that remains for differentiation is the palpation of the different contours felt on the spinous processes (e.g., C5 and C6) or by locating the first rib, which leads to the transverse process and ultimately to the T1 spinous process (Loyd et al., 2014).

There are various ways for reliably marking the T1 spinous process:
- Locating the spinous processes using cervical extension
- Locating the spinous processes using cervical rotation
- Posterior shift
- Locating the first rib

Location of the Spinous Processes Using Cervical Extension

One or two finger pads are placed over the middle of the posterior lower cervical spine. The anterior hand controls the position of the head (▶ Fig. 12.22).

12

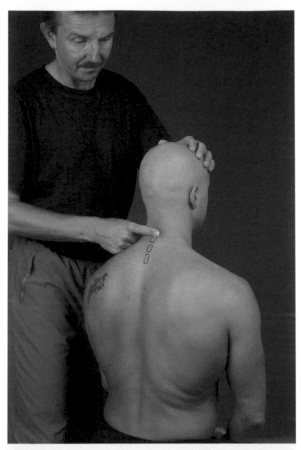

Fig. 12.22 Cervicothoracic palpation in the sitting starting position.

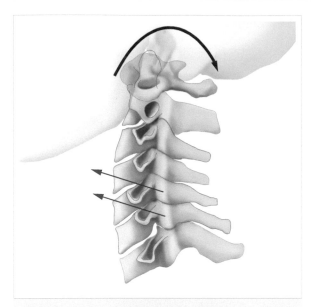

Fig. 12.23 Paradoxical translation of C5 and C6.

The position of the C6 spinous process can often be recognized by simply feeling its shape. When using moderate pressure to palpate from superior to inferior along the cervical mid-line, the therapist often feels the finger pads moving down onto a type of platform. The sides of the fingers come from a superior position and encounter the C6 spinous process. The finger pads are then lying on top of the C5 spinous process. As this method of location is not reliable enough, another aid is needed to confirm that it is correct.

Confirmation with Movement

The anterior hand is in contact with the patient's head and facilitates cervical extension by tilting the head backward. The C5 and C6 spinous processes behave typically during this movement. The upper cervical vertebrae move posteriorly during cervical extension. C5 and C6 shift anteriorly (▶ Fig. 12.23). C5 starts moving when extension is minimal, C6 at the end of the extension. These movements are clearly perceived as a spinous process disappears beneath the palpating finger pads.

The index finger pad remains on the assumed location of the C5 spinous process (▶ Fig. 12.24) and feels it

disappearing anteriorly when extension is minimal (▶ Fig. 12.25). The middle finger pad palpates the next inferior spinous process, most likely that of C6.

Cervical extension is repeated thoroughly (▶ Fig. 12.26). It is only at the end of extension that the spinous process moves anteriorly underneath the middle finger pad (▶ Fig. 12.27). This is the method used to precisely determine the position of the C6 spinous process.

The C7 spinous process is sought. It demonstrates a sudden decrease in movement during extension. The C7 spinous process remains more immobile in comparison to C5 and C6. Accordingly, the next inferior spinous process belongs to T1. This method enables the therapist to locate C5, C6, C7, and T1. However, this requires the patient to be able to extend the cervical spine without aggravating pain.

Locating the Spinous Processes Using Cervical Rotation

The movement pattern of the lower cervical spine is always composed of lateral flexion associated with ipsilateral rotation. This coupling is very strong and develops independent of the facilitation of rotation or lateral flexion.

These movements continue onto the upper thoracic spine, to approximately T4–T5. Extensive rotation or lateral flexion in the cervical spine can therefore be used to palpate movement at the cervicothoracic junction.

End-range cervical rotation or lateral flexion to the right always results in all spinous processes down to and including T4 rotating to the left. This occurs to different degrees. T1 and the vertebrae inferior to it are fixed by the ribs and the range of motion is reduced. It is therefore

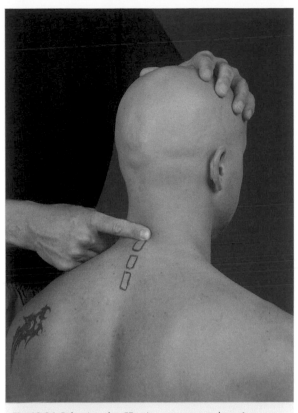

Fig. 12.24 Palpating the C5 spinous process—phase 1.

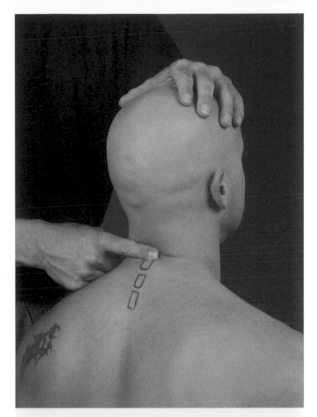

Fig. 12.25 Palpating the C5 spinous process—phase 2.

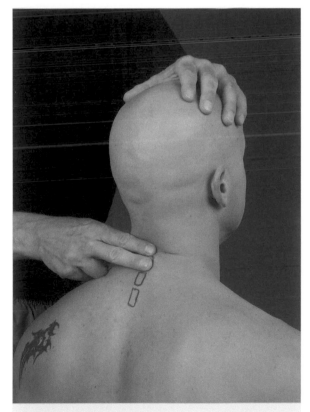

Fig. 12.26 Palpating the C6 spinous process—phase 1.

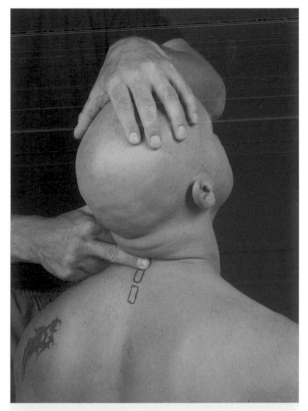

Fig. 12.27 Palpating the C6 spinous process—phase 2.

12

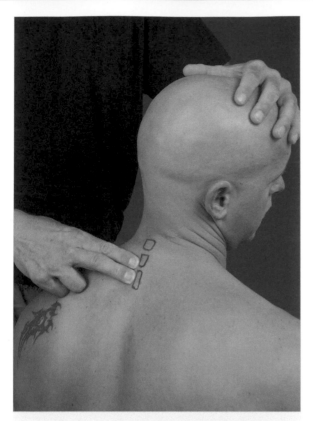

Fig. 12.28 Palpating the C7 and T1 spinous processes.

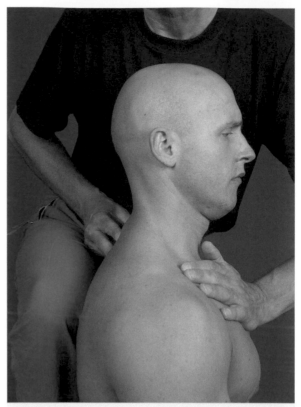

Fig. 12.29 Palpating T1 using posterior shift.

expected that rotation can only be detected down to the C7 spinous process.

The therapist is positioned next to the patient. When the therapist wishes to facilitate cervical rotation or lateral flexion to the right, two palpating fingers must be placed paravertebrally to the left of the cervicothoracic region.

They are placed against the left side of the assumed C7 and T1 spinous processes. When rotation or lateral flexion is facilitated, C7 is expected to move significantly further than the more slowly reacting T1 spinous process (▶ Fig. 12.28).

Locating T1 Using a Posterior Shift

So far, T1 has been characterized as a rigid vertebra with little mobility. The following differentiation method uses the intensive contact between T1 and the first rib ring segment. A translation movement of the first rib applied from anterior is felt posteriorly on the spinous process (▶ Fig. 12.29).

Two finger pads are placed posteriorly in the C7/T1 and T1/T2 interspinous spaces. The thenar eminence of the anterior hand applies a posterosuperiorly directed pressure onto the manubrium. This pressure is transmitted onto T1 via the first rib. The return movement of the T1 spinous process is palpable. The C7 spinous process tends to remain still. Up to three spinous processes move in flexible patients, with T1 moving the furthest.

Projection of the T1 Transverse Process

The T1 spinous process is located using the previously described options available for differentiation. Its inferior edge is marked on the skin. Starting from the inferior edge of the spinous process, the therapist now measures a patient's index finger width in a superior direction and approximately one patient's index finger length laterally (▶ Fig. 12.30).

This usually corresponds to the width of the T1 transverse process. The width of both T1 transverse processes is comparable to the distance between the tips of both C1 transverse processes (see the palpation techniques in the cervical spine).

Tip

The tip of the transverse process is always found in a muscular gap formed by the descending and transverse parts of the trapezius. The muscles (e.g., levator scapulae) nevertheless prevent direct contact with the transverse process and the rib.

However, therapists should always ensure that they are not mistakenly on the superior angle of the scapula by slightly elevating the scapula (see the section "Superior Angle of the Scapula" in Chapter 2).

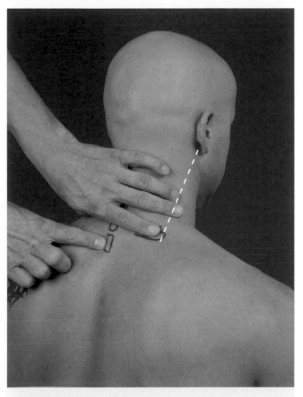

Fig. 12.30 Projection of the T1 transverse process.

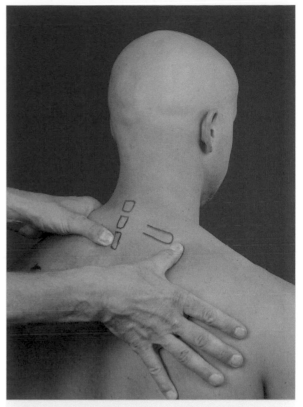

Fig. 12.31 Confirming the position of the T1 transverse process.

Locating the First Rib from Posterior

On the posterior aspect, the first rib can only be found directly adjacent to the assumed tip of the T1 transverse process. It changes its course from here onward, moves anteriorly, and cannot be palpated any more posteriorly. It can only be palpated through a layer of muscles by placing a thumb directly adjacent to the tip of the T1 transverse process.

Confirmation Using the Assessment of Consistency and Movement

▶ **Aim.** The junction between the tip of the transverse process and the first rib can only be correctly identified by assessing the end feel of both structures.

▶ **Criteria.** The thumb applies pressure onto the first rib and the T1 transverse process in an anterior and slightly medial direction. The first rib feels less firm than the transverse process. Naturally, the spinous process moves more clearly when pressure is applied onto the transverse process compared with pressure on the first rib. Some energy is absorbed by the costovertebral joints here.

Start by applying pressure very carefully. A blocked first rib can be very sensitive to direct pressure!

▶ **Procedure.** A thumb is placed over the T1 transverse process (right here). The other thumb braces itself against the T1 spinous process from the left side (▶ Fig. 12.31). Pressure on the transverse process rotates T1 to the left and the spinous process to the right. This is clearly felt as a decrease in pressure at the spinous process.

When the thumb is placed adjacent to the tip of the transverse process on the first rib and posteroanterior pressure is applied again, the therapist will feel the structure yielding slightly to pressure and resisting movement, not as firmly as is felt when pressure is applied to the transverse process. Associated T1 spinous process movement is still felt to a small extent.

12

Tip

Firm pressure must be applied to a layer of muscle that is frequently sensitive to pressure when this technique is used for differentiation. This difficulty is only slightly reduced by pressure being applied to the gap in the trapezius and the fact that the muscle layer is not particularly thick.

This differentiation technique requires a minimal amount of mobility in the costotransverse joint of the first rib.

Locating the First Rib Over Projections

Based on their specimen study, Loyd et al. (2014) described a highly precise way to locate the first rib, and in turn, the T1 transverse and spinous processes. They described the identical structural span (distance between the tips of the transverse processes) of C1 and T1. Furthermore, the vertical fall line of the mastoid process meets the costal tubercle of the first rib. The distance between the end of the transverse process of T1 and the first rib is approx. 1 cm (▶ Fig. 12.32).

For this reason, the IAOM teaching group recommends using these stable anatomical interconnections as the most reliable technique for determining the T1 processes.

- In the vertical fall line of an earlobe the body of the first rib can be directly palpated in the supraclavicular fossa.
- For palpation, this fall line is followed with vertical pressure of a thumb applied from a sagittal to a posterior direction (until behind the muscle belly of the descending part of the trapezius). This place corresponds to the transition from the mid to posterior third

of a sagittal line extending from the clavicle up to the level of the superior angle of the scapula, which is also located in the vertical fall line below the earlobe.

- As soon as the rib can no longer be felt from above and the palpating finger slides off in a caudal direction, the relationship between the level of the transverse process and T1 can be established. This point should coincide with the vertical fall line of the mastoid process. In slim individuals, if significant downward pressure is applied, the tip of the transverse process can even be palpated.
- The tip of the transverse process should coincide with the vertical fall line of the tip of the C1 transverse process.
- The T1 spinous process is located 1 finger width of the patient's finger in a further caudal direction (▶ Fig. 12.33).

From this point, all other thoracic spinous processes can be reliably reached in the sitting SP.

Tips for Assessment and Treatment

Restrictions in First Rib Mobility—Assessment

Painful restrictions in mobility in the joint between T1 and the first rib affect the expected end feel. The end feel is harder and is perceived as painful in most cases. Restrictions in the first rib joint mobility are the frequent cause of a persistently tensed trapezius.

Another well-established test—the springing test—can confirm restriction in mobility during inhalation (▶ Fig. 12.34).

▶ **Aim.** The springing test assesses movement in the first rib in the supraclavicular fossa with a sitting SP.

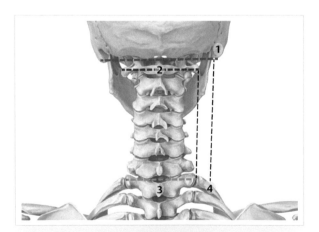

Fig. 12.32 Vertical projections on the patient according to Loyd et al. (2014). 1 = line connecting the two mastoid processes, 2 = line connecting the tips of the C1 transverse processes, 3 = line connecting the tips of the T1 transverse processes, 4 = vertical fall line of the mastoid process (ear lobe) meets the first rib.

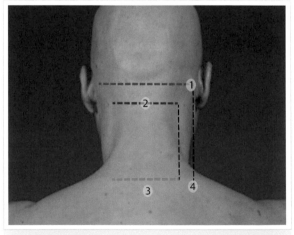

Fig. 12.33 Vertical projections on the model according to Loyd et al. (2014). 1 = line connecting the two mastoid processes, 2 = line connecting the tips of the C1 transverse processes, 3 = line connecting the tips of the T1 transverse processes, 4 = vertical fall line of the mastoid process (ear lobe) meets the first rib.

▶ **Procedure.** The therapist stands behind the sitting patient. An elbow controls the upper body. The hand is used to position the head. In the next step, the descending part of the trapezius is relaxed by slightly laterally flexing the neck to the ipsilateral side, allowing easier access to the rib. The second metacarpophalangeal joint of the palpating hand is placed to the side of the neck region and pushes in an inferior direction with the forearm strongly pronated. The first rib has been reached when the index finger feels significant resistance.

▶ **Criteria.** Repeated pressure indicates how much inferior movement is possible and how the rib resists movement as it springs up and down. The first rib is expected to have a firm-elastic feel. The rib only moves slightly, or not at all, when the rib is blocked in a position of inhalation. It resists movement very strongly. In most cases, the patient indicates that their symptoms are being aggravated during this procedure.

Restrictions in First Rib Mobility—Treatment

▶ **Aim.** To relieve pain or mobilize the costovertebral joints between T1 and the first rib in a neutral supine position.

▶ **Procedure.** The T1 transverse process is located in the supine position. The junction to the first rib is identified once again by assessing tissue consistency. The index finger is strongly flexed and its proximal interphalangeal (PIP) joint is placed on the posterior aspect of the first rib. The other fingers are also flexed and support the index finger. The thumb may be placed anteriorly but should not apply pressure. The PIP of the index finger is now found in the gap in the trapezius, superior to the superior angle of the scapula in most cases. To ensure that the fingers are not mistakenly in contact with the superior angle, the therapist assesses the location by moving the scapula into elevation and depression (▶ Fig. 12.35). No movement is expected to be felt beneath the index finger joint. Otherwise, the location must be assessed again.

The PIP joint of the index finger now applies pressure in an anterior and slightly medial direction. The necessary strength is obtained by abducting the wrist. The therapist may feel slight movement anteriorly on the first rib on some patients. To feel this, the therapist places the fingers of the second hand anteriorly over the first. The force used and the speed of movement depend on the aims of treatment:
- *Pain relief:* oscillations are used with quick, very small movements that should not provoke pain.
- *Mobilization:* pressure is applied until the tissue becomes taut. Pressure is repeatedly applied using small intensive movements every second for several minutes.

Tip

Mobilization can be further optimized and enhanced as follows:
- Using contralateral cervical rotation (here to the left) and the associated coupled lateral flexion (here to the left) would allow T1 to move along to a lesser extent with caudal pressure on the first rib and more energy of the mobilization to reach the joints of the first rib.
- If the first rib is blocked during inhalation, causing stretching of the lower parts of the brachial plexus, arm activities can additionally be used to induce caudal mobilization of the first rib.

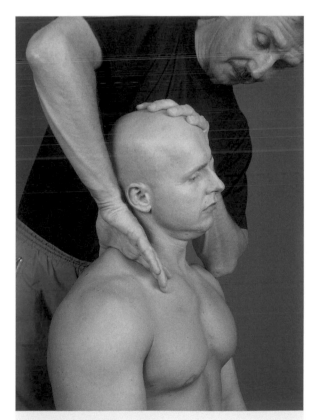

Fig. 12.34 Springing test.

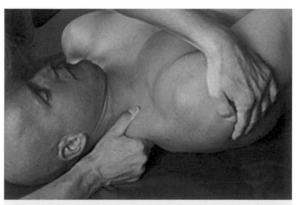

Fig. 12.35 Treating the first rib—phase 1.

12

Functional Massage of the Descending Part of the Trapezius

The functional massage in side-lying is one of the most effective methods available to reduce tension in the frequently tense descending part of the trapezius. This technique is integrated into massage therapy after large surface techniques (stroking and kneading) have been used. As changing position can be troublesome for patients, only one technique should be conducted per treatment. The technique combines a longitudinal stretch (shoulder girdle movement) with a transverse stretch (pressure applied by the hand).

▶ **Starting position.** The patient lies on the stomach and slides to the side of the treatment table, then rolls over into side-lying and moves as far as possible toward the edge of the treatment table, with the back to its edge. The therapist stands at this edge and stabilizes the patient with the body (▶ Fig. 12.36).

▶ **Preparation.** The technique starts with the passive movement of the shoulder girdle, for which both hands are placed on the shoulder. This exercise is used to help the patient learn to perceive movement in the shoulder girdle and to relax their muscles. This is possibly all that will be achieved in the first treatment session. The shoulder girdle is facilitated first into elevation and depression as well as protraction and retraction. Diagonal movements follow.

▶ **Variation 1—with depression and retraction**
- *Hand placement:* one hand is placed on top of the shoulder joint and facilitates the shoulder girdle. The second hand holds onto the descending part of trapezius using a palmar grip.
- *Technique:* the muscle is approximated somewhat by slightly elevating and protracting the shoulder girdle

("scapula moves forward and upward"). The thenar eminence is used to push the muscle anteriorly without allowing the hand to slide over the skin. The shoulder girdle is facilitated into extensive depression and retraction (scapula moves downward and backward) (▶ Fig. 12.37). The stretch should be stopped if the muscle belly slides out from underneath the hand.

Tip

If the base of the hand constantly rubs against the superior angle of the scapula during the previously described technique, extensive external rotation of the scapula can be used to move the superior angle inferiorly out of the way. This is achieved by elevating the arm extensively through flexion of the shoulder joint. This position must be maintained. There is then more space for the molding hand over the trapezius (▶ Fig. 12.38).

This technique is more effective when the cervical spine is positioned in lateral flexion away from the side to be treated (by lowering the head-end of the treatment table or by not using a pillow). This results in the muscle being placed in a position of high preliminary stretch, improving the stretching effect considerably. *Caution:* The patient must be able to laterally flex without aggravating pain. This must be assessed before applying the technique.

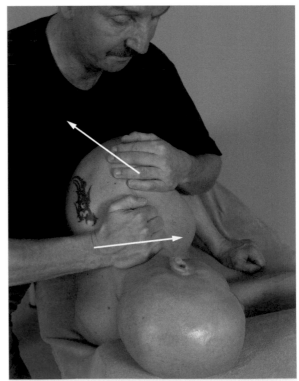

Fig. 12.37 Functional massage of the trapezius—variation 1.

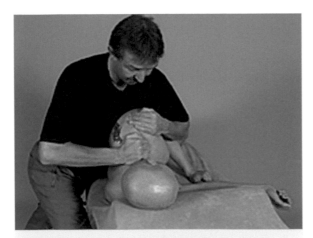

Fig. 12.36 Functional massage of the trapezius—starting position.

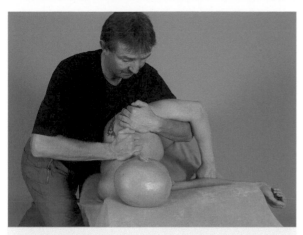
Fig. 12.38 Functional massage of the trapezius—variation in the starting position.

▶ **Variation 2—with depression and protraction**
- *Hand placement:* the same hand placement is used here as with variation 1.
- *Technique:* the muscle is approximated somewhat by slightly elevating and retracting the shoulder girdle (scapula moves backward and upward). The slightly flexed fingers pull the muscle posteriorly without allowing the fingers to slide over the skin. The shoulder girdle is facilitated into extensive depression and protraction (scapula moves forward and downward) (▶ Fig. 12.39). The stretch should be stopped if the muscle belly slides out from underneath the hand. The therapist should exercise caution when using the fingertips to palpate, as sensitive structures are found in the supraclavicular fossa (brachial plexus and vessels). This technique variation can also be conducted by initially positioning the cervical spine in lateral flexion.

12.7.2 Cervicothoracic Junction in the Prone Starting Position

If more precise assessment or treatment is going to be conducted in the prone position, it makes sense to also differentiate the vertebrae in the cervicothoracic junction in this SP. When switching to the prone position, it is not advisable to use the marks on the skin showing the spinous processes found during the palpation in sitting. The skin is subject to the effects of gravity and sags in sitting. This is different in the prone position. If the therapist were to use the markings from sitting in the prone position, the markings would be approximately one segment too high!

Location of the T1 Spinous Process Using Posterior Shift

The previously described location techniques using cervical extension and rotation or lateral flexion are difficult

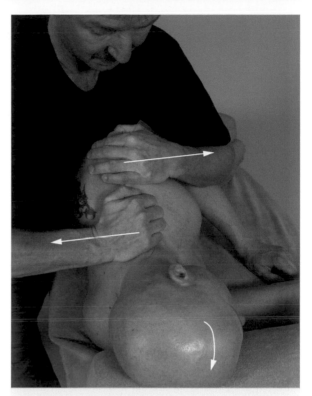
Fig. 12.39 Functional massage of the trapezius—variation 2.

to conduct in the prone position. The technique of choice is the anteroposterior pressure via the manubrium. The procedure and criteria basically correspond to the description for sitting.

Without the weight of the head, the applied pressure results in a larger and significantly more palpable posteriorly directed movement in the T1 spinous process. This technique is therefore a recommended method for location.

It is only in cases of severe restrictions in segmental mobility in this region that the use of this method for location will not be successful. If the C6 platform can be felt in sitting or in the prone position (see above), the inferior edges of the C6–T1 spinous processes can be counted.

Tip

Only a few finger pads can be used to apply the very local pressure onto the manubrium. Therapists should ensure that they are not pushing against the patient's throat. Patients often hold their sternum and shoulders in a posterior position, even when the pushing fingers have taken up their position. If necessary, the patient must be instructed to relax the shoulders and upper body and rest them on the treatment table.

12

Projection of the T1 Transverse Process in the Prone Position

The T1 transverse process is found 1 index finger width superior to the spinous process. The inferior edge of the T1 spinous process is located first and 1 finger width is measured superior to the tip of the spinous process. Here too, the length of the transverse process corresponds with the vertical fall line of the tip of the C1 transverse process.

Locating the First Rib from Posterior

The tip of the T1 transverse process is marked on the skin. The accessible section of the first rib lies immediately lateral to this. The junction between the transverse process and the rib can only be palpated on very slim people. This is also the case in the sitting SP. The position of the structures projected onto the skin must therefore be assessed (▶ Fig. 12.40). Again, the tissue resistance felt on direct pressure and the associated movement of the T1 spinous process play decisive roles. When the therapist applies pressure alternately to the assumed position of the first rib and the T1 transverse process (▶ Fig. 12.41), they realize again that the transverse process responds with considerably more resistance than felt in the first rib. By placing the thumb of the second hand on the other side of the T1 spinous process, the therapist can feel that the spinous process moves further away from the thumb when pressure is placed on the transverse process compared with when pressure is applied to the rib.

> **Tip**
>
> The costotransverse junction is usually found to be more superior than the superior angle of the scapula. It is nevertheless recommended that therapists passively move the shoulder slightly to ensure that their palpating hand is not mistakenly positioned over the angle of the scapula.

Locating the Other Thoracic Spinous Processes

There are principally three methods available to determine the position of the thoracic spinous processes:
- Identifying the level by using the structures of the scapula for orientation.
- Palpating from an inferior position by correctly locating the lumbar spinous processes or locating T11 via the 12th rib (see the section "Local Bony Palpation" in Chapter 10).
- Palpating from a superior position by locating the position of the spinous processes at the cervicothoracic junction (see the section "Cervicothoracic Junction in the Prone Starting Position" above).

When locating the spinous processes, the use of scapular bony landmarks for orientation is fairly unreliable as the size and position of the scapula vary between individuals. It is nevertheless suitable for rough orientation (▶ Fig. 12.42). The following classifications are recommended by Hoppenfeld (1992), Kapandji (1985), and Winkel (2004):
- The T1 spinous process and the second rib are found at the level of the superior angle of the scapula.
- The base of the spine of the scapula is found at the level of the T3 spinous process.
- The inferior scapular angle is found at the level of the T7 spinous process.

These classifications only apply to the vertical body posture. They do not apply to patients positioned in lying.

The palpatory process following the location of T1 is called the superior access. All further thoracic spinous processes can be located from here. The individual spinous processes are followed inferiorly. The lower edge of the processes should be used if the therapist wishes to correctly mark the location of the spinous processes on the skin.

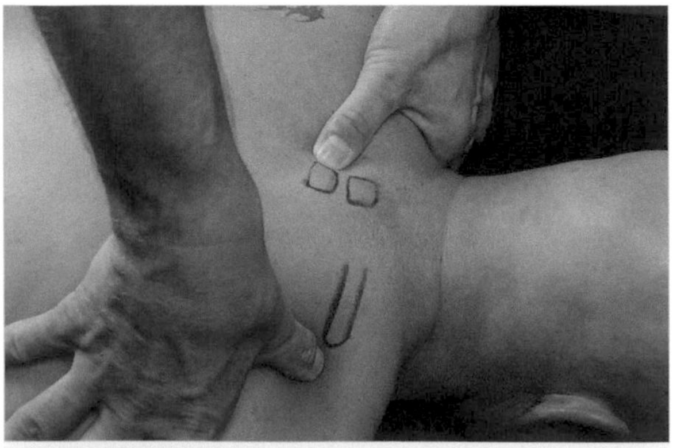

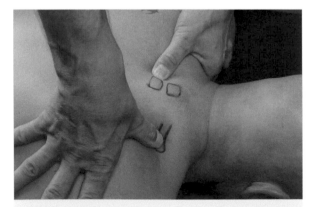

Fig. 12.40 Locating the first rib.

Fig. 12.41 Confirmation by assessing the consistency.

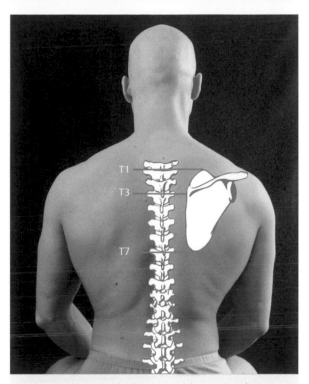

Fig. 12.42 Using scapular structures to locate a level.

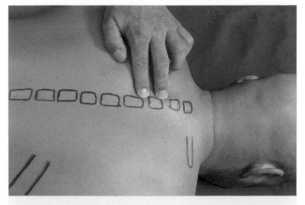

Fig. 12.43 Locating the levels using palpation starting from a superior position.

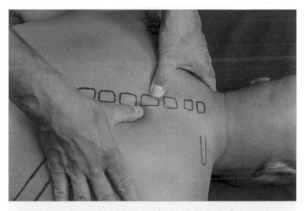

Fig. 12.44 Alternating palpation from the left and the right.

▶ **Starting position.** It is possible to palpate in sitting, in the prone position, and in side-lying. The prone and side-lying Ps are easier for palpation than the sitting SP. The tension in the intrinsic muscles near the mid-line (especially spinalis) makes it more difficult to gain access to the bony contour of a spinous process in the sitting SP.

Lowering the head-end of the treatment table significantly should be avoided when positioning the patient in prone position, as this places the interspinous ligaments under too much tension and makes location more difficult. Prepositioning in a slight kyphosis approximates the spinous processes and also hinders the palpation.

▶ **Technique.** The fingertips are placed perpendicular along the inferior edge of the spinous process. It is recommended that the interspinous space be found again using palpation. Interspinous spaces can be most skillfully palpated from the side and not from posterior (▶ Fig. 12.43). The tensed supraspinous ligament, covering the interspinous space, often makes it more difficult to palpate the contours of the spinous processes. Once the interspinous space has been palpated, the inferior edge of the more superiorly located spinous process can be marked with certainty.

All spinous processes can be marked using this method. This technique is reliable at the thoracolumbar junction when the area is accessed from an inferior position. Furthermore, it is helpful to know what changes are to be expected in the shape of the spinous processes. Once the therapist has

reached L1, the pointed and rounded forms of T11 and T12 change into long processes with larger dimensions.

Tip

The interspinous space can be palpated from both sides if the therapist needs further reassurance that the correct structure is being palpated. The most reliable method is to search for the interspinous spaces alternately from the left and the right (▶ Fig. 12.44). With this method, the palpating finger from one hand maintains contact with the correctly located interspinous space until the next inferior interspinous space has been located.

Difference in Height between the Spinous Process and Transverse Process of a Vertebra

The aim is to locate a spinous process in the mid-thoracic spine and its corresponding transverse process. The

12

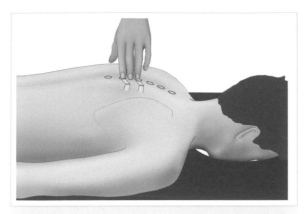

Fig. 12.45 Using the finger rule.

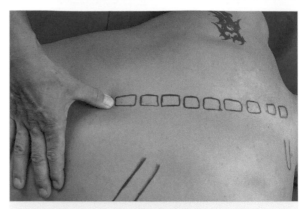

Fig. 12.46 Locating the T8 spinous process.

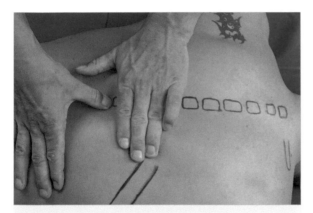

Fig. 12.47 Searching for the transverse process.

following exercise provides therapists with more confidence in their ability to exactly locate at every thoracic level.

It is typical for the thoracic vertebrae that there is a difference in height between the spinous process and the transverse process. The extent almost varies from segment to segment. This method of palpation uses the width of the patient's index finger in an attempt to specify the difference in height.

When the therapist wishes to access the transverse process of a specific vertebra, they calculate the superior distance using a certain number of finger widths from the spinous process (▶ Fig. 12.45). The transverse process and its corresponding rib are found at the same height. The procedure described here can therefore also be used to correctly locate the ribs.

▶ **Finger rule**
- T1, T2 spinous processes: plus 1 finger width in a superior direction.
- T3, T4 spinous processes: plus 2 finger widths in a superior direction.
- T5–T8 spinous processes: plus 3 finger widths in a superior direction.

- T9, T10 spinous processes: plus 2 finger widths in a superior direction.
- T11, T12 spinous processes: plus 1 finger width in a superior direction.

▶ **Starting position.** The palpation is conducted in the prone position but can also be conducted in sitting or side-lying.

▶ **Technique.** A spinous process is located, demonstrated here on T8, by marking its inferior edge (▶ Fig. 12.46). Three fingers are placed superior to the spinous process across the vertebral column. The corresponding transverse process and the eighth rib should be located at the level of the third finger (▶ Fig. 12.47).

Tip

The width of the fingers used should correspond to the patient's fingers. Measurements should be made to be on the safe side.

The correct location is confirmed using the corresponding palpable rib found at the same level. After using the finger rule, the rib is searched further laterally with a transverse palpation technique. The transverse process is found at the level of the most medial palpable aspect of the rib (angle of the rib). A step can often be felt between the rib and the tip of the transverse process when using the fingertips to palpate perpendicular to the skin (▶ Fig. 12.48).

Confirmation Using the Assessment of Consistency and Movement

The link between the spinous process and the transverse process can be observed during segmental movement. This involves applying pressure to the transverse process while palpating the corresponding spinous process from

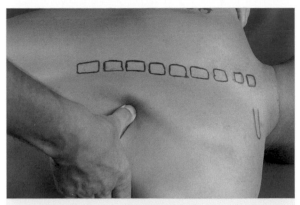

Fig. 12.48 Palpating the tip of the transverse process.

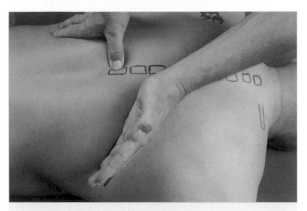

Fig. 12.49 Confirmation using movement.

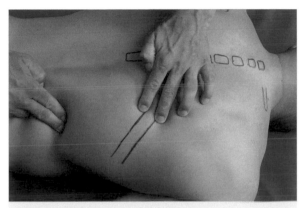

Fig. 12.50 Palpating the ribs from inferior.

the opposite side. The palpating finger can also be placed in an interspinous space. Posteroanterior pressure applied to the transverse process rotates the vertebra, for example, using the medial edge of the hand (▶ Fig. 12.49). The corresponding spinous process then rotates to the side of pressure and moves away from the palpating finger. It is recommended that pressure be released quickly as the return movement is often easier to feel than the movement into rotation.

The transverse process can be differentiated from the rib using the same technique. In this case, the medial border of the hand is placed more laterally on the rib and posteroanterior pressure is repeated. The rib demonstrates an elastic form of resistance, the movement in the spinous process is somewhat delayed and smaller than was previously seen when pressure was applied to the transverse process.

Confirming the Palpation of the Ribs from an Inferior Position

The reverse process can also be successfully used (locating a spinous process from the rib via the transverse process). The ribs are palpated one by one from the 12th rib upward (▶ Fig. 12.50), the level for the corresponding

transverse process is located, and the finger rule is used in an inferior direction to find the respective spinous process. This method is recommended for use in the area between approximately T7–T12. The scapula covers a large part of the ribs more superiorly.

12.7.3 Tips for Assessment and Treatment

There are a large number of options for treating the thoracic spine. Tactile perception and very exact anatomical orientation are of great use. The following section includes several descriptions of thoracic spine and costovertebral joint assessment and treatment techniques frequently seen in the daily clinical practice. This listing is certainly not complete.

Segmental Assessment of the Thoracic Spine

One example of a local segmental assessment technique is the assessment of mobility combined with a coupled pattern of movement. Contralateral rotation (left) and lateral flexion (right) are coupled here in combination with extension.

Technique in the Side-lying Starting Position

The patient lies in neutral side-lying (here, on the right) near the side of the therapist. The therapist places one hand on the upper-lying side of the thorax. The other hand is used to palpate the thoracic spine (▶ Fig. 12.51). The middle finger applies pressure from an inferior direction into the interspinous space. If necessary, the index finger may be used to support the middle finger (▶ Fig. 12.52). The original functional section of the thoracic spine is being tested here (T4/T5–T9/T10).

▶ Aim. The therapist attempts to assess the segmental mobility by feeling the movement in the spinous processes during rotation of the trunk.

12

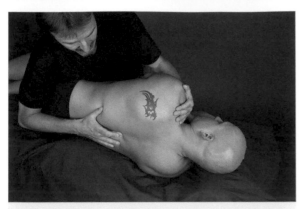

Fig. 12.51 Segmental mobility test, thoracic—starting position in side-lying.

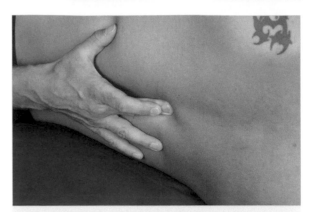

Fig. 12.52 Position of the palpating fingers.

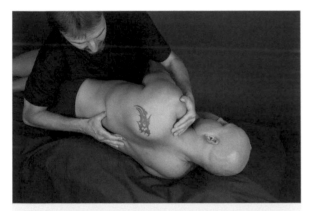

Fig. 12.53 Segmental mobility test, thoracic—final position.

▶ **Criteria.** It should only be determined whether movement occurs or not. The range of motion is not assessed.

▶ **Procedure.** The vertebral column is in a neutral position. The therapist first palpates interspinally from an inferior position and assesses the shape and alignment of the spinous processes compared with each other. Therapists should remind themselves at this point that the spinous processes may deviate up to half a centimeter from the midline due to a normal variation in shape. The position of the spinous processes should therefore only be palpated at this stage and not evaluated further.

The therapist facilitates rotation of the trunk from superior until the movement reaches the palpating finger (▶ Fig. 12.53). The therapist immediately repeats palpation of the position of the spinous processes in this segment. The upper body is then returned to a neutral position. Next, the palpating finger locates the inferior segment. The test is repeated.

▶ **Interpretation.** Segmental mobility is classified as normal in this test when the superior spinous process in the segment first moves (spatially downward) and the inferior spinous process remains immobile. The palpating finger feels a clear step between both spinous processes. In cases of restricted segmental mobility, no step is formed and both spinous processes move simultaneously.

Technique in the Sitting Starting Position

This mobility test can also be conducted in a position with loading, that is, in sitting. Compared with side-lying, this SP has considerable advantages and disadvantages. One advantage is that segmental mobility under loading is more obvious in this position. A disadvantage is that the patient is not relaxed and the paravertebral muscles are permanently active to a small extent. As the intrinsic thoracic muscles are found directly adjacent to the row of spinous processes (spinalis) at times, the access to the interspinous space can only be obtained by palpating with firm pressure (▶ Fig. 12.54). This makes the palpation not as exact. *Conclusion:* therapeutically more useful, but palpation is significantly more difficult.

The aims, criteria, procedure, and interpretation are the same as for the previous description. The procedure described here involves the same coupling of lateral flexion (here left) and rotation (here right) in opposite directions combined with the extended position. The palpating thumb is placed over the interspinous space on the therapist's side (here the left side). The spinous processes rotate to this side. The other hand facilitates the upper body from a neutral and upright sitting position into rotation and lateral flexion (▶ Fig. 12.55).

> **Tip**
>
> To facilitate thoracic extension, the therapist can additionally grasp below the patient's folded arms. The arm elevation additionally created during the movement of the upper body supports the achievement of thoracic extension.

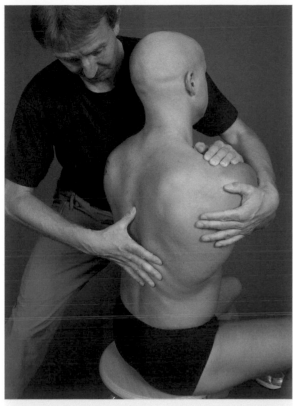

Fig. 12.54 Segmental mobility test, thoracic—starting position in sitting.

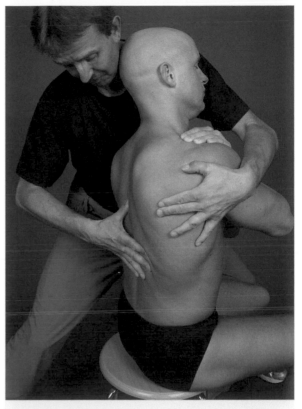

Fig. 12.55 Segmental mobility test, thoracic—final coupled position in extension.

Brismée et al. (2005) studied the interrater reliability of the palpation of intervertebral motion in the mid-thoracic spine with the patient in sitting position. With the patient in a passive extension position with lateral flexion and contralateral rotation, the change in the position of the spinous processes was examined manually. The extent of this segmental motion was compared with the extent achieved with the second lateral flexion. The average correlation between the three experienced testers yielded a kappa score of 0.41 and thus shows moderate reliability. This method therefore appears to be suitable for determining coupling of the mid-thoracic spine in extension.

Treatment of the Thoracic Spine

A variety of physical therapy methods form the basis for techniques that treat thoracic symptoms and are applied directly onto the thoracic spine. The total technique incorporates the entire thoracic section of the vertebral column. Local segmental techniques focus more on a single segment. All variations are based on the exact location of affected segments that cause pain or are responsible for restrictions in mobility.

Axial Traction

One of the total techniques is the axial traction (longitudinal technique) (▶ Fig. 12.56). The therapist applies a longitudinal traction in a superior direction to the vertebral column superior to the affected segment.

▶ **Procedure.** The therapist's sternum is in direct contact with the vertebra that forms the superior boundary to the affected segment. A folded towel may be placed between sternum and the vertebra, if needed. Both arms pull the thorax toward the therapist. By extending both legs, the therapist lifts the patient up slightly and the affected segment is relieved of load. This technique is successfully used to treat symptoms arising directly from the intervertebral disk (e.g., acute internal intervertebral disk rupture).

Local Segmental Treatment Techniques

Local segmental treatment techniques of manual therapy are used to relieve pain and increase mobility, especially in the ZAJs. The variations in these techniques are enormous. A traction technique is described here as an example (▶ Fig. 12.57).

12

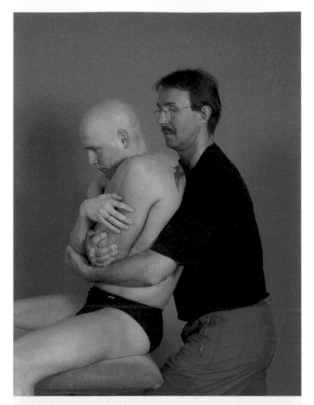

Fig. 12.56 Axial traction.

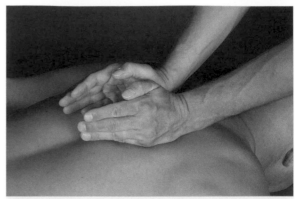

Fig. 12.57 Segmental traction.

▶ **Procedure.** The patient is positioned in prone, taking their kyphosis into account. The transverse processes of the vertebra forming the inferior boundary to the affected segment are located. The pisiform on the medial border of the hand rests on the transverse process. Gentle, rhythmical pressure is applied in an anteroinferior direction to relieve pain. This results in the articular surfaces of the inferior vertebra separating from the superior vertebra. A small gap is formed between the articular surfaces.

Assessment of the Costovertebral Joints

By precisely locating each rib, the therapist is able to assess the costovertebral joints for mobility and pain. The common symptoms patients complain of are based on a painful restriction in mobility with blocking in a neutral, expiration, or inhalation position. The assessment aims to determine whether symptoms are actually caused by a costovertebral joint, whether there is a change in mobility, and whether the thorax is blocked in an end position of movement.

Assessing the Position of the Ribs

▶ **Aim.** To determine whether a rib is fixed in a position of inhalation or expiration.

▶ **Procedure.** The vertebral column is placed in end-range flexion with rotation and lateral flexion away from

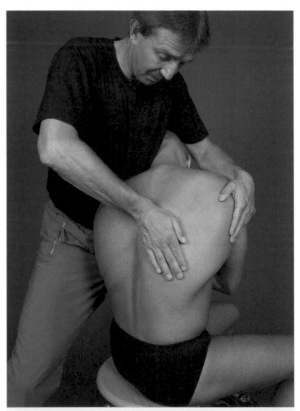

Fig. 12.58 Assessing the position of the ribs.

the side to be palpated. The shoulder girdle is protracted on the side of palpation (▶ Fig. 12.58). The therapist can then easily access the ribs while movement in the vertebral column is reduced. The flattened hand is used to gently palpate the thorax at the level of the 2nd–10th ribs and attempts to feel the contours of the ribs. The patient moves the thorax into the end range of movement using forced inhalation and expiration. All ribs should move in the same manner.

The side of the thorax is palpated from superior to inferior and back at the end range of forced respiration.

▶ **Criteria.** We speak of a normal rib position when a regular gap between the ribs and intercostal spaces can be felt and each rib has almost the same contour. Winkel (2004) describes the expected feeling as a "regular wave-shaped pattern."

▶ **Interpretation.** The therapist can start by developing a sense of whether the intercostal spaces are generally very narrow or very wide. When the intercostal spaces are generally narrow, the thorax may be in expiration position. A constantly widened gap indicates that the entire thorax is in inhalation position. This interpretation is based on a fair amount of experience, as no concrete specifications exist. The therapist should also keep in mind that all intercostal spaces are already widened on the side to be palpated due to the position of the upper body in flexion combined with lateral flexion and rotation to the opposite side.

Furthermore, the therapist can reach very concrete conclusions regarding the position of the individual ribs. Dautzenroth (2002) describes this as "position diagnosis."

A rib is fixed in a **position of expiration** when an edge is palpated during forced inhalation. In this case, the rib is fixed in an expiration position and it cannot move as required for inhalation. This results in an edge being clearly palpable. Further evidence for this fixed position can be found in changes in the neighboring intercostal spaces. When the eighth rib is fixed in an expiration position, the distance to the ninth rib decreases and the space to the seventh rib increases. This can be clearly palpated once the therapist has practiced a little.

A rib is fixed in a **position of inhalation** when an edge is palpated during forced expiration. In this case, the rib is fixed in a position of inhalation. It cannot move as required for expiration, which results in an edge being clearly palpable. The intercostal spaces also change in a typical manner. When the eighth rib is blocked in an inhalation position, the intercostal space to the seventh rib is narrower while the space to the ninth rib is wider.

> **Tip**
>
> Individual variations are also seen in the shape of the ribs. Stroking the thorax with the flattened hand may demonstrate that the ribs are protruding posteriorly in an almost odd manner on one or both sides. The palpatory results should only be viewed as pathological when these ribs are painful under pressure (see the section "Springing Test for One Rib" below) or when changes are felt in the intercostal spaces.

Springing Test for All Ribs

▶ **Aim.** Pain provocation and mobility test.

▶ **Procedure.** The patient is positioned in the same SP and the therapist uses the same hand position. The therapist does not palpate with a flattened hand, but rather applies firm pressure to the rib using the thenar eminence or the hypothenar eminence (see ▶ Fig. 12.58). The hand is placed along a line from superomedial to inferolateral running along the costal angle.

▶ **Criteria.** Does pressure provoke pain? Do the ribs move anteriorly when pressure is applied?

▶ **Interpretation.** The test results are viewed as normal when the hand applies pressure and the ribs yield somewhat in an anterior direction, and when the ribs are not sensitive to pressure. A blocked rib cannot yield to pressure and the pressure may cause pain.

Springing Test for One Rib

It is not always possible to clearly identify the affected rib during the first springing test as the hand moves over the entire thorax. A variation of this test is therefore needed to find the affected rib. It is also important for the documentation to precisely identify which level is affected, for example, whether the ninth rib is involved.

▶ **Aim.** To precisely locate the level of a rib and to confirm its position using the medial side of the hand to apply local pressure to a rib.

▶ **Procedure.** The patient is in the same SP and the medial border of the hand is now used to emphasize the pressure on one rib (▶ Fig. 12.59). Firm, anterolateral-directed pressure is applied rhythmically to the rib. End feel is assessed.

▶ **Criteria.** Pain provocation and end feel.

▶ **Interpretation.** Again, the rib normally moves somewhat anteriorly when local pressure is applied to it. A blocked rib cannot move. Its end feel is hard. Firm and elastic resistance is normally felt here.

> **Tip**
>
> Altering the recommended SP (see ▶ Fig. 12.58) by adding contralateral lateral flexion (here to the right) results in a locked position in the vertebral column. If the springing test provokes pain, this variation can be used to better exclude the involvement of thoracic segments.

Treatment of the Costovertebral Joints

Traction of the costovertebral joint is described here as an example of one of the many techniques available to treat

12

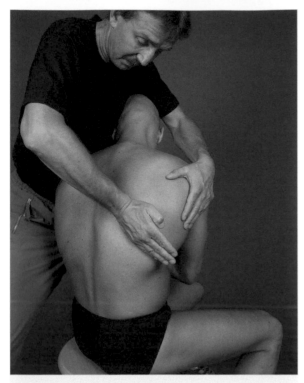

Fig. 12.59 Springing test for a single rib.

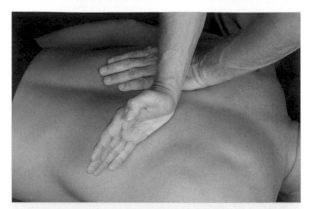

Fig. 12.60 Traction at the costotransverse joint.

the costovertebral joints. It is used to assess joint play and also to relieve pain or improve mobility.

▶ **Procedure.** The patient is in a neutral prone SP. The medial side of the hand is placed over the affected rib. The other hand stabilizes the vertebral column on the opposite side at the level of the transverse process (▶ Fig. 12.60). The medial side of the hand always applies pressure perpendicular to the thoracic spine's convexity. This generally means that pressure is applied in an anterolateral direction for the 2nd to 6th ribs and an additional, slightly superior direction for the 7th to 10th ribs.

The 11th and 12th ribs do not possess a costotransverse joint and therefore do not have to be treated.

This technique can be used as a traction test using the same criteria as described in the springing test for a single rib in the sitting SP. It can be used to relieve pain using oscillating movements and to improve mobility when the technique is conducted with force.

> **Tip**
>
> It is wise to position the vertebral column so that it moves as little as possible during treatment and so that the mobilizing force remains in the costotransverse joint. A good form of immobilization can be reached

through lateral flexion on the same side (here, on the right), for example, over the upper body. This positions the associated thoracic segments in rotation (here, on the right), which is opposed to the movement tendency upon pressure on the rib.

12.8 Anterior Palpation Techniques

The aim of this palpatory procedure is to systematically search for the most important accessible bony landmarks. The positions of these structures will be clarified to create the technical basis for the assessment of movement in the thorax or in each individual rib during respiration and movements of the arm. This is followed by several treatment examples related to thoracic palpation. Of course, the palpatory procedure can also be conducted with the patient in supine.

12.8.1 Anterior Palpation in the Sitting Starting Position

Jugular Notch

This shallow depression forms the superior boundary of the sternum. It is bordered by both tendons of the sternal sections of the sternocleidomastoid bilaterally and by both of the SC joints. The tendons can also be placed under tension by rotating the cervical spine extensively. The medial end of the clavicle and the SC joint space are found immediately lateral to these tendons (see Chapter 2).

The jugular notch can be palpated using two different methods (▶ Fig. 12.61): the first method involves sliding the flattened finger pads superiorly from the middle of the sternum until a depression is reached after palpating a rounded edge. The second method involves sliding the

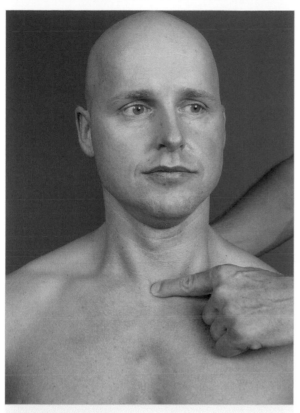

Fig. 12.61 Jugular notch.

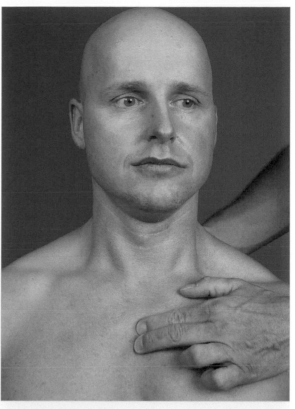

Fig. 12.62 Sternal angle.

finger pads inferiorly from the larynx using less pressure until the therapist encounters the distinctly palpable edge of the manubrium.

Sternal Angle

The therapist uses one or two finger pads to palpate from the jugular notch inferiorly onto the surface of the manubrium. A transverse bulge is felt after a distance of 2 to 3 finger widths. This is the sternal angle, the point where the manubrium is connected to the body of the sternum. The bulge is palpated transversely in a superior and inferior direction using small finger movements to register

the total size of the angle (▶ Fig. 12.62). The angle is the most reliable point of orientation to start the palpation of the anterior ribs and intercostal spaces (ICSs).

Locating the Second Rib

The second rib's costal cartilage is always fixed on the junction between the manubrium and the body of the sternum. The palpation is conducted using two vertically positioned fingers (e.g., using the index- and middle-finger pads) and palpating laterally from the sternal angle onto the superior and inferior edges of the costal cartilage (▶ Fig. 12.63). The index finger is then positioned in the first ICS and the middle finger in the second. When locating the second rib for the first time, therapists are generally surprised at how inferiorly it is positioned. The entire course of the second rib can now be visualized. It extends posteriorly from the superior angle of the scapula to the height of the sternal angle.

12

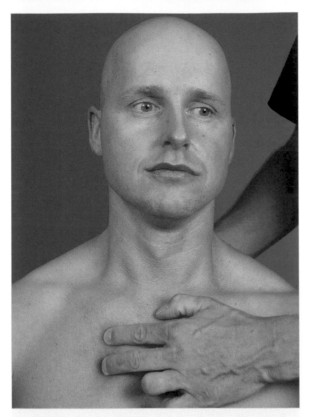

Fig. 12.63 Second rib.

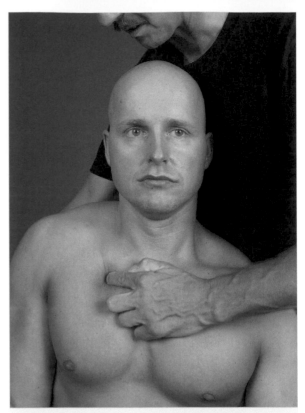

Fig. 12.64 First rib.

The correct location of the first two ICSs enables the therapist to search for all inferior-lying ICSs that are accessible on the anterior side of the body. This should be possible down to approximately the sixth ICS. The therapist palpates directly adjacent to the sternum as the ribs and the space between them are most clearly palpable here.

> **Tip**
>
> Swelling of the costosternal joints, especially at the second and third ribs, can indicate the presence of a Tietze syndrome. Diethelm (2005) has described the Tietze syndrome in his review on chest pain: "Its symptoms are hard to define. Its etiology has not been explained and it has a benign, self-limiting course with symptoms disappearing again mostly within one year." Patients with costochondritis, an alternative label for Tietze syndrome, frequently complain of acute chest pain (Freeston et al., 2004). This set of symptoms is seen quite frequently (Wise et al., 1992; Disla et al., 1994). It is, alongside coronary disease and breast cancer, one of the most important differential diagnoses in the medical examination of patients who

have not been subject to trauma. Diagnostics are based on direct provocation in particular, using palpation to produce the typical pain felt in this disorder.

Locating the First Rib

The only accessible anterior section of the first rib is found in the triangle formed by the clavicle and the manubrium. It is generally not possible to clearly locate the first rib as the rib disappears directly posteriorly beneath the clavicle after only a short distance.

Initially, the second rib and the first ICS, directly superior, are located. The palpating fingertips point in a slightly superior direction and push against the rib.

> **Tip**
>
> The length of the rib that can be palpated is increased by passively elevating the shoulder girdle
> (▶ Fig. 12.64).

The entire length of the first rib can be correctly visualized by looking at the location of the first rib combined with the results of the springing test.

12.8.2 Anterior Palpation in the Supine Starting Position

Intercostal Palpation during Respiration

The location of the ICS is used diagnostically to assess its constant opening and closing during thorax movements with forced respiration and large arm movements. As the upper thorax lifts up anteriorly during inhalation, the intercostal movements will also follow this movement anteriorly. This palpation can also be conducted with the body placed in an upright position. Extensive arm movements with movement in the thorax are easier to conduct in the supine position, as the inhibitory action of gravity is less.

The palpation is conducted using two or more finger pads, which are first placed adjacent to the sternum in the ICS. The second rib and the superior two ICSs are located first to ensure that the orientation is reliable (▶ Fig. 12.65). The finger pads can be placed parasternally down to the sixth ICS (▶ Fig. 12.66). The opening to the

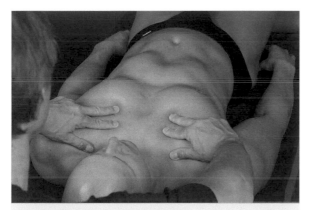

Fig. 12.65 Palpating the second rib.

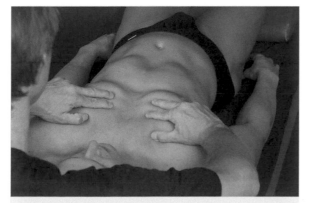

Fig. 12.66 Palpating the third to fourth intercostal spaces.

inferior ICSs in the inferior thorax is found more on the side. Therefore, the palpating finger pads are placed on the side of the thoracic cage as well (▶ Fig. 12.67).

The patient is now instructed to breathe deeply into the anterior section of the thorax five to six times before taking a break and breathing normally. The ICSs are expected to open and close uniformly. This applies when comparing the left and right sides and when comparing neighboring spaces on one side of the body. Mobility is limited in one or more ribs when the opening and closing movements cannot be felt at all or the movement is only minimal.

> ### Tip
>
> Tension in all three sections of the pectoralis major can be identified in this SP by using the transverse finger friction technique. A global increase in tension in several fiber bundles is an indication for manual treatment, including the use of functional massages (see the section "Tips for Assessment and Treatment" below).

Intercostal Palpation with Arm Elevation

The aim here is to use extensive arm elevation to assess the transmission of movement onto the thorax and therefore the mobility of the costovertebral joints using palpation. The superior ICSs are assessed by flexing the arm in supine. Again, two fingers are placed intercostally to feel the opening movement during extensive passive shoulder flexion and the closing movement when the arm returns to the neutral position (▶ Fig. 12.68 and ▶ Fig. 12.69). All ICSs accessible on the anterior side of the body are examined in this manner.

12.8.3 Thoracic Palpation in the Side-lying Starting Position

The use of arm elevation to widen the inferior thorax is not practical. It is significantly more favorable to use

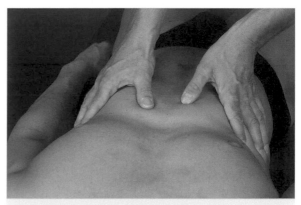

Fig. 12.67 Palpating the inferior intercostal spaces.

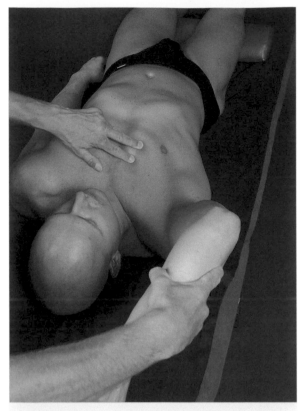

Fig. 12.68 Palpation of the anterior ribs during movement—initial position.

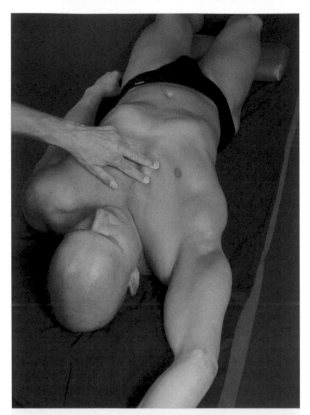

Fig. 12.69 Palpation of the anterior ribs during movement—end position.

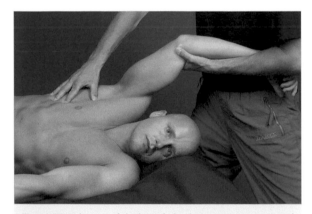

Fig. 12.70 Palpation of the lateral ribs during movement—initial position.

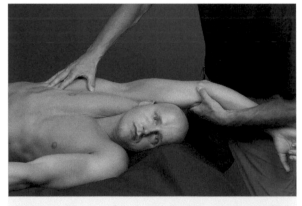

Fig. 12.71 Palpation of the lateral ribs during movement—final position.

extensive elevation of the arm to the side (abduction). It is recommended that the patient be placed in a neutral side-lying position to easily reach all ICSs. One of the therapist's hands facilitates the patient's arm; several finger pads from the other hand are placed in the ICS. The arm is positioned in moderate abduction (▶ Fig. 12.70) and then moved into extensive elevation until the movement is transmitted onto the ribs (▶ Fig. 12.71). The ICSs are expected to open uniformly as the arm moves more into elevation and close uniformly as the arm is returned to the SP. The interpretation of results is the same as previously described: mobility is limited in one or more ribs when the opening and closing movements cannot be felt at all or the movement is only minimal.

Tip

The mobility required for arm elevation must naturally be pain-free in the kinematic chain of the neck-shoulder-arm region. It is therefore very important to assess these movements beforehand. Based on experience, the movement is quickly completed when the arm is facilitated directly along the frontal plane of the patient. The range of motion is larger when the arm is facilitated slightly in an anterior direction during elevation.

12.8.4 Tips for Assessment and Treatment

Manual Techniques in Respiratory Therapy

Respiratory therapy techniques are divided according to their effect on the patient. These divisions include exercises with verbal instructions, the adoption of more advantageous body postures, and the use of manual techniques with different aims of treatment. The following section is an overview of techniques emphasizing the importance of good manual orientation on the thorax, the assessment of resistance and consistency, and the evaluation of the position of the ribs.

Tissue Release Methods

All manual interventions that decrease the resistance of skin and muscles are found in this group. This refers to the intrinsic muscles of the thoracic wall. Adhesions or increased muscular tension in the extrinsic, large muscles mainly belonging to the movement complex of the shoulder tend to be released using other manual techniques such as classical or functional massage.

The areas of skin with excessive turgor are stretched; the therapist's hand releases adhesions with the body's

fascia using lifting, rolling, displacement, and circular movements (Ehrenberg, 1998). These techniques result in a decrease in the elastic resistance to respiration and patients can inhale significantly more easily after these forms of treatment have been applied. These techniques are used in patients with restrictive respiratory disorders and with patients who have developed a large amount of tension in their respiratory muscles due to difficulty breathing. The latter causes increased tension in skin and muscles, or the development of reflex zones of skin with low elasticity.

▶ **Skin rolling.** Skin rolling (▶ Fig. 12.72) is a dynamic technique. It is conducted in an identical manner to the skin rolling used in the palpatory assessment of turgor in the Swedish massage (see Chapter 8, "Palpating the Quality of the Skin [Turgor],"). An example of this in the supine SP is grasping a skin fold along the anterior axillary line and rolling it toward the sternum along the course of the ribs.

▶ **Intercostal stroking.** Intercostal stroking (▶ Fig. 12.73) can be conducted in a variety of ways depending on the quality of the patient's tissues and the indications. On the one hand, it is known as the Swedish massage stroking technique along the course of the ICS. On the other hand, it is recommended in literature that local intensive tensile movements be applied that are more along the lines of the stroking technique used in connective-tissue massage (Ehrenberg, 1998). One or two fingers pull intensively in the ICS. This is the only really intensive manual technique that reaches the intercostal muscles. The other hand may have to keep the skin under tension if adhesions are affecting the skin or if treatment aims to affect the reflexes by using connective-tissue massage.

▶ **"Hold-grasp" techniques.** Hold-grasp techniques (▶ Fig. 12.74) are sustained techniques. They are conducted in a similar manner to the skin-lifting technique used for the palpatory assessment of skin consistency in the Swedish massage (see Chapter 8, "Palpating the

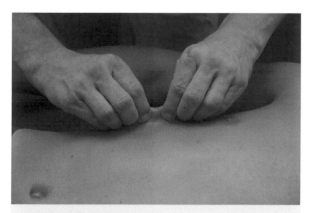
Fig. 12.72 Skin rolling.

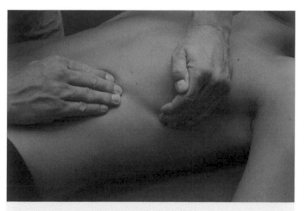
Fig. 12.73 Intercostal spaces (ICS) stroking.

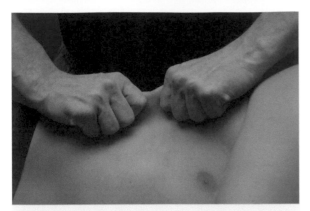

Fig. 12.74 Hold-grasp technique.

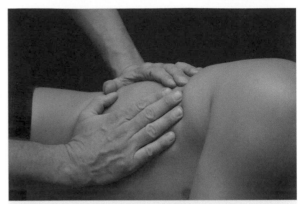

Fig. 12.75 Vibration with the diamond grip.

Quality of the Skin [Turgor]"). Both hands are used to lift up sections of the skin and pull the skin strongly away from the thorax while the patient breathes in and out several times. With regard to the SP, it is important that the therapist can easily access the tight sections of the skin. Lying or sitting positions can be used.

Interventions to Loosen Secretions

▶ **Vibration.** To mobilize and transport secretions and to affect the reflex-based increase in tension in the smooth muscles. This includes the treatment of obstructive bronchial diseases. The technique is applied for several minutes over different sections of the thorax:
- Superior thorax = subclavicular, sternal, between the scapulae.
- Inferior thorax = lateral, posterior (▶ Fig. 12.75).

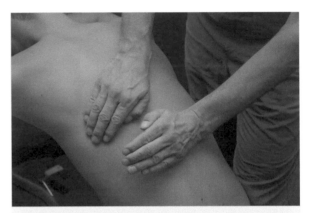

Fig. 12.76 Percussion with cupped hands.

The optimal frequency is stated as 8 to 12 Hz in the literature (Edel, 1999). Vibration is often combined with postural drainage, for example, lowering the head-end of the treatment table (Dautzenroth, 2002).

▶ **Percussion with the fist or cupped hands.** Tapotement (tapping) techniques are used to mobilize and loosen secretions. A loose fist or a firmly cupped hand moves downward at the wrist onto the thorax (▶ Fig. 12.76). The use of this technique must first be clarified using palpation. The therapist has to identify the area to be treated and the area that is not allowed to be percussed. The following structures must be palpated: spinous processes, edges of the scapula, inferior costal arch, xiphoid process. This technique should not be applied to the spinous processes in the kidney region (in the angle between the 12th ribs and the intrinsic back muscles), or the upper abdomen.

Contact Breathing

This is used to facilitate inhalation and to improve the relationship between ventilation and perfusion. Manual contact is used in respiratory therapy to train body awareness so that breathing can be directed to areas of low ventilation, for example, following operative interventions in the thorax. Once patients have practiced abdominal breathing, they are taught how to use thoracic movements during respiration to include areas of the lungs that have previously not been reached well and to ensure that all sections of the lung are evenly ventilated. The therapist positions the hands flat and applies only gentle pressure. The pressure is increased as the patient inhales so that the patient is aware of the direction of resistance. While breathing in, the patient tries to increase lung excursion toward the therapist's hands. The points of contact are:
- Sternum → costosternal direction for respiration (▶ Fig. 12.77).
- Epigastric angle → costoabdominal direction of respiration.
- Anterolateral on the inferior thorax → costolateral direction of respiration.
- Posterolateral on the inferior thorax → costoposterior direction of respiration.

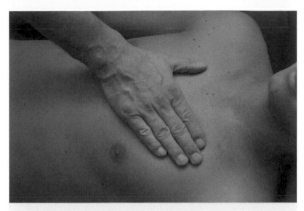

Fig. 12.77 Costosternal contact breathing.

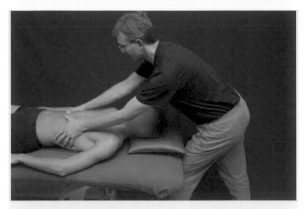

Fig. 12.78 Thorax compression.

Contact breathing is especially effective when the patient is instructed to adopt different SPs in terms of repositioning or atelectasis prophylaxis.

Mobilization of the Thorax

A mobile thorax guarantees sufficient respiratory minute volume with the deep drawing of the breath. Self-applied postural drainage and supportive interventions to loosen secretions can only be successful when the thorax is sufficiently mobile. Exercises can be used to improve mobility, for example, using stretching positions, where the thoracic spine is placed in a specific position and the large thoracic wall muscles are stretched. This alters the ability of the intercostal spaces to open up. Manual techniques can also be used, though in a much more differentiated fashion, to selectively treat affected areas. Palpation aims to identify movement disorders in the region of the thorax and to restore mobility using targeted techniques.

▶ **Thorax compression.** (▶ Fig. 12.78): In this technique, both hands are placed on the same area as during contact breathing. However, pressure is significantly increased during expiration (the "expiratory thorax compression" according to Ehrenberg, 1998). This technique supports the transportation of secretions and mobilizes the thorax, for example, when the respiratory muscles do not function properly or when inflammatory pleuritis is present. Thorax compressions act regionally on the costovertebral joints and the connection to the sternum but have no mobilizing effect on the ICSs.

▶ **Mobilization of the costovertebral joints.** As described before ("Tips for Assessment and Treatment") these techniques act on the joints between the ribs and the vertebrae. It is easiest to affect the costotransverse joints. The techniques also affect the joint of the head of the rib. The advantage of this manual therapy technique is the very selective treatment of individual malfunctioning movements of the ribs. The disadvantage is that improving the mobility of the entire thorax takes an enormous amount of time.

Functional Massage

A variety of soft-tissue mobilization techniques can be successfully used to specifically support the treatment of restrictions and to improve arm elevation. Techniques will be presented that relieve muscle tension and loosen adhesions:
• Latissimus dorsi.
• Teres major and minor.
• Pectoralis major (sternal and abdominal heads).

Latissimus Dorsi

The positioning and handling is almost identical to the thoracic palpation in side-lying (see the section "Thoracic Palpation in the Side-lying Starting Position" above). The palpating hand merely emphasizes the different muscle groups. The technique starts with a moderate approximation of the latissimus dorsi (▶ Fig. 12.79) and finishes with a stretch (▶ Fig. 12.80). The flat, free hand rests inferiorly on the scapula, covers the muscle, and pushes the muscle against the thorax. The arm is brought into extensive arm elevation until tension can be felt in the muscle belly of the latissimus dorsi beneath the hand. As with all functional massages, contracting a certain part of the muscle isometrically lengthens the section of the muscle found between the joint and the hand opposing the movement. The technique is conducted in a slow rhythm and frequently repeated.

Teres Major and Minor

To emphasize the teres major and minor on the lateral edge of the scapula, the inferior hand is placed closer to the shoulder joint laterally on the edge of the scapula. Initial and final positions (▶ Fig. 12.81 and ▶ Fig. 12.82) remain the same as described previously. This technique generally requires less mobility to effectively stretch the tissue.

12

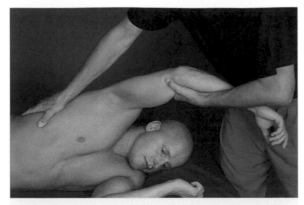

Fig. 12.79 Functional massage of the latissimus dorsi—initial position.

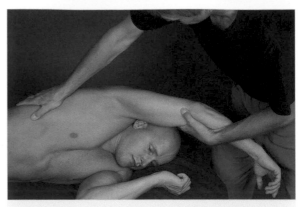

Fig. 12.80 Functional massage of the latissimus dorsi—final position.

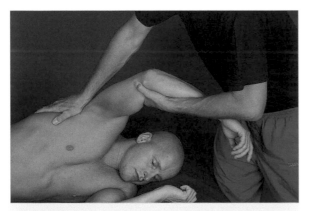

Fig. 12.81 Functional massage of the teres major and minor—initial position.

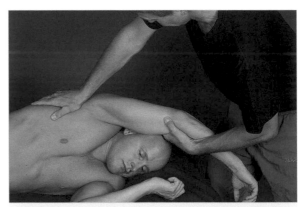

Fig. 12.82 Functional massage of the teres major and minor—final position.

Tips

- Classical massage techniques in the prone position should be used in this region first to optimize the effectiveness of the functional massage.
- It is important that the inferior hand does not slide over the skin while the muscle is being stretched further as this may cause unpleasant skin reactions.
- If the latissimus dorsi is already quite flexible, extensive arm flexion may not be sufficient to stretch the muscle further. If the therapist wishes to intensify the effect, they should stretch the muscle from its inferior side before starting with the above functional massage. This can be achieved by placing a large amount of padding underneath the thorax. The hip and knee joints can also be flexed to 90°. The lower legs then hang over the edge of the treatment table. Both of these methods result in contralateral lateral flexion of the thoracic spine or the lumbar spine.
- The latissimus dorsi, teres major, and teres minor can be stretched by elevating the arm with abduction or flexion. Therapists must find out for themselves which of these movements is the most effective during treatment.
- The side-lying SP lends itself to this technique. The muscles are easy to reach in this position and the thorax offers good support for the different parts of the muscles that are opposing movement. The therapist can take advantage of this and apply vertical pressure to the thorax with the hand. The muscles are also accessible in the prone position (▶ Fig. 12.83). However, the required arm movement cannot be performed well in this position. If the therapist wishes to make the latissimus dorsi and teres major and minor visible, the patient is instructed to move the arm from a slightly elevated (abducted) position toward the body. By conducting this maneuver isometrically with significant force, at least the outer borders of the muscles can be seen and followed for some distance inferiorly using palpation.

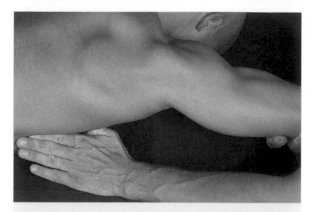

Fig. 12.83 Palpating the latissimus dorsi in the prone position.

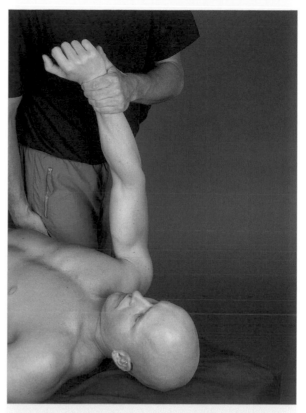

Fig. 12.84 Sternal head of the pectoralis major—contraction.

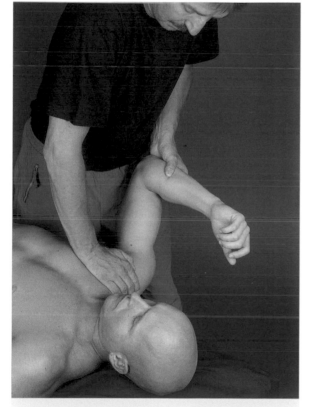

Fig. 12.85 Functional massage of the sternal head of the pectoralis major—initial position.

The Sternal Head of the Pectoralis Major

The pectoralis major is a muscle that develops a lot of tension and low elasticity when painful or persistent symptoms are present in the shoulder joint, when the shoulder girdle is held in a habitual posture of protraction, and when a variety of respiratory system symptoms are present. The position of this section of the muscle can often be made visible or palpable by using isometric contraction (horizontal adduction and internal rotation) when the muscle is strongly approximated (▶ Fig. 12.84).

The previously described principles for functional massage remain the same:
- Moderate approximation of the muscle (▶ Fig. 12.85).
- Manually opposed isometric contraction of specific muscle groups.
- Passive stretching.

To stretch the muscle, the shoulder is positioned first in external rotation and the arm is moved in horizontal adduction until the build up of tension is felt in the therapist's opposing hand (▶ Fig. 12.86). All the information provided for the procedure involved in the previously described functional massage techniques applies here as well. It is advantageous to position the patient near the edge of the treatment table so that the shoulder joint hangs somewhat freely over the edge. Only slight movement is needed for stretching when the isometric contraction is targeting muscles near the joint. The required mobility in the shoulder joint increases when the therapist's hand moves toward the sternum.

The Abdominal Head of the Pectoralis Major

To make the abdominal head of the pectoralis major more prominent, the muscle is moderately approximated and the patient is asked to isometrically contract into

12

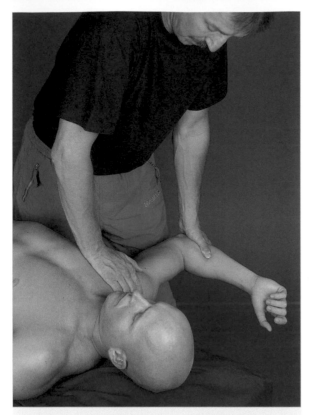

Fig. 12.86 Functional massage of the sternal head of the pectoralis major—final position.

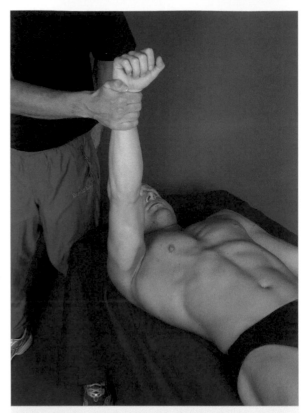

Fig. 12.87 Abdominal head of the pectoralis major—contraction.

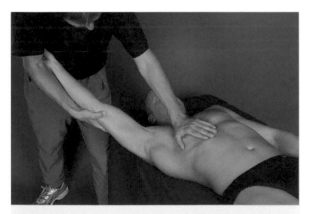

Fig. 12.88 Abdominal head of the pectoralis major—initial position.

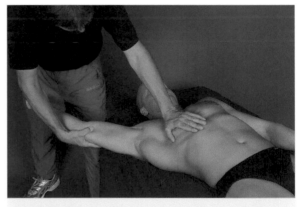

Fig. 12.89 Abdominal head of the pectoralis major—final position.

shoulder extension combined with adduction and internal rotation (▶ Fig. 12.87).

Before starting the functional massage, the pain-free range of motion is assessed to ascertain how much arm elevation is possible in the functional massage procedure.

The arm is positioned in moderate approximation or in a position of slight stretch and the therapist again places one hand over a specific part of the muscle (▶ Fig. 12.88). The muscle-fiber bundle is stretched between the

therapist's hand and the joint. The parts of the muscle found beneath the hand or closer to its origin are excluded from the stretch.

The hand placement is maintained, and the arm is moved further toward the maximal range of arm elevation until the muscle is in danger of sliding away from underneath the therapist's opposing hand (▶ Fig. 12.89). The arm elevation can be stopped here. Further stretch is not possible. The technique is repeated several times slowly and rhythmically. Different parts of the abdominal head of the muscle are accentuated. All other previously described tips for functional massage also apply here.

Bibliography

Brismée JM, Atwood K, Fain M, et al. Interrater reliability of palpation of three-dimensional segmental motion of the lumbar spine. J Manual Manip Ther. 2005; 13:216–221

Cui XG, Cai JF, Sun JM, Jiang ZS. Morphology study of thoracic transverse processes and its significance in pedicle-rib unit screw fixation. J Spinal Disord Tech. 2015; 28(2):E74–E77

Dautzenroth A. Cystische Fibrose. Stuttgart: Thieme; 2002

Diethelm M. Brustschmerz – nicht vom Herz. Schweiz Med Forum. 2005; 5:51–58

Disla E, Rhim HR, Reddy A, Karten I, Taranta A. Costochondritis. A prospective analysis in an emergency department setting. Arch Intern Med. 1994; 154(21):2466–2469

Dvořák J. Manuelle Medizin. Bd. 1, Diagnostik. Berlin: Springer; 1998

Edel H. Atemtherapie. 6. Aufl. München: Urban & Fischer; 1999

Ehrenberg H. Atemtherapie in der Physiotherapie/Krankengymnastik. München: Pflaum; 1998

Freeston J, Karim Z, Lindsay K, Gough A. Can early diagnosis and management of costochondritis reduce acute chest pain admissions? J Rheumatol. 2004; 31(11):2269–2271

Hoppenfeld S. Klinische Untersuchung der Wirbelsäule und Extremitäten. 2. Aufl. Stuttgart: Fischer; 1992

International Academy of Orthopedic Medicine. https://iaom-us.com

Kapandji IA. Funktionelle Anatomie der Gelenke. 4. Aufl. Stuttgart: Thieme; 2006

Lanz T von, Wachsmuth W. Praktische Anatomie, Rücken. Berlin: Springer; 2004

Loyd BJ, Gilbert KK, Sizer PS, et al. The relationship between various anatomical landmarks used for localizing the first rib during surface palpation. J Manual Manip Ther. 2014; 22(3):129–133

Migliore M, Signorelli M, Caltabiano R, Aguglia E. Flank pain caused by slipping rib syndrome. Lancet. 2014; 383(9919):844

Sapkas G, Papadakis S, Katonis P, Roidis N, Kontakis G. Operative treatment of unstable injuries of the cervicothoracic junction. Eur Spine J. 1999; 8(4):279–283

White AA, Panjabi MM. Clinical Biomechanics of the spine. 2nd ed. Philadelphia: Lippincott; 1990

Winkel D. Nichtoperative Orthopädie und Manualtherapie, Teil 4/2. Stuttgart: Fischer; 1993

Winkel D. Nichtoperative Orthopädie und Manualtherapie. Anatomie in Vivo. 3. Aufl. Urban & Fischer bei Elsevier; 2004

Wise CM, Semble EL, Dalton CB. Musculoskeletal chest wall syndromes in patients with noncardiac chest pain: a study of 100 patients. Arch Phys Med Rehabil. 1992; 73(2):147–149

12

Chapter 13

Cervical Spine

13 Cervical Spine

13.1 Significance and Function of the Cervical Spine

The cervical spine supports the head (approximately 10% of the weight of the body). The head's center of gravity is found at the level of the sella turcica (▶ Fig. 13.1) and is therefore positioned slightly anterior to the C0/C1 and C1/C2 joints so that the neck muscles are always slightly tensed when in an upright posture (Kapandji, 2006).

The cervical spine assists the sense organs (eyes, ears, nose) by positioning the head in space and should always keep the line connecting the eyes horizontal. Penning (2000) commented on this: "The head is continually moving in relation to the trunk in the awake state so that the eyes, ears, nose, and skin sense organs can take in the surroundings."

The cervical spine is particularly designed for rotation. During evolution, the cervical spine became vertical and resulted in rotation being the most important movement for human beings and the movement with the largest range. In comparison, the most important movement for quadrupeds is lateral flexion. The human head has to turn very precisely and often quickly. This requires fine coordination as well as strength to accelerate and decelerate movements.

The cervical region has other functions in addition to these extremely mechanical tasks. The superior vertebral canal protects vitally important centers in the elongated spinal cord. Hollow, pipelike organs (pharynx, larynx, trachea, and esophagus) are found anterior to the cervical spine. These organs belong to the digestive system and the upper respiratory tract. According to Hoppenfeld (1992), the cervical spine also protects the vertebral arteries.

13.2 Common Applications for Treatment in this Region

In addition to the lumbar spine, the cervical spine is the most frequent symptomatic region seen in physical therapy practices. Cervical structures cause differing degrees of pain and neurological symptoms in the periphery (shoulder and arm), as well as direct symptoms in the cervical spine. Similar observations have already been made in the thoracic and lumbar spines. New to this is a set of symptoms that is only seen in this section of the vertebral column and is consolidated in the general term "cervicocephalic symptoms":

- Headache.
- Tinnituslike symptoms.
- Difficulty swallowing.
- Vegetative disorders in the face.
- Nausea and dizziness.

The neuroanatomical relationship between the nuclei of various cranial nerves and the enormous proprioceptive innervation of the upper cervical muscles and joints is an essential aspect linking the cervical spine to symptoms in the head.

Symptoms associated with the cervical spine are a special challenge for therapists when planning and conducting treatment. Therapists must be well versed in anatomy and biomechanics if they wish to work professionally and effectively.

Manual therapeutic assessment and treatment of this region is divided into global and local techniques, as is also the case in the other sections of the vertebral column. Local examination techniques that provoke pain and assess mobility are of great importance in the cervical spine due to the difficulties in relating, for example, a restriction in rotational mobility to the proper level.

Long-term irritation of a facet joint causes pain felt in other areas (referred pain). It is not possible to link the patient's reported area of referred pain with a specific level in the cervical spine. In 1994, Dreyfuss et al. wrote that referred pain arising from the C0/C1 segment can extend quite a way up onto the occiput (▶ Fig. 13.2).

A good knowledge of topography and the ability to palpate reliably are the basis for confident hand placements during local assessment and treatment.

In addition to the manual techniques for the cervical joints, a range of cervical soft-tissue treatment techniques also exists. Classical massage and functional massage (▶ Fig. 13.3) are important forms of treatment used to obtain localized and general relaxation. Neck, head, and face massages belong to the most effective manual techniques available for relaxation. Functional massage is the first, and often initially the only, form of treatment that can be applied to a painful neck.

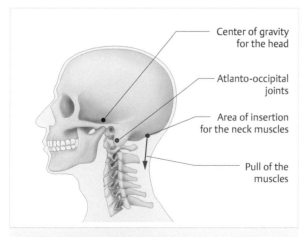

Center of gravity for the head

Atlanto-occipital joints

Area of insertion for the neck muscles

Pull of the muscles

Fig. 13.1 Center of gravity for the head.

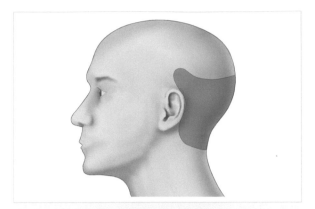

Fig. 13.2 Referred pain arising from the C0/C1 segment.

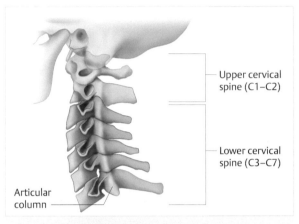

Fig. 13.4 Sections of the cervical spine.

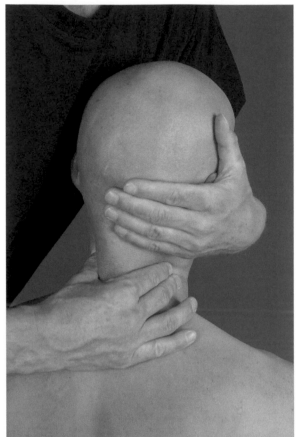

Fig. 13.3 Functional massage of the lower cervical spine.

Manual lymphatic drainage targets the large number of lymph nodes in the head and throat region. It can be used to generally stimulate the motor function in lymph vessels or to drain fluid in the neck, face, and head. The sterno-cleidomastoid, the descending part of the trapezius, and the supraclavicular fossa are important guiding structures here.

13.3 Required Basic Anatomical and Biomechanical Knowledge

13.3.1 Sections of the Cervical Spine

Due to its morphology, biomechanics, and the presence or absence of intervertebral disks, the cervical spine is divided anatomically and functionally into (▶ Fig. 13.4):
- Upper cervical spine:
  ○ anatomically: atlas and axis;
  ○ functionally: C0/C1 and C1/C2 segments; also called the segments without intervertebral disks.
- Lower cervical spine:
  ○ anatomically: C3–C7;
  ○ functionally: C2/C3 to T3/T4 segments; also called the segments with intervertebral disks.

13.3.2 Anatomy of the Lower Cervical Spine

The physiological curvature of the cervical spine is lordotic, with the C3/C4 segment usually positioned horizontally (White and Panjabi, 1990).

The vertebral body's end plate is very narrow, favoring rotation. The vertebral foramen is very large due to the long laminae of the vertebral arches. The spinal cord only occupies approximately 50% of the vertebral foramen's very wide diameter. The large vertebral foraminae provide the dural sac with a generous amount of space to move in during large cervical movements (White and Panjabi, 1990).

The wide laminae are well developed (being approximately as wide as an index finger) and can be palpated underneath the muscles. They are located at the level of the spinous processes. The articular processes protrude from the end of the laminae.

The zygapophysial joints (ZAJs) form the "articular column" (see ▶ Fig. 13.4) that is almost as wide as the row of transverse processes. The vertebrae, as a whole, have very wide bases due to the extremely lateral position of the joints, which results in the lower cervical spine not being particularly ideal for movement into lateral flexion. A narrow base (less distance between the left and right ZAJs), as is seen in the lumbar spine, is more conducive to lateral flexion.

The spinous processes are bifurcated down to C6. The bifurcation at C2 is very large and extremely asymmetrical. The spinous processes decrease in size down to C6. A large spinous process is seen again at C7 and is not bifurcated at this level. The asymmetrical bifurcations in the spinous processes interlock during extension and optimize the range of motion for the lordosis.

The transverse process is composed of two tubercles that connect laterally and form a hole at one point. This foramen transversarium has a diameter of approximately 4.5 to 5 mm, which almost corresponds to the diameter of the vertebral artery.

The anterior tubercle is a rudiment of a rib, while the posterior tubercle represents the actual transverse process. These two tubercles turn the transverse process into more of a groove than a process. The groove runs diagonally and is oriented anterolaterally (▶ Fig. 13.5).

The groove is at its narrowest in its medial section and is bordered by bones on all sides. The uncinate process forms the anterior border; the superior articular process of the ZAJ the posterior border.

The artery and the ventral ramus of the spinal nerve cross paths at this bony constriction (▶ Fig. 13.6). Both of these conductive pathways can be compressed and irritated by protruding osteophytes associated with severe degenerative changes in the segment. Of all the sections of the vertebral column, stenosis of the intervertebral foramen most often irritates nerves in the cervical spine.

The uncinate process (also called the uncus of body) deserves a special mention. This process forms the side rim of the vertebral body's end plate and its size increases in the more superior vertebrae. The uncinate processes are the largest on the C3 end plate. They develop between the ages of 2 and 24 and later form the uncovertebral joint with the more superiorly positioned vertebral body. During this development, the intervertebral disks tear on the outer sides from approximately the age of 10 onward (▶ Fig. 13.7). This can lead to bisection of the disk (Rauber and Kopsch, 2003). When this occurs, the contents of the nucleus pulposus neither leak out nor does the segment become thinner. This bisectioning is complete between the ages of 45 and 50. This is a natural adaption of the intervertebral disks in response to the large translation of the vertebra during cervical spine flexion and extension. The uncinate processes act as rails and guide this translation movement. The bisectioning of the disk is the reason why whiplash can cause height to increase by up to 2.5 cm (abnormal ability to separate) within seconds and is especially seen in the C2/C3 segment.

How Does this Affect Palpation?

In the cervical spine, a relatively large number of bony structures, joints, and muscles can be reached and differentiated from one another using palpation. Important reference points include the accessible spinous processes (C2, C5–C7) and the laminae of every cervical vertebra inferior to C2. The fact that the spinous process and laminae of a vertebra are located at the same level is very convenient for palpatory orientation.

This is of assistance when the exact level of structures, for example, the ZAJ and the transverse process, is being determined. The laminae can be used to fix a vertebra during certain manual therapy techniques.

When all accessible ZAJs (articular column) are palpated from superior to inferior, the protruding processes and the more concave sections between the processes have an undulating shape (▶ Fig. 13.8).

The cervical transverse processes are aligned diagonally in an anterolateral direction so that the ventral rami

13

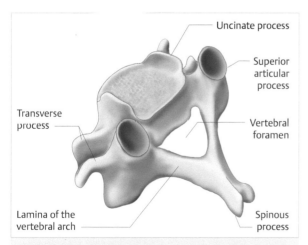

Fig. 13.5 Typical vertebra in the lower cervical spine.

Uncinate process
Superior articular process
Transverse process
Vertebral foramen
Lamina of the vertebral arch
Spinous process

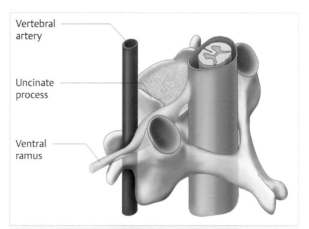

Fig. 13.6 Neurovascular cross.

Vertebral artery
Uncinate process
Ventral ramus

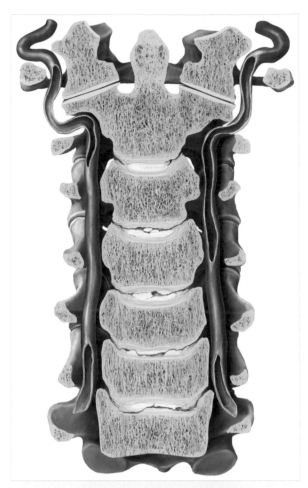

Fig. 13.7 Formation of horizontal tears in the cervical intervertebral disk.

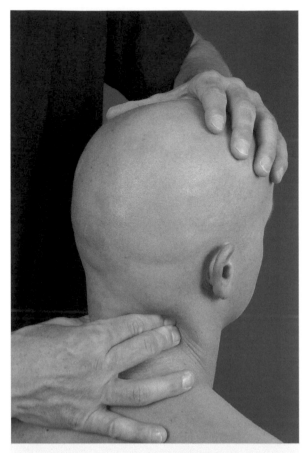

Fig. 13.8 Palpating a zygapophysial joint (ZAJ).

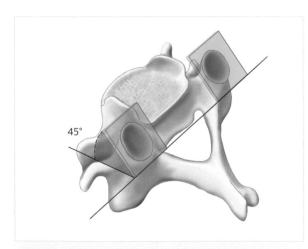

Fig. 13.9 Alignment of the zygapophysial joints (ZAJs) in the sagittal plane.

and the brachial plexus can be palpated between the sternocleidomastoid and the descending part of the trapezius (see "Supraclavicular Triangle of the Neck" below).

13.3.3 Lower Cervical Spine Biomechanics

The range of motion in the cervical spine is dependent on age and gender (Penning, 2000). Young women are the most mobile. The largest range of motion is seen with rotation, followed by flexion and extension. Lateral flexion has the smallest range of motion. Lateral flexion is quite complicated in the cervical spine and is mainly used in association with rotation (coupled movement).

The alignment of the ZAJ surfaces is crucial for determining how rotation and lateral flexion are conducted. The joint surfaces are large and flat and are aligned at an average angle of 45° anteriorly and superiorly toward the end plate (▸ Fig. 13.9; Dvořák et al., 1998). Penning (2000) reported a large variation in angles. In connection with cervical lordosis, therapists can note that the joint surfaces are generally aligned anteriorly and superiorly toward the eye socket.

Almost all lower cervical joint spaces are aligned horizontally in the frontal plane. Only the C2/C3 segment is angled in a superior direction (▶ Fig. 13.10).

Due to the alignment of the joint surfaces, rotation is inevitably coupled with lateral flexion and the axis of rotation is tilted (▶ Fig. 13.11). Corresponding to this, rotation to the right is accompanied by lateral flexion to the right, regardless of whether the cervical spine is positioned in flexion or extension. Lateral flexion to the right is also accompanied by rotation to the right. The range of the coupled motion is surprisingly large in the cervical spine. Lysell (1969) stated that approximately 8° of lateral flexion at the C2/C3 segment is connected with approximately 6° of coupled rotation.

During lateral flexion to the right and the associated ipsilateral rotation, the joint surfaces on the right glide together (convergence), just as they do during extension. The joint surfaces on the left glide away from one another

(divergence), similar to the movement during flexion (▶ Fig. 13.12).

How Does this Affect Palpation?

Therapists use the two previously described relationships to their advantage when palpating the lower cervical facet joints (inferior to C2/C3) during movement: the degree of coupling and the movement of the joint surfaces as they converge.

Therapists aim to feel the posteroinferiorly directed swaying of the joint processes as the ZAJ moves (see "Facet Joints" below). They therefore facilitate lateral flexion with rotation to the right when they are palpating the right side, so that the joint process moves toward the palpating finger. Movement is facilitated via lateral flexion and causes the segment to rotate extensively. If rotation was facilitated first, it would take quite a while for C1/C2 to reach end-range rotation and for rotation to be transferred onto the inferior segments.

Penning (2000) has explained the kinematics during flexion and extension very well. His study results describe the momentary rotation axes for flexion and extension and were radiologically determined for every 5° of movement. The investigators discovered a relationship between the superior joint processes and the end plate, which determines the position of the axis for rotation. In the upper intervertebral disk segments the axis is located in the inferior vertebra and results in the superior vertebra undergoing a large translation movement in addition to tilting during flexion and extension (▶ Fig. 13.13). In the lower intervertebral disk segments, the axis is found near the intervertebral disk. The tilting movement is therefore very large and the translation minimal (▶ Fig. 13.14).

The large translation, for example, in the C2/C3 segment, produces strong shear forces that act on the intervertebral disk. These forces must be seen as having a

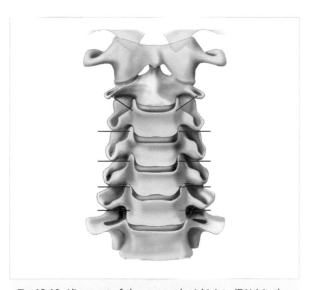

Fig. 13.10 Alignment of the zygapophysial joints (ZAJs) in the frontal plane.

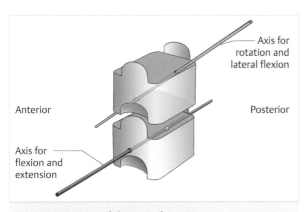

Fig. 13.11 Position of the axes of rotation.

Axis for rotation and lateral flexion

Anterior

Posterior

Axis for flexion and extension

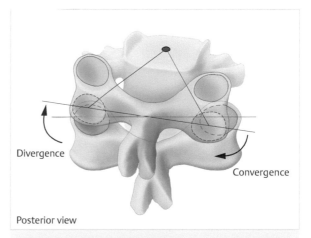

Divergence

Convergence

Posterior view

Fig. 13.12 Movement of the joint surfaces during lateral flexion and rotation to the right.

13

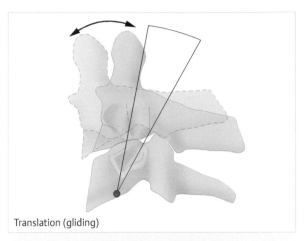

Translation (gliding)

Fig. 13.13 Position of the rotation axis for flexion and extension at C2/C3.

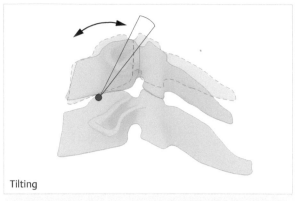

Tilting

Fig. 13.14 Position of the rotation axis for flexion and extension at C6/C7.

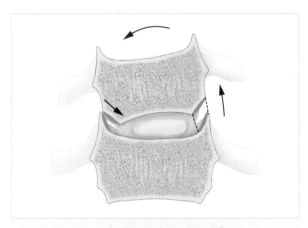

Fig. 13.15 Uncovertebral joints during lateral flexion.

direct relationship with the bisectioning of the intervertebral disk and the development of the uncinate process.

The uncovertebral joints control lateral flexion and ensure that the coupling of segmental rotation and lateral flexion is transferred quickly onto the next inferiorly located segment (▶ Fig. 13.15). As joints that develop with age, the uncovertebral joints can also cause local lateral cervical symptoms during lateral flexion when disorders are present.

13.3.4 Anatomy of the Occiput and the Upper Cervical Spine

The upper cervical spine is responsible for supporting the sense and balance organs (Herdman, 2000), for example, by coupling eye and head movements (cervico-ocular reflex) with the aim of stabilizing the field of vision.

The upper cervical spine "contains the most complex, unique, and highly specialized structures" in the vertebral column (White and Panjabi, 1990). Anatomy varies

greatly at the junction between the head and the cervical spine. These deviations from the norm affect the expected results of the local palpation of bony structures to a limited extent only. The effect of some anatomical variations is so extreme, and even pathological, that they are described as deformities. The following deformities directly influence palpation:

- Minimal development of the occipital condyles causes the dens to protrude into the inner skull. The malformations are labeled "primary basilar impressions" (von Lanz and Wachsmuth, 1979) and may result in neurological deficits. When condyles have a flattened form, it is difficult to palpate the transverse process of the atlas as the process is found directly underneath the occiput.
- When the atlas and occiput are fused together, the C0/C1 segment is immobile (occipitalization; present in less than 1% of the population).

Occipital Bone

The occiput is composed of two large areas:
- Posterior section: squamous part of the occipital bone.
- Inferior section: lateral and basilar parts.

The squamous part of the occipital bone (▶ Fig. 13.16) is the rounded posterior region of the roof of the skull. It is connected to the parietal bones via the lambdoid suture and the temporal bones via small lateral sutures. It is divided into two flat areas called the occipital plane and the nuchal plane. Each area has a different function. The nuchal plane is covered by the neck muscles and is separated from the occipital plane by the superior nuchal line. The transverse lines and ridges, protrusions, and areas found on the nuchal plane can be palpated particularly well.

The external occipital protuberance is the most prominent point. It represents the end of a medium-sized crest that travels in a posterosuperior direction from the

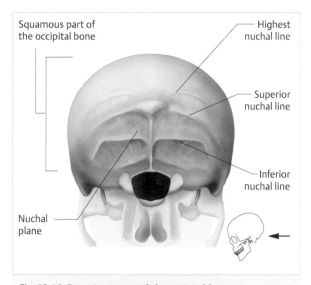

Fig. 13.16 Posterior aspect of the occipital bone.

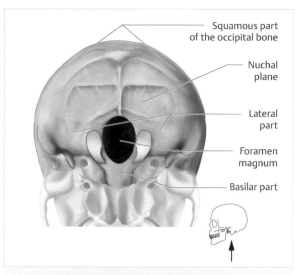

Fig. 13.17 Inferior aspect of the occipital bone.

foramen magnum and also marks the site of insertion for the ligamentum nuchae. Von Lanz and Wachsmuth (1979) describe this reference point very precisely. The shape of the protuberance varies greatly and it often tapers downward. It is only well developed in approximately 11% of all individuals. The point protruding the most is called the "inion." This elevation is more developed in pets (e.g., dogs and cats) than in humans. This is due to larger loads being applied to the ligamentum nuchae of these animals, which in turn places more tension on the site of insertion.

The position of the three transverse ridges can be described in relation to the protuberance:

- **Highest nuchal line.** This convex line starts directly on the protuberance and extends laterally and somewhat superiorly. It is the line of insertion for the extensive mimic muscles that are able to move the scalp and the ears to some extent. It is rarely well developed and may also be completely absent.
- **Superior nuchal line.** This widely arched, convex line also travels laterally, extending from a position slightly inferior to the protuberance. Von Lanz and Wachsmuth (1979) estimate that approximately 37% of all superior nuchal lines are well developed. The large intrinsic muscles are noticeable directly below this line: semispinalis cervicis, splenius capitis, and the descending part of the trapezius.
- **Inferior nuchal line.** This line is found 1 finger width inferior to the protuberance. It first travels transversely and later bends anteriorly, almost at a right angle. The transverse section meets with the superior nuchal line laterally. Together, both of these lines can form a palpable elevation: the retromastoid process (von Lanz and Wachsmuth, 1979). The inferior nuchal line marks the site of insertion for the deep neck muscles (rectus and obliquus muscles).

The inferior aspect of the occipital bone is divided into two sections (▶ Fig. 13.17). The lateral part is characterized by the area surrounding the foramen magnum. With its diameter of 3 to 3.5 cm and its bulging rim, the foramen magnum forms a passage for the spinal cord and other structures. Two biconvex condyles are found laterally and are divided into two separate parts in 5% of the population (Rauber and Kopsch, 2003). The division of the joint cartilage is an indication of the different types of loading applied to the cartilage surfaces during flexion and extension at the C0/C1 segment. As already mentioned, anatomy also varies considerably here. The condyles are aligned so that they converge anteriorly. The basilar part is similar to a wedge-shaped piece of bone and is connected to the sphenoid bone anteriorly.

Atlas

The atlas has the special function of an adaptor or intermediate plate by transmitting the predominant movements of flexion and extension in the C0/C1 segment onto the C1/C2 segment in the form of rotation.

The first cervical vertebra consists of a ring with delicate anterior and posterior arches (▶ Fig. 13.18). The earlier C1 vertebral body is now the C2 dens. The dens forms a joint with the anterior arch and is fixed at this point by a strong transverse ligament. The atlas also does not possess a spinous process. Only an anterior and a posterior tubercle can be found on the ring of the atlas. The atlas supports two very well-developed bony blocks on the lateral section of the ring, which support inferior and superior joint surfaces. The superior joint surfaces are biconcave and together with the occipital condyles form the upper cervical joints (C0/C1). Approximately 30% of the cartilage coating here has variable gaps in it. The occipital and atlantal articular surfaces have similar radiuses

13

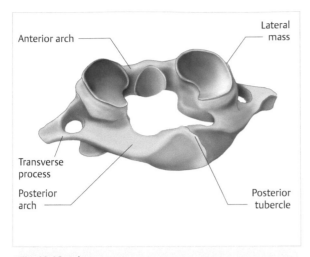

Fig. 13.18 Atlas.

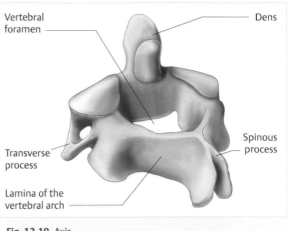

Fig. 13.19 Axis.

of curvature, which results in the high congruency and structural approximation seen in this segment. The inferior joint surfaces are rounded and the bone concave.

A special feature of the atlas is its wide transverse processes. This makes the atlas the widest of all cervical vertebrae. Von Lanz and Wachsmuth (1979) state that the distance between the tips of the transverse processes in male Central Europeans amounts to approximately 8.5 cm. This distance is approximately the same as the distance between the T1 transverse processes (Loyd et al., 2014). The tip of a transverse process can be felt between the mastoid process and the ramus of the mandible. The variations in shape and length of the transverse processes can lead to incorrect conclusions when sides are compared during palpation. Dörhage et al. (2004) have once more confirmed the large variation in the anatomy of the upper cervical region in a large radiological study: "We evaluated 212 X-rays of the entire vertebral column and assessed the upper cervical joints and the cervical spine of test subjects who reported being free of symptoms. The asymmetrical position of the participating joint partners varied considerably. Symmetrical positioning of the occiput, atlas, and axis in relation to each other could only be observed in 6% of all cases." They also discovered that the difference in cervical mobility to the left and the right "did not correlate with the anatomical position of the upper cervical joints as radiologically determined." Naturally, this knowledge also influences the results expected when palpating the C1 transverse process. It is not expected that the transverse processes will be of the same length on both sides and should not be classified as abnormal without further assessment of movement.

Axis

The second cervical vertebra is the transitional vertebra (▶ Fig. 13.19). Its superior section belongs to the vertebrae of the upper cervical spine, while its inferior side has a similar shape to vertebrae found in the lower cervical spine. The dens of C2 is 1.5 cm long on average, has a rounded tip, and is tilted 11 to 14° posteriorly in relation to the vertebral body (von Lanz and Wachsmuth, 1979). It is the most reliable bony orientation point in radiographs of the upper cervical spine. The axis for extensive rotation at C1/C2 is found here.

The anterior side of the dens articulates with the anterior arch of the atlas. Its posterior side articulates with the transverse ligament of the atlas. The superior joint surfaces are found directly adjacent to the dens. They have a biconvex shape and, together with the inferior joint surfaces of the atlas, form the lateral atlantoaxial joints, the real facet joints of C1/C2. The most important feature of the axis for palpation is its particularly prominent bifid spinous process. This is the most important reference point in the upper cervical region. It is found at the level of the laminae of the vertebral arches and the vertebral body. The transverse processes are considerably shorter when compared with the atlas.

The vertebral foraminae of the atlas and axis are large and offer a large amount of space for the dural sac and the spinal column to move in during extensive cervical movements. The dural sac is located near the axis for rotation at C1/C2 and is therefore only mildly deformed during large rotational movements and is not compressed by bone (White and Panjabi, 1990).

13.3.5 Ligaments of the Cervical Spine

Of the large number of ligamentous structures in the cervical spine, only a few ligaments are of crucial importance in this context.

Ligamentum Nuchae

This long ligament extends from the C7 spinous process to the occipital protuberance and assumes the role of the

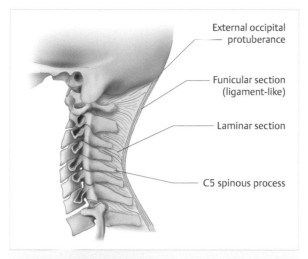

Fig. 13.20 Ligamentum nuchae.

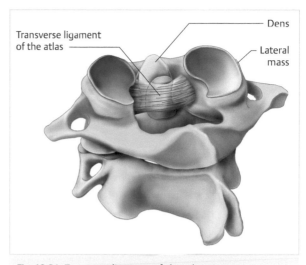

Fig. 13.21 Transverse ligament of the atlas.

supraspinous ligament (▶ Fig. 13.20). It has deep laminar and superficial funicular (ligament-like) sections and connects the occiput directly with the C5–C7 spinous processes. The laminar section is a thin partition (septum) made of elastic fibers. The funicular, thin, superficial section is shaped like a ligament. It is formed by the following muscles as they merge to form an aponeurosis:

• Trapezius.
• Splenius capitis.
• Serratus posterior superior.
• Rhomboid minor.

It can be palpated during extensive cervical flexion. The ligamentum nuchae pulls the head back slightly when the cervical spine is maximally flexed, preventing the upper cervical joints from moving into their maximal end position. This presumably helps to protect the spinal cord. It is also placed under tension when the head is retracted and pulls the more inferior vertebrae posteriorly so that real extension is produced.

Transverse Ligament of the Atlas

This ligament forms the transverse part of a cross-shaped ligament (▶ Fig. 13.21). It originates from the inner side of the lateral mass of the atlas and is 2 cm long. It is approximately 2 mm thick in the middle and approximately 1 cm in height. It is made of very taut connective tissue and is very firm. In the past, anatomists have performed studies demonstrating that this ligament has a tensile strength of approximately 130 kg (Macalister, 1893 in von Lanz and Wachsmuth, 1979). It is covered by thin hyaline cartilage on its anterior side and forms part of the median atlantoaxial joints with the dens.

It is found on the posterior aspect of the dens in a circular depression beneath the tip (similar to a scarf

wrapped around the neck). The dens is therefore positioned in an osteofibrotic funnel that tapers downward. Even massive tensile forces (up to 40–50 kg) are not able to separate C1 from C2 when the ligament is intact. This means that it is impossible to apply traction therapeutically at this joint.

The main function of the ligament is to keep the dens away from the dural sac (with the spinal cord). Physical therapists are familiar with several tests assessing the stability of this important ligament. The ligament also controls the biomechanics between the atlas and axis during flexion and extension and stabilizes the atlantoaxial joints by approximating the joint surfaces with the strength of its tissues.

Alar Ligaments

The four alar ligaments are also very firm (stiff and rigid) and are mostly comprised of type I collagen. The ligamental columns are divided into two groups (▶ Fig. 13.22):

• **Alar ligaments, occipital sections.** These sections directly connect the posterior upper side of the dens with the occiput. They are 11 to 13 mm long, 3.5 to 6 mm thick, and approximately 8 mm wide (Dvorak and Panjabi, 1987). These sections transfer lateral flexion of the head directly onto C2.
• **Alar ligaments, atlas sections.** These are found at the level of the transverse ligament of the atlas. They connect the side of the dens with the anterior arch and are therefore only approximately 3 mm long.

Their functions include moving the dens during cervical flexion and extension, limiting the atlantoaxial rotation, and passing lateral flexion of the head onto the axis by rotating C2. The alar ligaments therefore control the central biomechanics in the upper cervical region.

13

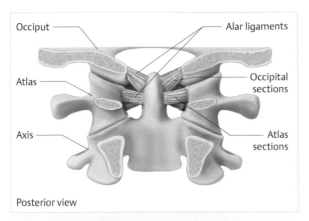

Occiput — Alar ligaments

Atlas —

— Occipital sections

Axis —

— Atlas sections

Posterior view

Fig. 13.22 Alar ligaments.

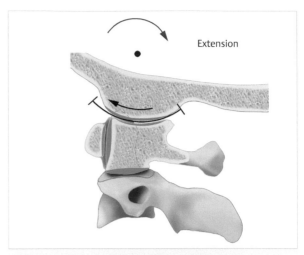

Extension

Fig. 13.23 Movement in the atlanto-occipital joints.

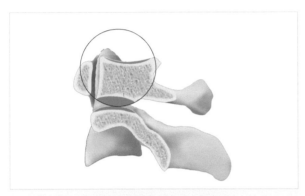

Fig. 13.24 Lateral atlantoaxial joints.

13.3.6 Biomechanics of the Upper Cervical Spine

Atlanto-occipital Joints (C0/C1)

The atlanto-occipital joints mainly move in the sagittal plane (▶ Fig. 13.23). The range of flexion and extension amounts to approximately 27° (Panjabi et al., 2001). This range can be further divided into 7.2° flexion and 20.2° extension. C0/C1 should be viewed as an extensor. Approximately 5° of rotation and lateral flexion is possible to each side. Another sideways movement is also possible: an "offset" of the atlas. When the upper cervical spine laterally flexes, the atlas shifts a few millimeters to the same side. This offset can be assessed using palpation and provides information on the mobility of C0/C1 (see the section "Tips for Assessment and Treatment" below).

Lateral Atlantoaxial Joints

The lateral osseous atlantoaxial joint surfaces tend to be either flatter in the sagittal plane or have a concave shape (▶ Fig. 13.24). The cartilage is particularly thick in the middle, forming two convexities that face each other and only come into contact with each other in places. This

unstable position results in low friction and allows movements to be performed quickly. However, tissues must be quite strong to maintain joint surface contact. The joint capsule is very large as a whole, allowing all movements to be performed. The incongruent joint surfaces are balanced out by the meniscal invagination of the joint capsule.

It is well known that axial rotation is the main movement performed at the C1/C2 segment. Details regarding axial rotation and lateral flexion vary in the literature. When C2 is fixed, approximately 20° of rotation is available to each side. When C2 is free to move, the range of motion amounts to approximately 40°.

The range of flexion and extension adds up to approximately 20°, with this range being evenly divided between flexion and extension. If this were not the case, the range of rotation would differ. The documented range of lateral flexion varies between 0° and 6.5°.

Coupling of Movements during Lateral Flexion of the Upper Cervical Spine

Lateral flexion to the left initially places the occipital section of the right alar ligaments under tension (▶ Fig. 13.25). This causes the posterior side of the dens to move simultaneously and the axis rotates immediately to the left. This transmission of movement is the strongest form of coupling in the musculoskeletal system. It can be recognized by observing the C2 spinous process as it moves to the right. The movement of the spinous process is used to assess the stability of the alar ligaments (see the section "Test for the Alar Ligaments" below).

However, the overall movement range over C0 to C2 does not allow conclusions to be drawn about the motion ranges of the individual segments. The coupling of lateral flexion and rotation is individual here and must therefore be assessed on each patient separately. The variable

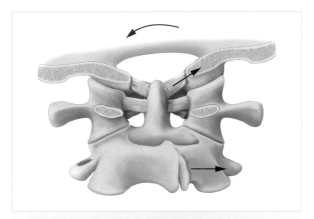

Fig. 13.25 Functions of the alar ligaments, posterior view.

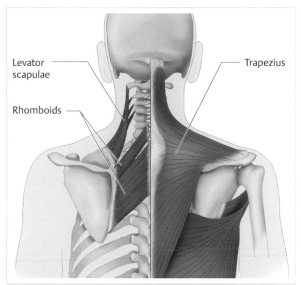

Fig. 13.26 Extrinsic muscles of the neck.

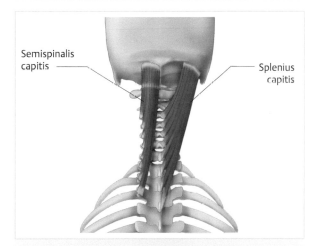

Fig. 13.27 Semispinalis capitis and splenius capitis.

anatomical shape of the joint surfaces is the presumed cause of these differences.

13.3.7 Posterior Muscles

The medial tract intrinsic muscles are the most important stabilizers and mobilizers in the cervical spine and protrude from the bony depression located between the transverse process and the spinous process (e.g., semispinalis cervicis and capitis).

Extrinsic Muscles

The extrinsic muscles of the cervical spine are also defined as muscles that can no longer be found in their original position and are supplied by the ventral rami of the spinal nerves.

The following muscles are of importance (▶ Fig. 13.26):

- **Descending part of the trapezius.** Extends from the superior nuchal line and ligamentum nuchae onto the lateral third of the clavicle.

- **Levator scapulae.** Extends from the C1–C4 transverse processes onto the superior angle of the scapula.
- **Scalenus muscles.** See the section "Anterior and Lateral Muscles" below for a description of their course.
- **Sternocleidomastoid.** Extends from the mastoid process to the manubrium of the sternum and to the medial third of the clavicle.

Intrinsic Muscles

When considered from an evolutionary point of view, we observe that a number of elementary muscles also exist in the cervical spine, which are innervated by the dorsal rami of the spinal nerves.

The following large intrinsic muscles (cervical or occipital) are of importance:

- **Semispinalis cervicis and capitis** (▶ Fig. 13.27). The course of the semispinalis capitis: from the C3–T3 transverse processes to the insertion between the superior and inferior nuchal lines. According to von Lanz and Wachsmuth (1979) this area is approximately 3 cm wide and 2 cm high.
- **Splenius cervicis and capitis** (▶ Fig. 13.27). The course of splenius capitis: from ligamentum nuchae and the C3–T3 spinous processes to the superior nuchal line.
- **Longissimus cervicis and capitis.** The course of the longissimus capitis: transverse processes of the lower cervical spine and the upper thoracic spine up to the mastoid process.
- **Longus colli and capitis.** See the section "Anterior and Lateral Muscles" below for a description of their course.

13

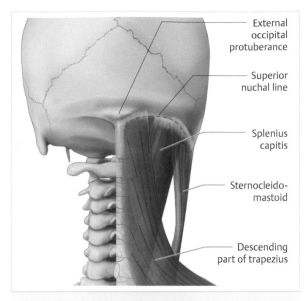

Fig. 13.28 Posterior view of the superficial muscles of the neck.

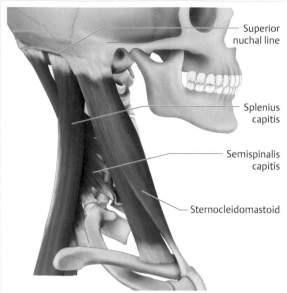

Fig. 13.29 Lateral view of the superficial muscles of the neck.

How Does this Affect Palpation?

An entire group of muscles is encountered when therapists use palpation for orientation. The superficial muscles are the only muscles that can be palpated reliably (▶ Fig. 13.28). Therapists are able to do this by orienting themselves either immediately adjacent to the row of spinous processes or on the edge of the occiput and by instructing their patients to tense the appropriate muscle to confirm its position.

The multisegmental muscle belly of the **semispinalis** is found near the spinous processes and is one of the oblique intrinsic muscles. It occupies the space between the midline and the laminae of the vertebrae. Its insertion is located immediately inferior to the superior nuchal line, where half of its width is covered by the **descending part of the trapezius** before it attaches itself onto the superior nuchal line. The anterior edge of the muscle can be palpated by starting at its insertion on the clavicle and moving in a superomedial direction. The insertion of the semispinalis capitis occupies approximately a third of a widely curved line on the edge of the occiput between the mid-line and the tip of the mastoid process.

The **splenius capitis** inserts into the middle third of this line. This strong rotator and extensor belongs to the superficial layer of the intrinsic muscles of the back. The lateral third of the line is occupied by the **sternocleidomastoid.** This muscle not only inserts onto the mastoid process, but also somewhat posterior to it. This can be easily recognized in the lateral view of this region (▶ Fig. 13.29). The sternocleidomastoid aids orientation when the C1–C3 transverse processes are being palpated. The C1 **transverse process** is usually found anterior to the muscle, the C2 transverse process directly posterior to the muscle, and the C3 transverse process along its posterior edge. This muscle is a helpful guiding structure for therapists who wish to correctly locate the transverse processes. The sternocleidomastoid must often be pushed to the side so that therapists can palpate closer to the transverse processes.

Upper Cervical Muscles

The following deep, short suboccipital muscles are of importance:
- **Rectus capitis posterior major and minor:**
  - Rectus capitis posterior major extends from the C2 spinous process and travels obliquely in a superior direction where it inserts into the inferior nuchal line.
  - Rectus capitis posterior minor extends from the C1 posterior tubercle to the inferior nuchal line.
- **Obliquus capitis inferior and superior:**
  - Obliquus capitis inferior extends from the anterior surface of the C2 spinous process, travels in a superior and quite lateral direction, and inserts onto the C1 transverse process.
  - Obliquus capitis superior extends from the C1 transverse process in an almost lateral direction in the sagittal plane and inserts into the inferior nuchal line (retromastoid process, see the section "Anatomy of the Occiput and the Upper Cervical Spine" discussed above).
- **Rectus capitis lateralis and anterior:**
  - See the section "Anterior and Lateral Muscles" below for a description of their course.

The upper cervical muscles (▶ Fig. 13.30 and ▶ Fig. 13.31) are supplied by a very large proprioceptive innervation

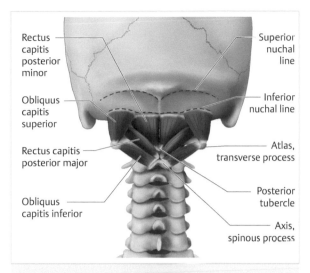

Fig. 13.30 Suboccipital muscles, posterior view.

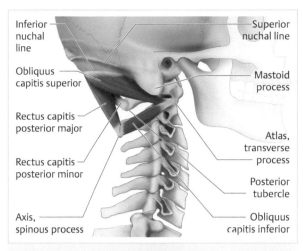

Fig. 13.31 Suboccipital muscles, lateral view.

and are important for the fine control of upper cervical movements. These muscles, in combination with the short anterior muscles, form the upper cervical spine's own muscle apparatus. This muscle apparatus takes advantage of the special anatomical features (e.g., using the long lever of the C1 transverse process and the C2 spinous process) and the special biomechanics found in the upper cervical region, and ensures that the upper cervical joints are approximated using the strength of their tissues. Together with the mechanoreceptors in the C0/C1 to C2/C3 joint capsules, the muscle spindles of these muscles form the third organ for balance.

How Does this Affect Palpation?

The upper cervical muscles are covered completely by superficial muscles, making it difficult to reliably locate these structures using palpation. The deep transverse deformation of the functional massage techniques (see the section "Functional Massage" below) can be used to easily access the muscles and to relieve tension.

13.3.8 Anterior and Lateral Muscles

The anterior muscles in the cervical spine are divided into two systems according to their position:
• Superficial prevertebral muscles found anterior to the organs of the throat.
• Deep prevertebral muscles found directly anterior to the vertebral bodies.

The **superficial prevertebral muscles** are further divided topographically into the following:
• **Suprahyoid muscles:** these muscles are found in the floor of the mouth and connect the hyoid bone with the

mandible. They belong functionally to the muscles of mastication (Rauber and Kopsch, 2003).
• **Infrahyoid muscles, also called the strap muscles:** these muscles connect the hyoid bone with the larynx (thyroid cartilage) and the sternum. According to Rauber and Kopsch (2003), they participate in complex actions such as "chewing, swallowing, and phonation."

From a mechanical point of view, they form a kinematic flexor chain when the mouth is closed and the jaw closers (masseter and temporalis) are active, producing some strength when the cervical spine is flexed.

How Does this Affect Palpation?

The correct location of the hyoid bone and the prominent sections of the larynx is used to confirm the level of the cervical vertebrae. The palpation of posterior structures is very difficult in the supine position, for example, when locating the exact position of the C4 lamina. The anterior structures are used as a further aid here.

The hyoid bone is mostly found deep in the angle between the floor of the mouth and the vertical surface of the throat, at approximately the level of C3. Its position varies a lot. It is quite often found at the level of the mandible and is then difficult to reach. Please refer to the section "Anterior Palpation Techniques" below..

The **deep prevertebral** muscles include:
• Rectus capitis lateralis and anterior:
  ○ Rectus capitis lateralis extends superiorly from the C1 transverse process onto the lateral part of the occiput.
  ○ Rectus capitis anterior extends in a superomedial direction from the anterior aspect of the C1 transverse process to the basilar part of the occiput.
• Longus colli and capitis:
  ○ Course of longus colli: this muscle is divided into several sections. Its vertically and transversely oriented

13

fibers extend from approximately T3 to the atlas and rest against the vertebral bodies on both sides.

○ Course of longus capitis: from the C3–C6 transverse processes, traveling in the depression between the transverse process and vertebral bodies, and inserting onto the basilar part of the occiput.

The rectus muscles and longus capitis, in combination with the short posterior muscles of the neck, ensure that the upper cervical joints are approximated. These muscles should be trained when the upper cervical region is unstable.

The longus group of muscles is known clinically as the stabilizers of the cervical spine. Physical therapy treatment for instability, particularly in the lower cervical spine, should aim to recruit the longus colli muscle. Falla et al. (2004) proved in their electromyographic (EMG) study how important the longus colli and longus capitis muscles (deep flexors of the neck) are. These muscles were shown to be less active during craniocervical flexion in patients with chronic cervical symptoms compared with people who were free of symptoms. The patients' symptoms responded positively to the training of these muscles.

The deep prevertebral muscles (▶ Fig. 13.32) cannot be palpated. They have only been included in this chapter due to their great importance in clinical practice.

• **Scalenus muscles.** According to Rauber/Kopsch (2003), these muscles belong to the deep lateral muscles of the neck and are the continuation of the intercostal muscles in the cervical region. Due to this, the scalenus muscles

also originate on the anterior tubercle of the transverse process, the rudiments of the cervical ribs. Their muscle bellies form a cone-shaped covering over the pleural dome, with nerves and vessels being able to pass through two gaps in the muscles (scalenus gaps) (▶ Fig. 13.33). It is obvious that their suitability as respiratory aid muscles is based on their position and their site of origin:

○ Course of scalenus anterior: extends anterolaterally from the C3–C4 transverse processes onto the first rib. The phrenic nerve accompanies it for part of its course.

○ Course of scalenus medius: from the C3–C7 transverse processes down onto the first rib.

○ Course of scalenus posterior: travels more posteriorly from the C5–C7 transverse processes down onto the second rib.

The scalenus muscles can be reached well using palpation. They cover the anterolateral region of the throat and are only partially covered by the sternocleidomastoid.

The **anterior scalenus gap** (▶ Fig. 13.34) is formed by the sternocleidomastoid and scalenus anterior. The subclavian vein and the phrenic nerve pass through here.

The **posterior scalenus gap** (▶ Fig. 13.34) is formed by the scalenus anterior and scalenus medius. The subclavian artery and the brachial plexus pass through this gap. The constriction of these structures as they pass through this gap in the muscles is known as scalenus syndrome or a form of thoracic outlet syndrome.

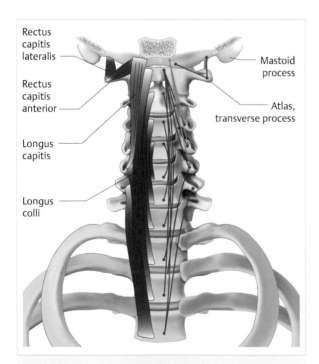

Fig. 13.32 Deep prevertebral muscles.

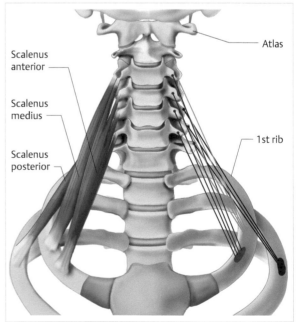

Fig. 13.33 Scalenus muscles.

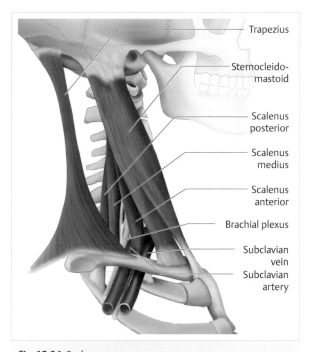

Fig. 13.34 Scalenus gaps.

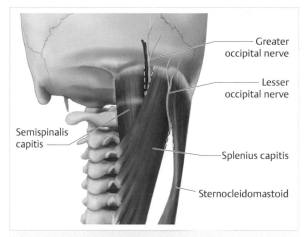

Fig. 13.35 Nerves and blood vessels at the occiput.

13.3.9 Nerves and Blood Vessels

The nuchal fascia extends superiorly from the upper edge of the serratus posterior superior. In contrast to the thoracolumbar fascia, the nuchal fascia is generally weak. It encloses the intrinsic muscles, lying on top of the semispinalis capitis and splenius, and, together with these muscles, is noticeable along the superior nuchal line. It merges with the ligamentum nuchae medially and is connected anteriorly with the deep layer of the cervical prevertebral fascia that surrounds the scalenus muscles, longissimus cervicis, and longissimus capitis. A stabilizing action, as seen in the corresponding fascia in the lumbar spine, has not been attributed to the nuchal fascia.

A variety of neural and vascular structures travel posteriorly, through the superficial neck muscles and the posterior fascia (nuchal fascia and the trapezius fascia), and onto the skull, where they supply the posterior aspect of the head (▶ Fig. 13.35).

Splenius capitis is the **guiding** structure used to comprehend the course of the vessels and nerves in this region.

The lesser occipital nerve emerges from an **angle** formed by the lateral edge of splenius capitis and the posterior edge of the sternocleidomastoid and travels up onto the posterior aspect of the head. It is a branch of the cervical plexus and therefore has an anterior origin.

The occipital vessels (occipital artery and accompanying veins) and the greater occipital nerve exit the fascia of the neck via a **triangle** formed by the medial edge of the splenius capitis, the lateral edge of the semispinalis, and

the occiput. They emerge on the surface and also travel to the occiput. The greater occipital nerve passes through the muscle bellies of the semispinalis capitis and the descending part of the trapezius beforehand (von Lanz and Wachsmuth, 2004a).

The position of the nerves and blood vessels mentioned here appears to be variable as common anatomy textbooks describe and illustrate their position and course quite differently.

How Does this Affect Palpation?

The clinical consequence of neural structures passing through fascia and muscles in the limbs is known as compression neuropathy (entrapment neuropathy). Similar pathological conditions have also been described for the pathway of the greater occipital nerve, which lead to pain and dysesthesia at the occiput. Symptoms increase when the nerve is provoked by palpation.

Brachial Plexus

The muscles in the neck and throat region are innervated by the cervical plexus and the cranial nerves. Parts of the brachial plexus innervate the shoulder girdle and arm muscles.

The anterior branches of the C5–T1 spinal nerves unite at the brachial plexus via three trunks and cords and form a number of peripheral nerves. The main peripheral nerves that innervate the arm muscles are well known: the median, ulnar, and radial nerves. Due to the alignment of the transverse processes, the branches that merge into the brachial plexus travel anteriorly at an angle. Together with the subclavian artery, they pass through the scalenus muscles at the posterior scalenus gap and follow the artery through the subsequent narrow gap between the clavicle and the first rib (▶ Fig. 13.36). They can be palpated at the scalenus gap by moving the

13

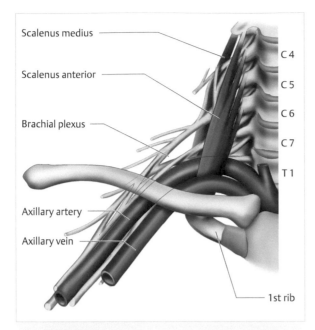

Fig. 13.36 Brachial plexus.

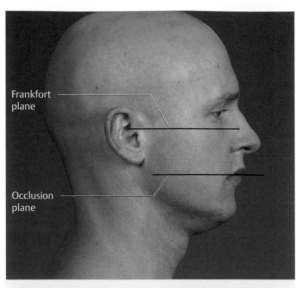

Fig. 13.37 Neutral starting position in unsupported sitting.

arm and placing the branches under tension (see the section "Supraclavicular Triangle of the Neck" below).

13.4 Overview of the Structures to be Palpated

The aim of palpation is to lay the technical foundations for the local assessment and treatment of the cervical spine. Therapists concentrate on the cervical region as a whole. Instructions are provided individually for the posterior, lateral, and anterior sections of the cervical spine. The anatomical division of the upper and lower cervical spines is not practical enough for the palpatory procedure.

13.5 Summary of the Palpatory Process

The palpation of the **posterior** side is the first of the four palpatory procedures that will be conducted. Protrusions and contours from the occiput to the mastoid process will become distinct first. In addition, all bony and muscular structures on the line connecting the occiput to the C7 spinous process will be located as well as possible. The posterolateral ligaments and the ZAJs (facet joints) are palpated next. We finish by returning to the occiput and locating the accessible muscles, nerves, and blood vessels.

Palpation of the **lateral** aspect allows therapists to locate the C1–C3 transverse processes. Additionally, the location of structures will be described, varying from the

soft tissues in the posterior triangle of the neck to the structures found in the posterior scalenus gap.

The **anterior** structures allow therapists to determine the level of individual vertebrae with great certainty. It is for this reason that the hyoid bone and the larynx are included in the palpatory orientation.

It is necessary to discuss the starting positions (SPs) beforehand to ensure that the same conditions are present for each and every palpation.

13.6 Starting Position

It is recommended that patients be positioned in neutral, unsupported sitting when the cervical spine is being palpated. The advantage of this SP is that all posterior, lateral, and anterior structures can be easily reached. The slight resting tension in the neck muscles is acceptable. The positioning of the cervical spine in neutral is described very precisely. This position should always be used, except when mobility is clearly restricted or when the patient's current symptoms do not allow this position:

- The head is not shifted forward (protraction) or backward (retraction) in relation to the trunk. In other words, the occiput (most posterior aspect) should be found in the same plane as the upper thoracic spine.
- The cervical spine is also placed in neutral lateral flexion and rotation. Therapists should check the distance between the ears and the upper part of the shoulders as well as the position of the nose in the sagittal plane.
- The upper cervical spine should be positioned in neutral flexion/extension (▶ Fig. 13.37):
  - **Option 1—Frankfort plane.** This reference plane is ascertained using the upper edge of the bony outer

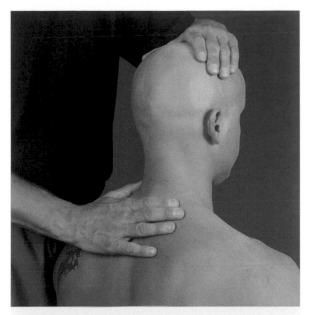

Fig. 13.38 Therapist position and handling—variation 1.

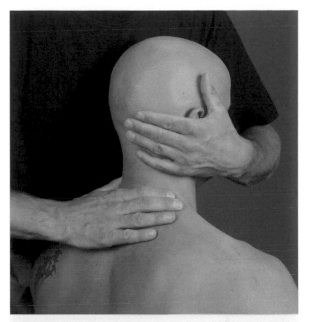

Fig. 13.39 Handling—variation 2.

opening of the ear (external acoustic aperture or pore) and the most inferior part of the eye socket (orbit) (Greiner, 2000, Williams, 2009). Penning (2000) used the term orbitomeatal plane. It is very easy for therapists to place the head in a neutral position.

○ **Option 2—optimal occlusion.** When the head is raised and lowered repeatedly in an upright sitting position, the two rows of teeth come into contact when the head is found at a certain position. This is the point of occlusion: the neutral flexion/extension position for the upper cervical spine. This method of positioning in neutral is not particularly practical for therapists.

The therapist usually stands next to the patient. The palpating hand comes from anterior. The other hand controls the patient's head position by placing a flattened hand on the top of the head (▶ Fig. 13.38). Only slight effort is needed to move the head into a neutral position when using this method. Small and large movements can be facilitated very easily.

Another option is to use the therapeutic ring. The therapist's hand comes from anterior and encircles the patient's head. The edge of the small finger rests on the occiput, unless low cervical segments need to be emphasized. If this is the case, the edge of the small finger is placed lower in the neck (▶ Fig. 13.39). The therapist should make sure that the hands do not compress the patient's ear or mandible excessively. The patient's head rests against the therapist's sternum or ipsilateral shoulder. A folded towel can be placed between the head and the sternum or shoulder so that the therapist does not have to bend forward too

much to reach the patient's head and to maintain the neutral position.

The advantage of this handling technique is the extensive control of the head. Small movements can be facilitated precisely. Furthermore, the therapist can apply compression or traction along the longitudinal axis of the cervical spine when needed.

Tip

As simple as this hand placement technique may appear, therapists are tempted to move the cervical spine out of the neutral position by pulling the patient's head toward them instead of moving themselves toward the head. It is therefore helpful for therapists with little experience to initially practice this technique in front of a mirror.

The therapist must change position when palpating anteriorly. This SP will be described in the section "Anterior Palpation Techniques" below. Please read the section "Neutral Starting Position: Sitting," Chapter 13.10, for further information on the SP in unsupported sitting.

13.6.1 Difficult and Alternative Starting Positions

Several treatment techniques require patients to be positioned in the supine or prone SP. Cervical spine techniques in side-lying are rare. In the lying SPs, the cervical spine should also be positioned as neutral as possible

13

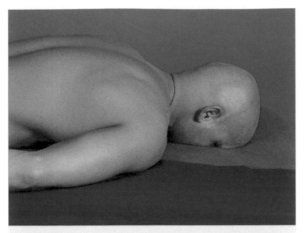

Fig. 13.40 Neutral starting position (SP) in prone position.

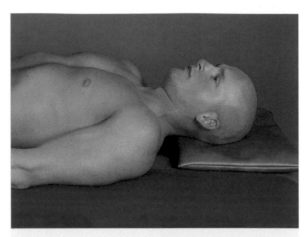

Fig. 13.41 Neutral starting position (SP) in supine position.

providing the patient's symptoms do not require another position.

Prone-lying

The prone SP has already been described extensively in Chapter 8. The position of the body on the treatment table is crucial for the positioning of the cervical spine when the nose is positioned in the table's face hole, as is usually the case. Once again, the patient should lie in the middle of the treatment table so that the cervical spine is not positioned in lateral flexion. The thoracic spine is placed in a kyphosis when the head-end of the treatment table is slightly lowered. The extent of cervical lordosis can be altered by sliding a little toward the foot-end or head-end of the table. If the cervical spine cannot be positioned in neutral, as described above, it must at least be placed in the position seen when the patient is upright (► Fig. 13.40).

Supine Position

This starting position has not yet been discussed. The patient usually lies on the treatment table with the arms placed next to the body. Their knees are slightly flexed and rest on padding. For the assessment and treatment of the cervical spine, it is important that the patient is positioned as near to the head-end of the treatment table as possible so that the distance between the therapist and the cervical spine is not too large. The cervical spine is often positioned in too much flexion by using too much padding. This places the posterior soft tissue under passive tension and positions the lower and upper cervical joints in flexion. This in turn reduces the range of a variety of movements and changes the results of local assessment. It is therefore recommended not to use padding underneath the occiput or to use only a small amount of padding if the lordosis is too extreme (► Fig. 13.41). In

addition, it must be kept in mind that rolling the head causes rotation and lateral bending.

Memorize

Place padding only under the occiput and not under the cervical spine!

Certain pathological conditions are painful, for example, an acute wry neck (torticollis), and require other positions. Of course, the patient's perception has priority over the desire to position the cervical spine in neutral.

13.7 Posterior Palpation Techniques

13.7.1 Occiput

The finger pads of the second and third fingers are placed flatly over the occiput. Using a palpation technique with slightly circular motion, the therapist searches for the raised part of the occiput that corresponds to the dimensions and shape of a well-developed tubercle: the external occipital protuberance (► Fig. 13.42). The ligamentum nuchae attaches firmly to this point.

Tip

The protuberance is often found higher than expected.

The uppermost line of the neck, the highest nuchal line, can be visualized from this point by placing a finger across the occiput immediately above the protuberance (► Fig. 13.43). The line extends laterally from here in a large arch and is only rarely felt as a raised ridge.

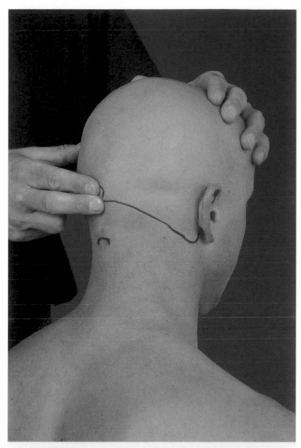

Fig. 13.42 Palpating the external occipital protuberance.

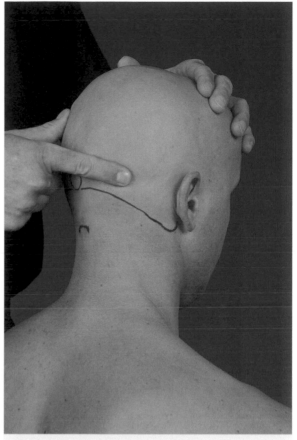

Fig. 13.43 Highest nuchal line.

The actual palpation of the edge of the occiput starts now. Starting at the external occipital protuberance, the therapist palpates more inferiorly and laterally until the rounded edge of the occiput can be clearly felt. A perpendicular palpatory technique is used here with the pads of the index fingers pushing against the edge of the occiput from an inferior position (▶ Fig. 13.44).

From an anatomical point of view, the fingers are at approximately the level of the superior nuchal line. According to von Lanz and Wachsmuth (1979), the muscles of this area are coarse, with the degree of coarseness depending on the individual. This coarseness bulges out (torus occipitalis) in athletes who have to lean forward and hold their head upright (speed skaters, cyclists).

The insertions of the semispinalis capitis and the descending part of the trapezius (▶ Fig. 13.44) are found medial and directly inferior to this point. As the therapist moves laterally, the edge of the occiput can be palpated more clearly at two points. These points correspond to the gaps between neighboring muscles and allow the therapist to access deeper-lying structures. More detailed information can be found in the section "Muscles, Suboccipital Nerves, and Blood Vessels" below.

A slightly rounded elevation can be felt further laterally (▶ Fig. 13.45). The superior and inferior nuchal lines meet at this retromastoid process. The obliquus capitis superior attaches here.

Finally, the palpating finger encounters the posterior aspect of the mastoid process as it moves laterally (▶ Fig. 13.46). The edges of the mastoid process are palpated to measure its dimensions. This process is no longer found on the occipital bone. Instead, it is positioned on the temporal bone. The suture connecting the occipital and the temporal bones runs immediately posterior to the mastoid process.

13.7.2 Suboccipital Fossa and Ligamentum Nuchae

The therapist returns to the external occipital protuberance. The pad of the index or middle finger is placed flat on the surface of the skin for palpation.

The occiput is palpated by starting at the protuberance, then moving inferiorly. The palpating finger is pressed repeatedly against the bone during this process, enabling the therapist to palpate the shape and course of the occiput.

13

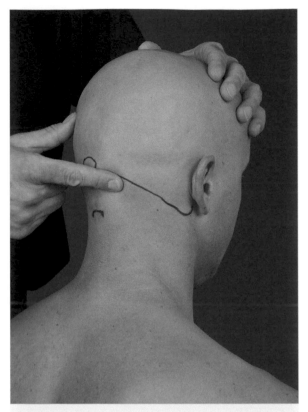

Fig. 13.44 Superior nuchal line; medial.

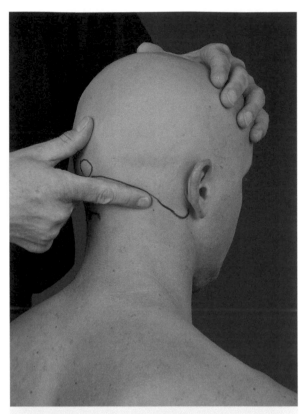

Fig. 13.45 Superior nuchal line; lateral.

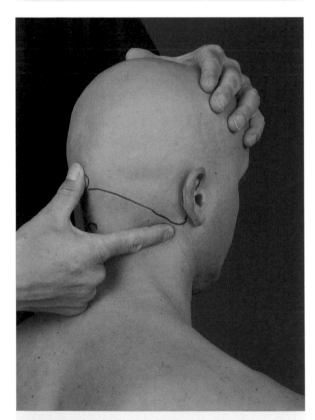

Fig. 13.46 Palpating the mastoid process.

Memorize

Important

The therapist should pay special attention to the neutral position of the cervical spine. Every nodding movement, no matter how small, makes it more difficult to palpate the edge of the bone.

When the last point of bony contact with the occiput is felt, the palpating finger pad is located in a large fossa approximately 1 cm in size (▶ Fig. 13.47), which is bordered by a variety of structures (▶ Fig. 13.48):

- The occiput forms the superior boundary, as has already been palpated.
- The C2 spinous process forms the inferior boundary.
- The strong muscle bellies of the semispinalis capitis and the descending part of the trapezius form the lateral boundaries.
- The ligamentum nuchae forms the anterior boundary.

The therapist feels an extremely elastic form of resistance when applying posteroanterior pressure using the finger pad. By moving the cervical spine into extensive flexion or extension, the therapist can feel the increase and decrease in tension in the ligamentum nuchae more clearly.

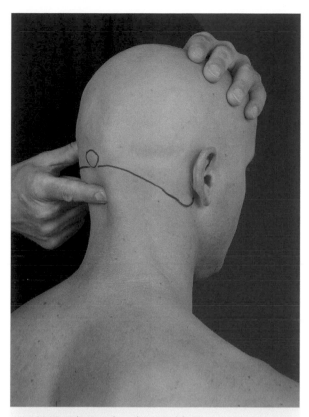

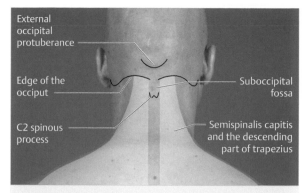

External
occipital
protuberance

Edge of the
occiput

C2 spinous
process

Suboccipital
fossa

Semispinalis capitis
and the descending
part of trapezius

Fig. 13.48 Boundaries to the suboccipital fossa.

Fig. 13.47 Palpating the suboccipital fossa.

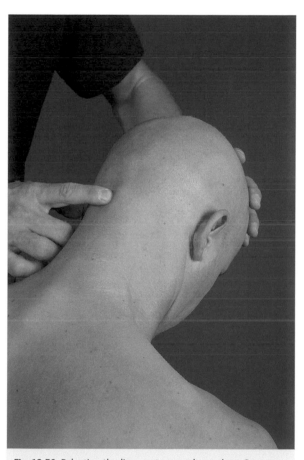

Fig. 13.50 Palpating the ligamentum nuchae—phase 2.

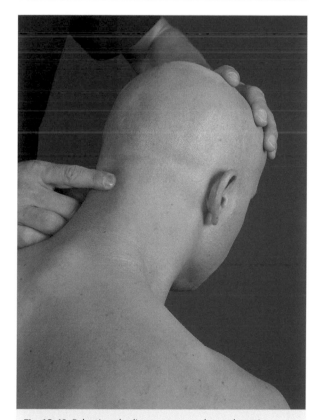

Fig. 13.49 Palpating the ligamentum nuchae—phase 1.

Ligamentum Nuchae

The therapist continues to palpate the suboccipital fossa, applying gentle pressure, and moves the cervical spine into full-range flexion (▶ Fig. 13.49).

The upper cervical spine is then moved into alternating extension and flexion (▶ Fig. 13.50). The patient can help by moving their chin forward or by making a double chin.

13

Expectations

When the head is retracted, the whole ligament is placed under tension and pushes the palpating finger out of the fossa (▶ Fig. 13.50). During active extension, the therapist can feel the tense muscle bellies of both semispinalis capitis muscles on the right and left side.

The therapist can follow the ligamentum nuchae as it extends superiorly up to its point of attachment on the skull by alternately placing the ligament under tension and relaxing it. This method is ultimately used to verify the exact position of the external occipital protuberance.

13.7.3 C2 Spinous Process

The cervical spine is again placed in a neutral position. The palpating finger is positioned in the suboccipital fossa and pushes inferiorly. The hard, bony resistance of the C2 spinous process can be felt immediately. The thumb and index finger are used to palpate the posterior aspect of the asymmetrical bifurcated spinous process (▶ Fig. 13.51).

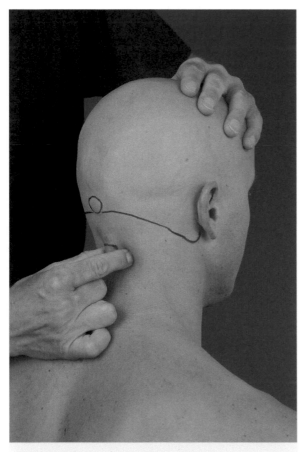

Fig. 13.51 Palpating the C2 spinous process.

The C2 spinous process has to be palpated precisely and even be fixed for local assessment and treatment techniques in the upper cervical region. Fixation is only possible laterally via the laminae of C2 (see the section "Test for the Alar Ligaments" below).

13.7.4 Spinous Processes of the Lower Cervical Spine

The identification of the spinous processes at the cervicothoracic junction has already been described in detail in Chapter 12.7. The methods involved are therefore only summarized here.

In general, it is not possible to accurately identify the C3 and C4 spinous processes. Occasionally, the spinous processes can be felt in patients whose cervical spines have an extremely reduced lordosis. Again, it is not possible to precisely locate the level here. If the therapist wishes to locate the C2/C3 segment, for example, the corresponding posterolateral laminae are used to help define the level. Only the spinous processes from C5 to C7 can be felt reasonably well and can be differentiated from one another.

Unreliable Method

The position of the C5 spinous process can often be recognized by simply feeling the shape of the C6 spinous process. When the therapist uses moderate pressure to palpate along the cervical mid-line from superior to inferior, the finger pads can be felt moving down onto a type of platform (▶ Fig. 13.52). The medial side of the fingers encounters the superior aspect of the C6 spinous process. The C5 spinous process is reached by applying gentle posteroanterior pressure with the finger pad. Since this method is not reliable enough, another aid is needed to improve reliability.

Reliable Method

The patient's cervical spine is placed in a lordosis by tilting the head backward (▶ Fig. 13.53). During this movement, the C5 and C6 spinous processes typically translate anteriorly. This phenomenon has already been commented on in Chapter 12.7.

The C5 spinous process first moves in an anterior direction, moving clearly away from the palpating finger after

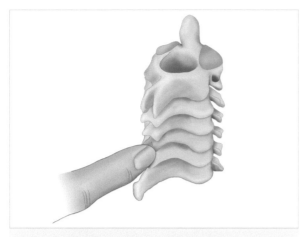

Fig. 13.52 C6 spinous process—unreliable method.

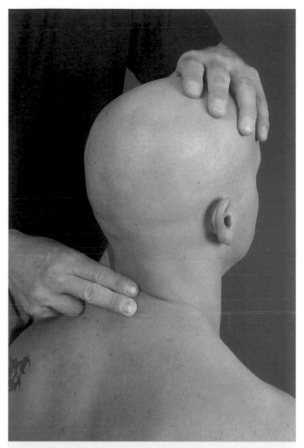

Fig. 13.53 Palpating the spinous processes of the lower cervical spine.

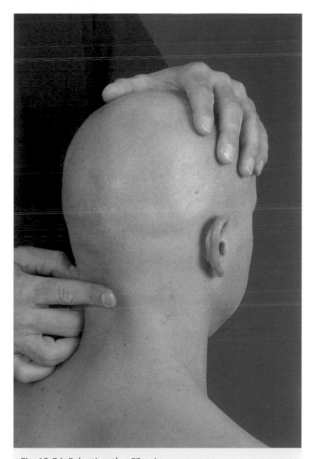

Fig. 13.54 Palpating the C2 spinous process.

only slight lordosis has been achieved. The C6 spinous process is then sought. The movement into cervical lordosis is repeated and conducted over a large range. The C6 spinous process starts moving anteriorly at the end of the lordotic range. In contrast, the C7 spinous process tends to remain stationary. It is a prerequisite that the patient or study partner can extend the neck over a large range without feeling pain.

13.7.5 Facet Joints

The ZAJs, the precise anatomical term for the facet joints, can only be clearly identified in the cervical section of the vertebral column. They are located for diagnostic and therapeutic purposes. Restrictions in joint mobility can be palpated, and irritated capsules are very sensitive to the pressure of palpation.

The following palpatory procedure emphasizes the steps involved when locating the ZAJ between C2 and C3 (see ▶ Fig. 13.54):

- C2 spinous process.
- C2 lamina.
- C3 lamina.
- C3 superior articular process.
- Posterior tubercle of the C3 transverse process.
- Palpating movement in the C2/C3 ZAJ.

13

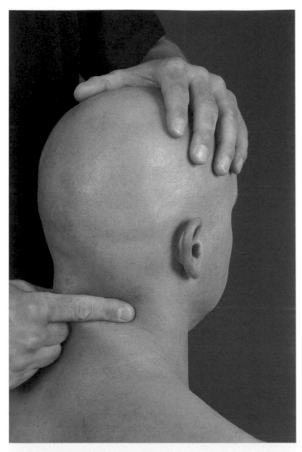

Fig. 13.55 Palpating the lamina of C2.

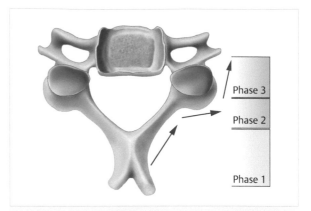

Fig. 13.56 Phases during the palpation of the zygapophysial joint (ZAJ).

Locating the Articular Column

The lamina of C3 is located (▶ Fig. 13.57). The palpating finger increases the pressure applied to the lamina and follows its course further anterolaterally (▶ Fig. 13.57, phase 1). After a short distance, the palpating finger encounters increased resistance and the palpation changes in a more lateral direction (▶ Fig. 13.57, phase 2). The superior articular process, the C3 component of the articular column, is located here.

Confirming the Correct Location

Three methods are available to confirm the correct location of the C2/C3 ZAJ:
- The articular column's undulating shape can be felt underneath the palpating finger as the finger moves extensively in a superior and inferior direction. The ZAJ bulges out posteriorly. The area between neighboring ZAJs is somewhat flatter. Irritated joint capsules are sensitive to pressure when the technique is performed as a provocating palpation.
- The palpation is continued in a lateral direction. The bony resistance decreases and the finger moves anteriorly, with the finger movement depicting a sudden curve (▶ Fig. 13.56, phase 3). The finger has now slid down laterally from the articular column and is located on the posterior boundary of the transverse process (posterior tubercle).
- Confirmation with movement. The finger moves back onto the articular column (▶ Fig. 13.58). The finger pad is located slightly inferior to the C2/C3 ZAJ. This joint is formed by the C3 superior articular process and the C2 inferior articular process. By moving the joint at a very local level, it is possible to feel joint movement as the articular surfaces glide together or glide apart:
  ○ Convergence—gliding together (▶ Fig. 13.59). The movement preferred here is a very localized lateral flexion toward the side of palpation, with the head

Identifying a Level via the Laminae

To find the C2/C3 ZAJ, the palpating finger must first be placed over the lamina of C3.

The C2 spinous process is located next (▶ Fig. 13.55). This has already been successfully achieved in previous palpations. Starting at the spinous process, the therapist palpates in an anterolateral direction around the semispinalis capitis. The paravertebral muscles are pushed out of the way posteromedially and posteroanterior pressure is applied. The tissue responds with very firm resistance. The therapist is now palpating the lamina of C2 (▶ Fig. 13.56). The laminae of each further cervical vertebra are found approximately 1 index finger width (of the patient) inferiorly.

Tip

All cervical vertebrae can be identified with high reliability when this rule is followed. Reliability can be further increased by identifying the level anteriorly (see section "Anterior Palpation Techniques" below).

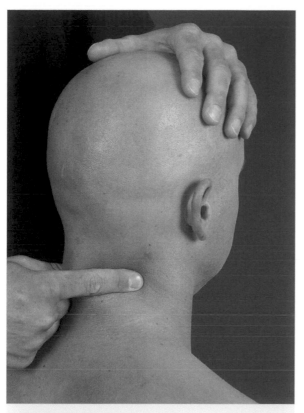

Fig. 13.57 Palpating the lamina of C3.

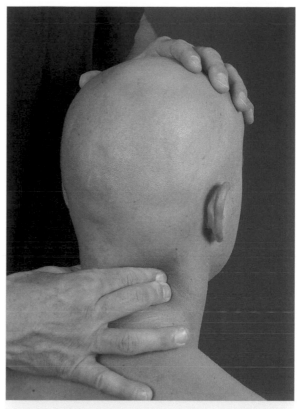

Fig. 13.58 Palpating the C2/C3 zygapophysial joint (ZAJ).

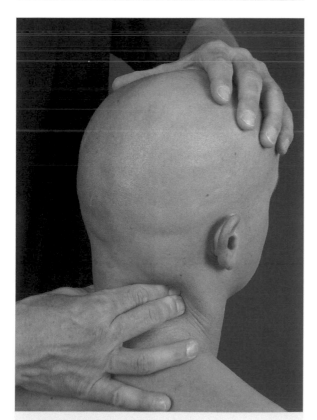

Fig. 13.59 Confirmation with movement.

being used to facilitate this movement. The therapist can also introduce rotation by rotating the C1/C2 segment for approximately 40° until the movement is passed onto the target segment of C2/C3. When the therapist introduces slight lateral flexion, C2 rotates immediately toward the side of lateral flexion. Movement can be felt at the C2/C3 ZAJ rather quickly.

○ Divergence—gliding apart. C2 moves away from the finger pad during contralateral lateral flexion and, if necessary, slight flexion.

Tip

The resistance felt by the finger pad is expected to increase when pressure is applied to the inferior articular process of C2. If the expected resistance is not immediately felt, the procedure must be repeated several times. When the therapist places the joint at its end range via lateral flexion and/or rotation and uses the finger pad to apply rhythmical pressure toward the orbit (parallel to the alignment of the joint space), a firm-elastic resistance is expected. This maneuver can also be conducted for all further ipsilateral ZAJs as the springing test. Joints with local restrictions in mobility resist pressure with an almost hard resistance.

13

13.7.6 Muscles, Suboccipital Nerves, and Blood Vessels

Muscles insert into three lines on the occiput (▶ Fig. 13.60):
- Highest nuchal line: extends superiorly and laterally from the external occipital protuberance.
- Superior nuchal line: extends laterally from the external occipital protuberance in a large arc.

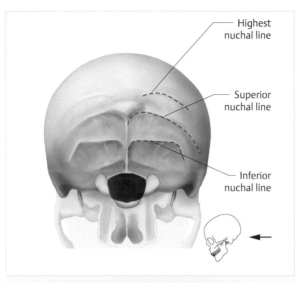

Fig. 13.60 Posterior aspect of the occipital bone.

- Inferior nuchal line: the deep neck muscles insert into this difficult-to-reach line.

The accessible superficial muscles are evident on the superior nuchal line approximately 2 finger widths superior to the palpable edge of the occiput. The predominant muscles in this region are semispinalis capitis, splenius capitis, and sternocleidomastoid.

The position of the muscles, the intermuscular gaps, and the neural and vascular structures passing through these gaps will be clarified in the following palpation.

Semispinalis Capitis and the Descending Part of the Trapezius

The palpation starts in the suboccipital fossa. This is bordered on both sides by the semispinalis capitis and trapezius muscles. The muscles are activated to make their position and dimensions clearer.

The pads of the thumb and two fingers are first used to grasp the muscle mass directly parallel to the vertebral column (▶ Fig. 13.61).

The patient then bends the head forward completely. This results in flexion of the lower cervical spine in particular. This is followed by active upper cervical extension where the patient pushes against the therapist's hand (▶ Fig. 13.62). It is very helpful to instruct the patient to move the chin forward during this step.

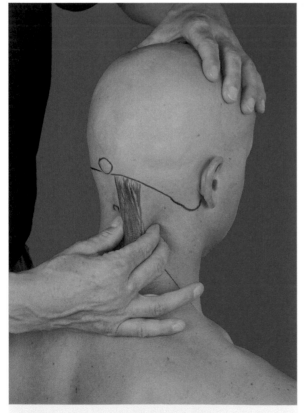

Fig. 13.61 Palpating the semispinalis capitis.

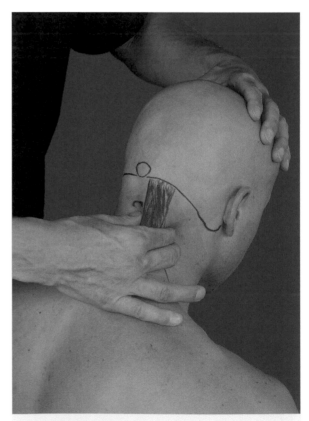

Fig. 13.62 Contraction of the semispinalis capitis.

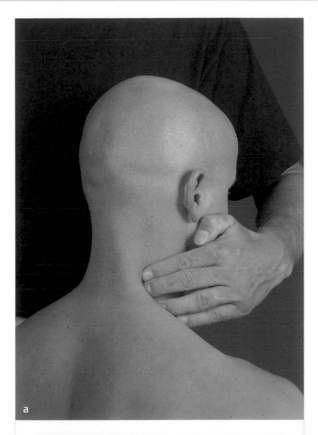

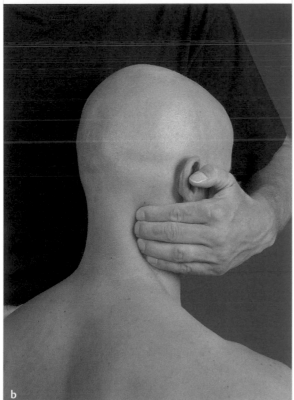

Fig. 13.63 Palpating the descending part of the trapezius.
a Phase 1. **b** Phase 2.

The semispinalis capitis can now be palpated and observed as a firm, distinct muscle mass directly adjacent to the vertebral column. Its course can be followed up to the superior nuchal line when the muscle remains active.

The anterior edge of the descending part of the trapezius forms the posterior boundary for the fossa superior to the clavicle. Its position is generally well known and it is easy to palpate its anterior edge. The palpatory technique involves placing the tips of the fingers perpendicular to the edge of the muscle (► Fig. 13.63a, phase 1).

Gentle pressure is applied and the edge of the muscle is followed superomedially. The palpating finger then encounters the superior nuchal line exactly in the middle of the insertion of the semispinalis capitis (► Fig. 13.63b, phase 2).

Sternocleidomastoid

The position and the edges of the sternocleidomastoid can be clearly identified. If the muscle cannot be easily recognized in upright sitting, the muscle must be contracted to make its position more distinct. A suitable method to activate the muscle is for the therapist to place a hand on the patient's head and resist contralateral isometric rotation or ipsilateral isometric lateral flexion (► Fig. 13.64a, phase 1).

The posterior edge is followed superiorly until the insertion directly posterior to the mastoid process at the level of the superior nuchal line is reached (► Fig. 13.64b, phase 2). The same technique is used to palpate the anterior edge of the sternocleidomastoid, that is, by palpating perpendicular to the edge of the muscle. The anterior edge ends at the anterior edge of the mastoid process.

To aid orientation during the next steps, the therapist marks the edges of the muscles that have already been palpated on the skin (► Fig. 13.65): semispinalis capitis, the descending part of the trapezius, and sternocleidomastoid. The therapist can additionally transfer their knowledge of the topography of nerves and vessels in this region onto the drawing (► Fig. 13.65).

Splenius Capitis

Another strong muscle can be located in the neck region: the splenius capitis. This muscle belongs to the superficial layer of the intrinsic muscles of the back and extends from the cervical spinous processes up onto the superior nuchal line. It can be observed directly lateral to the semispinalis capitis and directly medial to the mastoid process and sternocleidomastoid. It is not as easy to accurately locate this muscle compared with the location of the sternocleidomastoid. The muscle often has to be strongly contracted to make its position clear. Its muscle belly becomes distinct during extensive active movements of the cervical spine into extension, rotation, and lateral flexion toward the side being palpated.

13

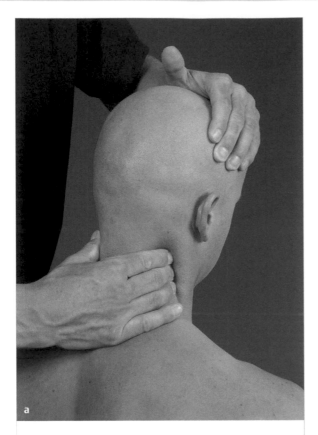

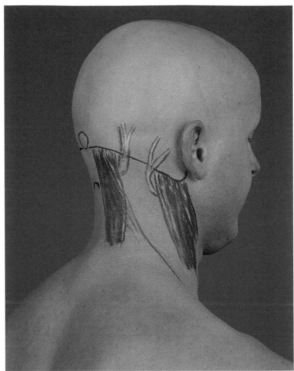

Fig. 13.65 Drawing of the edges of the muscle, nerves, and blood vessels on the skin.

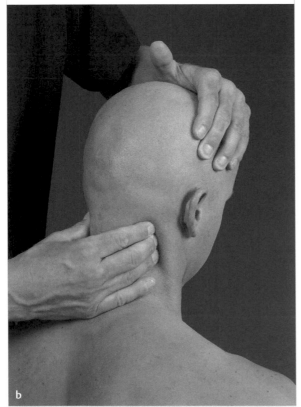

Fig. 13.64 Palpating the sternocleidomastoid.
a Phase 1. b Phase 2.

The patient's cervical spine is positioned in neutral and the therapist places the finger pads flat over the edge of the occiput in the space between the semispinalis capitis and sternocleidomastoid (▶ Fig. 13.66a, phase 1). The therapist then positions the cervical spine in slight extension, rotation, and lateral flexion toward the side to be palpated (▶ Fig. 13.66b, phase 2). The patient is now looking over the therapist's shoulder. The patient pushes the head further in this direction, while the therapist's hand opposes this movement. The splenius, in particular, provides the necessary strength and its muscle belly can be clearly felt as it pushes against the palpating fingers.

Suboccipital Nerves and Blood Vessels

As already discussed in the section on anatomy, two nerves and one artery pass over the edge of the occiput as they travel toward the head: the occipital artery and the greater and lesser occipital nerves. The position of these structures is very variable. The most accurate description of their course can be found in von Lanz and Wachsmuth (1979). The course described in this book represents the accepted average. These structures can be identified very precisely using palpation once therapists have practiced a lot and gained experience. Two areas on the occiput exist that are covered by less-firm muscles. These areas will be named the intermuscular gaps on the occiput in the following text; they aid therapists in locating the nerves and

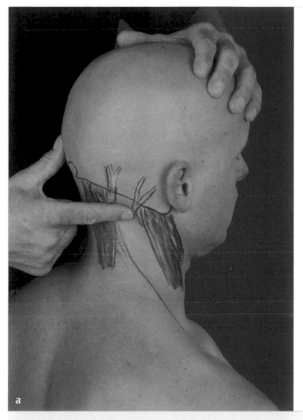 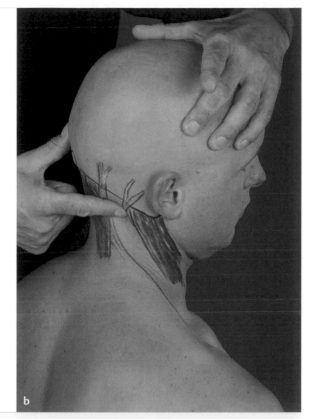

Fig. 13.66 Palpating the splenius capitis. **a** Phase 1. **b** Phase 2.

the artery. These intermuscular gaps can be clearly felt at two points when palpating from medial to lateral along the occiput. Each gap is located in the space between two neighboring muscles (▶ Fig. 13.67):

- *Medial intermuscular gap*: lateral edge of the semispinalis capitis and medial edge of the splenius capitis. The occipital artery and the greater occipital nerve pass through the fascia at this point and travel subcutaneously onto the occiput. At this point, the posterior arch of the atlas can be indirectly reached when firm pressure is applied. This is of great importance for a variety of mobility and stability tests as well as for manual therapeutic treatment techniques targeting the C0/C1 segment.
- The *lateral intermuscular gap* is found between the lateral edge of the splenius and the posterior (medial) edge of the sternocleidomastoid. The lesser occipital nerve passes over the edge of the occipital bone here. It juts out from behind the sternocleidomastoid around the level of C2 and travels in a straight line up onto the occiput.

To locate the **occipital artery**, a finger pad is gently placed flat over the edge of the occiput at the level of the medial intermuscular gap (▶ Fig. 13.68). It usually takes a while before the arterial pulse can be felt. If the pulse cannot be felt, the therapist should continue palpation more medial or lateral to this point.

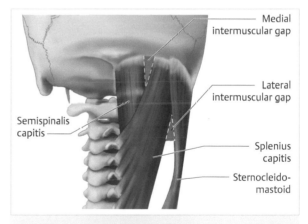

Fig. 13.67 Suboccipital intermuscular gaps.

Medial intermuscular gap

Lateral intermuscular gap

Splenius capitis

Sternocleido-mastoid

Semispinalis capitis

13

The **greater occipital nerve** is found directly adjacent to the artery. To locate the nerve, the correct technique involves holding the finger vertically and using the fingertip for palpation (▶ Fig. 13.69). A peripheral nerve can be plucked especially well on top of this hard underlying surface. This is similar to plucking a guitar string and is achieved by applying firm pressure and quickly moving the finger back and forth. The nerve rolls underneath the fingertip during this movement.

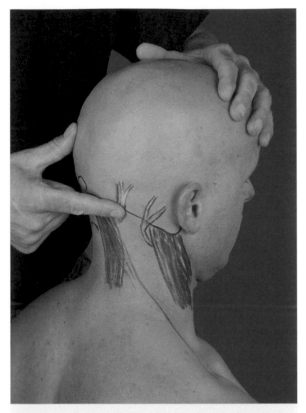

Fig. 13.68 Palpating suboccipital nerves; occipital artery.

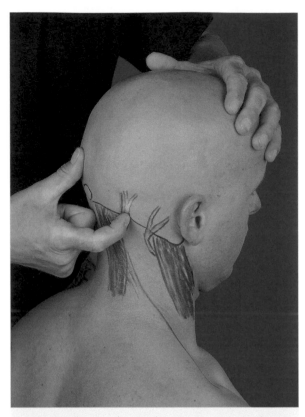

Fig. 13.69 Palpating suboccipital nerves: Greater occipital nerve.

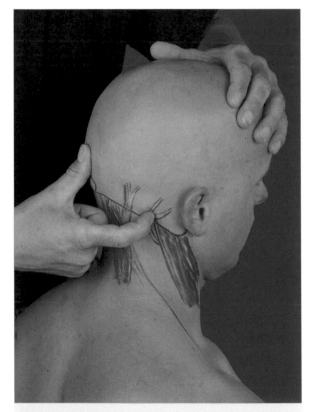

Fig. 13.70 Palpating suboccipital nerves: Lesser occipital nerve.

The therapist attempts to find the **lesser occipital nerve** in the lateral suboccipital intermuscular gap using the same technique (▶ Fig. 13.70).

13.8 Tips for Assessment and Treatment

These first palpations on the posterior aspect of the cervical spine have shown options that can be implemented well when working with patients. The level of structures can now be determined reliably. Posterior muscles and posterolaterally positioned ZAJs can be palpated well.

The groundwork for the local mobility tests at the ZAJ has been laid. The "Facet Joints" section above has already described how movement is felt in the ZAJs. The springing test is one of the quickest and most conclusive tests available to assess the mobility of a ZAJ. A variety of manual therapy techniques use the laminae to influence segmental mobility (traction and gliding). Therapists should refer to specialist literature on this topic.

The sections below present the following:

- First, alternatives for functional massage of the descending part of the trapezius muscle.
- Second, three techniques that are of importance within and outside the field of manual therapy and focus primarily on assessment of upper cervical stability.

In addition to the tests assessing the stability of the transverse ligament of the atlas, testing of the alar ligaments belongs to the crucial skills providing information on the important ligaments of this region (see the section "Test for the Alar Ligaments" below).

In the lower cervical spine, age-related degenerative processes in the movement segment play an important role. A simple technique is used for the important provocation of the affected segment and to determine its level (see the section "Identifying the Level of Chronically Irritated Intervertebral Disks" below).

This section finishes with an extremely pleasant, functional, and effective type of muscle technique that is used to relieve muscle tension. All therapists can carry out these functional massages on the paravertebral muscles with some aptitude. These techniques are often used as the initial treatment of painful symptoms or to prepare patients for local assessment or treatment (see the section "Functional Massage" below).

13.8.1 Functional Massage of the Trapezius in Supine Position

A technique in the supine position provides the therapist with another option to lower the tension in the descending part of the trapezius and paravertebral neck muscles. It essentially differs from the technique in side-lying through its use of cervical rotation and simple shoulder depression. The range of pain-free cervical rotation must therefore be assessed before applying the technique.

Starting Position

The patient lies toward the head-end of the treatment table in a neutral supine position. The back of the head should actually extend somewhat over the edge of the treatment table. It is supported with some padding, for example, with a folded towel.

Caution

Do not place padding underneath the cervical spine!

The patient's forearm on the side to be treated is placed on the abdomen and held onto by the other hand (variation according to Oliver Oswald). This facilitates the necessary movement of the scapula.

The therapist's body is in contact with the side of the patient's head. One hand facilitates the shoulder girdle and the other hand grasps the trapezius and molds the muscle. The therapist's forearm rests against the side of the patient's head.

Technique

The hand close to the head molds the muscles (trapezius and neck muscles) by stretching the trapezius transversely in an anterior direction and stretching the paravertebral muscles more to the side. The therapist's forearm facilitates the head into cervical rotation while the therapist slightly moves their body out of the way. The other hand leads the shoulder girdle into depression. The deformation of muscles and the depression are eased again as the therapist's body brings the patient's head back into a neutrally rotated position.

- **Variation 1** (▶ Fig. 13.71): More emphasis is placed on the trapezius, forced shoulder girdle depression, and less cervical rotation. The grip is more to the side.
- **Variation 2** (▶ Fig. 13.72): More emphasis is placed on the paravertebral neck muscles using less depression and significant rotation. The grip is therefore more medial.

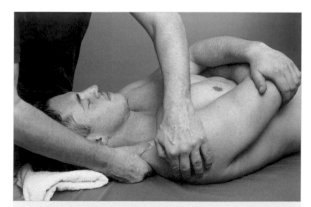

Fig. 13.71 Functional massage of the trapezius in supine position—variation 1.

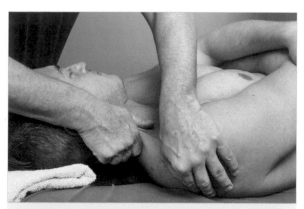

Fig. 13.72 Functional massage of the trapezius in the supine position—variation 2.

13

13.8.2 Test for the Alar Ligaments

Several local upper cervical assessment and treatment techniques require the C2 spinous process to be well palpated and, in some cases, even fixed. The test for stability in the occipital parts of the alar ligaments demonstrates how important local palpation is for assessment techniques.

Aim

To assess the stability of the occipital parts of the alar ligaments.

Criteria

C2 moves immediately when the upper cervical spine moves into slight lateral flexion (bending the head to the side). Hard end feel when the elasticity of the ligaments is tested.

Procedure

The following procedure is taught at the IAOM manual therapy study group and the VPT (German Physical Therapy Association) Academy in Fellbach, Germany. The test is performed on both sides and for both occipital alar ligaments.

▶ **Preparation.** The C2 spinous process is first located and held onto by the thumb and the index finger. Contact is made with the laminae on both sides (▶ Fig. 13.73). The head is then stabilized in the therapeutic ring and the index finger is removed from one of the laminae (right in ▶ Fig. 13.74). The thumb should now clearly be in contact with the side of the lamina of C2.

▶ **Phase 1—Mobility Test.** Using gentle axial pressure, the head is now facilitated into slight local lateral flexion (to the right in this example) away from the therapist (▶ Fig. 13.75). Because of the direct coupling of movements, C2 immediately rotates to the right with C2's spinous process moving to the left. This result is expected when the alar ligaments are intact and C2 is able to move freely on C3. The spinous process movement is perceived immediately as an increase in pressure against the thumb.

▶ **Phase 2—Mobility Cross-check Test.** An attempt is now made to laterally flex the cervical spine when the spinous process is being fixed. The pressure on the spinous process is increased again so that the process can no longer move. The therapist applies slight axial traction to the cervical spine and attempts to facilitate lateral flexion using the therapeutic ring. Normally no movement occurs.

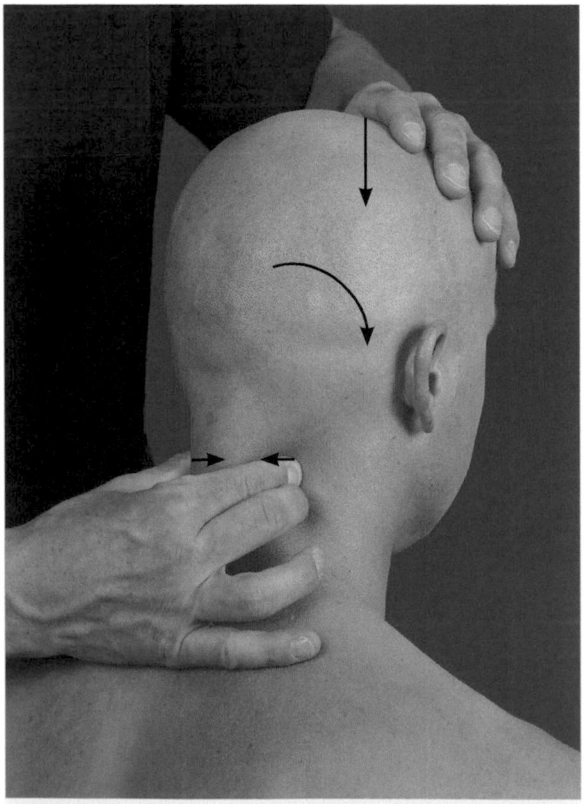

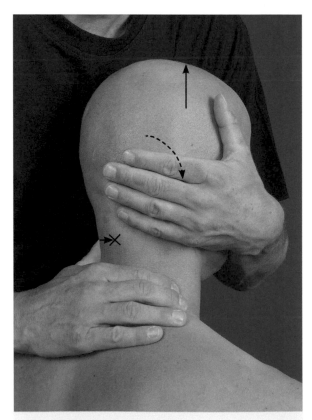

Fig. 13.73 Test for the alar ligaments. Locating the laminae of C2.

Fig. 13.74 Fixating one of the laminae.

▶ **Phase 3—Test for End Feel.** Finally, a quick test for the elasticity of the ligaments is conducted. Slight lateral flexion is first facilitated. The thumb resting on the spinous process allows this movement. The head is then held in this position and the thumb applies short but intensive pressure onto the rotated spinous process, pushing it back in a medial direction. A hard end feel proves that the ligament is intact.

Interpretation

▶ **Phase 1.** The test is positive when the rotation of the spinous process is delayed for even a minimal amount of time. The hand placement at the spinous process is therefore the most essential component of this test. The most common mistake when conducting this test is that too little contact is made with the spinous process. This means that movement cannot be felt immediately and results in false positives that are interpreted as a laxity in the ligament. Limited mobility between C2 and C3 can also limit rotation at C2. It is therefore recommended that the mobility of the C2/C3 segment be first assessed using the springing test (see Chapter 13.7.5 "Facet Joints").

▶ **Phase 2.** Ligamental laxity is also confirmed when the C2 spinous process is being fixed and lateral flexion is possible. It is important that movement of the hand via

the skin of the face moving against the skull should not be mistaken for lateral flexion.

▶ **Phase 3.** The alar ligaments are only proven to be intact when the end feel is hard. The test is positive when the thumb pushes on the spinous process and an elastic end feel is felt.

Therapists may only claim that the alar ligaments are stabile when all three of these tests do not demonstrate laxity of the ligament on both sides. If the alar ligaments are lax, treatment techniques may not be used where strong cervical traction is applied or where large rotational movements are conducted.

13.8.3 Identifying the Level of Chronically Irritated Intervertebral Disks

Another good example of the use of surface anatomy in the posterior cervical spine is an extremely simple test that is used to identify the level of chronically irritated intervertebral disks in patients suffering from persistent neck symptoms (▶ Fig. 13.76).

The cervical intervertebral disks control the translation movement occurring in the vertebra above during real extension (tilting the head backward with the chin pulled

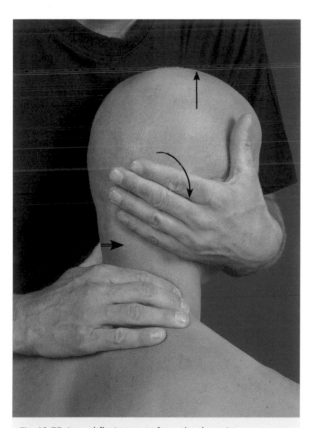

Fig. 13.75 Lateral flexion away from the therapist.

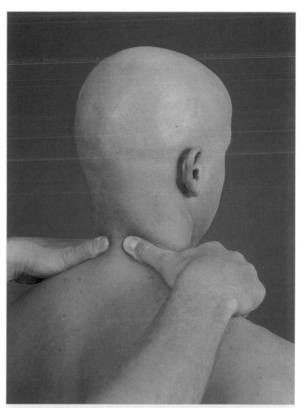

Fig. 13.76 Identifying the level of a chronically irritated intervertebral disk.

13

in). This movement is painful when an intervertebral disk is irritated. The irritated intervertebral disk segment must be located before it can be treated locally. The principle of this test is to stabilize the lamina of the lower vertebra in the segment and conduct real extension above this point.

Aim

To locate the irritated segment.

Criteria

Patient reporting pain.

Procedure

Starting at the C2 spinous process, the lamina of C2 is located, followed by the lamina of C3. This is the first intervertebral disk segment. Both thumbs are placed flat over the laminae. They hold onto the laminae tightly and by applying pressure in an anterior direction they prevent movement in a posterior direction. The patient extends the lower cervical spine by tilting the head backward and pulling the chin in (real extension). C3 cannot move as it is fixed by the thumbs. Extension only takes place at the C2/C3 level. If the test is negative, the next inferiorly located laminae are stabilized and the test is repeated.

Interpretation

The test is positive and the segment found when the patient indicates their typical type of pain. The test is expected to be positive in the lower intervertebral disk segments, if anywhere, as these segments, similar to the lowermost lumbar segments, are expected to suffer from intervertebral disk degeneration more often.

13.8.4 Functional Massage

Several types of functional massage in the sitting SP will also be demonstrated here to supplement those presented at the end of Chapter 8. To successfully relieve tension in the neck muscles, it is important that the head is held securely in the therapeutic ring so that the patient can allow the therapist to support the majority of the weight of the head.

The technique aims to displace the muscles transversely and is combined with a longitudinal stretch via movement in the cervical spine. One hand is placed over the neck and is used for the massage by transversely displacing tissue. Movement is controlled via the therapeutic ring. In the illustrated example, the paravertebral neck muscles are held in a wide V-grip and displaced posteriorly while the head is being flexed.

The cervical spine is placed in a neutral SP and one hand grasps around the area just above the region to be treated. This means that the following flexion movement does not need to be too large to stretch the tissue longitudinally (▶ Fig. 13.77a, Phase 1). The massage hand is placed posteriorly over the neck muscles with the thumb splayed out widely. The hand comes into contact with the underlying muscles and pinches the muscles, pulling them medially and posteriorly. This transverse stretch is maintained and a longitudinal stretch is added by flexing the cervical spine (▶ Fig. 13.77b, Phase 2).

This functional massage can be varied in several ways:
- Slowly repeating the stretch rhythmically or stretching statically.
- Repeating the transverse displacement at one segment or working systematically from superior to inferior along the entire neck musculature.
- Wider V-grip = semispinalis, trapezius, splenius, and longissimus (▶ Fig. 13.78).
- Narrower V-grip = semispinalis and trapezius.
- Moving the cervical spine symmetrically into flexion and stretching the muscles evenly on both sides, or coupling flexion with lateral flexion and rotation toward the therapist while stretching the muscles more on the opposite side.

13.9 Lateral Palpation Techniques

The sternocleidomastoid crosses the side region of the neck diagonally. In the area above the muscle belly, only the location of the C1 transverse process is of interest for palpation. All other accessible structures are located inferior to the muscle, in the posterior triangle of the neck, and superior to the supraclavicular fossa. When practicing locating these structures, the most suitable SP is once again the neutral sitting position. Other SPs (e.g., supinelying) can also be selected later on.

The position of the transverse processes must be viewed in relation to the sternocleidomastoid in particular. The C1 transverse process is found anterior to the sternocleidomastoid, the C2 transverse process directly beneath the muscle, and the C3 transverse process more posterior to the muscle belly (▶ Fig. 13.79). The shape expected to be felt is also crucial:
- The C1 transverse process is very long and varies greatly in length and form. In rare cases it can point posteriorly or be positioned close to the occiput. The variation in shape and length of the transverse process can lead to incorrect conclusions being made when comparing sides using palpation. Making a diagnosis based on the position of structures alone is therefore very unreliable.
- All transverse processes inferior to and including C2 tend to be shorter. It is therefore expected that when the palpating finger moves down from the tip of the C1 transverse process it will slide deep into the tissue until the transverse process of C2 is reached. Again, topographical anatomy and expectations related to

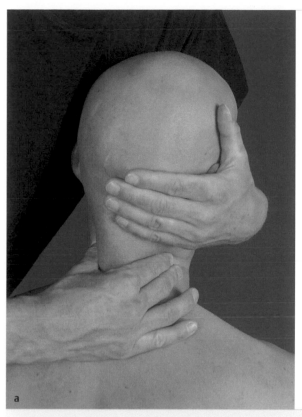

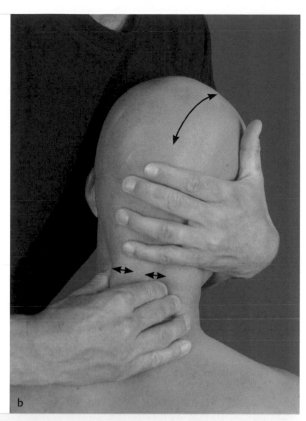

Fig. 13.77 Paravertebral functional massage. **a** Initial position. **b** Final position.

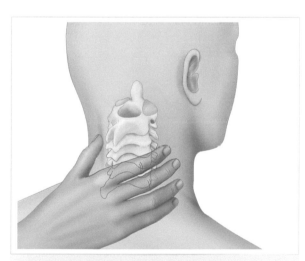

Fig. 13.78 Functional massage using a wide V-grip.

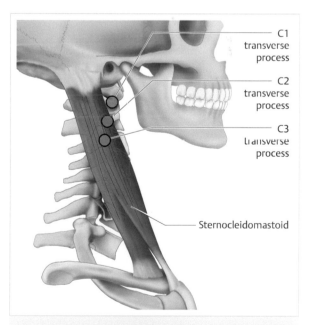

C1 transverse process

C2 transverse process

C3 transverse process

Sternocleidomastoid

Fig. 13.79 Transverse processes and the sternocleidomastoid.

consistency and shape form the foundations for precise palpation.

13.9.1 Angle of the Mandible

The edge of the occiput is followed laterally until the mastoid process is reached. A perpendicular technique is applied using one or two fingertips so that the fingers push against the posterior aspect of the mandible (▸ Fig. 13.80a). The patient can open and close the mouth

13

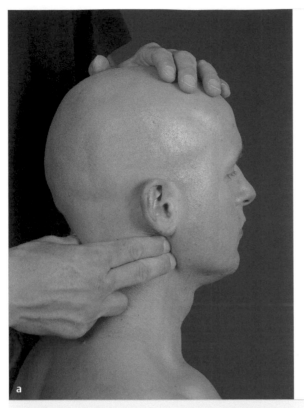
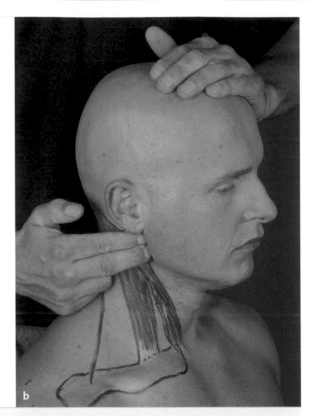

Fig. 13.80 Angle of the mandible. **a** Palpatory technique. **b** Alternative view.

slightly if the therapist is unsure of the position. The angle of the mandible pushes against the palpating finger when the mouth opens. The most important bony reference points for this region have now been found. The search for clinically relevant structures can begin. The palpating finger is always positioned anterior to the sternocleidomastoid at this stage (▶ Fig. 13.80b).

13.9.2 C1 Transverse Process

The transverse process of the atlas is surrounded by the following structures (▶ Fig. 13.81):
- Posteriorly by the sternocleidomastoid.
- Anteriorly by the angle of the mandible.
- Superiorly by the cartilage of the auricle. The temporomandibular joint (TMJ) is found anterior to this.

The distance from the inferior tip of the mastoid process to the posterior border of the angle of the mandible is measured. The C1 transverse process is found about halfway along the slightly sloping line connecting both of these reference points and is always located anterior to the sternocleidomastoid. Palpability varies according to the individual. Its tip is rounded.

A circular technique with the pad of the index finger is used for the palpation (▶ Fig. 13.82). The hand should rest

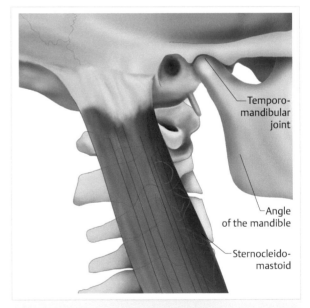

Fig. 13.81 Position of the C1 transverse process.

on the patient's cervical spine and/or occiput so that the finger pad can palpate smoothly and surely. The therapist should always expect to feel hard resistance deep in the tissue when applying direct pressure.

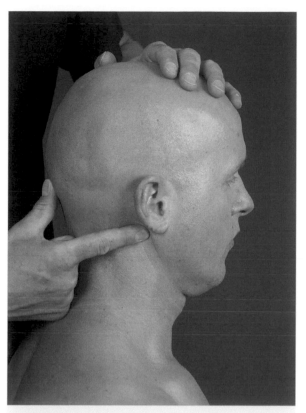

Fig. 13.82 Palpating the C1 transverse process.

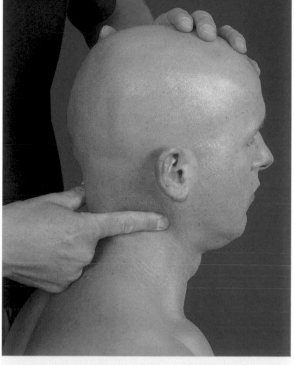

Fig. 13.83 Palpating the C2 transverse process.

Differences between the sides are easily recognizable in an individual. The length of the C1 transverse process can vary, as can the shape of its tip and the location of the surrounding bony structures. It is important to know that differences between the sides do not imply segmental malpositioning in the segment between the atlas and the axis.

13.9.3 C2 and C3 Transverse Processes

The C2 transverse process is considerably shorter than the C1 transverse process. It is found in a depression 1 finger width inferior to the C1 transverse process. As it lies underneath the sternocleidomastoid, it is difficult to palpate directly. To reach the process, the muscle belly is moved posteriorly (or anteriorly) and the pressure applied deep into the tissues is increased (▶ Fig. 13.83). The C2 transverse process can now be clearly palpated.

The tip of the C3 transverse process is expected to be found 1 finger width further inferior. The sternocleidomastoid can partially cover the process when the muscle is well developed. To be on the safe side, the muscle belly is shifted slightly in an anterior direction before applying

more pressure deep into the tissue (▶ Fig. 13.84a, b). This transverse process is expected to be rather short. The time it takes to push deep into the tissue until bone is felt depends on the thickness of the tissue.

The following points should be considered to aid orientation: all spinal nerves in the mid-cervical spine are reached anterior to the respective transverse process and posterior to the sternocleidomastoid. The facet joints are found posteromedial to the corresponding transverse process.

13.9.4 Boundaries of the Posterior Triangle of the Neck

The lateral region of the neck posterior and inferior to the sternocleidomastoid has a triangular form with the base of the triangle located inferiorly. This triangle is named the "posterior triangle of the neck" in the following sections (▶ Fig. 13.85). The following structures form its boundaries:
• Posterior: anterior edge of the descending part of the trapezius.

13

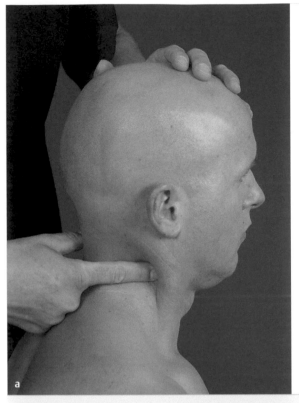

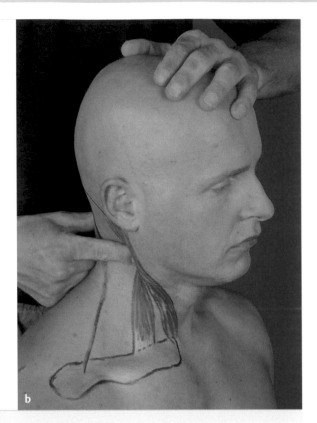

Fig. 13.84 C3 transverse process. **a** Palpation. **b** Alternative view.

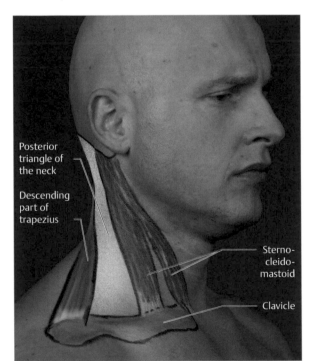

Posterior triangle of the neck

Descending part of trapezius

Sterno-cleido-mastoid

Clavicle

Fig. 13.85 Posterior triangle of the neck.

- Inferior: superior edge of the clavicle.
- Anterior: posterior edge of the sternocleidomastoid.

It is necessary to subdivide this region into the upper (occipital) and lower (supraclavicular) triangles of the neck for the following descriptions (see also ▶ Fig. 13.94). The bellies of the following muscles are found in the occipital triangle:
- Levator scapulae.
- Scalenus posterior.

The flattened depression directly superior to the clavicle forms the supraclavicular triangle of the neck and is anatomically labeled the supraclavicular fossa. The following structures are found here:
- Scalenus anterior and medius.
- First rib.
- Subclavian artery.
- Brachial plexus.

Sternocleidomastoid

Usually, this strong muscle can be easily found in the lateral region of the neck. The sternal head on the right side becomes prominent when the head rotates to the left over a large range. The posterior edge of the muscle is

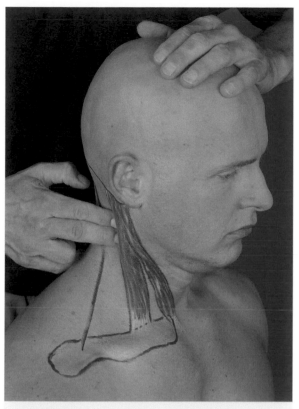

Fig. 13.86 Posterior edge of the sternocleidomastoid.

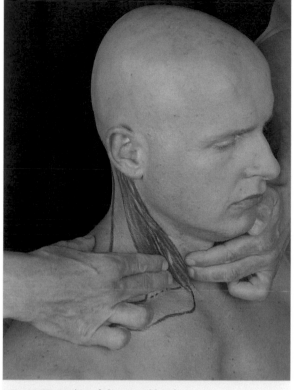

Fig. 13.87 Borders of the sternal head.

followed inferiorly until the insertion is reached. A perpendicular palpatory technique is used with two fingertips resting against the posterior aspect of the mastoid process, the site of muscular insertion (▶ Fig. 13.86).

From the mastoid process, the posterior edge of the muscle is followed inferiorly and anteriorly until the tips of the fingers feel the tendon and eventually land on the manubrium of the sternum. Its relationship to the sternoclavicular joint is described in Chapter 2.6.

The anterior edge of the muscle belly can be felt by palpating the tendon of the sternal head from inferior to superior. Finally, the edges of the sternal head can be visualized to determine how wide the muscle is (▶ Fig. 13.87).

The muscle belly of the clavicular head is often only visible when the muscle isometrically contracts into ipsilateral lateral flexion. It is notably wider, but also weaker, than the sternal head. Using the same perpendicular palpatory technique, the therapist begins again at the mastoid process and follows the muscle inferiorly until its insertion into the middle third of the clavicle (▶ Fig. 13.89). Its posterior edge forms the anterior boundary of the posterior triangle of the neck.

The gap between the two heads can be felt, and even observed, in the inferior region when the muscle is strongly contracted or when the therapist has gained some experience. It enables the therapist to palpate the anterior edge of the clavicular head and to visualize its width (▶ Fig. 13.90).

Clavicle

The borders of the clavicle are most clearly felt in the middle third, where the convex bone bends anteriorly (▶ Fig. 13.91). In addition to the shape of the clavicle, the presence of a superior and inferior soft-tissue depression aids palpation here: the supraclavicular and infraclavicular fossae. The supraclavicular fossa forms the inferior section of the posterior triangle of the neck, while the infraclavicular fossa is formed by the gap between the clavicular head of the deltoids and pectoralis major.

13

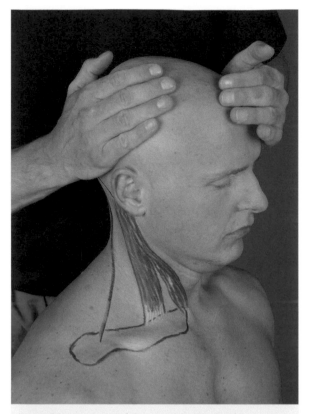

Fig. 13.88 Contraction of the sternocleidomastoid.

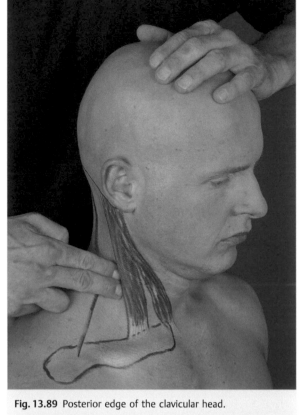

Fig. 13.89 Posterior edge of the clavicular head.

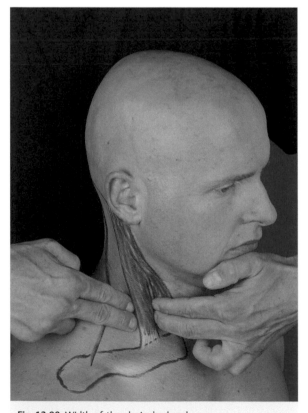

Fig. 13.90 Width of the clavicular head.

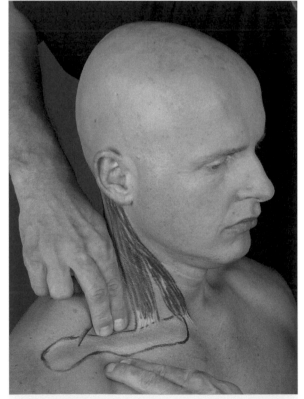

Fig. 13.91 Borders of the clavicle.

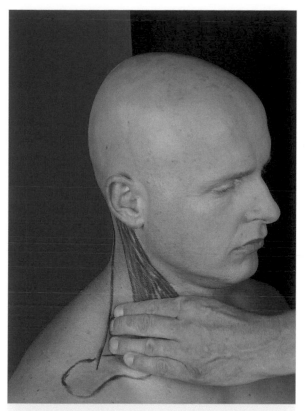

Fig. 13.92 Anterior edge of the descending part of the trapezius.

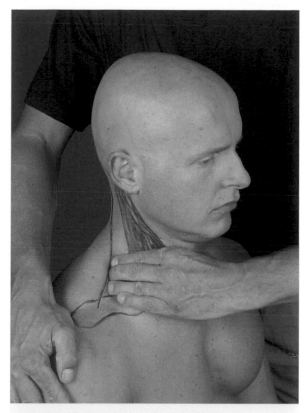

Fig. 13.93 Palpating with muscle contraction.

The superior and inferior edges can be followed very easily in a medial and lateral direction. The posterior edge is covered laterally by the belly of the descending part of the trapezius and is the only section that is difficult to palpate.

The upper border of the middle third of the clavicle marks the wide inferior border of the posterior triangle of the neck and the supraclavicular fossa in particular.

Tip

When the contours of this pipelike bone are drawn onto the skin, the borders of this three-dimensional structure are transferred onto a two-dimensional drawing. This often results in drawings that appear strangely large but are nevertheless technically correct.

Descending Part of the Trapezius

The descending part of the trapezius must now be identified to locate the borders of the posterior triangle of the neck. The perpendicular palpatory technique with two fingertips is used once again, with the fingertips resting against the anterior edge of the muscle (▶ Fig. 13.92): starting at the muscle's insertion on the clavicle, the

therapist follows the edge posteriorly and superiorly until reaching the superior nuchal line again. The anterior edge of this muscle forms the last and lateral boundary of the posterior triangle of the neck. This edge can be palpated in the supraclavicular fossa very easily, where it extends transversely in a medial direction. Its course then changes in a superior and slightly medial direction.

Tip

If the edge of the muscle cannot be clearly felt, the palpation can be conducted in conjunction with an isometric contraction of the muscle (▶ Fig. 13.93). The free hand is used to resist shoulder movement and the patient is instructed to push the shoulder behind the ear in a posteriorly directed elevation.

13.9.5 Occipital Triangle of the Neck

Levator Scapulae

This thick muscle belly is found anterior to the descending part of the trapezius at the point where its medially directed course changes in a superior direction (▶ Fig. 13.94). The same technique is used as for locating the edges of the trapezius, the only difference being that

13

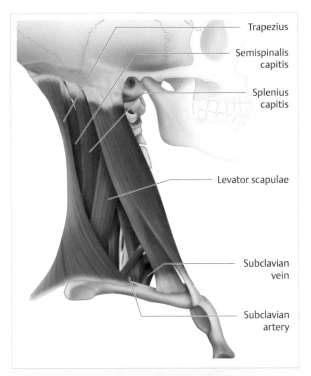

Fig. 13.94 Muscles in the occipital triangle of the neck.

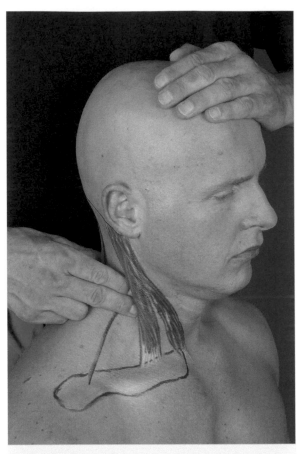

Fig. 13.95 Scalenus posterior.

the finger pads now palpate deep into the tissue. To confirm that the location was correct, the patient should elevate the shoulder girdle and move it anteriorly. The contraction in the muscle belly can now be felt clearly. While maintaining this tension, the muscle can be followed superiorly and anteriorly all the way to its insertion at the transverse processes. The inferior section of the muscle covers the transverse processes of the lower cervical spine. These processes can also be palpated when the muscle is relaxed.

Tip

The levator scapulae is differentiated from the descending part of the trapezius by tensing the muscle and following its course superiorly and posteriorly. Directly superior to the muscle belly of the levator scapulae is the splenius capitis. This muscle has already been located in the palpation of the posterior aspect.

Scalenus Posterior

The scalenus posterior is found directly inferior to the muscle belly of the levator scapulae, with both muscles traveling in almost the same direction. The location begins in the triangle formed by the inferior border of the

levator scapulae and the posterior border of the sternocleidomastoid. When the palpating finger is positioned in this triangle, the finger automatically rests on the scalenus posterior. This muscle is approximately as wide as one finger (▶ Fig. 13.95). The muscle is also easier to palpate when contracted. This is achieved by inhaling deeply or by using isometric lateral flexion to the same side.

Tip

To differentiate this muscle from the levator scapulae and sternocleidomastoid, the muscle bellies are again made more prominent using muscle contraction:
- Levator scapulae: isometric elevation and protraction of the shoulder girdle.
- Sternocleidomastoid: isometric rotation of the neck to the opposite side.

It is difficult to differentiate this muscle from the scalenus medius because both muscles are positioned very close to one another.

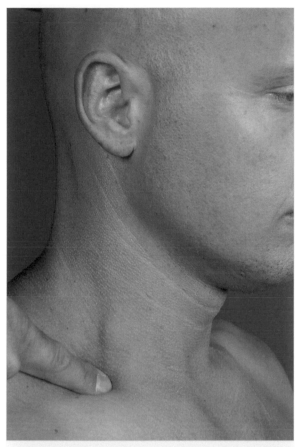

Fig. 13.96 Scalenus anterior.

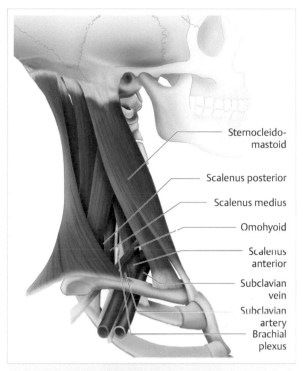

Fig. 13.97 Position of the first rib.

13.9.6 Supraclavicular Triangle of the Neck

Scalenus Anterior

The sternocleidomastoid covers most of the scalenus anterior. It can first be easily palpated in the supraclavicular fossa. The muscle belly and its insertion on the first rib can be palpated directly lateral to the clavicular insertion of the sternocleidomastoid.

The therapist starts by clarifying the insertion and palpates laterally from this point so that the finger is positioned in the angle formed by the borders of the clavicle and the sternocleidomastoid (▶ Fig. 13.96).

Tip

The therapist should not feel a distinctly pulsating artery here. If this is the case, the finger is positioned too posteriorly. This finger-wide muscle belly also becomes distinct during forced inhalation or an isometric contraction into lateral flexion to the same side. The anterior scalenus gap is found between the scalenus anterior and sternocleidomastoid.

First Rib

After finding the muscle belly of the scalenus anterior, the therapist follows the muscle inferiorly until a hard structure is felt. This is the first rib, just before it disappears underneath the clavicle and later attaches onto the manubrium. Its position has already been described in the thoracic spine chapter, where its flexibility was tested using the springing test (see the "Tips for Assessment and Treatment" in Chapter 12.7). Moving from the insertion of the scalenus anterior, the entire posteriorly extending portion of the rib can be directly palpated on its superior aspect. Its position separates the occipital and supraclavicular triangles (▶ Fig. 13.97).

Subclavian Artery and Scalenus Medius

The therapist begins searching for the posterior scalenus gap at the insertion of the scalenus anterior on the first rib. Moving from here, the therapist palpates approximately 2 cm posteriorly, applies gentle pressure, and very quickly feels the pulsating subclavian artery, confirming the correct location of the posterior scalenus gap. The brachial plexus accompanies the artery as it passes through this intermuscular gap. The almost vertical muscle belly of the scalenus medius is found immediately posterior to this.

13

Brachial Plexus

The branches of the brachial plexus can be palpated in the area surrounding the artery and immediately superior to it. These thin strands can be felt using a transverse palpation, even without the use of extra aids. When the branches have been correctly located, they can typically be rolled back and forth underneath the palpating finger, similar to the plucking of a very loose guitar string.

Tips

If it is impossible to find the plexus using the above-mentioned method, the following aids are recommended to place the plexus under tension and enable the branches to be felt more clearly. The therapist's hand palpates in the posterior scalenus gap and the other hand facilitates movement in the ipsilateral arm of the patient.

The following section describes the steps used to position the arm and the cervical spine so that more tension is placed on the median nerve, which makes the plexus more prominent. Each of the phases described places the nerves under tension, enabling easy palpation of the plexus. The therapist need not be afraid of palpating the plexus or conducting this maneuver as peripheral neural structures are usually insensitive to moderate direct pressure that is applied slowly:

- Phase 1: The ipsilateral arm is extensively abducted in the frontal plane (90° is optimal) and rests on the therapist's thigh. The elbow is slightly bent and the hand almost positioned in neutral.
- Phase 2: The elbow and wrist are extended. This places the median nerve under considerable tension. The correct location of the plexus can be confirmed by alternately tensing and relaxing the plexus and is achieved by extending and flexing the hand and elbow.
- Phase 3: If the plexus still cannot be palpated, tension can be further increased by laterally flexing the cervical spine to the opposite side. Further tension can only be achieved by depressing the shoulder girdle.

13.10 Anterior Palpation Techniques

Anterior structures allow therapists to identify the level of individual vertebrae with more confidence. It is for this reason that the hyoid bone and the larynx are included in the palpatory orientation. If it is difficult to locate the lamina of a vertebra and the therapist wants to ensure that structures have been correctly located, an anterior structure of the same level can be located. It is impossible to identify the level of a vertebra using the usual

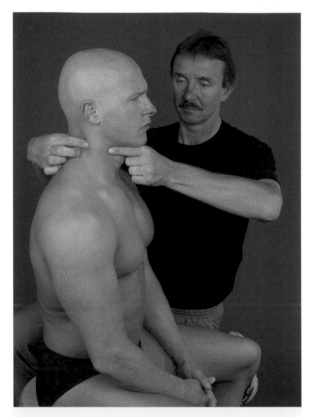

Fig. 13.98 Patient and therapist starting positions.

techniques (in the sitting SP) when treating the patient in supination. Palpation of the anterior aspect can now be used as a crucial aid in identifying the vertebra being sought.

The patient is positioned in erect sitting with the cervical spine in neutral (see the section "Starting Position," Chapter 13.6). The therapist is positioned next to the patient at eye level with the anterior region of the neck. One hand is used for local palpation and the other hand for the identification of posterior structures (▶ Fig. 13.98). The therapist proceeds slowly and with caution when approaching this region. Many patients indicate that they feel uncomfortable when these structures are palpated. The therapist will frequently notice clear signs of increased sympathetic activity, for example, general agitation, swallowing more often than usual, an increased pulse rate, or distinct perspiration. Palpation is terminated in this case.

13.10.1 Anatomy

The anterior structures of the neck needed for the following palpations are described here in more detail, supplementing the information provided in the anatomy section for the cervical spine (▶ Fig. 13.99). Some

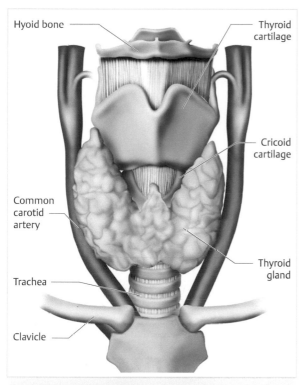

Fig. 13.99 Anterior anatomy.

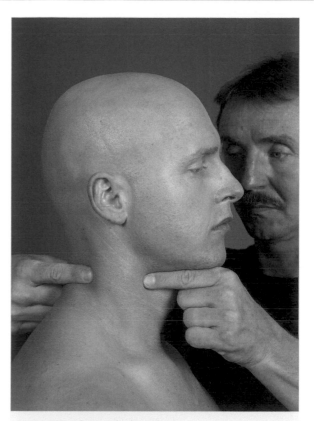

Fig. 13.100 Palpating the hyoid bone.

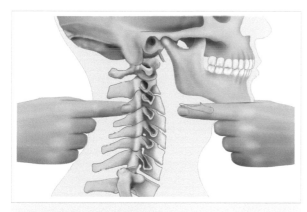

Fig. 13.101 Identifying the level of C3.

structures can be accessed easily, listed here from superior to inferior:
• Hyoid bone.
• Thyroid cartilage (laryngeal prominence).
• Cricoid cartilage (cricoid).
• Carotid tubercle.
• Jugular notch and fossa.

The following palpation describes how these structures clarify the identification of the cervical vertebral level. Hoppenfeld (1992) and Winkel (2004) have already described this classification. These structures are always found at the same level in each person, with only one exception: hyoid bone—lamina C3.

Hyoid Bone—Lamina C3

The thumb and index finger are spread wide apart and slide along the floor of the mouth. Both fingers attempt to hold onto a firm structure in the angle between the floor of the mouth and the neck by pinching slightly. The consistency is expected to be firm and more elastic than the resistance felt when pressing on bone. To confirm the correct location, the therapist carefully attempts to move the hyoid bone to the left and right using both fingers. The firm lateral edges are palpated and are felt to curve slightly outward. When the patient swallows, the therapist feels the hyoid bone moving up and down, as is the case with all structures that will be sought in this palpation.

Observed from the side, the index finger of the other hand rests against the posterolateral aspect of the cervical spine and applies gentle pressure (▶ Fig. 13.100). When the index fingers of both hands are located at the same level, the therapist can be fairly sure that they have found the level of the C3 lamina (▶ Fig. 13.101). Compared with the other anterior structures, the position of the hyoid

13

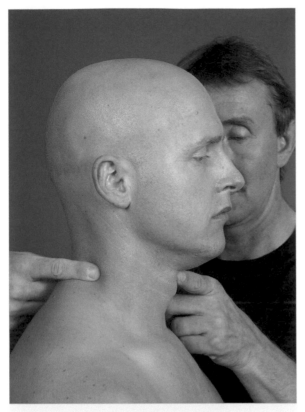

Fig. 13.102 Palpating the indentation.

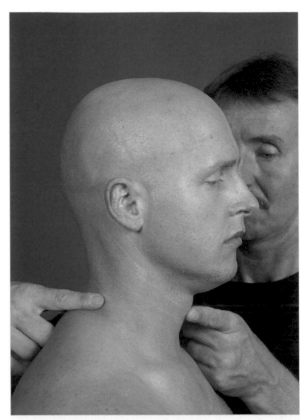

Fig. 13.104 Palpating the larynx.

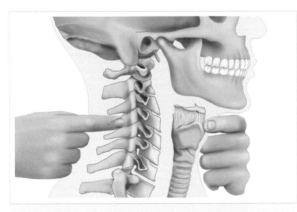

Fig. 13.103 Identifying the level of C4.

bone varies considerably. It can be found somewhat more superior or inferior to the floor of the mouth, meaning that there is no exact determination of the level of C3.

Thyroid Cartilage (Indentation)— Lamina C4

The therapist continues the palpation using the pad of one finger. The anterior, most prominent edge of the larynx is sought first. This point is used for orientation and the palpation continues by moving superiorly a short

distance until a distinct indentation can be felt that opens up superiorly. This indentation is found directly superior to the prominent tip commonly known as the Adam's apple and is particularly noticeable in men. When the posterior index finger is placed at the same height, the level of the C4 lamina has been marked (▶ Fig. 13.102 and ▶ Fig. 13.103).

Tip

If the hyoid bone could not be found using the previously described technique, it can be alternatively identified by palpating superior to this indentation. The hyoid bone and the thyroid cartilage are only separated from each other by a ringshaped depression.

Thyroid Cartilage (Lateral Surfaces)— Lamina C5

The palpating finger slides inferiorly again for a short distance onto the middle of the anterior ridge of the thyroid cartilage. Two lateral surfaces can be felt from this point. When the finger pads are positioned in the middle of these surfaces, this corresponds to the level of the C5 lamina (▶ Fig. 13.104 and ▶ Fig. 13.105).

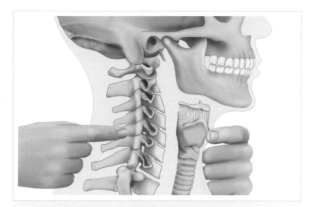

Fig. 13.105 Identifying the level of C5.

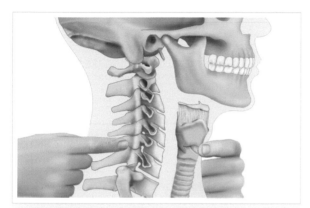

Fig. 13.107 Identifying the level of C6.

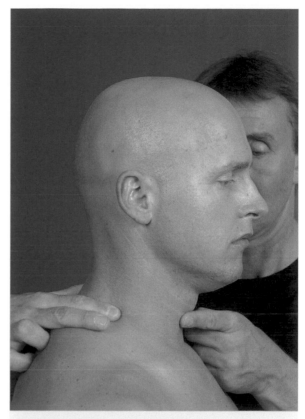

Fig. 13.106 Palpating the cricoid cartilage.

Cricoid Cartilage—Lamina C6

Starting from the anterior ridge of the thyroid cartilage, the palpation continues in an inferior direction. The finger pad slides into a depression that is bordered inferiorly by the cricoid cartilage (cricoid) (▶ Fig. 13.106). The therapist is now palpating the uppermost boundary of the trachea, which is the only complete ring of the cartilage clasp surrounding the trachea. The correct location of the cricoid cartilage is characterized by its typical convex form when it is palpated in a superior/inferior direction. It is found at the height of the lamina of C6 (▶ Fig. 13.107). The tracheotomy incision site is found superior to the cricoid. Good knowledge of anatomy is critical when applying first aid at accident sites. The thyroid gland is found on both sides of the cricoid and can rarely be felt as a structure in its own right due to its very soft consistency.

Carotid Tubercle

The common carotid artery and the anterior tubercle of the C6 transverse process (carotid tubercle) can be easily

reached lateral to the cricoid. For this purpose, a finger pad palpates the anterior aspect of the cricoid and moves posteriorly over the cricoid, applying pressure with care. Once the finger pad loses contact with the cricoid, the fingertips apply more pressure in a posterior direction. The anterior border of the sternocleidomastoid is reached here and can be moved to the side during this palpation. The pulse of the common carotid artery can already be felt at this location. The carotid tubercle is found approximately 2 to 3 cm away from the cricoid and has been correctly reached when the fingertip feels a distinctly hard structure (▶ Fig. 13.108 and ▶ Fig. 13.109).

Caution

Only one side may be palpated at a time to make sure that both carotid arteries are not pinched off simultaneously! Additionally, the palpation must not be conducted on people over 60 years of age when the person is suspected or known to suffer from arteriosclerosis. Otherwise, there is the risk of the sclerotic plaques found on the walls of the artery detaching and causing a cerebral embolus.

13

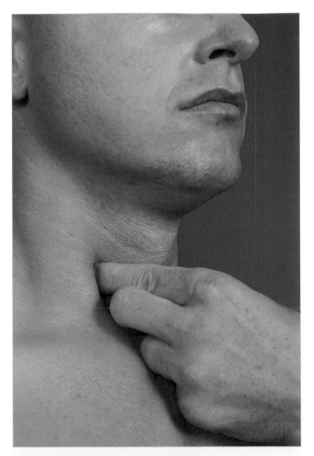

Fig. 13.108 Palpating the carotid tubercle.

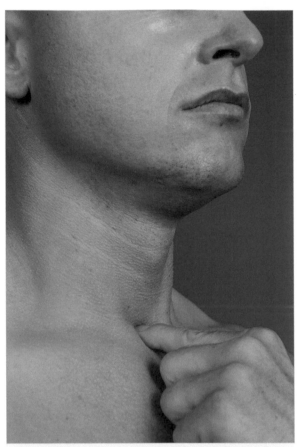

Fig. 13.110 Jugular notch and fossa.

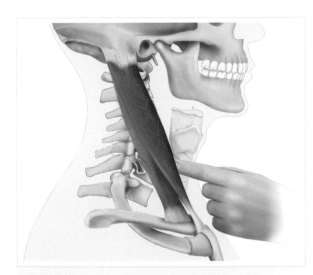

Fig. 13.109 Identifying the level of the carotid tubercle.

Jugular Notch—T2 Spinous Process

Starting at the anterior aspect of the cricoid, the finger palpates inferiorly for approximately 2 finger widths until it reaches the superior border of the manubrium. This point is bordered bilaterally by the sternocleidomastoid tendons and the protruding medial ends of the clavicles. This fossa corresponds to the level of the T2 spinous process. The fingertips extend into the superiorly lying soft-tissue fossa (jugular fossa) when a finger pad rests on the superior aspect of the jugular notch. Further sections of the trachea can be reached by carefully applying pressure deeper into the tissue (▶ Fig. 13.110).

Bibliography

Dörhage K, Knopf H, Graumann-Brunt S, Koch L. Asymmetrie der Kopfgelenke – Physiologische Lateralität. Manuelle Medizin. 2004; 42:122–128

Dvořák J. Manuelle Medizin. Bd. 1, Diagnostik. Berlin: Springer; 1998

Dvořák J, Panjabi MM. Functional anatomy of the alar ligaments. Spine. 1987; 12(2):183–189

Falla DL, Jull GA, Hodges PW. Patients with neck pain demonstrate reduced electromyographic activity of the deep cervical flexor muscles during performance of the craniocervical flexion test. Spine. 2004; 29(19):2108–2114

Greiner P. Die Frankfurter Horizontale. Eine anatomisch-röntgenkephalometrische Untersuchung zur Lageveränderung von Porion und Orbita während des Wachstums [Dissertation]. Marburg: Philipps-Universität Marburg; 2000

Herdman SJ. Vestibular Rehabilitation. 2nd ed. Philadelphia, USA: F.A. Davis; 2000

Hoppenfeld S. Klinische Untersuchung der Wirbelsäule und Extremitäten. 2. Aufl. Stuttgart: Fischer; 1992

Kapandji IA. Funktionelle Anatomie der Gelenke. 4. Aufl. Stuttgart: Thieme; 2006

Lanz T von, Wachsmuth W. Praktische Anatomie. Teil 1A, Kopf – Übergeordnete Systeme. Berlin: Springer; 2004

Lanz T von, Wachsmuth W. Praktische Anatomie. Teil 1B, Kopf – Gehirn- und Augenschädel. Berlin: Springer; 1979

Loyd BJ, Gilbert KK, Sizer PS, et al. The relationship between various anatomical landmarks used for localizing the first rib during surface palpation. J Manual ManipTher. 2014; 22(3):129–133

Lysell E. Motion in the cervical spine. An experimental study on autopsy specimens. Acta OrthopScand. 1969; 123

Osmotherly PG, Rivett DA, Mercer SR. Revisiting the clinical anatomy of the alar ligaments. Eur Spine J. 2013; 22(1):60–64

Panjabi MM, Crisco JJ, Vasavada A, et al. Mechanical properties of the human cervical spine as shown by three-dimensional load-displacement curves. Spine. 2001; 26(24):2692–2700

Penning L. Hals- und Lendenwirbelsäule. München: Pflaum; 2000

Rauber A, Leonhardt H, Eds. Anatomie des Menschen: Lehrbuch und Atlas. Bd. 1, Bewegungsapparat. Stuttgart: Thieme; 1987

Shabshin N, Schweitzer ME, Carrino JA. Anatomical landmarks and skin markers are not reliable for accurate labeling of thoracic vertebrae on MRI. Acta Radiol. 2010; 51(9):1038–1042

White AA, Panjabi MM. Clinical Biomechanics of the spine. 2nd ed. Philadelphia: Lippincott; 1990

Williams PL. Gray's anatomy. 40th ed. Edinburgh: Churchill Livingstone; 2009

Winkel D. Nichtoperative Orthopädie und Manualtherapie. Anatomie in Vivo. 3. Aufl. München: Urban & Fischer bei Elsevier; 2004

13

Chapter 14

Head and Jaw

14

14 Head and Jaw

Wolfgang Stelzenmüller

14.1 Introduction

Of all the structures in the head region, physical therapists are best able to treat the jaw (temporomandibular joint or TMJ) and the atlanto-occipital joint, which have already been described in Chapter 13.3.6. The special feature of the TMJ is that one joint never moves alone and the interaction with the contralateral joint must always be considered.

Symptoms arising in the head/jaw/facial region are integrated into the general term craniomandibular dysfunction (CMD). This literally describes the suboptimal functioning of the cranium (condylar path on the skull) and the mandible (the head[s] of the lower jaw) joint partners. The term temporomandibular joint disorder (TMD) is more commonly used in English. It more precisely describes the suboptimal functioning of the head of the mandible (including the articular disk located in the joint) and the temporal bone and names the bones that contribute anatomically to the TMJ.

Many craniomandibular symptoms present as different types of headache or as ear, tooth, jaw, or face pain. This frequently involves referred pain arising from structures such as muscle trigger points (where pain is projected from sections of muscle into other regions).

In addition to the systematic subjective and objective assessments, precise palpation of the muscles and, as much as possible, the articular structures is of importance. This enables the therapist to differentiate symptoms arising from referred pain (from muscular trigger points) and other causes, such as arthrotic changes in a joint or articular damage.

14.1.1 Significance and Function of the Temporomandibular Joint

The TMJ is not only needed for the function of mastication, it is also used for speaking, singing, yawning, kissing, etc. These are generally movements involving the opening and closing of the mouth.

The biomechanics of the TMJ enable movement in all three spatial axes (vertical, transverse, sagittal). Mandibular movements are never purely translational or purely rotational.

The main movements in the mandible are the following:
- Elevation and depression (opening/closing the mouth).
- Protrusion and retrusion (translation movement of the mandible anteriorly and posteriorly).
- Lateral and medial deviation (movement of the mandible to the side away from or toward the median plane).

14.1.2 Common Applications for Treatment in this Region

As with other joints in our body, the TMJ also suffers from the following:
- Capsular and noncapsular restrictions in mobility.
- Hypermobility or instability.
- Pathological conditions in the disk-condyle complex (the relationship between the head of the lower jaw and the buffering articular disk as well as the opposing joint surface).
- Injuries to ligaments or ligamental overuse syndromes.
- Injuries to muscles or muscular overuse syndromes.
- Arthrotic changes.

In dental literature, TMDs are commonly subdivided as follows:
- Myogenic, that is, symptoms originating in the muscles.
- Arthrogenic, that is, direct joint symptoms.
- Myoarthropathic symptoms, that is, a combination of muscular and joint symptoms.

It is difficult to directly differentiate the above-mentioned symptoms in practice, as a TMD arising from muscular symptoms is usually directly followed by the involvement of articular structures.

14.1.3 Required Basic Anatomical and Biomechanical Knowledge

Often, there is not enough time available in physical therapy training to intensively address the head and the TMJ, in particular. A summary of the fundamental (palpable) structures is included in sections 14.6.1 and 14.6.2 to improve anatomical orientation. Therapists should initially practice on a plastic skull to obtain more confidence, before palpating the corresponding structures on patients.

> **Tip**
>
> When studying the biomechanics of the TMJ, rubber bands or a TheraBand can simulate and illustrate the pull of muscles very well.

14

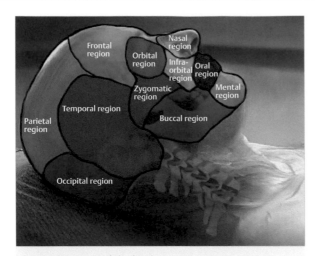

Fig. 14.1 Regions of the head.

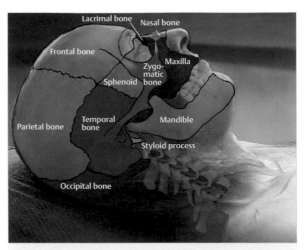

Fig. 14.2 Palpable bony structures of the head.

14.2 Anatomy of the Bony Skull

14.2.1 Dividing the Head into Regions

To aid orientation, the skull is divided into 11 regions (▶ Fig. 14.1):

- Frontal region.
- Parietal region.
- Occipital region.
- Temporal region.
- Zygomatic region.
- Orbital region.
- Infraorbital region.
- Buccal region.
- Mental region.
- Oral region.
- Nasal region.

The following 11 bony structures found in these regions can be palpated well (▶ Fig. 14.2):

- Occipital bone.
- Parietal bone.
- Frontal bone.
- Lacrimal bone.
- Nasal bone.
- Temporal bone.
- Styloid process.
- Sphenoid.
- Zygomatic bone.
- Maxilla.
- Mandible.

Now that rough anatomical orientation is possible, the more specific palpation of bony structures on the skull follows.

14.2.2 Overview of the Frontal Aspect of the Viscerocranium

The viscerocranium is divided into the following:
- The upper face with the squamous part.
- The middle face, mainly characterized by the maxilla (upper jaw).
- The lower face, dominated by the mandible (lower jaw).

The following structures are found in the viscerocranium:
- Orbits.
- Nasal cavities.
- Paranasal sinuses.
- Oral cavity.

14.3 Palpation of the Bony Skull

14.3.1 Frontal Aspect of the Viscerocranium

Overview of the Structures to be Palpated

In addition to the structures mentioned above, prominent, palpable bony structures include the following (▶ Fig. 14.3):
- Pressure points of the trigeminal nerve:
  - supraorbital foramen: exit point for the lateral branch of the supraorbital nerve (first pressure point of the trigeminal nerve) (1);
  - infraorbital foramen: exit point for the infraorbital nerve (second pressure point of the trigeminal nerve) (2);
  - mental foramen: exit point for the mental nerve (third pressure point of the trigeminal nerve) (3).

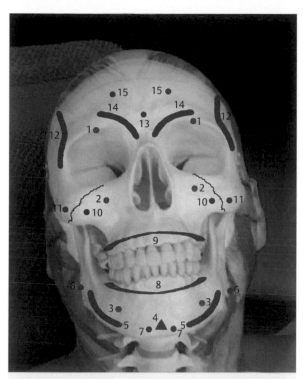

Fig. 14.3 Additional prominent, palpable bony structures of the head.

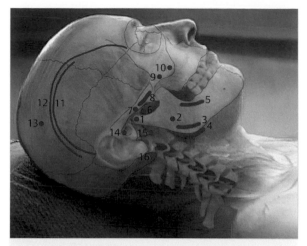

Fig. 14.4 Additional prominent, palpable bony structures of the lateral aspect of the head.

- The structures that can be palpated via the lower jaw (mandible) include the following:
  - mental protuberance (4).
  - body of the mandible (5).
  - angle of the mandible (6).
  - mental tubercle (7).
  - alveolar part of the mandible (8).
  - alveolar process of the maxilla (9).
  - zygomatic process of the maxilla (10).
  - zygomatic bone (11).
  - temporal line (12).
  - glabella (13).
  - superciliary arch (14).
  - frontal tuber (15).

14.3.2 Lateral Aspect of the Skull

The dominating section of the lateral skull is formed by the side wall of the skull, the parietal bone. The temporal bone is the central bone in the lateral skull. Its surface forms a joint with the articular disk and the head of the mandible, forming the TMJ.

Overview of the Structures to be Palpated

Once again, orientation begins with the mandible (▶ Fig. 14.4):

- Head of the mandible (1).
- Ramus of the mandible (2).
- Masseteric tuberosity (3).
- Angle of the mandible (4).
- Oblique line (5).
- Articular tubercle (eminence) (6).
- Zygomatic process of the temporal bone (7).
- Zygomatic arch (8).
- Temporal process of the zygomatic bone (9).
- Lateral surface of the zygomatic bone (10).
- Inferior temporal line (11).
- Superior temporal line (12).
- Parietal tuber (13).
- Suprameatal spine (14).
- Styloid process (15).
- Mastoid process (site of insertion for the sternocleido-mastoid) (16).

14.4 The Jaw—Temporomandibular Joints

Compared with other joints such as the knee, many of the ligamentous and bony structures in the TMJ cannot be palpated directly and therapists must use a variety of knacks to test these structures. It is important that therapists have good spatial sense as well as comprehensive knowledge in biomechanics of one or, more precisely, both TMJs, as movement in one TMJ causes simultaneous movement in the other.

In actual fact, the jaw should be called the temporo-(disco)mandibular joint, as the temporal bone and the mandible do not articulate with one another alone.

14

14.4.1 Required Basic Knowledge of Topography and Morphology

The articular disk, the meniscus or joint buffer, divides the jaw into superior and inferior compartments. The superior compartment, otherwise known as the upper joint, is formed by the temporal bone and the articular disk (discotemporal), while the inferior compartment or lower joint is the articulation between the mandible and the disk. The superior compartment functions as a gliding joint, while the inferior compartment acts as a mobile hinge joint.

The basic shape of the articular disk is similar to a horizontal figure eight. It is thinnest in the middle, approximately 1 to 2 mm thick, and can be approximately 3 to 4 mm thick at the ends. It is made of taut connective tissue, with cartilaginous cells still found at the edges. The disk is fibrocartilaginous in the area lying over the head of the mandible, where it resembles a cap (▶ Fig. 14.5a, b).

The true function of the disk is to even out existing differences in articulating surfaces, namely the condylar path (temporal bone) and the head of the mandible. During movements of the jaw, rotation of the head of the mandible and the pull from the lateral pterygoid muscle causes the disk to move along the path formed by the temporal bone. The disk could therefore also be labeled a mobile joint socket.

14.4.2 Biomechanics of the Temporomandibular Joint

TMJ movements essentially consist of combined rotation and gliding. When the mouth is opened, a hingelike rotation occurs around a transverse axis running through both condyles. This is accompanied by translation in a sagittal direction, moving anteroinferiorly when the mouth is opened and posterosuperiorly when the mouth closes.

We primarily differentiate between:
- movements associated with the opening and closing of the mouth; and
- the required grinding movements associated with mastication.

Let us now take a more precise look at the movements that occur when the mouth is opened. The rotational-translational movement pattern at the TMJ is flowing, but will be divided here into three phases to make the complex biomechanics easier to understand.

Opening the Mouth

Muscles: Presented simply, mouth opening involves rotation initiated by the pull of the lateral pterygoid and the suprahyoid muscles and controlled by the mouth closure muscles that decelerate movement.

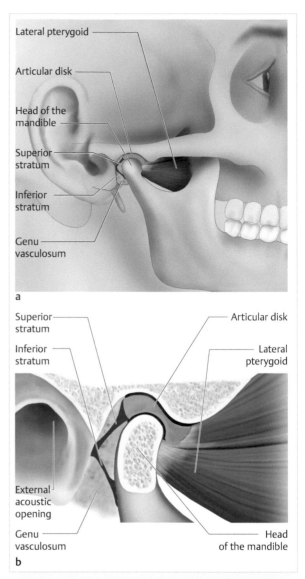

Fig. 14.5 a, b Overview of the temporomandibular joint (TMJ). **a** Overview. **b** Enlarged sectional view.

Joint: In **phase 1** (**first phase of rotation**), the condyles in the inferior compartment rotate slightly. This movement is initiated by the pull of the lateral pterygoid and the suprahyoid muscles and acts to overcome the occlusion of the teeth. This causes the head of the mandible to briefly rotate anteriorly. Following the mobile joint socket principle, the articular disk ideally moves in an anterior direction along the condylar path in a similar manner to the action of a pasta machine. Its movement is decelerated by the superior stratum of the bilaminar zone and the posterior fibers of the temporalis muscle and the lateral ligament. The inferior stratum, secured onto the condyle, relaxes (▶ Fig. 14.6a).

The first phase flows over into **phase 2**, where more gliding occurs at the head of the mandible. The lateral

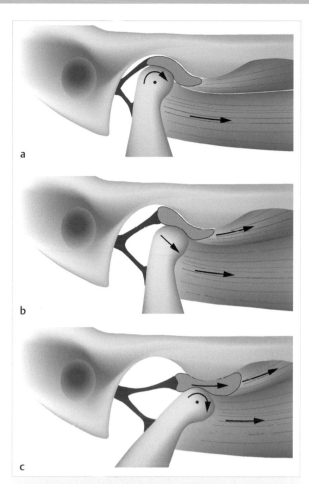

Fig. 14.6 a–c Phases of opening the mouth.
a Phase 1: rotational phase/opening phase.
b Phase 2: gliding phase.
c Phase 3: second rotational phase.

pterygoid muscle pulls the disk, acting as a mobile joint socket, in an inferoanteromedial direction beneath the articular tubercle. This is also defined as protrusion. This movement is produced by the pull of the lateral pterygoid, assisted and controlled by the muscles mentioned above, and is essentially decelerated by the **superior stratum of the bilaminar zone,** the posterior fibers of temporalis, and the lateral ligament (▶ Fig. 14.6b). To open the mouth as wide as possible, the condyles must rotate once again at the end of the condylar path in **phase 3 (second phase of rotation).**

The disk was pulled underneath the articular tubercle in the second phase and is now pulled along anteriorly, as the head of the mandible rotates, and pulled up onto the articular tubercle with the assistance of the lateral pterygoid muscle and the above-mentioned muscles. Only then can the mouth open up fully by further rotating. The movement of the disk is decelerated again by the superior

stratum of the bilaminar zone. The inferior stratum, secured onto the condyle, is now placed under tension (▶ Fig. 14.6c).

Closing the Mouth

The closure movement will now be addressed. The returning rotation of the head of the mandible moves the disk back to its original position (posterior direction of rotation for the head of the mandible) (▶ Fig. 14.7).

The disk moves posteriorly at the same time and its movement is decelerated by the lateral pterygoid muscle.

Grinding Movements

The movements associated with mouth opening involve simultaneous contraction of the respective muscle groups and result in a relatively symmetrical and simultaneous movement of the two joints in the same direction. In comparison, grinding movements require muscles and joints to act differently.

While the chin remains in the median plane when the mouth is opened or closed, the tip of the chin moves to the right or the left during grinding movements. We differentiate between the working side and the balancing side. Food is reduced to small pieces on the working side while the other side (balancing side) carries out the required anteroinferior translation.

Therapists can only recognize, interpret, and treat abnormalities when they understand the biomechanics discussed above.

14.4.3 Assessing Deviations from the Mid-line during Mouth Opening

As not all structures of the jaw can be palpated directly, therapists have to use a variety of tests when palpating the bony and capsular-ligamentous structures of the jaw and the articular disk to recognize possible pathological conditions in these structures.

The two TMJs are always observed at the same time, making significant deviations from the mid-line, during mouth opening for example, immediately apparent.

> **Memorize**
>
> Deflection = deviation of the incisor point (or the middle of the tip of the chin) to one side when the lower jaw opens the mouth without returning to the median plane.
> Deviation = deviation of the incisor point (or the middle of the tip of the chin) to one side when the lower jaw opens the mouth with a return movement to the median plane.

14

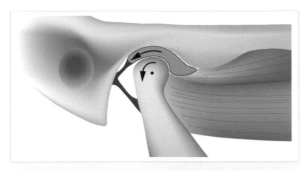

Fig. 14.7 Jaw closure.

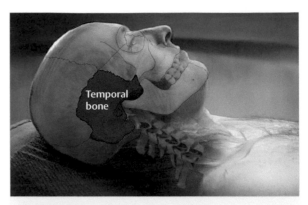

Temporal bone

Fig. 14.8 Position of the temporal bone.

Technique: Test for Active Mouth Opening

The first test used to assess the presence of deviations or deflections is active mouth opening. It provides information on eventual restrictions in mobility caused by, for example, problems in the capsule or a unilateral blocking in the condylar path (opposing joint surface formed by the temporal bone). To assess active mouth opening, the patient is requested to open their mouth as wide as possible. This instruction is repeated several times as the mouth usually opens up more when the movement is repeated. The maximal mouth opening possible (incisal edge distance, IED) is measured using a caliper or a ruler where the scaling starts with 0 directly at its edge and this value is added to the vertical anterior teeth overbite. Once the symmetry and the degree of mouth opening possible have been determined, the clicking phenomenon will be assessed using palpation and is described in the following section.

Tip

According to the Helkimo index, normal mouth opening amounts to ≥ 40 mm. If this is not possible, possible deviations to the side can be discovered by measuring the degree of respective mandibular lateral deviation. If a deviation is not present, that is, with a lateral deviation to the right and left side of, for example, 10 mm, the 10 mm of lateral deviation is multiplied by 3 and 4 and the mouth is expected to be able to open up approximately 30 to 40 mm. If lateral deviation to one side (e.g., to the left) is not possible, a mechanical blocking of the right TMJ is the most likely cause, possibly due to anterior displacement of the disk. If the movement to one side is restricted, but nevertheless possible (e.g., only 5 mm to the left, but 10 mm to the right), the shorter distance is multiplied by 3 and 4 and the expected amount of mouth opening is calculated.

14.5 Palpating the Temporomandibular Joints

14.5.1 Overview of the Structures to be Palpated

- Temporal bone.
- Head of the mandible.
- Articular disk (indirectly palpable via the clicking sound).

14.5.2 Summary of the Palpatory Process

The structures of the disk-condyle complex are palpated as the mouth is being opened as follows (▶ Fig. 14.8, ▶ Fig. 14.9, and ▶ Fig. 14.10).

14.5.3 Assessment of the Clicking Phenomenon during Active Mouth Opening

Starting Position

The patient either lies on a treatment table in a relaxed position with the head slightly elevated or sits in a treatment chair. The therapist sits at an 11–12 o'clock position at the head-end of the patient.

Technique

During mouth opening, the therapist palpates the indentation of the TMJ approximately one finger-width anterior and inferior to the auditory canal. In some cases, clicking or crepitation can be felt underneath the fingertips as the mouth actively opens. This can occur:
- Initially, as the mouth starts to open;
- Intermediately, when the mouth has opened approximately halfway to maximal opening;
- At the end of movement, just before maximal mouth opening is reached.

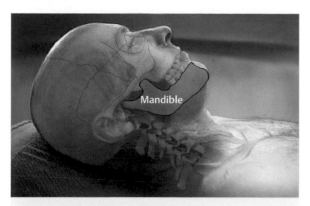

Fig. 14.9 Position of the mandible.

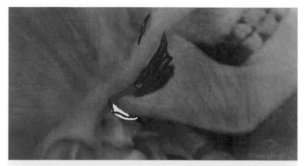

Fig. 14.10 Disk-condyle complex.

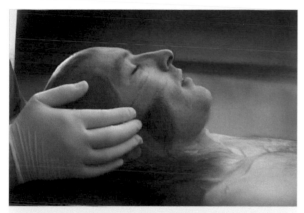

Fig. 14.11 Palpating the temporomandibular joint (TMJ) indentation with the mouth almost closed.

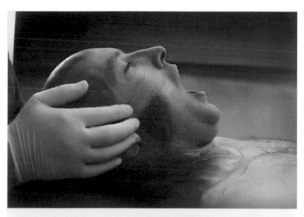

Fig. 14.12 Palpating the temporomandibular joint (TMJ) indentation with the mouth opened wide.

This describes the suspected position of the disk on the head of the mandible (► Fig. 14.11, ► Fig. 14.12, and ► Fig. 14.13).

Tip

As already mentioned, the TMJ essentially consists of the temporal bone and the head of the mandible. It is divided into the superior and inferior compartments by the articular disk. The articular disk ideally lies on top of the head of the mandible as a horizontal figure of eight. If the condyle strongly compresses the posterior pole of the disk, this can result in morphological changes in the disk and cause the disk to displace anteriorly. The attached superior stratum is then overstretched and the clicking phenomenon occurs. The previously described biomechanics of the disk-condyle complex worsen the pathological situation when the disk is displaced anteriorly and the jaw starts to click.

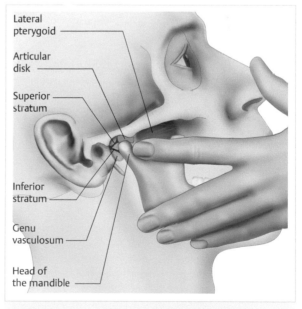

Lateral pterygoid

Articular disk

Superior stratum

Inferior stratum

Genu vasculosum

Head of the mandible

Fig. 14.13 Position of the palpating fingers on the jaw.

14

14.6 Palpatory Examination of the Jaw Muscles

14.6.1 Overview of the Structures to be Palpated

- Masseter.
- Medial pterygoid muscle.
- Lateral pterygoid muscle.
- Temporalis.
- Anterior and posterior bellies of the digastric.

14.6.2 Summary of the Palpatory Process

Practical aspects should also be considered when deciding how to proceed with the palpation. The orofacial muscles can be palpated intraorally and extraorally. It is recommended that gloves be removed or at least cleaned after the intraoral palpation is completed before continuing with the extraoral palpation. To aid understanding, the palpation of the muscles will be presented based on the action of the muscles.

> **Tip**
>
> It is essential that therapists wear gloves and especially a mask to protect themselves and their patients. This may be uncommon in a physical therapy practice, but is nevertheless necessary due to an increased risk of infections during the treatment of CMD patients due to the direct contact with patients' saliva and, in some cases, blood. This also offers therapists and patients additional protection from airborne infections. As muscles are palpated extraorally (on the face) and intraorally (in the oral cavity), the esthetic question is raised as to whether the fingers, obligatorily gloved and moistened with the patient's saliva, should immediately continue to palpate extraorally on the patient's face. It is also not pleasant for patients when the intraoral palpation is conducted after the extraoral palpation on their face if they wear make-up.

14.6.3 Masseter

The masseter muscle is one of the most distinct and easy-to-palpate muscles of the masticatory system and is also frequently visible to the naked eye. It is divided into a superficial part and a deep part. It originates on the zygomatic arch and extends over a large area onto the masseteric tuberosity on the angle of the mandible.

It forms a muscle sling at the angle of the mandible together with the medial pterygoid muscle. These muscles are responsible for approximately 55% of mouth closure.

Starting Position

The patient either lies on a treatment table in a relaxed position with the head slightly elevated or is sitting in a treatment chair. The therapist sits next to the patient's head on the side to be assessed.

Technique

The palpation is conducted intraorally with the index or middle finger placed on the buccal side (inside of the cheek) and the thumb on the outer side of the cheek. The muscle can also be palpated extraorally on the outer side of the cheek. The masseter muscle is palpable intraorally just under the skin on the side of the ramus of the mandible. Its bulge during contraction can be seen on the side at the angle of the mandible. The patient can be requested to gently press the teeth together to facilitate differentiation of the individual structures. By doing so, the contracting sections of the masseter are easy to palpate and differentiate (▶ Fig. 14.14, ▶ Fig. 14.15, ▶ Fig. 14.16, and ▶ Fig. 14.17).

14.6.4 Tips for Assessment and Treatment

Ear and tooth pain in the lateral area of the teeth can be caused by referred pain originating in trigger points, for example, in the masseter (▶ Fig. 14.18, ▶ Fig. 14.19, ▶ Fig. 14.20, and ▶ Fig. 14.21).

14.6.5 Medial Pterygoid Muscle

The medial pterygoid muscle originates in the pterygoid fossa, extends almost parallel to the masseter found on the outer side of the jaw, and inserts into the angle of the mandible. It attaches to the pterygoid tuberosity here.

Together with the masseter, it forms a muscle sling at the angle of the mandible. Both of these muscles are responsible for approximately 55% of mouth closure.

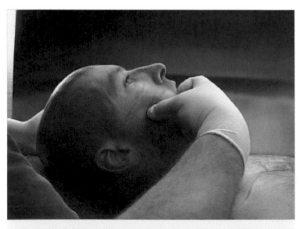

Fig. 14.14 Palpating the superficial part of the masseter.

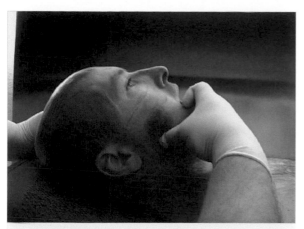

Fig. 14.15 Palpating the deep part of the masseter.

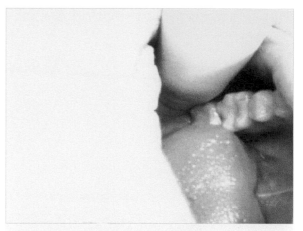

Fig. 14.16 Intraoral palpation of the masseter.

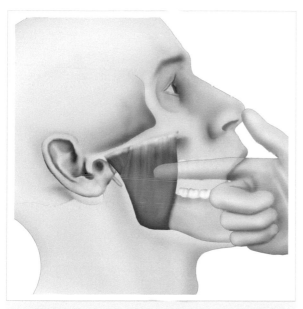

Fig. 14.17 Schematic illustration of the intraoral palpation of the masseter.

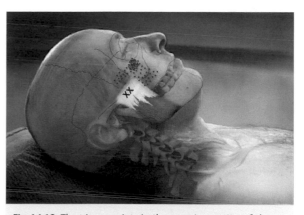

Fig. 14.18 The trigger points in the superior section of the superficial part of the masseter refer pain to the upper molar region and the maxillary sinuses.

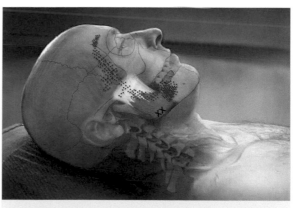

Fig. 14.20 Myofacial pain arising directly in the angle of the mandible, where the superficial part of the masseter is noticeable, is referred to the horizontal section of the mandible and the temples.

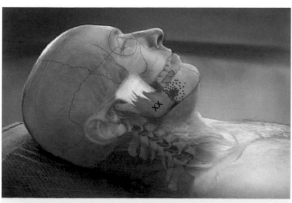

Fig. 14.19 Myofacial pain arising in the inferior section of the superficial part of the masseter is referred to the lower molar region and the horizontal section of the mandible.

14

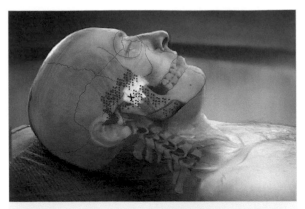

Fig. 14.21 The trigger points in the deep part of the masseter refer pain mainly to the ear and the preauricular region.

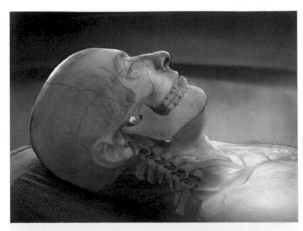

Fig. 14.22 Position of the medial pterygoid muscle.

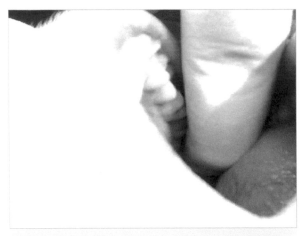

Fig. 14.23 Intraoral palpation of the medial pterygoid muscle.

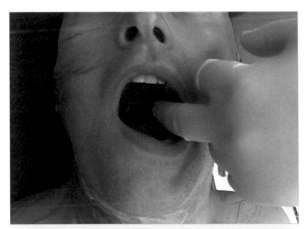

Fig. 14.24 Palpation route, view from above.

Tip

The intense loading on the TMJ is obvious when observing the pressure applied during mastication. The pressure of mastication can amount to 700 to 950 N when biting, but may also be stronger. The teeth and bite can be changed or damaged in patients who clench their teeth together or grind their teeth (bruxism); this is due to the intense pressure applied during mastication. The muscular dysbalances seen here can also cause pain in the face and other symptoms, for example, in the sacroiliac (SI) joint, by affecting the entire statics of the body.

Starting Position

The patient either lies on a treatment table in a relaxed position with the head slightly elevated or sits in a treatment chair. The therapist sits next to the patient's head on the side to be assessed.

Technique

The palpation is conducted intraorally and lingually by placing the index or middle finger on the medial side of the ramus of the mandible at the point where the ramus extends from the maxillary tuberosity to the angle of the mandible. It can also be palpated extraorally via the inner side of the medial tip of the angle of the mandible (▶ Fig. 14.22, ▶ Fig. 14.23, ▶ Fig. 14.24, and ▶ Fig. 14.25).

Tips for Assessment and Treatment

The trigger points in the medial pterygoid muscle can refer pain to the preauricular region (▶ Fig. 14.26).

14.6.6 Lateral Pterygoid Muscle

The superior head of the lateral pterygoid muscle originates on the infratemporal crest of the sphenoid bone. The inferior head comes from the lateral plate of the pterygoid process. The superior head is attached to the articular disk, pulls the disk anteriorly, and initiates mouth opening. The inferior head inserts onto the condylar process of the mandible. When acting alone, it displaces the lower jaw to the contralateral side (medial deviation). When the two inferior heads act together, they move the lower jaw anteriorly (protrusion).

The kinematics initiated by the lateral pterygoid muscle continue with the suprahyoid muscles. Recent studies (Schindler, 2004) have shown that the lateral pterygoid muscle is involved in almost all movements of the TMJ in one way or another.

The lateral pterygoid muscle is one of the muscles of the jaw that causes the most pain. As it was not clear whether this muscle could be palpated at all, we conducted our own study (Stelzenmüller et al., 2004) and proved for the first time that it is possible to palpate this muscle. This is necessary as this muscle can only be specifically treated when direct digital palpation of the quality of muscular tissue, the assessment of pain, and the following functional massage (opening and closing the mouth while palpating with the fingers) is possible. The inclusion criterion for the study was that patients had to have healthy TMJs. The palpation was confirmed beyond doubt using MRI and EMG. The method for palpation was simulated on five anatomical specimens with differing dimensional relationships. Prerequisite for this palpation is that therapists are familiar with the exact palpatory method and have the necessary experience (▸ Fig. 14.27, ▸ Fig. 14.28, and ▸ Fig. 14.29).

Starting Position

The patient either lies on a treatment table in a relaxed position with the head slightly elevated or sits in a treatment chair. The therapist sits next to the patient's head on the side to be assessed.

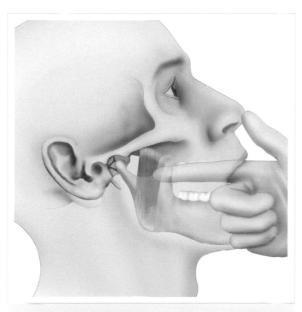

Fig. 14.25 Schematic illustration of the intraoral palpation of the medial pterygoid muscle.

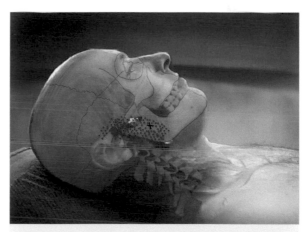

Fig. 14.26 The trigger points in the medial pterygoid muscle can refer pain to the preauricular region.

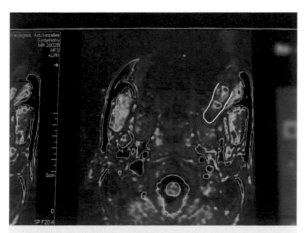

Fig. 14.27 Illustration of the access path on an MRI. Red: lateral pterygoid muscles. Yellow: palpating finger.

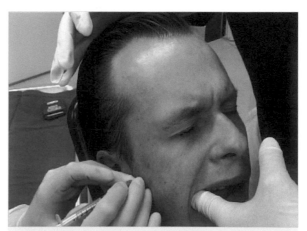

Fig. 14.28 Palpating the lateral pterygoid muscle with EMG monitoring.

14

Technique

The digital palpation of the lateral pterygoid muscle takes place intraorally in the cheek using either the small or the index finger. The patient deviates the mandible laterally (shifts the lower jaw sideways, away from the midline) toward the side to be assessed. The therapist's small or index finger palpates along the oral vestibule parallel to the superior section of the alveolar process of the maxilla, onto the maxillary tuberosity, and further, until the lateral plate of the pterygoid process is reached. The palpation crosses over the superior section of the medial pterygoid muscle during this step. The final part of the palpation moves in a superomedial direction.

This muscle can also be tested isometrically outside the mouth. This test is not as informative as the digital palpation. To conduct this test, the patient is instructed to open their mouth slightly and then move their lower jaw to the side, for example, to the left. This movement is decelerated using submaximal resistance applied to the left side of the mandible. This tests the strength and presence of pain in the right lateral pterygoid muscle.

Up until the palpation of the lateral pterygoid muscle was proven, this technique was also used as treatment to relax the lateral pterygoid muscle using the contract-relax technique (▶ Fig. 14.30, ▶ Fig. 14.31, and ▶ Fig. 14.32).

Tips for Assessment and Treatment

Trigger points in the lateral pterygoid muscle refer pain to the jaw. This can be confused with arthrogenic problems and maxillary sinuses symptoms (▶ Fig. 14.33).

14.6.7 Temporalis

The temporalis is divided into three segments: the anterior, medial, and posterior parts. Palpatory assessment of this muscle is essential due to its extensive size and the different actions of the individual muscle parts and their referral of pain (▶ Fig. 14.34, ▶ Fig. 14.35, ▶ Fig. 14.36, ▶ Fig. 14.37, ▶ Fig. 14.38, ▶ Fig. 14.39, ▶ Fig. 14.40, ▶ Fig. 14.41, and ▶ Fig. 14.42). It originates on the temporal line of the squamous part of the temporal bone and the parietal bone. It inserts into the coronoid process of

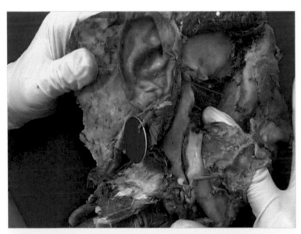

Fig. 14.29 Illustration of the access path on an anatomical specimen. Red outline: lateral pterygoid muscle. Blue outline: medial pterygoid muscle.

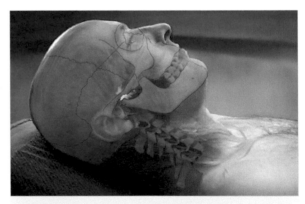

Fig. 14.30 Position of the lateral pterygoid muscle.

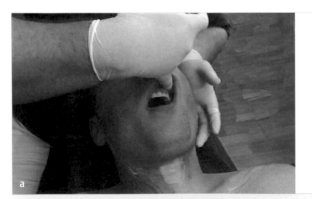
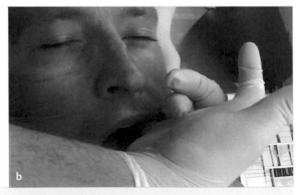

Fig. 14.31 The mandible is laterally deviated and the lateral pterygoid muscle then palpated intraorally.
a The small finger moves parallel to the superior section of the alveolar process here and
b then moves along the oral vestibule onto the maxillary tubercle, followed by the lateral plate of the pterygoid process.

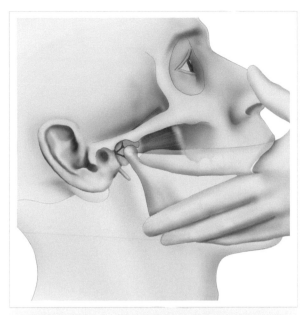

Fig. 14.32 Schematic illustration of the intraoral palpation of the lateral pterygoid muscle (orange: articular disk).

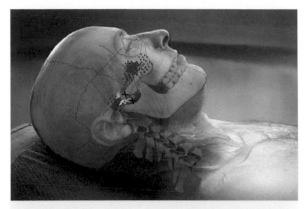

Fig. 14.33 Trigger points in the lateral pterygoid muscle cause referred pain in the jaw. This can be confused with arthrogenic problems and symptoms in the maxillary sinuses.

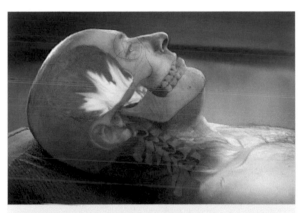

Fig. 14.34 Position of the temporalis.

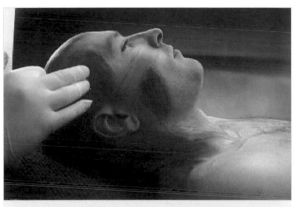

Fig. 14.35 The extraoral palpation starts in the anterior region of the temples.

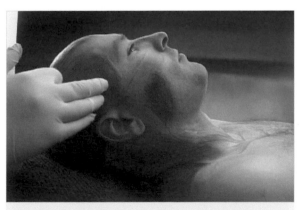

Fig. 14.36 Continuing to palpate the medial part of the temporalis muscle.

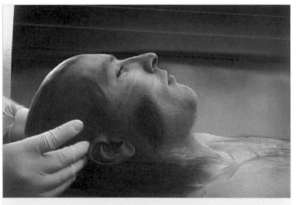

Fig. 14.37 Palpating the posterior part of the temporalis.

the mandible. When both temporalis muscles are active, they produce approximately 45% of mouth closure. The posterior section of the mandible moves posterosuperiorly at the coronoid process during this. The anterior parts contribute to protrusion and opening of the mouth.

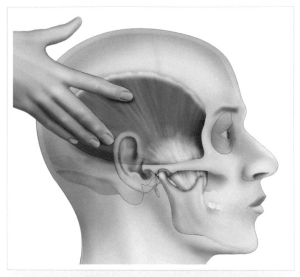

Fig. 14.38 Schematic illustration of the area of palpation for the temporalis.

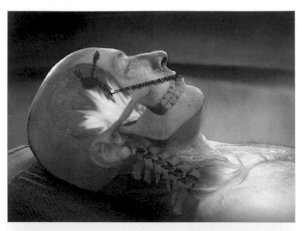

Fig. 14.39 The trigger points in the anterior part of the temporalis refer pain to the upper front teeth.

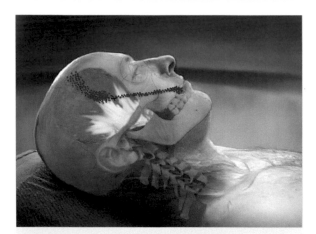

Fig. 14.40 The trigger points in the medial part of the temporalis radiate symptoms into the canine teeth and the premolars.

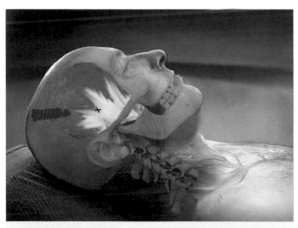

Fig. 14.41 Myofascial pain originating in the medial part of temporalis can radiate into the middle region of the parietal bone.

Starting Position

The patient either lies on a treatment table in a relaxed position with the head slightly elevated or sits in a treatment chair. The therapist sits at an 11 to 12 o'clock position at the head-end of the patient.

Technique

The extraoral palpation starts in the anterior region of the temples. The therapist starts palpating with moderate pressure perpendicular to the course of fibers. The palpation of the anterior part begins on the temporal line of the temporal squamous part of the parietal bone. The therapist palpates this part of the muscle from anterior to posterior, then continues toward the muscle's insertion at the zygomatic arch. This method is especially necessary to locate trigger and/or tender points in the different parts of the muscle segments. The medial and posterior segments are palpated in a similar manner.

It can be helpful when the patient is instructed to briefly open the mouth or press the teeth together during

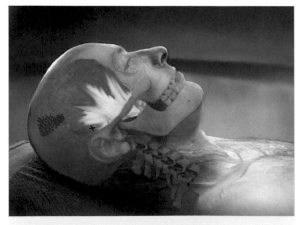

Fig. 14.42 Myofascial pain originating in the posterior part can be referred onto the parietal bone.

palpation to facilitate differentiation of the individual structures. The index, middle, or ring finger can be used for palpation in the temple region of the patient.

14.6.8 Anterior and Posterior Bellies of the Digastric

The posterior belly of the digastric originates on the mastoid notch of the temporal bone and, together with the anterior belly, is connected to the lesser horn of the hyoid bone via the intermediate tendon. The anterior belly inserts into the digastric fossa.

One of the most important actions of the digastric is to raise the hyoid bone during swallowing. It also helps to open the mouth.

Tip

The therapist should always assess the floor of the mouth for pain and/or changes at specific intervals in all patients suffering from head/jaw symptoms. The motor activity in the tongue is assessed by instructing the patient to try and place the tip of the tongue on the nose, on the point of the chin, and to move the tongue as far as possible to the left and to the right. If these motor function tests demonstrate differences between the sides, further examination of the floor of the mouth and the tongue region should be performed by dentists, oral surgeons, oral and maxillofacial surgeons, or neurologists. These deviations may simply be due to a lack of body awareness or may be caused by changes in the floor of the mouth, for example, an ulcer in the mouth (aphthous ulcer), swelling in the lymph nodes, a stone in the salivary gland (sialolith), tumors, organic processes arising in the brain, etc. The complete floor of the mouth is therefore palpated (taking care that only minimal pressure is applied intraorally as this region is very sensitive to pain).

Starting Position

The patient either lies on a treatment table in a relaxed position with the head slightly elevated or sits in a treatment chair. The therapist sits next to the patient's head on the side to be assessed.

Technique (Intraoral)

The middle or index finger is used to palpate sublingually (underneath the tongue) in the floor of the patient's mouth. The therapist's intraoral finger pushes the anterior belly of the digastric lightly into the floor of the mouth and the muscle can now be easily palpated intraorally and extraorally.

To better differentiate the anterior belly of the digastric from the other suprahyoid muscles in the floor of the mouth, it has proven useful to oppose mouth opening with slight resistance applied to the point of the chin. The V-form of the anterior belly of the digastric then becomes distinct as it travels to the point of the chin.

Technique (Extraoral)

The extraoral technique used to palpate the posterior belly of the digastric is an alternative to the intraoral procedure. The therapist grasps around the angle of the mandible and palpates the soft tissue posterior to the ramus of the mandible.

The posterior belly of the digastric can be felt in the soft tissue as the hand grasps around the angle of the mandible and gentle pressure is applied posterior to the ramus of the mandible.

Ideally the patient is asked to briefly swallow during the palpation. The posterior belly of the digastric then slides directly against the palpating finger. The intraoral treatment of the anterior belly of the digastric should take priority (▶ Fig. 14.43, ▶ Fig. 14.44, ▶ Fig. 14.45, and ▶ Fig. 14.46).

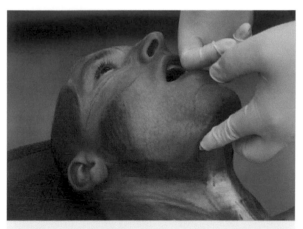

Fig. 14.43 Intraoral palpation of the anterior belly of the digastric.

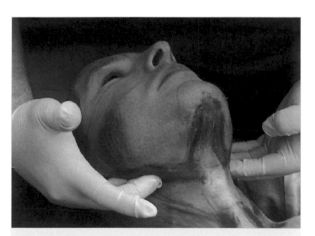

Fig. 14.44 Extraoral palpation of the posterior belly of the digastric.

14

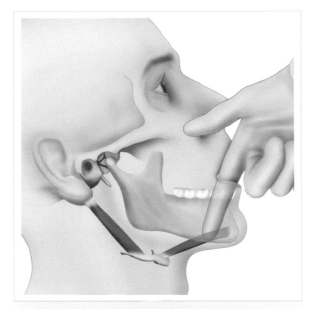

Fig. 14.45 Schematic illustration of the intraoral palpation of the anterior belly of the digastric.

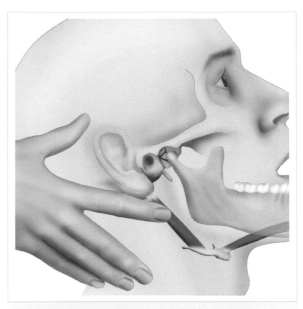

Fig. 14.46 Schematic illustration of the extraoral palpation of the posterior belly of the digastric.

Tip

Suprahyoid muscles: the suprahyoid muscles include the digastric, as well as stylohyoid, mylohyoid, and geniohyoid. Geniohyoid, mylohyoid, and the anterior belly of the digastric help to form the floor of the mouth. The suprahyoid muscles are involved in mastication and swallowing as well as articulation when speaking and singing. When the mandible is fixed, the mylohyoid can elevate the base of the tongue, pushing it against the roof of the mouth. The hyoid bone and the larynx are then pulled anterosuperiorly. When the infrahyoid muscles fix the hyoid bone, the mylohyoids participate in mouth opening and the sideways movement of the mandible (Rauber and Leonhardt, 1987).

Bibliography

Rauber A, Leonhardt H, Eds. Anatomie des Menschen: Lehrbuch und Atlas. Bd 1. Bewegungsapparat. Stuttgart: Thieme; 1987

Schindler HJ. Vortrag auf der 37. Jahrestagung der Arbeitsgemeinschaft für Funktionsdiagnostik und Therapie (AFDT). Bad Homburg; November 2004

Stelzenmüller W, Weber D, Özkan V, Umstadt H. Is the lateral pterygoid muscle palpable? A pilot study for determining the possibilities of palpating the lateral pterygoid muscle. Best awarded poster presentation. AFDT der DGZMK (Deutsche Gesellschaft für Zahn-, Mund- und Kieferheilkunde). 28.11.2004. Int Poster J Dent Oral med 2006; 8: 301. http://ipj.quintessenz.de; accessed: 28.08.2017

Index

Note: Page numbers set *italic* indicate headings or figures, respectively.

.